Public Health
Preparedness

CASE STUDIES IN POLICY AND MANAGEMENT

Public Health Preparedness

CASE STUDIES IN POLICY AND MANAGEMENT

EDITED BY
Arnold M. Howitt
Herman B. "Dutch" Leonard
David W. Giles

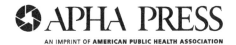

AN IMPRINT OF **AMERICAN PUBLIC HEALTH ASSOCIATION**

American Public Health Association
800 I Street, NW
Washington, DC 20001-3710
www.apha.org

Georges C. Benjamin, MD, FACP, FACEP (Emeritus), Executive Director

Printed and bound in the United States of America
Book Production Editor: Maya Ribault
Typesetting: The Charlesworth Group
Cover Design: Alan Giarcanella
Printing and Binding: Sheridan Books

Library of Congress Cataloging-in-Publication Data

Names: Howitt, Arnold M., 1947- editor. | Leonard, Herman B., editor. |
  Giles, David W., editor. | American Public Health Association, issuing
  body.
Title: Public health preparedness : case studies in policy and management /
  editors, Arnold M. Howitt, Herman B. "Dutch" Leonard, David W. Giles.
Other titles: Public health preparedness (Howitt)
Description: Washington, DC : American Public Health Association, [2016]
Identifiers: LCCN 2016027527 (print) | LCCN 2016028178 (ebook) | ISBN
  9780875532837 (print) | ISBN 9780875532844 (ebook)
Subjects: | MESH: Disaster Planning–organization & administration | Public
  Health Administration | Terrorism | Civil Defense | Disease Outbreaks |
  Organizational Case Studies | United States | Canada
Classification: LCC RA645.9 (print) | LCC RA645.9 (ebook) | NLM WA 295 | DDC
  362.1068/4–dc23
LC record available at https://lccn.loc.gov/2016027527

Table of Contents

Acknowledgments

Every book ever published owes much to people whose names do not appear as authors or editors. Certainly this collection of case studies is no exception. The case authors and the editors owe our greatest debt to the many dozens of individuals who consented to be interviewed about their experiences so that we could write the 15 case studies that appear in this volume. They were generous with their time, patient in answering detailed questions, and often candidly spoke about mistakes as well as expressed pride at the accomplishments they and colleagues made under difficult circumstances. The case studies and ultimately this book literally could not have been produced without the collaboration of our interviewees.

The editors are extremely thankful for an exceptional team of case authors—John Buntin, Daniel J. Collings, Kirsten Lundberg, Esther Scott, Wendy Robison, and Pamela Varley—with whom it was a pleasure to work during the conception, research, and writing of the case studies. They are true professionals who performed these tasks with imagination, diligence, persistence, and high standards.

These cases have been used in a number of teaching venues at Harvard, as well as being individually available to faculty at other universities worldwide through the Harvard Kennedy School (HKS) Case Program. During the Executive Session on Domestic Preparedness at HKS from 1999 to 2003, Arnold Howitt, Richard Falkenrath, and Juliette Kayyem explored issues of bioterrorism with an extremely thoughtful group of federal, state, and local officials and Harvard colleagues concerned with the threat of terrorism against the United States. Since 2002, these cases have been featured in the HKS Executive Education programs that Arnold Howitt and Dutch Leonard have led and taught in: Leadership in Crises, Crisis Leadership in Higher Education, the General and Flag Officers Homeland Security Executive Seminar, Leadership in Homeland Security, China Crisis Management, and the National Preparedness Leadership Initiative. Both Howitt and Leonard have taught these cases as well in various graduate degree program courses at Harvard Kennedy School, Harvard Business School, and Harvard Extension School. We have benefited tremendously from the thoughtful insights of our students and executive education participants during discussion of these materials.

The editors owe considerable gratitude to the funders of our case research and writing. The Robert Wood Johnson Foundation, through the Association of State and Territorial Health Officials (ASTHO), has supported the development of the majority of these case studies as part of the Robert Wood Johnson Foundation's and ASTHO's State

Health Leadership Initiative. We thank especially ASTHO's former executive director Paul Jarris and senior staff members Ramon Bonzon and Lacy Fehrenbach for their help in suggesting case topics and overall support for the case writing project.

A number of the case studies in this volume were developed for the Executive Session on Domestic Preparedness, generously funded by the US Department of Justice, Office of Justice Programs, and sponsored at Harvard by the Robert and Renee Belfer Center for Science and International Affairs and the Taubman Center for State and Local Government. We are very thankful for the backing of Graham Allison at Belfer and Alan Altshuler at Taubman.

In addition, the Centers for Disease Control and Prevention, through funding for Harvard's National Preparedness Leadership Initiative, also provided financial support for case writing. We thank the National Preparedness Leadership Initiative's Leonard Marcus and David Gergen for making this possible.

The US Department of Transportation also provided funding for parts of this volume through the New England University Transportation Center, based at the Massachusetts Institute of Technology, and through its Volpe National Transportation Systems Center. We thank in particular the Massachusetts Institute of Technology's Joseph Coughlin, Paula Magliozzi, and Karen van Nederpelt.

Many individuals have provided intellectual and personal support for our work. Present and past HKS faculty and staff colleagues in the Program on Crisis Leadership—Juliette Kayyem, Doug Ahlers, Chelsea Lei, David Tannenwald, and Arrietta Chakos—have provided ideas, constructive criticism, and friendship throughout the years in which this project has developed. Several student research assistants have provided important contributions too, notably Rene Vollenbroich, who conducted background research on public health emergency preparedness, and Molly Finlayson, who took meticulous care in helping to prepare the manuscript for publication.

The Program on Crisis Leadership is jointly sponsored by two HKS research centers, the Roy and Lila Ash Center for Democratic Governance and Innovation and the A. Alfred Taubman Center for State and Local Government. We have benefited tremendously from the support of the directors of these centers—Tony Saich at Ash; Alan Altshuler, Edward Glaeser, and Jeffrey Liebman at Taubman—and from their former executive directors—Marty Mauzy at Ash and Sandra Garron at Taubman. Our many past and present colleagues at the Ash Center and the Taubman Center have provided intellectual stimulation and friendship, both of which have influenced the work in this volume in too many ways to enumerate.

The Harvard Kennedy School case program and its parent Strengthening Learning and Teaching Excellence program have been supportive initial publishers of these cases and generous representatives of HKS in facilitating publication of this volume. We note particularly staff members Laura Madden, Christy Murphy, and Rebecca Loose, as well as former directors Carolyn Wood, Anne Drazen, and Howard Husock.

At HKS, Executive Education programs have long been instrumental in sponsoring much of the curriculum development at HKS and, as already noted, the materials in this volume have benefited significantly from programmatic support in Executive Education. We thank our current and past colleagues there—Debra Iles, Christine Letts, Peter Zimmerman, Sheila Burke, Annette Wilson, Horace Ling, Laura Simolaris, Anna Shanley, the late Jane Latcham, Maryellen Smyth, and Neal Duckworth—for exceptional comradeship. We have also benefited from a productive partnership in executive education with faculty colleagues at Harvard's Graduate School of Education—Judith McLaughlin, James Honan, and Joseph Zolner.

The President and Fellows of Harvard College (the Harvard Corporation), which owns the original copyrights to the cases in this volume, generously allowed us to seek their publication as a book.

As this volume has taken shape, the publications department of the American Public Health Association has been unflaggingly supportive and unbelievably patient. We thank the American Public Health Association's executive director Georges Benjamin for his enthusiasm as the project was launched and Ashell Alston, Brian Selzer, David Hartogs, and Maya Ribault for their staunch support as the manuscript was prepared and readied for publication.

Throughout our lives' journeys, we have received strength and unconditional support from our parents Mildred and Wilfred Howitt, Margery and Charles Leonard, and Elizabeth and Patrick Giles. Although it is impossible to properly acknowledge and thank them for the legacies they so lovingly handed down to us, we are conscious of drawing on them every day.

During the years in which these cases and this volume were germinating, we have depended on, have been inspired by, and have often been happily diverted by our wives—Maryalice Sloan-Howitt and Kathryn Angell—to whom we dedicated a previous book. Their contributions to this volume are no smaller, but with them we now dedicate this one to the next generations: to Arn and Maryalice's children and their spouses—Mark, Alexandra and Lee, Molly and Aurel, and Matt and Melissa—and grandchildren—Celeste, Emery, Jessica, and Allison; to Dutch and Kathy's children—Whitney and Dana; and to David's nephews—Nico, Alec, and Elliot.

To conclude with what should not need saying: notwithstanding our debts to these individuals and organizations, all errors of omission and commission in this volume remain the responsibility of the editors and case authors.

Arnold M. Howitt, Herman B. "Dutch" Leonard, and David W. Giles
Cambridge, MA, August 2017

Abbreviations

ACIP	= Advisory Committee on Immunization Practices	**EPA**	= US Environmental Protection Agency
AFCS	= Advanced Facer Canceller System	**E-prep**	= emergency preparedness Web site
AMI	= American Media, Inc.	**FBI**	= Federal Bureau of Investigation
APHL	= Association of Public Health Laboratories	**FDA**	= US Food and Drug Administration
		FDNY	= Fire Department of the City of New York
ASPR	= Assistant Secretary for Preparedness and Response	**FEMA**	= Federal Emergency Management Agency
ASTHO	= Association of State and Territorial Health Officials	**FRP**	= Federal Response Plan
BiPAP	= bilevel positive airway pressure	**GAO**	= US Government Accountability Office
BLD	= Bukas-Loob Sa Diyos Covenant Community	**GDEM**	= Governor's Division of Emergency Management
BPHC	= Boston Public Health Commission	**GDPH**	= Georgia Division of Public Health
BRT	= biological response team	**GEMA**	= Georgia Emergency Management Agency
CDC	= Centers for Disease Control and Prevention	**GPHL**	= Georgia Public Health Laboratory
CEDS	= Communicable and Environmental Disease Services	**GPS**	= Global Positioning System
		GTA	= Greater Toronto Area
CIA	= Central Intelligence Agency	**H1N1**	= a type of influenza A
Cipro	= ciprofloxacin	**hazmat**	= hazardous materials
CMT	= Crisis Management Team	**HGAC**	= Houston–Galveston Area Council
COO	= Chief Operating Officer	**HHS**	= US Department of Health and Human Services
CPHC	= Cambridge Public Health Commission		
CPR	= cardiopulmonary resuscitation	**HIPAA**	= Health Insurance Portability and Accountability Act
DBCS	= Delivery Barcode Sorter	**HMS**	= Harvard Medical School
DCHHS	= Dallas County Health and Human Services	**HPAC**	= Harvard Public Affairs and Communications
DEC	= Department of Environmental Conservation (NY)	**HR**	= Human Resources
		HSDM	= Harvard School of Dental Medicine
DEM	= Division of Emergency Management	**HSPH**	= Harvard School of Public Health
DHH	= Department of Health and Hospitals (LA)	**HUDS**	= Harvard University Dining Services
		HUENS	= Harvard University Emergency Notification System
DHS	= Department of Homeland Security	**HUHS**	= Harvard University Health Services
DMAT	= Disaster Medical Assistance Team	**ICS**	= Incident Command System
DOA	= dead on arrival	**ICT**	= incident command team
DOH	= Department of Health (DC, NYC)	**ICU**	= intensive care unit
DSHS	= Department of State Health Services (TX)	**IOM**	= Institute of Medicine
		iPHIS	= Integrated Public Health Information System
DSS	= Department of Social Services (LA)	**ISD**	= Independent School District
EAP	= Employee Assistance Program	**IST**	= Incident Support Team
ED	= emergency department	**LAPT**	= Learning, Analysis and Perspective Team
EMS	= Emergency Medical Services		
EMT	= emergency medical technician		
EOC	= Emergency Operations Center	**LEEP**	= Louisiana Emergency Evacuation Plan

LEMT	= Local Emergency Management Team	**PKEMRA**	= Post-Katrina Emergency Management Reform Act
LRN	= Laboratory Response Network	**PPE**	= personal protective equipment
MABAS	= Mutual Aid Box Alarm System	**POC**	= Provincial Operations Centre
MAC	= Medical Advisory Committee	**POD**	= point of distribution
MACC	= multiagency coordination center	**ProMED**	= Program for Monitoring Emerging Diseases
MAG	= Ministry Action Group	**PUI**	= person under investigation
MCHC	= Metropolitan Chicago Healthcare Council	**RFID**	= Radio Frequency Identification
MDH	= Minnesota Department of Health	**SAC**	= Science Advisory Committee
MDPH	= Massachusetts Department of Public Health	**SARS**	= severe acute respiratory syndrome
MEMS	= Modular Emergency Medical System	**SITREP**	= situation report
		SHOC	= State Health Operations Center
MERS	= Middle East respiratory syndrome	**SLE**	= St. Louis encephalitis
MessageME	= an emergency messaging system	**SNETS**	= Special Needs Evacuation Tracking System
NACCHO	= National Association of County and City Health Officials	**SNS**	= Strategic National Stockpile
		SOC	= State Operations Center
NCID	= National Center for Infectious Diseases	**SOSTF**	= State of Ohio Security Task Force
NCP	= National Contingency Plan	**TALHO**	= Texas Association of Local Health Officials
NDMS	= National Disaster Medical System		
NEFRLS	= National Emergency Family Registry and Locator System	**TAKS**	= Texas Assessment of Knowledge and Skills
NMETS	= National Mass Evacuation Tracking Systems	**TB**	= tuberculosis
		TDEM	= Texas Division of Emergency Management
NICU	= neonatal intensive care unit	**TEA**	= Texas Education Agency
NIMS	= National Incident Management System	**TEMA**	= Tennessee Emergency Management Agency
NIP	= National Immunization Program	**TMOSA**	= Temporary Medical Operations and Staging Areas
NOC	= National Operations Center		
NVSL	= National Veterinary Services Laboratory	**TPH**	= Toronto Public Health
NWS	= National Weather Service	**TWIS**	= Tennessee Web Immunization System
ODH	= Ohio Department of Health		
OEM	= Office of Emergency Management (NYC)	**UICC**	= Unified Incident Command Center
OEP	= Office of Emergency Preparedness (MN)	**USAMRIID**	= US Army Medical Research Institute of Infectious Diseases
OSHA	= Occupational Safety and Health Administration	**USMBHC**	= United States–Mexico Border Health Commission
OSI	= Office of Strategy and Innovation (in CDC)	**USPS**	= US Postal Service
		VP	= Vice President
PCR	= polymerase chain reaction	**WHO**	= World Health Organization
PHPPO	= Public Health Practice Program Office	**WIC**	= Women, Infants and Children (a federal program)

I. CHALLENGES IN PUBLIC HEALTH EMERGENCY PREPAREDNESS

Public Health Emergencies: Preparedness and Response

Arnold M. Howitt, Herman B. "Dutch" Leonard, and David W. Giles

We live in an era when, by historical standards, public health resources are rich and robust. But it is also an era in which billions of lives across the globe interconnect in complex ways, in which public health threats can be transported from one place to another at great speed, and in which biological technologies can be used with evil intent. As this book shows, the United States and other countries must therefore prepare for a significant range of public health emergencies. That requires institutions and leaders who have prepared themselves effectively.

The narrative case studies presented here reveal some of the challenges that public health faces in our times, but the identification of these problems is hardly new. The voluminous public health and medical literature is a highly valuable source of insights. What is distinctive about this volume is a focus on telling the full story of these events in a comprehensive way by highlighting the sequence and flow of events, the interrelationships among stakeholders, and the institutional relationships that structure their actions. Day-to-day media coverage captures some of these elements but often comes up short in reporting on the full picture, while long-form journalism frequently focuses on the human-interest dimensions of emergencies. By contrast, the cases in this volume provide data about the leadership styles and responsibilities of senior leaders, the dilemmas of decision making, the capacity constraints of key organizations, the pressures exerted by stakeholders, the refinement of scientific knowledge and response strategies in the face of novel challenges, and the problems of implementation and coordination that arise as plans solidify and action is needed. It is these problems of leadership, management, and expertise that we seek to highlight.

This introductory chapter has three purposes: we briefly explore the goals and use of teaching case studies, preview the specific topics that the case studies in this volume cover, and introduce a conceptual framework that may prove useful for readers as they read and analyze the cases. Whether a reader of this volume is a public health professional, a specialist in a related field, a student, or a concerned citizen, our hope is that the book will contribute in modest measure to society's preparation for the challenges that public health faces.

STIMULATING ANALYSIS AND DISCUSSION WITH CASE STUDIES

How can case studies of public health emergencies help current and future professionals, as well as thoughtful opinion leaders and citizens, understand the challenges of crisis response and frame and implement improvements in professional practice? Of course, case analysis through hospital rounds is a major way of training medical practitioners. In addition, written case studies designed for teaching purposes have long been used in other fields in the training of both aspiring professionals and experienced practitioners seeking to enhance their views and skills—most notably in business administration, public management and policy, urban planning, and, in a different way, law.

Broadly, we can think of a case study, such as the ones in this volume, as a collection of information selected and organized as a narrative to stimulate discussion of management problems, policy issues, or specific decisions that a leader or manager must make. Case method teaching does not discount the value of textbooks or journal articles and indeed often utilizes these resources alongside case studies. In contrast with a textbook or a journal article, however, case studies designed for teaching purposes do not provide analytic conclusions; rather, analysis is meant to emerge in classroom discussion or in dialogue among peers. Case study teaching seeks to make readers become more than passive recipients of others' ideas. Through preclass preparation and in-class discussion, it requires readers to assess the events described, consider the varying perspectives of different stakeholders, analyze the wisdom and efficacy of the actions taken, consider whether other approaches to the problems of the case might have been advisable, and ponder how these might have been implemented more effectively. Hopefully, our readers will find the cases interesting as well as useful in framing ideas about public health under emergency conditions.

ORGANIZATIONAL PLAN OF THE BOOK

The case studies in this volume seek to illuminate public health in action and, by conveying realistic information about how our institutions protect the public's health in difficult circumstances, point toward system characteristics to be sustained, capacities to be developed, and problems to be rectified.

Challenges in Public Health Emergency Preparedness

The first section of the book provides a close look at two pressing contemporary problems in public health preparedness: the control of potentially lethal infections that stoke public fears and the provision and sustainment of health services in the wake of major natural disasters. "Fears and Realities: Managing Ebola in Dallas" examines how the West African Ebola epidemic made its way to the United States by way of a man who contracted the disease in Liberia but traveled to Texas before his infection had manifested itself. Initially sent home from a Dallas hospital when his illness was misdiagnosed, he soon returned with a full-blown case that ultimately proved fatal. Confronting the possibility of a more extensive outbreak, Texas authorities at the city, county, and state levels worked with the Centers for Disease Control and Prevention (CDC) to identify, isolate, and monitor individuals who had come in contact with the patient; but just as it seemed that a broader outbreak had been avoided, two nurses, who had followed CDC infection control guidelines while caring for the patient, tested positive for Ebola, setting off increased concerns of more widespread infection.

"Surviving the Surge: New York City Hospitals Respond to Superstorm Sandy" deals with a very different form of public health challenge—that is, a severe natural disaster that knocked major health care institutions out of commission and created danger for hospitalized patients who could not receive the care and services they needed. This case study looks at the experience during Superstorm Sandy in 2012 of three New York City hospitals located close to the East River and hence vulnerable to flooding. In the days before the storm struck, facing increasingly dire predictions about the potential impact of the approaching hurricane, the hospitals made different decisions about how to cope. One evacuated its patients, while the other two, feeling confident about their preparedness, chose to shelter in place. The storm surge generated by Sandy proved even worse than the forecasts, however. Both of the latter hospitals were inundated, lost power, and were forced to undertake a harrowing evacuation of patients under extremely hazardous conditions.

Emergent Infectious Disease

The book's second section follows on the Ebola case study by examining how outbreaks of several other novel infectious diseases have strained the public health system after striking North America. Infectious disease today may originate in one part of the world but, more rapidly than ever before, leap to distant locales via transcontinental air travel. The three-part case series "The West Nile Virus Outbreak in New York City" describes the discovery of the first cases of West Nile in this country and the successful identification of the virus after an initial misidentification as St. Louis encephalitis. But discovery of the nature and cause of the viral outbreak, as important as it was, did not constitute a sufficient response to the emerging West Nile outbreak. It soon became necessary for the city to initiate mosquito spraying—initially in one borough but soon in all five boroughs of the city—to control the vector by which the disease was transmitted. Although nominally in charge, the city's health department turned to the city's Office of Emergency

Management, which had the skills and relationships with other city agencies to implement the complex spraying campaign.

Concern with emergent infectious disease would only increase. Severe acute respiratory syndrome, known widely by its acronym SARS, began causing grave illness and death in southern China in late 2002. Even before China had fully recognized the threat, SARS had traveled around the world in February 2003 to Toronto, Canada, carried by an elderly woman returning home from a visit to Hong Kong. The three-part case study "Emergency Response System Under Duress: The Public Health Fight to Contain SARS in Toronto" details the struggle to contain the disease during a major outbreak that followed in the spring. The majority of Toronto's cases of SARS were actually directly or indirectly contracted in hospitals where people seeking emergency care for respiratory distress transmitted it to other patients or hospital staff. The typical infection controls in emergency departments proved wholly inadequate to protect against a disease more contagious than other respiratory illnesses usually presenting there.

The challenges of dealing with SARS were not entirely medical. The epidemic strained the operational capacities of even a major city health system. Institutions struggled to scale up activities in many ways, managing heavy caseloads of highly contagious, hospitalized individuals at a time when some sister institutions had to shut down because of contamination. At times the system seemed to totter on the edge of collapse.

The SARS crisis was an alert for public health leaders worldwide to develop stronger defenses against a possible global pandemic of infectious disease, most likely a new strain of influenza. In 2005, President George W. Bush and CDC launched a national effort to improve preparations for pandemic disease, perhaps resulting from mutating avian flu or another pathogen. "X-treme Planning: Ohio Prepares for Pandemic Flu" describes how one state fulfilled the national mandate to develop a plan for preventing or responding to a lethal epidemic. Although the elements of flu defense were well established, the difficulties of implementing a strategy in a large state like Ohio were daunting. Using World Health Organization estimates of a 25% infection rate, Ohio could expect 2.8 million cases during a pandemic, a number drastically beyond the normal capacity of the health care system. At a time when other states would most likely be experiencing similar outbreaks and therefore be unable to help, Ohio had to find a way of surging resources and facilities—and adopting unconventional means—to meet the demand for treatment and other forms of help.

SARS and pandemic planning proved to be dress rehearsals for an actual pandemic. In 2009, a worldwide epidemic of novel H1N1 influenza A, sometimes called swine flu, did arise—a terrifying one in its early manifestations when reports from Mexico indicated initially that death rates were very high. Fortunately, H1N1 ultimately proved only about as lethal as seasonal flu, or a little less—a serious disease with severe consequences for some but not the extreme tragedy that some feared. However, the experience of the H1N1 response provides both signs of how improved preparedness over the course of the previous decade had paid off and revealing hints about what a worldwide pandemic of a more lethal strain of influenza might require.

In three H1N1-focused case studies, we explore the response from several perspectives. As the case study "On the Front Lines of a Pandemic: Texas Responds to 2009 Novel H1N1 Influenza A" describes, during the early stages of the epidemic, the state had to improvise its response at a time when the extent and severity of the disease were still being discovered and when preventive tactics and mass treatment methods were being developed. Knowing that it could be months before an H1N1 vaccine could be developed, tested, manufactured, and distributed in quantity, Texas implemented social distancing strategies that it hoped would minimize transmission of the virus. To distribute antiviral medications that could moderate the impact of the flu for people who contracted H1N1, Texas authorities had to completely revamp its previously developed antibiotic distribution system, which they realized was ill-suited to the very different needs of distributing medications for H1N1.

At Harvard University, some of the earliest cases of H1N1 in Massachusetts tested that institution's crisis management plans. As the case study "H1N1 at Harvard" describes, in the spring of 2009, the outbreak originated among students at the medical area campus, many of whom worked in clinics at the major teaching hospitals in Boston. If they contracted H1N1, they could conceivably infect patients. The university had to make many decisions under considerable time pressure, including temporary closure of its medical, dental, and public health schools on the medical area campus. A previously developed university-wide pandemic plan proved useful as a basic template for many necessary actions, but it had to be adapted and altered for unanticipated or distinctive features of the H1N1 situation.

The final case study in the H1N1 series, "Tennessee Responds to the 2009 Novel H1N1 Influenza A Pandemic," concerns a state that experienced an initial burst of cases in the spring and then a second-wave outbreak in the fall of 2009. Over the summer when the volume of H1N1 cases temporarily subsided, state health officials reoriented their response, getting ready for the availability of vaccine expected in the early fall. During this period, Tennessee's health department developed data about likely demand, demographics, and geography that enabled it to more confidently make critical decisions about vaccine distribution priorities and to allow local health care providers and institutions to preorder their supplies. Tennessee was thereby able to apply lessons learned from its own and other states' experience in the spring, refine some of the methods that others had used, and develop innovative response elements of its own.

Bioterrorism

In the third section of this book, several case studies examine the potential of biological weapons being used by terrorists. By the late 1990s, terrorism had become a matter of urgent public concern in the United States. The possibility of a domestic chemical or biological weapons attack was all too realistic in the aftermath of the first attack on New York's World Trade Center in 1993, as well as the Oklahoma City bombing and the sarin attack by the cult Aum Shinrikyo in the Tokyo subway system in 1995. Such attacks continue to pose difficult problems of prevention as well as response. Even the *threat* of intentional harm to public health—whether it turns out to be a hoax, a false alarm, or a real attack—taxes the coping capacity of the public health system.

"Anthrax Threats in Southern California" examines the wave of anthrax hoaxes that broke out in 1998 and 1999. These incidents were usually triggered by a telephoned warning that anthrax had been placed in a public place or by agitated calls from business people, government workers, or individuals who had come across white powders that they suspected could be anthrax. In this period, all of these events proved to be hoaxes or alarms with no substance. But often-sensational media coverage aroused the general public's fears, and the publicity may have created incentives for others to engineer similar incidents. These events, in turn, generated great pressure on public safety and health officials who then had to devote personnel time and effort to the response—often erring on the side of public safety even when the probability seemed very small that the threat was real. The case describes their efforts to develop sound risk assessment and decision-making practices and protocols that could guide the people who had to deal directly with these incidents, so that valuable resources would not be wasted.

But could such protocols definitively determine the risk of a real attack? "Charting a Course in a Storm: US Postal Service and the Anthrax Crisis" depicts that possibility becoming reality. Only a few weeks after the 9/11 terrorist attacks on the World Trade Center and the Pentagon and just after the United States began a retaliatory war in Afghanistan, a series of anthrax-laden letters began arriving at news media and government offices in Florida, New York City, and Washington, DC. To reassure the public, the secretary of the US Department of Health and Human Services initially declared the first anthrax death a naturally occurring event, not terrorism. But when that soon proved wrong, law enforcement and public health officials had to mobilize on an unprecedented scale to deal with both the reality of the attacks and the fear spreading across the country. The response was greatly complicated by the fact that events were outstripping scientific knowledge and predictions about how anthrax behaved and therefore what steps were necessary for exposed individuals to avert illness and death and for others to avoid exposure.

The postal service was hard hit. Its mail services had served as the vector for the anthrax attacks, and, notwithstanding unwitting assurances about safety from high-level postal service leaders, several of its workers contracted anthrax and died after spores escaped from letters into the air at postal processing facilities in Washington, DC, and New Jersey. Moreover, charges of racism arose over the difference in treatment of white Congressional staff, exposed in Capitol Hill offices, who were quickly offered prophylactic medication and of black postal workers whose exposure at the Brentwood mail processing center in Washington, DC, was not recognized until too late. The case study examines how, as the emergency expanded, senior postal officials organized and searched for a way in which the massive postal system could cope with the consequences and future possibilities of the anthrax crisis.

Meanwhile, as reports mounted of anthrax deaths in several states along the eastern seaboard and as new instances of anthrax hoaxes arose, the American public became increasingly alarmed. The result was an explosion of anxious calls to local public health, fire service, Emergency Medical Services, and law enforcement agencies all over the country about suspicious white powders that the callers feared might be deadly.

"White Powders in Georgia: Responding to Cases of Suspected Anthrax After 9/11" examines what happened in one state that found not a single spore of anthrax among the suspicious powders generating many hundreds of hazmat alarms. The case study highlights the interdependencies among the law enforcement, emergency response, and public health professionals—relationships that spanned federal, state, and local agencies—who had to deal with suspected anthrax. It describes how under the pressure of ballooning demand for hazmat response, they had to develop new protocols for action; forge closer cooperative bonds across professions, jurisdictions, and levels of government; train hundreds of young first responders who had not gone through full hazardous materials education on how to protect themselves when responding to a suspected anthrax call; cope with a host of practical operational problems; and accomplish all this while adapting to the rapidly changing guidance from federal public health sources about how to secure anthrax safely.

By late 2001 and early 2002, the United States was on high alert against potential threats in the aftermath of the 9/11 attacks and the anthrax letters. To many, the country was dangerously vulnerable to a possible bioterror attack, and a number believed that the most serious vulnerability was a smallpox attack. "When Prevention Can Kill: Minnesota and the Smallpox Vaccination Program" examines a strategic debate that raged both inside and outside the Bush Administration about whether the United States should inaugurate a precautionary smallpox vaccination program. But how great was the risk of a smallpox attack? How many and who should be vaccinated if a plan went forward? 50,000 public health workers? 500,000 public health and public safety personnel? All Americans? Giving pause was the fact that a relatively small percentage of Americans, but a large aggregate number, could experience deadly side effects because of adverse reactions to the vaccine itself or because of the weakness of their immune systems.

In December 2002, President Bush formally proposed that 500,000 health workers be vaccinated through a program administered by the states. But the administration encountered a number of practical issues as it pressed for implementation. State participation was voluntary, and some hesitated because of fundamental concerns about the policy, including who bore legal liability for adverse outcomes and who would cover a variety of costs. In addition, as states went forward, a host of operational questions plagued the implementation process: training for health care workers who would administer the vaccinations, care for those who experienced reactions to the vaccine, adequacy of vaccine supply, and resistance from labor unions representing those who would receive vaccinations.

Public Health System Issues

The fourth section of the book examines several quite different but trying public health events that demanded changes in terms of how the system responded.

"The City of Chicago and the 1995 Heat Wave" describes the dilemmas of emergency response that arose in the course of five steamy days in July 1995 when 576 people died—mostly frail, elderly residents, many of them poor, living alone in non–air-conditioned apartments. It was an emergency that caught city and county government unaware until the increasing number of bodies of the deceased literally compelled realization that something unprecedented was happening. As the heat wave progressed, ambulance services were overwhelmed by call volumes, fire trucks were pressed into supplementary service, and the capacities of hospital emergency departments were severely strained. Chicago officials were slow to put together a clear picture of the circumstances they were confronting. By the time the city had declared a heat emergency on Day 4 and mobilized additional response, the heat wave was starting to abate. In the aftermath, a mayoral commission sought to understand why so many had died and made recommendations about how the city should deal with extremes of heat or cold.

Initially failing to recognize novel elements in a public health emergency can lead to insufficient, misguided, or counterproductive response as the anthrax and SARS in Toronto crises demonstrated. Explicitly recognizing this problem in the aftermath of the anthrax crisis, CDC began a concerted effort to create organizational practices and structures that would improve its ability to pick up such signals of novelty in future public health emergencies. "Keeping an Open Mind in an Emergency: CDC Experiments With Team B" describes how, over several years, CDC sought to find ways to supplement the intense work being done by crisis managers by bringing additional voices to the table and reaching outside of the organization for insight as events evolved. CDC tried a number of methods to accomplish this goal. Seeking the right configuration required finding a delicate balance between the perspective and intelligence that this newly formed Team B might provide during an emergency with the possibility that the members of Team B would be perceived by operational leaders as either competitors or second guessers.

Responding effectively to large-scale disasters may also require public and private institutions to develop complex systems and manage specialized cooperative relationships that cross jurisdictional and functional lines. "Moving People Out of Danger: Special Needs Evacuations From Gulf Coast Hurricanes" focuses on how evacuating special needs individuals—those who need assistance in relocating, such as hospital patients, nursing home residents, the homebound, the carless—adds layers of complications to the evacuation process. Following events in Louisiana, Arkansas, and Texas, the first part of the case study describes how health, social service, and public safety officials sought to protect vulnerable individuals from Hurricanes Katrina and Rita in 2005 while encountering enormous problems. The second part of the case study describes how in the next several years state and federal officials developed reformed practices for evacuating or sheltering special needs individuals, including new transport plans and tracking systems to make sure that evacuees did not get lost. Those systems were put to the test in 2008 when two storms, Gustav in the New Orleans area and Ike in Texas, again prompted mass evacuations.

A CONCEPTUAL FRAMEWORK FOR UNDERSTANDING THE CONTINUUM OF EMERGENCIES[1]

As these brief descriptions suggest, the case studies in this volume describe a rich set of events that can enhance our understanding of the forces operating in public health emergencies. Before examining these institutional and political forces in detail, it is useful to develop a conceptual framework about the nature of emergencies. This will provide grounding for readers in comparing and contrasting the events described in the case studies. We shall argue that public health leaders must understand and deal with a spectrum of emergency situations—ranging from what we will call *routine emergencies* through *crises*—a continuum characterized by increasing degrees of novelty in the emergency situation. In contrast with routine emergencies, crisis conditions often create distinctive challenges. Leaders and their organizations therefore must develop capacities for managing, in different ways, both routine emergencies and crises. In effect, they have to become managerially ambidextrous, mastering two distinctive modes of leadership rather than relying on a single skill-set or uniform organizational competences.

---

1. This section draws extensively on concepts presented in Arnold M. Howitt, Herman B. "Dutch" Leonard, and David W. Giles, "Leadership in Routine Emergencies and Crises: The Deepwater Horizon Accident," *Proceedings of the Marine Safety & Security Council* 74 (May–December 2017). See also: Leonard and Howitt, "In Desperate Peril: High Performance in Emergency Preparation and Response," in *Communicable Crises: Prevention, Response, and Recovery in the Global Arena*, ed. Deborah E. Gibbons (Charlotte, NC: Information Age Publishing, 2007), 2–25; Leonard and Howitt, "High Performance in Emergencies: Two Modes of Operation," in *Managing Crises: Responses to Large-Scale Emergencies*, ed. Howitt and Leonard (Washington, DC: CQ Press, 2009), 611–624; Leonard and Howitt, "Acting in Time against Disasters: A Comprehensive Risk Management Framework," in *Learning from Catastrophes: Strategies for Reaction and Response*, ed. Howard W. Kunreuther and Michael Useem (Upper Saddle River, NJ: Wharton School Publishing, 2010), 18–40; Leonard and Howitt, "Leading in Crisis: Reflections on the Political and Decision-Making Dimensions of Response," in *Mega-Crises: Understanding the Prospects, Nature, Characteristics, and the Effects of Cataclysmic Events*, ed. Ira Helsloot, Arjen Boin, Brian Jacobs, and Louise Comfort (Springfield, IL: Charles C. Thomas Publishing, 2012), 25–34.

Responding to Routine Emergencies

Over time, societies have developed specialized professions and organizations to deal with emergencies. These practitioners include emergency managers, police, urban and wildland firefighters, emergency medical technicians, emergency physicians, and, increasingly, public health professionals. By far the most common form of emergency they face is what we term "routine" emergencies. These situations are not necessarily small in any sense; they may be large, widespread, and dangerous. We call them routine not because of scale but because these *types* of hazards can be anticipated, even when their timing, size, and precise location cannot be predicted.

Routine emergencies occur frequently enough that organizations can frame and inform expectations about future incidents; experience teaches lessons that can be absorbed and applied to the next occurrence of the same general type of emergency. Examples in the public health or health care sphere include preparation for and operations during seasonal flu outbreaks or the protocols that emergency medical teams follow when responding to a suspected heart attack victim. It is this degree of predictability that allows society to prepare in advance and thereby reduce the harm that such emergencies might otherwise cause. This is highly significant because the vast majority of emergencies that arise are routine in this sense. The professionalization of various emergency services over the past century and more, which has made life safer in ways that earlier generations could never have dreamed of, has resulted in large part because organizational leaders take advantage of their ability to anticipate emergencies by type and effectively prepare to respond.

Most importantly, they prepare by framing plans to avert, minimize, or react to such events. Then they train, equip, and exercise individual responders so they will be ready when emergencies arise. To codify organizational experience with specific types of emergencies, response organizations develop standard operating procedures or protocols that encapsulate operational principles and action steps. These may be disseminated to rank-and-file responders through checklists or scripts that lay out the steps to be followed in dealing with these emergencies. To facilitate collaboration, they develop personal and organizational relationships, devise coordination methods, and practice implementation of response tactics in drills and exercises. They also strategically station critical resources (people, equipment, supplies) in appropriate places so that response can be launched expeditiously. As a result, when an anticipated emergency actually arises, they can deploy personnel and resources quickly and respond effectively. Ideally, over time and repeated occurrences, organizations, leaders, and individual responders develop experience with many types of emergencies and become highly proficient in handling them.

Public health professionals—frequently in collaboration with colleagues from other disciplines—deal with routine emergencies regularly, for example, conducting epidemiological analyses in disease outbreaks, advising relief workers how to protect water supplies in the wake of a natural disaster, and conducting public information campaigns on acute health issues. They can anticipate that such emergencies will reoccur and have developed standard practices for planning, getting resources in place, coordinating their own and their partners' work, and constantly assessing and refining the methods by which they respond to these types of emergencies. In this book's case study about the Southern California anthrax threats, for example, law enforcement and public health sought to develop workable protocols for circumstances that were rapidly becoming routine: determining whether suspicious powders or telephoned anthrax threats should be considered as hoaxes or, by contrast, as serious hazards that required decontamination or other forms of treatment. In the case about Ohio's efforts to get ready for a potential pandemic influenza epidemic, we can see a public health system working hard to improve its ability to handle a very large but anticipatable challenge.

As already noted, to say that an emergency is routine does not diminish the possibility that it may be quite hazardous and have substantial scale; nor does this terminology at all imply that the organizational capabilities that enable effective response are in some sense ordinary. To the contrary, it is a significant achievement for response organizations to develop, refine, and keep well honed the multiple capacities that enable them to deal with potentially tragic or costly occurrences. As related in the case study about hurricane evacuation in Louisiana and Texas, following the severe difficulties they experienced in Hurricanes Katrina and Rita, planners significantly improved their ability to evacuate and care for special needs patients during natural disasters. This demonstrates how experience can help responders transform potential crises into more manageable—even routine— emergency practices. In fact, the histories of each type of emergency response profession can importantly be told as narratives in which increasing numbers of previously unmanageable hazards were turned into tractable (i.e., routine) problems of response.

Novelty: The Distinguishing Feature of Crises

On the spectrum of emergencies, we differentiate a *crisis* from a *routine emergency* by one key trait that has many consequences. Crises involve substantial *novelty*—characteristics of the emergency that have not been previously encountered by the organizations or people involved.[2] As will be discussed, novelty often creates distinctive challenges for emergency responders that require very different modes of leadership when confronting crisis conditions.

The novelty that characterizes crises may stem from at least three sources, and the case studies in this book will provide a variety of examples. One particularly frequent

---

2. The perspective of novelty is thus a subjective one; "novel" means new to the people or organizations involved even if others have previously experienced it.

source of novelty is an event that, while anticipated by type, is so large in scale that it exceeds the planning frame and the resources ready to deploy in response. Response organizations may be prepared for this type of emergency, but its extraordinary size and the extent of its consequences can severely disrupt plans and be at least temporarily overwhelming. In this book, we will see a number of examples of this kind of situation: the severe shortcomings in special needs evacuations from Hurricanes Katrina and Rita, the inadequate preparations for flooding undertaken by several New York City hospitals facing Superstorm Sandy's unprecedented storm surge, the hazardous materials handling practices that were overwhelmed in Georgia by concern about possible anthrax attacks, and the city of Chicago's faltering response to the heat wave death toll.

A second source of novelty is an event that is truly unprecedented—something "new under the sun"—for which no plan has been prepared and which may require in response the improvisation of new tactics and resources. Several of our case studies describe public health authorities coping with just such situations, including the city of Toronto confronting a hospital-based outbreak of SARS, Dallas dealing with the appearance of Ebola, and the US Postal Service coping with the turmoil of anthrax-laden letters sickening and killing both its customers and workers.

Third, novelty may arise from a combination of emergencies that occur at virtually the same time. Each of these may have been prepared for separately, but the conjoined occurrence may confound what was planned or overload responders. In its struggle to deal with the anthrax attacks, the Postal Service had to deal with multiple dimensions of novelty. In addition to the uncertainties of how weaponized anthrax enclosed in letters behaved, it also had to address the business challenge of keeping the mail flowing, the environmental crisis of cleaning up many contaminated postal facilities, and dual political crises— reassuring customers that it was safe to use the mail and countering the perceived lack of concern for minority postal workers who were exposed to the anthrax letters.

STRESSES ON THE SYSTEM: THE CORE CHALLENGES OF CRISES[3]

Crises put enormous strain on the response system—on individuals, organizations, and engaged response groups. In a crisis, rank and file responders and their leaders may feel that events and consequences are beyond their usual operating capabilities or out of control, thus generating very high stress. The stress of crisis results, to a substantial degree, from several core challenges that frequently arise in such situations. These challenges, described below, are well illustrated by the case studies in this book.

---

3. This section draws on concepts developed in Arnold M. Howitt and Herman B. "Dutch" Leonard, "Prepared for the Worst? Dilemmas of Crisis Management," in *Managing Crises: Responses to Large-Scale Emergencies*, ed. Howitt and Leonard (Washington, DC: CQ Press, 2009), 1–12.

Recognizing and Responding to Novelty

Although by our definition all crises involve novelty, we can distinguish two distinct patterns by which novelty becomes manifest. The first is a *sudden* crisis: an event clearly beyond routine that occurs with dramatic visibility—for example, a no-notice natural disaster like an earthquake, a severe technology failure like Japan's Fukushima Daiichi nuclear accident, or a terrorist attack. Because significant novelty is absolutely clear from the beginning, high-level officials rapidly engage, senior professionals mobilize, and unusually high levels of resources become available to deal with the situation. The moment of diagnosis of Ebola in Dallas (after an initial failure to do so)—and its immediate aftermath—was a sudden crisis. That diagnosis triggered quick action from a wide range of public health professionals at the city, county, state, and federal levels and by elected political leaders (including the mayor, county judge, and governor), as well as intense media and public attention. All of these actors clearly believed that this was a crisis necessitating extraordinary response.

The second pattern of crisis generation is an *emergent* crisis. An event that at first appears to be a routine emergency transforms at some point, gradually or dramatically, into a novel occurrence that goes well beyond the plans and capacities designed for routine emergencies. At initial encounter, because novelty is not revealed or perceived, an emergent crisis may seem to show familiar characteristics that can be treated as so many others have been in the past. When novelty is actually present, however, responding as if to a routine emergency can lead to insufficient, misguided, or counterproductive response. Many examples in this book illustrate the point: Toronto's slow recognition of the nature of SARS, CDC and others only gradually grasping the full dimensions of the anthrax attacks in October 2001, and Chicago's failure to see the dangers of the 1995 heat wave until bodies literally piled up.

The Special Problems of Emergent Crises

Both sudden and emergent crises are difficult to deal with, but emergent crises pose special problems of recognition and response. The key to distinguishing an emergent crisis from a routine emergency—and putting in train the appropriate crisis management steps in response—is to perceive as quickly as possible *anomalous* features of the situation. Are there factors or conditions present that are different in significant degree from what would be happening in the more familiar situation that those involved think they are seeing? Failure to recognize that an emergent crisis is developing often stems from missing a crucial deviation—an anomaly—in the pattern that typifies the more routine situation. But several factors may make it difficult for the responders deployed to the scene to recognize the gradually evolving divergence between the characteristics of a routine emergency and the novel elements that constitute a crisis.

When a situation initially appears to be a routine emergency, the individuals and units deployed in response are those that are used to dealing with that form of routine emergency. Experienced practitioners may ignore or simply not perceive information that disconfirms their expectations. Human cognitive processing can easily miss signs of novelty. In Toronto, the majority of SARS cases were actually directly or indirectly contracted in hospitals where people seeking emergency care for respiratory distress transmitted it to other patients and hospital staff. For individual clinicians or the public health system as a whole, immersed in dealing with specific cases, it was difficult to see and recognize that they were facing a new illness rather than the more familiar illnesses with similar symptoms that they had frequently encountered and had already mastered. In such situations, practitioners, convinced that they understand what they are facing, may fail to recognize signs or data that disconfirm their expectations because they are not looking for such information. Expecting the kinds of situation they have often seen before, they bring the mindsets, training, skills, and operating procedures appropriate for those situations, all of which are anchored and reinforced by previous effectiveness in dealing with the routine circumstances. Moreover, past success with the methods that worked well in routine emergencies may blind responders to the shortcomings of that approach when deployed against an emergent crisis. In Toronto, the shortcut infection control techniques that, under ordinary circumstances, hospital emergency departments used to cope with the flow of patients with less contagious respiratory ailments proved seriously inadequate for protecting against SARS infection. But practitioners were slow to recognize this.

Failing to recognize novelty is more likely when normal circumstances—for example, the incidence of seasonal flu and pneumonia or other respiratory ailments—fluctuate within a relatively wide operating range. It is particularly problematic to spot a gradually emerging break in normal operating experience when there are normally significant swings in the caseload. Certainly SARS in Toronto demonstrated that difficulty; in this instance, it was an accumulation of cases of unusual respiratory illness.

Another factor sometimes makes it difficult to recognize or acknowledge novelty. Responders who expect to see a routine emergency may become personally invested in making a success of their first approach to the problem. They may be reluctant or refuse to perceive or admit that it falls short and therefore might require reinforcements or different tactics. They may also be concerned that changing course might be seen as failure, resulting in career damage or loss of control.

Improvisation in the Face of Novelty

Because any emergency response, even a relatively straightforward one, is different in some respects from all others, the standard operating procedures that develop for handling routine emergencies typically need some degree of customization to fit the circumstances of each incident. As already noted, however, as the degree of novelty increases and moves toward the range that might be called a crisis, there is considerable likelihood that established protocols will be insufficient or invalidated by the situation. As Presbyterian Hospital in Dallas discovered, the initial CDC advisories for dealing with an Ebola patient did not protect all of the personnel who ministered to the patient who contracted the disease in Liberia. If the novelty inherent in an emergency goes unnoticed, as may happen in emergent crises, there is an increased chance that inadequate, misguided, or counterproductive responses will be carried out, which is what also happened in Toronto's hospitals facing the SARS outbreak.

How are strategies and tactics for dealing with a true crisis crafted? Although responders may have experience with some aspects of a situation characterized by substantial novelties, no single leader or decision maker is a comprehensive expert on what is happening or how to respond. Unlike in routine emergencies where leaders can at least partially depend on standard operating procedures or checklists, under novel conditions they have quite limited scripts to rely on. As a result, strategy and response measures must be improvised in order to meet unprecedented demands. That is accomplished in part by piecing together existing plans and capacities in new combinations and in part by innovation. Plans and tactics may have to be adapted and re-adapted as the situation unfolds, perhaps in repeatedly unexpected directions.

We see such improvisation in both large and small ways in a number of the cases in this volume. As several hospitals in New York City flooded and lost power during Superstorm Sandy, they first had to cope with myriad complications in maintaining patient welfare on site, and ultimately they had to effect a safe evacuation of hundreds of patients, including some extremely fragile ones, with considerable aid from outside response organizations like the fire department and National Guard. At Bellevue Hospital Center, Guard members and others formed an ad hoc bucket brigade to deliver fuel to an emergency generator in a desperate effort to keep the hospital supplied with a minimal amount of power. Meanwhile, at NYU Langone Medical Center, doctors, nurses, and medical students formed teams to move newborns out of the hospital's neonatal intensive care unit (NICU). This was a highly unusual undertaking that culminated in what has been described as the largest forced evacuation of a NICU in US history. Also in New York City, when mosquito spraying was required citywide to stem the West Nile virus outbreak, the city health department and the mayor's Office of Emergency Management partnered in carrying out the first such effort in New York since early in the 20th century. This required, among many other things, acquiring spraying equipment, training personnel, routing and scheduling the spraying campaign, anticipating and assuaging public anxiety about the use of insecticide, and notifying individual communities when the spraying there would be done. In less expansive but nonetheless critical improvisations, the Toronto public health community, the Harvard University health services, and the emergency managers of Louisiana and Texas had to improvise specialized patient tracking systems for dealing with SARS, H1N1, and hurricane evacuation, respectively.

It is important to note that improvisation in crises does not mean undisciplined action. As Frank Barrett has noted, improvisation in a jazz ensemble is not simply a performer doing her own thing with little or no regard for the form of the music or the musical contributions of other players. Instead, the improvisational soloist is disciplined in her creativity. She fits innovative elements into the performance so as to complement the overall structure, rhythm, key, and playing of her colleagues. But this structure does not wholly constrain the jazz musician. Limited structure with substantial freedom to improvise, Barrett argues in comparing innovation in management to jazz improvisation, permits "guided autonomy," a collaborative generator of innovation.[4] So too is effective crisis improvisation a highly collaborative effort in which the capabilities of multiple response organizations are meshed in crafting crisis response tactics.

To the extent that improvised response tactics involve piecing together existing routines in new configurations, the work of some rank-and-file personnel may not deviate drastically from what they would do during a routine emergency, except perhaps in urgency. But improvisation in the face of crisis entails heightened risk—sometimes physical, sometimes operational. Under normal conditions, for reasons of effectiveness and safety, response organizations generally prefer to develop and execute new capabilities cautiously—only after careful planning, personnel training, and practice in implementation. In crises, that prudent approach is often not possible; improvised response may have to be launched with minimal preparation and trial runs. In our case studies, we see numerous examples of people striving to make necessary improvisation as careful and safe as possible. The New York City hospital evacuations posed severe risks to patients, to responders, and to the reputations and liabilities of the hospitals themselves. So it also was in Toronto during the SARS outbreak, in Georgia's efforts to cope with the huge wave of suspected anthrax powders, and during Hurricane Katrina in both the jurisdictions that had to evacuate special needs individuals and those that received them. Force of necessity makes responders undertake operations that ordinarily they would be loath to risk. The result may be ragged and imperfect, but the appropriate standards under crisis conditions can't be the same as they are for response to routine emergencies.

Developing and Maintaining Situational Awareness

In a routine emergency, achieving a comprehensive picture of current conditions and their future implications is far more straightforward than it is in a crisis. Because a routine emergency is familiar by type and because individual responders often have substantial previous experience with such conditions, they are aware of the critical dimensions of

---

4. Frank J. Barrett, *Yes to the Mess: Surprising Leadership Lessons From Jazz* (Boston, MA: Harvard Business Review Press, 2012), 67–92.

the emergency and know what kinds of information to gather and assess to shape their actions. By contrast, under crisis conditions, responders may be unsure of crucial elements of the situation, and, to the extent that novel elements go unrecognized in an emergent crisis, some important elements may be overlooked. In a crisis, therefore, achieving strong situational awareness needs to be a high priority for leaders and responders.

However, under crisis conditions simply gathering and assimilating basic information about current circumstances—the foundation of situational awareness—can be a very difficult task. In a disaster like a hurricane or earthquake, physical destruction often impedes the collection of critical data: debris and damaged transportation facilities make movement difficult, communications systems fail, and the people who normally report information may be stunned, injured, helping family and neighbors, or grieving. As the situation in New Orleans after Hurricane Katrina graphically demonstrated, reliable information about people stranded in the flooded city, and particularly about those who had special health needs, was exceedingly difficult to secure.

The novelty inherent in a crisis adds to the difficulties of achieving foundational situational awareness. In Chicago, as awareness of the toll taken by the 1995 heat wave dawned, the number of affected people only gradually emerged. Similarly, the US Postal Service faced major obstacles in determining which of its facilities were contaminated by the anthrax letter attacks. In both the West Nile and SARS situations, situational awareness was severely hampered by the initial inability of the health system to identify the illness.

Four Stages of Situational Awareness

Understanding what is happening in the moment creates the underpinning of necessary situational awareness—and this is what is often understood by that term. A second stage (which we term "situational anticipation"), however, is crucial: the ability to project forward the implications of what is happening in the current period into the future—to conceive of conditions the next day, week, or month. That second stage then feeds into a third stage of situational awareness ("situational analysis"): assessing current conditions and forecasting near-term and longer-term developments in order to develop a plan of action. Finally, a fourth stage ("situational action") is faced: using the devised plan to implement whatever actions are required.

Making well-grounded predictions about what is likely to happen is a prerequisite for responders to construct a plan of action; simply reacting to current conditions may put them well behind the curve of a developing crisis. Of course, because responders cannot be certain what will happen in the future, forecasts must be made with an appreciation for alternative possibilities, and contingency plans must be readied in case initial predictions prove wrong. Such concerns motivated public health and health care leaders facing H1N1 to use the summer months of 2009, after the first wave of the virus, to make detailed plans for how they would respond as an expected second wave emerged in the fall. In a much more concentrated time frame, emergency managers working with public health during the West Nile crisis in New York City built their plans for citywide mosquito spraying on forecasts about how the disease would likely spread.

Making forecasts of what will happen and then tracking those predictions against what actually happens is extremely valuable even if those events don't conform to what was expected. Any forecast is based on an underlying concept or theory about how a given set of circumstances will work out. If events turn out differently, that is a strong indication that the underlying theory—and hence the action plan based on it—requires revision. For example, the public health and health care systems in Toronto began their response to SARS with one set of assumptions and expectations about how the surge of flu-like illnesses would respond to their efforts. When the results did not match expectations and conditions significantly worsened, those managing the growing epidemic had to rethink their theory of what was happening and their plans for response.

Projecting future conditions, however, is greatly complicated by the fact that even expert understanding of novel challenges may prove fallible or require considerable time to develop. Situational awareness, moreover, may be greatly hampered by scientific uncertainties—as was true not only in the SARS case but also in the anthrax letter attacks and, especially early on, in the H1N1 pandemic as well. As better understanding developed, expectations changed and plans had to be adapted—sometimes repeatedly. Because of uncertainty, decision makers may have to weigh the risks of one kind of action against another (or Type 1 vs. Type 2 risks). New York City hospitals facing onrushing Superstorm Sandy had to make decisions about the risks of evacuating hospitalized patients in advance—which could be quite hazardous itself—against the risks of sheltering in place during the storm.

In a prototypical crisis, the multiple dimensions of situational awareness—to gather information and assess what is happening, project likely impacts forward, and conceive and implement appropriate actions in response—are very difficult to achieve in comparison to what happens in routine emergencies, when experienced responders are able to make well-formed judgments about how the emergency is likely to develop.

Mobilizing Surge Capacity

Crises frequently (but not always) involve events that are much larger in scale than routine emergencies. Even very well-prepared local governments or states may lack sufficient resources to cope with the demands of such situations. Indeed, it would not make sense for jurisdictions to bear the cost and have on hand all the people, equipment, and other resources needed to respond to the largest emergencies that could conceivably strike them; much of that capacity would be unused most of the time, and the full complement of resources might never be used during its useful lifespan. Inevitably, therefore, for emergencies of extraordinary scale, which exceed the size for which a given area has prepared, an affected jurisdiction must call on others for help. They must have plans for *surge capacity*—resources that can be quickly secured to deal with an emergency that outstrips the capacity routinely in place.

Mutual aid most frequently provides that support. In fact, for the fire service or emergency medical transportation services, mutual aid from surrounding communities is often a matter of routine, organized and structured in advance and utilized quite frequently. Less frequently employed but also structured in advance is help from state or federal authorities. The Emergency Management Assistance Compact, a congressionally authorized interstate agreement, creates a framework for mutual aid from one or more states to another in need.[5] Individual federal agencies may provide support to their state and local counterparts, as the Ebola case study shows with CDC assisting Texas and Dallas. More broadly, federal resources, coordinated by the Federal Emergency Management Agency, can be mobilized under the National Response Framework.[6]

But having a plan for surge capacity does not ensure that needs can be supplied quickly enough to deal with a crisis. Since aid resources may not be physically located where they are needed, the speed by which they can be provided depends on fulfilling legal authorizations in timely fashion, securing sufficient and appropriate transport, and making the journey to the location of the emergency. Cost may deter requests for or supply of resources. And, in a widespread emergency like an epidemic in which many or all jurisdictions are experiencing the crisis, resources may be in very short supply, and potential providers may not be able to share with others.

Our case studies offer many examples of how challenging it can be to scale up emergency response and mobilize surge capacity to meet vastly greater than normal needs. The Chicago heat wave strained ambulance capacity, overloaded hospital emergency departments, and created severe capacity strains on the medical examiner's operations. In Toronto, the SARS outbreak strained a variety of health care and public health resources, especially when several hospitals had to close or restrict admissions because of contamination. In Georgia, the explosive proliferation of suspected anthrax cases overwhelmed hazardous materials response capabilities and forced the development of improvised procedures for handling the volume of calls. And in Ohio, the pandemic planning process had to take account of a potential demand for health care capacity that far outstripped what the system could ordinarily provide.

---

5. FEMA, "Emergency Management Assistance Compact," https://www.fema.gov/pdf/emergency/nrf/EMACoverviewForNRF.pdf.
6. FEMA, "National Response Plan, Third Edition," https://www.fema.gov/media-library/assets/documents/117791.

Coordinating Multiple Organizations

In routine emergencies, a single, specialized response organization (a public health, law enforcement, or fire department, for example) is likely to have a well-defined, sole lead role. By contrast, however, in either sudden or emergent crises the stakeholder environment is likely to be far more complex than normal in a routine emergency. In crises, the number of key actors is likely to be much larger, including many types of agencies, not only from a local jurisdiction directly involved but also from other jurisdictions or levels of government providing help through mutual aid or dealing with the same conditions, such as a hurricane that also affects many areas. Not only other agencies but also other levels of government (local, state, federal) are likely to be involved in a crisis. Moreover, in public health emergencies, as in some other types, nonprofit and private sector entities are frequently critical players.

In this volume, we see the complexity of stakeholder engagement particularly clearly in the case studies of infectious disease outbreaks: West Nile virus in New York City, SARS in Toronto, H1N1 in Texas and Tennessee, and the Ebola outbreak in Dallas. But it appears as well in other situations, including Minnesota's experience with the Bush Administration's smallpox vaccination program, the white powder crisis in Georgia, and the special needs evacuations following Hurricane Katrina.

As a result, coordination of responders is crucial. The multiple response organizations involved in a crisis must find ways of collaborating effectively rather than overlapping, duplicating, or interfering with each other. But, while effective coordination and collaboration are situationally required, they may prove very difficult to achieve. The institutional lead, even when formally assigned, can often be ambiguous in practice. A response organization is likely to share legal authorities, not solely possess them, and operate parallel to other tactical units that it does not directly control. Unity of command will be an ideal that may be attained only by voluntary cooperation, not the exercise of authority.

The National Incident Management System (NIMS), mandated by Congress in 2002 for use by all emergency response organizations in the United States, is gradually providing a common operating framework for organizations involved as crisis responders, including public health. It provides an organizational template for leadership, whether centered on a single incident commander or on a collective unified command. It also establishes a framework for dividing up and managing the work of response, institutionalizes the achievement of situational awareness through operational planning, and provides for logistical and administrative support for operations. However, implementation of NIMS remains a work in progress in the United States even 15 years or more after the Congressional mandate; while used by many jurisdictions, others have only gradually (and, frequently, just partially) adopted and applied it.

The case studies in this book provide contrasting examples of interagency and interjurisdictional collaboration. On one side, there were the difficulties of achieving a cohesive response against SARS in Toronto (where there was skepticism about using incident management methods); on the other, there was the largely effective collaboration in Texas during the H1N1 epidemic and the Ebola outbreak and the use of NIMS principles in pandemic planning in Ohio.

Handoffs Across Boundaries

As action in a crisis scales up and becomes more complex, those who initially mobilize may find the responsibilities or leadership required too taxing or beyond their capabilities; the situation may demand different skills or broader authority and resources. Yet transfers of authority or responsibility can cause substantial friction between organizations or jurisdictions even when emergency plans or statutes theoretically provide for such transitions. Simply because procedures have been written into laws or plans or are part of the procedures of NIMS does not mean that transitions will be handled smoothly. Officials on either side may not know how to play their roles effectively, or conflicts may arise in interpreting laws intended to structure their relationships in emergency situations. These frictions can be most severe when the organizations involved are not part of a single hierarchical structure—that is, when they are at different levels of government; represent independent municipalities or institutions; or cross public-, private-, or nonprofit-sector lines.

The case studies in this volume capture some of those tensions (for example, in Toronto during the SARS outbreak and in New Orleans during Hurricane Katrina). However, these cases also report on situations where cross-boundary handoffs work well, if not perfectly, as in the relationship between the city of Dallas and Dallas County and between the city/county and the state of Texas during the Ebola crisis.

Tensions Between Operational and Political Leaders

Routine emergencies typically occur in a single jurisdiction, where political authority is clearly marked and understood. In these situations, political oversight of professional responders is likely to be minimal and restrained unless dysfunction occurs. Elected officials tend to defer to their professional response leaders in routine emergencies because responders' expertise is manifest and response tends to be relatively short-term.

In crises, by contrast, particularly those that spread across jurisdictional boundaries, there often are many overseers of action (for example, mayors of different municipalities, city councilors, state legislators, perhaps the judiciary) who frequently have too little clarity about responsibility and authority. The NIMS system prescribes roles for professional response organizations and other organizational entities, whether from the public, private, or nonprofit sectors, but it does not very clearly lay out the relationships among those professionals and various sorts of political overseers, especially when multiple jurisdictions are involved.

In crises, especially in extended duration events like those that frequently involve public health, political leaders are likely to come off the sidelines and become more deeply involved. Elected leaders or appointed officials directly responsible to elected leaders may have very different viewpoints on a crisis situation than career professionals. They have different experiences, see events from different perspectives, and perceive obstacles and feasibility in different ways. Their viewpoints are often more superficial but also broader than those of professional responders. They typically lack expertise in emergency practices but sometimes better understand stakeholder pressures and the problems of publicly communicating, mobilizing support, and helping the community cope with loss. Political leaders, quite importantly, also carry the legitimacy of having been elected to office and thereby having been chosen by their constituents to make critical decisions and value judgments, including in the face of crisis conditions. On the positive side, we see elected leaders playing key roles in several of the case studies in this volume (for example, New York City's Mayor Rudolph Giuliani during the West Nile outbreak; the mayor and county judge in Dallas during the Ebola crisis). On the other hand, we see less directly engaged political leaders in Toronto during much of the SARS crisis.

Sometimes sharp tensions emerge between operational chiefs and political leaders, and less visible but still significant stress is even more frequent. Political leaders may interfere with what operational leaders see as appropriate professional practice, and operational leaders may try to hold political leaders at arm's length even when important value choices must be made. Senior operational leaders ideally will work in tandem with political leaders, recognizing their distinctive competences, accommodating the perspectives and decisions that the community has elected them to make, as well as proffering and standing up for the professionals' own strategic and tactical viewpoints. But sometimes leaders of both types fail to recognize the legitimate roles of the other, which can exacerbate tensions.

Moreover, in a crisis, because goals and priorities may be unclear or conflicting, there may be contention among different political leaders—a president, governor, or mayor—who each have different responsibilities, have different bases of authority, or represent different constituencies. This can make managing in a crisis very difficult for the professional response leaders. The Minnesota smallpox vaccination case study shows some aspects of such problems.

EXCELLENCE IN ROUTINE EMERGENCIES AND CRISES

What constitutes *excellence* in preparing for and responding to routine emergencies, whether in public health or other domains of emergency response? Ideally, effective preparedness includes a robust set of contingency plans for anticipated scenarios, combined with people who have strong training, skills, practice, and actual operational experience. Coordination methods are well established and drilled. When routine emergencies occur, responders can quickly achieve high levels of situational awareness because they know what factors matter and therefore what to look for. As they determine what they are confronting, they typically trigger standard operating procedures that all experienced personnel have practiced and employed before. Of course, any emergency has distinctive features, and these are accommodated through some degree of real-time customization of standard operating procedures. But the basic approach to routine emergencies has been set in advance. When well prepared for routine emergencies—even very large or dangerous ones—response organizations can thus act with confidence, discipline, a sense of purpose, clarity about what needs to be accomplished, and the advantages of well-honed skills.

Public health has cultivated and groomed professional leaders who can deal effectively with such situations. Leadership in routine emergencies is expertise-driven and usually hierarchical. Leaders know what to do because they have trained for such situations and performed well before. Ideally, they are chosen for leadership positions because of their knowledge, effectiveness during prior events, and demonstrated capacity to function under pressure. They exercise authority directly and expect a high degree of compliance from their subordinates, who follow them because they have confidence in their leaders' proven judgment. In the aftermath of events, leaders are accountable for results; they are explicitly or implicitly evaluated by how those results compare with what has been achieved in similar events in the past. At their best, public health organizations, like other emergency response agencies, can aim for operational precision and high efficiency in confronting routine emergencies.

In contrast with what makes good leadership in routine emergencies, crises demand abilities and skills that are quite different from—or in addition to—those necessary for leading in routine emergencies. Leaders must be alert for novelty that could be easily missed, especially in an emergent crisis. They are effective not only because of their expertise and experience but to a great extent because of their ability to adapt flexibly to cope with the unexpected. Open to the realization that no one is a comprehensive expert in the face of novelty, they reach out to others who have useful expertise or varying experiences, as CDC attempted to do in some configurations of its Team B. To achieve situational awareness and generate ideas about response, leaders need to feel comfortable with a flattened organizational structure effective for drawing on information from all levels of their own organization and from very diverse sources outside. Hierarchical command may have to be relaxed not only to secure a broader perspective but also because action may need to engage many partners over whom no single leader has direct authority. Because improvised problem solutions may not work completely or at all on first try, strong leaders have to be ready to adapt their approach creatively to find better tactics; they have to be fault tolerant of themselves and their subordinates.

Dealing With Public Health Emergencies

The ideal is not always the real. Although the case studies in this book provide many examples of leaders performing well in these dimensions, they also provide examples in which leaders fall short of excellence in response to crises. Routine emergencies usually prove dominant in number and frequency. It is normal practice to optimize organizational competence for such emergencies. Getting response right for these types of anticipatable emergencies is certainly crucial and necessary for any response organization. Indeed, society benefits greatly when the range of routine emergencies is expanded, that is, when potential crises are transformed into routine emergencies by effective hazard recognition, planning, procedural development, training, and exercising.

But even though routine emergencies prove to be the dominant type of situation leaders of response organizations confront, they have to master a different set of skills in order to perform strongly in crises. Because the differences between routine emergencies and crises are profound, the question for leaders in emergencies, not least in public health, is whether they and their organizations can become truly ambidextrous. Will the next generation of leaders, as well as the current one, be ready to manage routine emergencies effectively but also be able to recognize novelty when it appears, manage in a different mode, prove highly adaptive, and improvise the responses necessary to deal with future crises?

We encourage those who read this book to see it as a dialogue between a conceptual perspective on emergencies, as outlined in this chapter, and the real world case studies that compose the main body of the text. The cases tell rich stories about many of the issues that frame preparation for both routine emergencies and crises in public health. In a sense, the events recounted here are limited by time and place, but many elements of these accounts reflect more general problems that contemporary public health practitioners must confront. For many readers, these cases will resonate with their own experiences and perhaps shed new light on analogous events through which they have lived. For others, these cases will shine light on the realities of professional practice in crisis conditions. There are many practical insights here into how leadership and management skills and substantive expertise must combine to deal with the pressures that the public health system faces.

Fears and Realities: Managing Ebola in Dallas

Kirsten Lundberg

EDITORS' INTRODUCTION

In 2014, an epidemic of Ebola—a form of hemorrhagic fever—spread rapidly in West Africa, concentrating in Guinea, Sierra Leone, and Liberia. Health officials in the rest of the world increasingly worried about the possibility of the disease appearing in their countries.

Ebola was hardly an unknown disease, but it was a greatly feared one with horrifying symptoms and a high death rate for people who contracted it by coming in contact with the bodily fluids of infected individuals. First identified in 1976 in Zaire (now the Democratic Republic of Congo), Ebola outbreaks had subsequently occurred with some regularity—24 outbreaks in nearly 40 years—typically in rural areas where it was possible to isolate affected populations until the outbreak burned out. But the current epidemic was dramatically different; it had migrated to cities where greater population density and the complex interactions of urban life led to an accelerating spread of the disease.

In the United States, the Centers for Disease Control and Prevention (CDC) issued guidelines in August 2014 on how a hospital should handle an Ebola case.

This case was written by Kirsten Lundberg for Dr. Arnold M. Howitt, Executive Director of the Ash Center for Democratic Governance and Innovation at the John F. Kennedy School of Government, Harvard University. Funds for case development were provided by the Robert Wood Johnson Foundation for use at the Harvard Kennedy School as part of its State Health Leadership Initiative, sponsored in conjunction with the Association of State and Territorial Health Officials. HKS cases are developed solely as the basis for class discussion. Cases are not intended to serve as endorsements, sources of primary data, or illustrations of effective or ineffective management.

These were less stringent than the guidelines under which Doctors Without Borders was operating in Africa; CDC assumed that any US hospital would be able to deal with an appearance of the disease if basic precautions were taken. In addition, several specialized US hospitals readied themselves to handle, under carefully controlled conditions, Ebola patients who had contracted the disease in West Africa. By September, these hospitals had treated four patients successfully.

On September 25, 2014, in Dallas, Texas, Thomas Eric Duncan was admitted to Texas Health Presbyterian Hospital (Presbyterian) with headaches, fever, and abdominal pains; after an examination, he was sent home with antibiotics. But three days later, he returned to Presbyterian by ambulance with high fever, abdominal pain, and diarrhea; soon after arrival he began vomiting. At this time, he related that he had recently come from Liberia but denied having had contact with any Ebola patients, which subsequently proved untrue. Tests revealed he had Ebola.

Quickly the alarm went out to CDC and the Texas Department of State Health Services (DSHS), and soon the White House, Texas, and Dallas-area elected officials were informed. A flurry of issues had to be confronted as the emergency apparatus of the state of Texas and the Dallas area were being mobilized and as approaches to Duncan's care and to protecting the public were being developed and coordinated with the federal government. Duncan's condition worsened, however, and he died on October 8.

The crisis then seemed to slacken, but two days later word came that one of Duncan's nurses had fallen sick; tests the next day confirmed she had Ebola. Then on October 13, another nurse complained of symptoms, was quickly tested, and was confirmed as being infected with Ebola as well. Something had clearly gone wrong with the precautions that Presbyterian, carefully following CDC guidelines, had taken in caring for Duncan. Would these new cases burgeon into a more widespread epidemic of Ebola in Dallas and elsewhere? How would Texas public health officials cope with this new challenge?

DISCUSSION QUESTIONS

1. What explains Presbyterian's mistakes in recognizing Ebola when Duncan first presented himself for care?
2. What issues—public health, organizational, and political—had to be accommodated in deciding on a structure for managing Ebola in Dallas?
3. How effective were the strategies developed for communicating about Ebola with the public health and health care communities in Texas? With the general public?

4. What role did elected leaders play during the Ebola crisis? In what ways did they help with the situation? In what ways, if any, did they hamper the efforts of health professionals? What should the role of elected leaders be in such a crisis?

*   *   *

In early 2014, an epidemic gathered force in West Africa largely unseen by the global community. By the time a second wave of the deadly hemorrhagic fever known as Ebola erupted in Sierra Leone, Liberia, and Guinea in May, it was spiraling out of control. On August 8, the World Health Organization (WHO) declared Ebola an urgent global health emergency. Other countries waited anxiously for the disease—which killed at least half of those infected—to reach their shores.

The United States did not have long to wait. On Tuesday, September 30, 2014, Thomas Eric Duncan—a patient at Texas Health Presbyterian Hospital (Presbyterian) in Dallas—was diagnosed with Ebola. A Liberian citizen, he had flown to the United States on a visitor's visa just days earlier. The Centers for Disease Control and Prevention (CDC) deployed a team of epidemiologists to Dallas that night. The hospital had already isolated Duncan in accordance with CDC guidelines on managing Ebola patients.

Meanwhile, public health authorities moved quickly to manage the wider response to the first case of Ebola in the United States. Texas was a home-rule state, meaning that city or county governments led the response to any crisis, including public health (the state took charge only if no local health department existed).[1] After some initial ambiguity, Dallas County Judge Clay Jenkins, the highest elected county official, took leadership. On the morning of Thursday, October 2, Jenkins, Dallas Mayor Mike Rawlings, and Texas Department of State Health Services (DSHS) Commissioner Dr. David Lakey activated a county Emergency Operations Center (EOC) in Dallas with representatives from relevant local, state, and national agencies.

Over the next two weeks, EOC members conferred daily on dozens of issues ranging from Duncan's medical status to the decontamination of the apartment he'd occupied. The EOC coordinated quarantine and lodging for Duncan's family and supplies of personal protective equipment (PPE) for medical personnel. It worked with schools worried about exposed children and dealt with waste disposal, both from the hospital and the apartment. Teams of epidemiologists tracked down anyone who had been near Duncan, including those who later rode in his ambulance, and monitored them for Ebola symptoms. Finally, the EOC oversaw media and communication with an increasingly anxious public.

---

1. For an explanation and comparison of public health governance structures, see: Eileen Salinsky, "Governmental Public Health: An Overview of State and Local Public Health Agencies," *National Health Policy Forum*, August 18, 2010, http://www.nhpf.org/library/background-papers/BP77_GovPublicHealth_08-18-2010.pdf.

Duncan died on October 8. As of Friday, October 10, it seemed there were no new cases. The team had been working around the clock, and all were ready to consider the worst over. But on Friday, a Presbyterian nurse who had treated Duncan felt ill. Late Saturday, a Texas state laboratory confirmed: Nina Pham had Ebola. On Tuesday, October 14, a second Presbyterian nurse—Amber Vinson—was diagnosed. Vinson had just flown twice on commercial airlines.

State Health Commissioner Lakey, Dallas County Judge Jenkins, and others on the frontlines were stunned. For two weeks, CDC and Texas public health officials had reassured the public that the situation was under control. But if nurses wearing the PPE that CDC recommended had contracted the disease, how many others might be infected? What good were CDC guidelines if they didn't work? What were the risks to others who had come into contact with Pham and Vinson? Was this the start of an epidemic? What should the public health leadership tell medical personnel at Presbyterian? What should they tell the public? The worst wasn't over after all.

EBOLA, 1976–2014

Ebola was first identified in 1976 by Dr. Peter Piot, then at the Institute of Tropical Medicine in Antwerp, Belgium, and a team working in then-Zaire (now the Democratic Republic of Congo).[2] They named the disease for the nearby Ebola River. The illness was thought to originate in fruit bats, which spread it to other animals either through their blood or fruit they touched. Humans in remote areas contracted it from infected animals.[3]

The disease proved highly dangerous to people. It started with fever, which rose to high levels, followed by vomiting, diarrhea, and eventually uncontrolled hemorrhaging.[4] In early outbreaks, the fatality rate was 90%. Fortunately, it was not as contagious as other infectious diseases such as malaria (carried by mosquitos) or tuberculosis (conveyed by airborne droplets). Among humans, Ebola spread only through direct contact with the bodily fluids of an infected person.

Before 2014, Ebola had appeared almost exclusively in remote forest villages in Central and East Africa, where quarantine had been able to contain it. As of late 2013, Ebola had killed 1,590 people, but that was in 24 separate outbreaks over four decades.[5] The disease had never before struck a dense urban area where people lived, worked, and played in close proximity to one another.

---

2. For more on Dr. Peter Piot, see: http://www.lshtm.ac.uk/aboutus/people/piot.peter.
3. WHO, "Ebola Virus Disease," no. 103 (January 2016), http://www.who.int/mediacentre/factsheets/fs103/en.
4. For Ebola symptoms, see: Mayo Clinic, "Ebola Virus and Marburg Virus," August 6, 2014, http://www.mayoclinic.org/diseases-conditions/ebola-virus/basics/symptoms/con-20031241.
5. For a comprehensive and continually updated list of Ebola cases, see: CDC, "Outbreaks Chronology: Ebola Virus Disease," April 14, 2016, http://www.cdc.gov/vhf/ebola/outbreaks/history/chronology.html.

GUINEA FIRST

But in January 2014, the country of Guinea in West Africa experienced a cluster of puzzling deaths. There had only ever been a single, nonfatal Ebola case in West Africa— in Ivory Coast. Guinea and its neighbors were among the poorest countries on earth; they lacked the resources or the infrastructure to deal with a disease outbreak of any size. Typically, WHO's Strategic Health Operations Center in Geneva coordinated the global response to infectious disease episodes wherever they occurred. Historically, it had taken some two months to recognize an Ebola outbreak and three weeks to mount an international response.

In early 2014, WHO had an overflowing agenda. It was managing an outbreak of the Middle East respiratory syndrome (MERS) virus in Saudi Arabia, avian influenza A in China, polio in Syria, and conflicts in the Central African Republic and South Sudan with public health repercussions. Moreover, as part of a broader funding crunch, its budget for African epidemic preparedness and response had been more than halved over the preceding five years, from $26 million in 2010–2011 to $11 million in 2014–2015. It had laid off 9 of 12 emergency response specialists in Africa.[6]

Nonetheless, WHO on March 23 confirmed that Ebola had erupted in Guinea and sent a team of 38 to handle it. There were some 49 suspected cases and 29 deaths. By late March, neighboring Liberia also reported some cases in its northwest region abutting Guinea. By mid-May, however, the worst seemed to be over and WHO reduced its staff.

Unhappily, it was only a temporary reprieve. In late May, Ebola reemerged with a vengeance—this time in Sierra Leone. In mid-June, the nongovernmental medical organization Doctors Without Borders sounded an urgent alarm.[7] By late July, more than 800 had died in Guinea, Liberia, and Sierra Leone. On August 8, WHO declared Ebola "a public health emergency of international concern," its top public-health threat level.[8]

It was not long before international medical and public health officials who had served in West Africa themselves became infected. On August 2 and 5, respectively, two American health workers (Dr. Kent Brantly and Nancy Writebol) were airlifted from Liberia to Emory University Hospital in Atlanta, Georgia, one of four hospitals in the United States equipped with a biocontainment unit for infectious disease patients.[9] Both patients received an experimental drug, ZMapp, but doctors were unable to say whether

---

6. Kevin Sack, Sheri Fink, Pam Belluck, and Adam Nossiter, "How Ebola Roared Back," *New York Times*, December 29, 2014, http://www.nytimes.com/2014/12/30/health/how-ebola-roared-back.html.
7. Associated Press, "Ebola Cases Rise in West Africa," *Daily News*, June 24, 2014, http://www.nydailynews.com/news/world/ebola-cases-rise-africa-doctors-sound-alarm-outbreak-article-1.1841389.
8. WHO, "Ebola Disease Virus Update—West Africa," August 8, 2014, http://www.who.int/csr/don/2014_08_08_ebola/en. For the full statement, see: http://who.int/mediacentre/news/statements/2014/ebola-20140808/en.
9. The other three hospitals were the Nebraska Medical Center in Omaha, the National Institutes of Health Hospital in Bethesda, MD, and St. Patrick's in Missoula, MT.

the drug contributed to their recovery. An infected Spanish priest flown from Liberia died August 12 in a Madrid hospital despite treatment with ZMapp.[10]

As of mid-September, two of the specialized US hospitals had treated four Ebola patients from West Africa, all successfully.[11] But on September 23, CDC warned that the number of Ebola cases in West Africa could reach 1.3 million by January.[12] CDC put doctors and hospitals across the country on alert for the first domestic case of Ebola.

CENTERS FOR DISEASE CONTROL AND PREVENTION

Based in Atlanta and part of the federal Department of Health and Human Services, CDC is the preeminent public health agency in the United States. The agency is authorized to "protect America from health, safety and security threats, both foreign and in the US."[13] But federal government funding for public health and hospital readiness had declined steadily in the decade before 2014; some 50,000 public health jobs had been eliminated.[14] The funding drop was part of a roller coaster for public health budgets dating back to the late 1990s when these budgets had begun to rise. Public health preparedness funding had increased further after the events of September 11, 2001, the anthrax letter attacks that immediately followed, and the severe acute respiratory syndrome scare of 2003, only to decline again.

CDC had no direct authority to mandate an outbreak response integrated across local, state, and federal levels. It could only advise or provide services on request from states. Even to impose quarantine required a state order, and state laws varied.[15] In general, a governor could quarantine any individual believed to pose a danger to others. Quarantine was used very sparingly, however, as it invariably raised questions of civil liberties.

As the Ebola crisis in Africa deepened, CDC worked with public health authorities across the country on readiness measures for containing the disease should it occur in

10. Matt Moffett, "Ebola Virus: Infected Priest Has Died in Spain," *Wall Street Journal*, August 13, 2014, http://www.wsj.com/articles/missionary-doctor-infected-with-ebola-dies-in-madrid-1407835487.

11. CNN Wire, "4th US Ebola Patient Arrives From Sierra Leone," *KTLA 5-TV*, September 9, 2014, http://ktla.com/2014/09/09/4th-us-ebola-patient-arrives-from-sierra-leone-for-treatment-in-atlanta.

12. Denise Grady, "Ebola Cases Could Reach 1.4 Million in 4 Months," *New York Times*, September 23, 2014, http://www.nytimes.com/2014/09/24/health/ebola-cases-could-reach-14-million-in-4-months-cdc-estimates.html?_r=0.

13. CDC, "Mission, Role and Pledge," April 14, 2014, http://www.cdc.gov/about/organization/mission.htm.

14. Felice J. Freyer, "Ebola Response Shows Flaws in US System," *Boston Globe*, January 3, 2015, http://www.bostonglobe.com/metro/2015/01/03/ebola-exposed-flaws-nation-ability-respond-dangerous-new-germs/K26m73JZ5zn4tEXKKvLMZJ/story.html.

15. Jeffrey Levi and others, "Outbreaks: Protecting Americans from Infectious Diseases," Trust for America's Health, Robert Wood Johnson Foundation, Issue Report (December 2014):18–19, http://healthyamericans.org/assets/files/Final%20Outbreaks%202014%20Report.pdf. The federal government, under authority from the Commerce Clause of the Constitution as well as section 361 of the Public Health Services Act, could impose quarantine if someone infected with certain diseases arrived in the United States from abroad or if an infected person traveled between states.

the United States. The chief tool would be tracing contacts: identify, locate, and monitor for 21 days (the incubation period) all individuals who had come into close contact with a confirmed Ebola patient. The monitoring was twofold—measure body temperature twice a day and watch for other symptoms such as headache or vomiting. If fever rose above 101.5°F and other symptoms were present, test for Ebola (Exhibit 2A-1).[16]

On August 1, 2014, CDC sent an initial advisory to hospitals nationwide on how to handle an Ebola case. The premise was that any major hospital could deal with it. Hospital personnel were told to isolate the patient and protect themselves: wear gloves, a fluid-resistant gown, shoe covers, eye protection, and a face mask.[17] If a patient had copious amounts of body fluids, CDC suggested the addition of double gloves, disposable shoe covers, and leg coverings.

CDC guidelines were less stringent than those Doctors Without Borders followed in Africa, which called for head-to-toe coverage. Its guidelines also differed from procedures at the four hospitals with biocontainment units, but those units were intended for all infectious diseases, most of them far more contagious than Ebola. There, workers entered special locker rooms to put on scrubs, a mask, and a pair of gloves. To tend a patient, they added shoe covers, a second pair of gloves, a full-body impermeable gown, a hood over head and neck, and a respirator. A colleague monitored each step to ensure equipment went on and off in the correct order. CDC considered US hospitals far safer environments than African field hospitals or biocontainment units and believed its guidelines were fully appropriate to the situation.

It was up to each individual hospital to determine how seriously to take CDC notices. Some hospitals trained personnel in how to don protective gear, posted signs about Ebola precautions, and even sent decoy patients into emergency departments (EDs) to sharpen disease detection procedures. Far more hospitals simply circulated handouts or posted notices—and little more.

TEXAS PUBLIC HEALTH

Public health authorities in Texas were among those making ready. Texas is the second largest state in the United States, both by population (25 million) and area (269,000 sq miles). It boasts several large, thriving cities, among them Houston, Dallas, San Antonio, and the capital, Austin. At the time of this writing, Texas had a hybrid state–local public health system with 64 local health departments, primarily in the more

---

16. For a copy of the CDC monitoring guidelines, see Exhibit 2A-1. Monitoring was not simple. Who should monitor, and how—a nurse? The patient? In person? By phone?

17. For a copy of the CDC health advisory, see: http://emergency.cdc.gov/HAN/han00364.asp. For the transcript of a CDC emergency preparedness and response August 5, 2014 national conference call, detailing what hospitals needed to prepare for Ebola, also see: http://emergency.cdc.gov/coca/transcripts/2014/call-transcript-080514.asp.

populous counties, and eight public health regions staffed by DSHS, mainly covering small towns and rural areas.[18] The state health commissioner since 2007 was Dr. David Lakey, an Indiana native specialized in infectious diseases.

DSHS was a large agency, employing some 12,000, with a budget of $3.2 billion and a mission "to improve health and well-being in Texas."[19] Not only did it deliver or oversee local public health services but among its goals were to "prevent and prepare for health threats" and to promote recovery for infectious disease patients. It gathered data on the health of Texas citizens; maintained birth, death, and other records; oversaw mental health and substance abuse programs; and issued health-related licenses and regulations. In a disease emergency, DSHS was authorized to support an existing local health authority if requested to do so and to coordinate state-level assistance. DSHS also kept the governor, legislature, and other state and national health officials informed in times of crisis.

Texas also had a state-level Division of Emergency Management (TDEM), part of the Texas Department of Public Safety. TDEM, says Director Nim Kidd, "is responsible but not in charge" of emergency logistics.[20] The division's role was to communicate, cooperate, and collaborate with local officials. It operated 24 disaster districts statewide. In an emergency, the authorized local leader would activate a local EOC. The appropriate local agency (for a disease, that meant the health department if one existed) would take the lead. The agency director, in turn, could appoint an emergency coordinator to run the logistical operation.

Home Rule

Importantly, Texas was a home-rule state, meaning that much policy and administrative authority rested with local officials. Across the state, different jurisdictions had different definitions for whom the chief administrative officer was—in cities, the mayor; in unincorporated areas, a so-called county judge. In Texas, the county judge was the highest elected official, who functioned much like a mayor and was head of disaster relief for a county. The term could be confusing to those outside Texas: the officeholder did not adjudicate in a courtroom and did not even have to be a lawyer. Rather, the county judge presided over a Commissioners Court of four elected officials, akin to a city council. Each of four local districts within a county elected one commissioner; all county residents voted for the position of county judge.[21]

---

18. For more detail on the Texas public health system, see: https://www.dshs.texas.gov/rls/RLHS042211.shtm.
19. See: https://www.dshs.texas.gov/about-DSHS.shtm; https://www.dshs.texas.gov/commissioner/biography.shtm.
20. TDEM Director Nim Kidd in phone interview with the author, March 10, 2015. All further quotes from Kidd, unless otherwise attributed, are from this interview.
21. For a description of the county judge office, see: https://county.org/texas-county-government/texas-county-officials/Pages/County-Judge.aspx. Also see: David B. Brooks, *Guide to Texas Law for County Officials* (Austin, TX: Texas Association of Counties, 2016).

Under this system, state and national agencies could participate in emergency response only by invitation from a local jurisdiction. Chapter 418 of the Texas Government Code stipulated that in an emergency, the presiding officer of the governing board of the jurisdiction was the emergency management director. Local public health agencies—those who managed any disease outbreak response—were also variously structured. In San Antonio, for example, the city employed public health workers and the department held contracts with the surrounding areas in Bexar County. In Dallas, it was the opposite; the county health department was contracted by the city to deliver public health services. In those rural areas that could not afford a dedicated health department, DSHS was the *de jure* local public health authority, conducting such routine services as vaccinations or public education campaigns. In the event of a public health crisis in those rural areas, the state health department sent an incident response team to manage the situation.

Dallas County Health and Human Services

The Dallas County Health and Human Services (DCHHS) department oversaw public health services in the county. It had a director, Zachary Thompson, as well as a medical director, Dr. Christopher Perkins. The director was a political appointee, selected by one of four commissioners on the Commissioners Court. The City of Dallas did not have a separate public health department but by contract outsourced those functions to the county.

Ebola was already on the state's radar. In August, the Department of Defense approved the Texas State Public Health Laboratory in Austin—already a member of the National Laboratory Response Network (LRN) for bioterrorism or infectious disease—as one of several labs nationwide to receive a test kit for Ebola. Both Dallas and Houston also had LRN labs, but the Department of Defense selected the Austin location for Texas. In the event of a suspected Ebola case, the DSHS infectious disease epidemiology unit required that a sample be sent first to the lab in Austin, and subsequently to CDC, which would confirm the diagnosis. "It was a system that was adding capabilities," recalls State Health Commissioner Lakey.[22]

But Ebola was far from a priority and was largely wrapped into a larger upper-respiratory, viral disease plan. "Like many things, when it's not near you, you don't treat it as in-depth as other things," recalls DSHS Assistant Commissioner for Regional and Local Health Services David Gruber. "We had an Ebola plan, but I think it's hard to say that it was really an operational Ebola plan."[23]

---

22. DSHS Commissioner Dr. David Lakey in phone interview with author, March 2, 2015. All further quotes from Lakey, unless otherwise attributed, are from this interview.
23. DSHS Assistant Commissioner for Regional and Local Health Services David Gruber in phone interview with author, March 3, 2015. All further quotes from Gruber, unless otherwise attributed, are from this interview. Gruber's department also had responsibility for health emergency preparedness.

EBOLA COMES TO DALLAS

On Monday morning, September 29, 2014, State Health Commissioner Lakey first learned that a patient at Presbyterian, one of the Texas Health Resources group of 24 hospitals, was being tested for Ebola. Duncan, 45, had come to the ED by ambulance the day before—Sunday, September 28—with a high fever, abdominal pain, and diarrhea; after admission, he began to vomit and exhibit other worrying symptoms.

Prior Emergency Department Visit

Doctors did not immediately realize that Duncan had already been at the ED on Thursday, September 25, with a headache, fever, and abdominal pain and been sent home with antibiotics for possible sinusitis. On Sunday, September 28, Duncan told doctors that he had come recently from Liberia but denied any exposure to an Ebola patient. He did confirm that he had left Liberia September 19 on a visitor's visa approved a month earlier and, flying via Brussels and Washington, DC, landed Saturday, September 20, in Dallas.[24] He had come to marry Louise Troh, the mother of his 19-year-old son, and went to stay with her at the Ivy Apartments in the Vickery Meadows neighborhood of Dallas. On Wednesday, September 24, Duncan began to feel sick.

After Duncan's admission to the ED on Sunday morning, the hospital had quickly isolated the patient. The doctor tending Duncan had called CDC, while the hospital's infection preventionist simultaneously notified the DCHHS epidemiologist on duty, who in turn contacted her boss, DCHHS Chief Epidemiologist Dr. Wendy Chung. Since Duncan denied any exposure to Ebola, he did not meet CDC criteria for Ebola testing.[25] But by afternoon, Chung found the latest test results increasingly disturbing; while some of Duncan's symptoms and lab results mimicked those of malaria, he did not test positive for malaria. "This is how it is in real life," she comments. "Pieces of information don't get presented all at once at the very beginning; they're trickling in through the day."[26]

---

24. For more on Duncan's personal history, see: Associated Press, "Thomas Eric Duncan Fled Liberian War Years Before Fatal Ebola Infection," *Guardian*, October 8, 2014, http://www.theguardian.com/world/2014/oct/08/thomas-eric-duncan-liberia-ebola-war-texas-family-obituary. Duncan applied for a visa to visit his sister, who lived in North Carolina.

25. CDC, "Health Advisory to Clinicians: Guidelines for Evaluation of US Patients Suspected of Having Ebola Virus Disease," August 8, 2014, http://emergency.cdc.gov/HAN/han00364.asp. The advisory based its testing threshold on a patient's stated exposure to Ebola.

26. DCHHS Epidemiologist Dr. Wendy Chung, in phone interview with the author, March 5, 2015. All further quotes from Chung, unless otherwise attributed, are from this interview.

Confirmed

Chung had followed events in West Africa and received the multiple notices from CDC. Now she wanted to test Duncan for Ebola, but the process was not straightforward. Under protocol, as an epidemiologist for the county, Chung had to request a test first from the authorized state lab in Austin (she learned only that day that Texas had acquired Ebola testing capacity) and then from CDC. Nor could she contact the state lab directly but had to make the request through the state's infectious disease epidemiology unit.

Once she got through to both agencies, Chung found she had to press her case. Without confirmed exposure to Ebola, Duncan's symptoms didn't meet CDC recommendations for a test. Chung persisted, however, and also argued for sending samples simultaneously rather than sequentially to the state and then CDC labs. On Monday, after considerable confusion over the protocol for shipping Ebola samples, two went out via FedEx—to Austin and Atlanta. Late Tuesday, September 30, first the state and then CDC confirmed: Duncan had Ebola.

Over the next two days, it would emerge that while still in Africa Duncan had in fact helped transport a young Liberian neighbor who died from Ebola.[27] Duncan had confided this late Sunday to a night nurse at Presbyterian who, like himself, was African— but she did not pass on the information until Tuesday.[28] The breaking news raised concerns about the reliability of the patient's prior reports. Chung on Tuesday decided to question Duncan herself to reconcile varying accounts of the timing and sequence of his initial symptoms. Typically, a public health official interviewed an infectious patient by proxy—by phone or through an attending doctor or family member. But Chung was at the hospital already and particularly wanted to confirm quickly and with some finality whether Duncan may have been ill even during his flight from Liberia.

At the hospital's direction, she donned a protective face shield, double gowns and gloves, and knee-high plastic boots and went in accompanied by an infectious disease doctor and a hospitalist. "I wasn't worried," she says. "I didn't touch anything. I didn't touch his table. I didn't touch him. I stayed right about three feet from him." Duncan assured her he'd had no symptoms in flight. While she was there, she also asked about the Liberian neighbor; Duncan denied any contact with an Ebola victim. Notes Chung: "Our entire exposure risk-classification system was predicated upon an individual's willingness or ability to self-disclose their exposure."

---

27. Manny Fernandez and Norimitsu Onishi, "U.S. Patient Aided Ebola Victim in Liberia," *New York Times*, October 2, 2014, http://www.nytimes.com/2014/10/02/us/after-ebola-case-in-dallas-health-officials-seek-those-who-had-contact-with-patient.html.
28. At the time, there were evolving accounts of who told whom what on Sunday night and of Duncan's initial visit to the hospital September 25.

In a sense, it no longer mattered. Regardless of how Duncan had contracted Ebola, Texas health authorities were now responsible for preventing its spread, most immediately to the Dallas County population of 2.5 million. Chung and her staff of seven epidemiologists started the process of tracing his contacts Sunday night. As typical for contact tracing, she had requested Presbyterian to compile a list of all medical personnel who had encountered Duncan on both ED visits. As Chung knew from past experience with measles exposures in hospitals, "getting together that list of contacts takes time."

She also learned that Duncan had been living in an apartment with Troh and three young male relatives (one a child), and on Monday, September 29, she found out there had been other visitors to the household. All were asked to monitor themselves for fever and other symptoms of illness, but their movement at first was not restricted. On Tuesday night, however, DCHHS at CDC's request asked that the child be kept home from school on Wednesday so that monitors could check him in person.

BREAKING THE NEWS

From Austin, State Health Commissioner Lakey followed developments closely. Starting Monday, September 29, he spoke frequently with CDC Director Dr. Thomas Frieden who was managing the case at the national level, with the White House, with state elected officials, and with authorities in Dallas. He also met with officials at the state lab.

Once Duncan's test results came in positive on the afternoon of Tuesday, September 30, Lakey on behalf of the state formally requested assistance from CDC. He already had close ties to CDC Director Frieden; they had worked in the past on an outbreak of the H1N1 virus and other issues. That relationship now paid dividends: "As I tell folks, the time to exchange business cards is not at the scene of the disaster," comments Lakey. "You need to have a trust and a relationship there."

Throughout Tuesday, Frieden and Lakey conferred repeatedly by phone on how to present the news that Ebola had come to the United States. In early afternoon, DSHS announced that it was "aware of the suspect Ebola case in Dallas and is coordinating with the CDC and local health officials."[29] A simultaneous CDC press release combined information about Ebola with public reassurance. It quoted CDC Director Frieden: "While it is not impossible that there could be additional cases associated with this patient in the coming weeks, I have no doubt that we will contain this."[30] A second DSHS press release that evening confirmed the positive diagnosis and reassured the public that the hospital had put in place infection control measures. In addition, Lakey joined a 5:30 p.m. CDC national teleconference hosted by Frieden to take questions from the press.

---

29. For the DSHS press release, see: https://www.dshs.texas.gov/news/releases/20140930a.aspx.
30. For the CDC press release, see: "CDC and Texas Health Department Confirm First Ebola Case Diagnosed in the U.S.," October 1, 2014, http://www.cdc.gov/media/releases/2014/s930-ebola-confirmed-case.html.

Meanwhile, at the Dallas County level, DCHHS Director Thompson and DCHHS Medical Director Perkins informed the Commissioners Court at its regular Tuesday 9 a.m. meeting about the possible Ebola case. They assured the elected officials that contact tracing had started. "We communicated to them that we were in the midst of doing what we prepare for all the time, be it tuberculosis or an STD," says Perkins.[31] That briefing was the first Dallas County Judge Jenkins had heard of a potential Ebola case in Dallas.

Emergency Operations Centers

Later Tuesday, DCHHS opened an EOC intended, says Director Thompson, to "stand up until state and federal [help] arrived." Thompson also put out a DCHHS press release that commended Perkins and county epidemiologists for their quick work so far in tracing Duncan's contacts; he added that "Dallas County residents should be aware that the public health is our number one priority."[32] Meanwhile, as dictated by the city's June 2011 Master Emergency Operations Basic Plan, the city of Dallas on Tuesday opened its own EOC at City Hall. That plan put the mayor in overall charge of an emergency, with specific responsibilities assigned to city agencies, including DCHHS.

Meanwhile, other players arrived in Dallas. On Tuesday evening, an epidemiological team, which CDC had dispatched immediately on getting Duncan's positive diagnosis, arrived. The team included three senior scientists, five epidemic intelligence service officers, a public health advisor, and a communications officer. The team's job was to help with contact tracing, disease containment, and public information.

Late Tuesday, Texas Governor Rick Perry contacted State Health Commissioner Lakey to request Lakey's presence at a press conference scheduled for Dallas on Wednesday afternoon. Lakey agreed and pulled together a small team: DSHS Assistant Health Commissioner Gruber, DSHS Communications Director Ricky Garcia, and State Epidemiologist Dr. Linda Gaul. On Wednesday morning, they left Austin for the three-hour drive to Dallas in time to arrive by 8 a.m. The plan was to return home that night.

THE LONGEST DAY

Wednesday, October 1, was a very long day. On arrival in Dallas, Lakey and his colleagues gathered early with representatives from the state, county, and city to discuss the situation and what they would say at the press conference scheduled for 1 p.m. at

---

31. DCHHS Director Zachary Thompson and DCHHS Medical Director Dr. Christopher Perkins in phone interview, March 5, 2015. All further quotes from Thompson and Perkins, unless otherwise attributed, are from this interview.
32. For the DCHHS press release, see: "Public Statement from DCHHS Director Zachary Thompson on First U.S. Diagnosed Ebola Case," September 30, 2014, http://www.dallascounty.org/department/hhs/press/documents/PressReleasePublicStatementonFirstU.S.DiagnosedEbolaCaseinDallas.pdf.

Presbyterian. On hand were a range of politicians from both parties: Governor Rick Perry (a Republican), Dallas Mayor Mike Rawlings (a Democrat), Dallas County Judge Jenkins (a Democrat), and several congressmen. Also lined up to speak were State Health Commissioner Lakey, DCHHS Director Thompson, and other officials, including the Dallas schools superintendent.

Those gathered held a variety of assumptions about who was in charge of the Ebola response. Mayor Rawlings, for one, thought he knew the answer: the White House, or maybe CDC. Recalls Rawlings: "For a naïve person like myself, I thought it would just go up the chain and ultimately the President of the United States makes the call."[33] For his part, Dallas County Judge Jenkins went to bed Tuesday, he says, "believing ... that [CDC] would be the people in charge." The CDC officials in Dallas, however, quickly made it clear that they were not in charge of incident response; they were epidemiologists. State Health Commissioner Lakey thought DCHHS was in charge. In a Texas public health emergency, he says, "it depends on where an event is occurring whether the state is the lead or the local health department is the lead.... Dallas has a wholly functional health department, so they are the lead in those situations." Typically, the state health department (DSHS) would send its regional health director to represent the state in a county (DCHHS)-run EOC.

At the morning meeting, it became clear that the ambiguity about authority had potentially serious implications. Governor Perry, recalls Mayor Rawlings, asked a lot of questions. Then Rawlings queried where the identified Duncan contacts were right now. They went around the room, and "it was obvious that no one knew that," he says.[34] In fact, it came as news to most of those in the room that one of the children at Duncan's apartment had gone to school Monday and Tuesday. The group noted the confusion caused by conflicting media reports—based on conflicting official sources—of the number of Duncan's contacts. Additionally, it emerged that DCHHS Wednesday morning mistakenly told a local TV news program that there was a second suspected Ebola case.[35] "And I said, well, no one's in charge," notes Mayor Rawlings.

The press conference went ahead at 1 p.m. with the prevailing message that state and local officials had the situation under control. But immediately afterward, Jenkins, Lakey, and a few others convened in a nearby hospital meeting room. Lakey says they called to invite DCHHS Director Thompson or his designated representative, but he was not free. In addition to urgent questions of what to do with Duncan's family and apartment, there were leadership issues. "It was exceptionally evident" at the press conference, says DSHS Assistant Health Commissioner Gruber, "that the response was not taking off the way it

33. Dallas Mayor Mike Rawlings in phone interview with author, March 20, 2015. All further quotes from Rawlings, unless otherwise attributed, are from this interview.
34. Dallas County Judge Clay Jenkins in phone interview with the author, March 4, 2015. All further quotes from Jenkins, unless otherwise attributed, are from this interview.
35. Eliana Dokterman, "Second Patient Monitored for Ebola in Texas," Time, October 1, 2014, http://time.com/3453093/ebola-texas-dallas-second-patient.

needed to…. It was just painful to watch." The two EOCs, at City Hall and DCHHS, were "not appropriate for the event," he adds, because they focused either too narrowly on traditional emergency management "guns and hoses" issues or on tracing contacts, rather than on the wider universe of practical, public health logistical needs. Moreover, so far the city and county EOCs were not integrated with each other or with the state health department.

West Nile Precedent

But what else could be done, and who would do it? Jenkins and Lakey had experienced a precedent for an alternative command structure. In 2012, Dallas County had experienced a severe outbreak of West Nile virus, which sickened 398 people and eventually killed 19. When the death toll stood at 10, the state took the controversial decision to spray mosquitoes from the air.[36] While DCHHS leadership had no objection to spraying by trucks, it opposed aerial spraying. But Mayor Rawlings, Dallas County Judge Jenkins, and State Health Commissioner Lakey had worked together to make it work, with the state picking up the cost of airplanes and chemicals. The operation was successful, and the three men grew to know one another well.

On Wednesday afternoon, Lakey and Jenkins called CDC Director Frieden to clarify once again the federal role. "This is the first time that you've had this disease in the United States, so what is the role of the CDC?" Lakey recalls asking. When Frieden reiterated that CDC did not have the capacity to act as incident response manager, Lakey and Jenkins decided the best course of action was to reconstitute the emergency management operation that had worked for West Nile.

COUNTY EMERGENCY OPERATIONS CENTER

Dallas County Judge Jenkins agreed to lead a Dallas County EOC if Lakey would agree to be onsite as medical advisor. While it would take Lakey away from Austin and his other statewide duties, he agreed. "There isn't always a clear understanding of home rule and what the role of the state is versus the local health department," he says. "How do you move things forward quickly is always something that you have discussions about…. You're at the very beginning of an event trying to figure out what exactly is going on." He adds: "My concern was that [DCHHS] was probably not big enough" to handle the Ebola response, "because this is an event that's going to transcend any one area."

---

36. For the prespraying death toll, see: DCHHS, "DCHHS Confirms Tenth West Nile Virus Related Death in Dallas County," August 13, 2012, http://www.dallascounty.org/department/hhs/press/documents/WestNile2012-10thDeath.pdf.

Lakey and Jenkins then drove to the Dallas County Administration Building on Elm Street, where they brought in the county director of emergency management, Doug Bass. On the spot, Jenkins and Lakey drew a rough Incident Command System (ICS) structure on a white board (Exhibit 2A-2). "Normally, you have an 'incident command in a box' for things like a hurricane or a tornado," notes Jenkins. "With this, we're literally writing it out on a whiteboard."

Bass agreed to run the EOC day-to-day. Jenkins, Lakey, and Rawlings would constitute an oversight policy group. They divided responsibilities into medical and public health (run by DSHS Assistant Health Commissioner Gruber), finance, logistics, operations, and planning. Under medical were grouped the epidemiologists (led by DCHHS Chief Epidemiologist Chung), Presbyterian, emergency services (e.g., ambulances), and the state laboratory. As Chung points out, "an ICS in and of itself isn't a cure-all. You need not just the ICS structure, but people who understand what it means, respect it, obey it and listen to it and support it." While the EOC geared up, Mayor Rawlings agreed to handle media for the first 48 hours.

The arrangement was unorthodox for a city with a mayor. Rawlings recognized that he could have declared a state of emergency, with himself in charge. But, he explains, "the county was the controlling authority on health issues," and Dallas County Judge Jenkins was the county executive. Moreover, a state of emergency carried psychological and economic costs that the situation did not yet warrant. "To me, that felt counterproductive when we could just partner and get through this," says Rawlings.

> I didn't want to create a perception in the public that the left hand was fighting with the right hand. We needed to say, we're all working together and we're focused on this disease and the patients, and you don't have to worry about the politics of this.

Jenkins, too, could have declared a disaster. That would have put him automatically in charge of the recovery effort. But a disaster had to be reauthorized after seven days by the Commissioners Court, and Jenkins could not be sure he had the votes. It seemed better to do without the disaster declaration.

Immediate priorities, the group agreed, were to keep the Troh family at home and under observation, relocate the family to a clean apartment, decontaminate the Troh apartment, remove waste from both the apartment and hospital, and identify and monitor Duncan's contacts. As of late Wednesday, October 1, epidemiologists were focused on contacts in the higher risk category, that is, those who had personal contact with Duncan and required in-person monitoring by the health department. The Dallas Fire and Rescue Department had already tracked down ambulance drivers and staff and had voluntarily isolated them. The hospital had also determined that no one in the waiting room when Duncan arrived had been within 3 feet of him. But others still had to be located—for example, the patients who had used the ambulance after Duncan but before he was diagnosed.

Control Order

Late Wednesday, October 1, Lakey and his Austin colleagues returned to the capital. But their work wasn't done; they had to address the report that the child from the Troh household had attended school the morning after his mother had been instructed not to send him and that another adult member of the household had left the premises despite a request from the monitoring team to stay put.

In Texas, the health commissioner by law could request an infectious disease contact to remain isolated via a so-called control order. The control order allowed authorities to post police outside the contact's residence but not to make arrests. The control order was not legally enforceable; but if the contact broke the order, the commissioner could apply for a judge's order for full quarantine, which was enforceable.

On the drive, Lakey and his team debated with the group in Dallas and lawyers in Austin how best to ensure the Troh family's seclusion for 21 days. They worried that full-out quarantine might discourage other contacts from coming forward. They decided instead to impose a control order instructing Troh family members to stay home.[37] "We made the decision because I couldn't get comfortable that they were following the rules that were being laid out for them to follow," recalls Lakey.

As Jenkins explains, the control order was a compromise and an example of how public health precepts sometimes conflict with public policy. While public health guidelines might dictate full quarantine for Duncan's contacts, an astute public policy would try to avoid the "bad outcomes if you place a large pool of people under some form of house arrest," says Jenkins. Likewise, public health might insist that contact tracing remain entirely private information, but public policy would dictate the release of certain information to avoid panic, such as parents pulling kids out of school. The challenge, he says, was "balancing people's personal liberties with the public's need to know that they're protected from an Ebola exposure."

Lakey and DCHHS Medical Director Perkins cosigned the control order for four individuals—Louise Troh, her 13-year-old son, Duncan's 21-year-old nephew, and a male friend. The order provided that they remain home without visitors (except by prior approval) until at least October 19. Thompson and Perkins delivered it to the apartment late Wednesday evening. "The apartment was very neat," recalls Thompson, contradicting press reports that it was strewn with vomit and feces. Troh had gathered all of Duncan's belongings in one room and closed the door. Thompson and Perkins had no hesitation going into the apartment. "We felt comfortable going in. We felt no threat," says Thompson.

---

37. For a fuller explanation of the legal framework behind control orders for quarantine in Texas, see: Allison N. Winnike, "Quarantine and Isolation Law in Texas," http://www.law.uh.edu/healthlaw/ebola/Winnike.pdf.

EMERGENCY MANAGEMENT

In Austin, Lakey slept a couple of hours, packed for a week, and, at 5 a.m. Thursday, October 2, set out again for Dallas with a new DHSH group in order to activate the new Dallas County EOC by 8 a.m. at the County Administration Building on Elm Street. Lakey and his staff took over direction of the health and medical component of the EOC. In general, Lakey handled relations with CDC, while Dallas County Judge Jenkins and Mayor Rawlings took responsibility for community and political relations. "We were embedded into the EOC basically from 8 o'clock in the morning until 10 o'clock at night every day," remembers Lakey. Jenkins early Thursday issued a press release about the EOC.[38]

Other EOC representatives came from DCHHS, the police, fire department, emergency services, the department of transportation, and other relevant city and county departments. Epidemiologists from the county as well as CDC and, in time, the state were there. The hospital sent a representative. By late Thursday, recalls DCHHS Chief Epidemiologist Chung, the epidemiology team had identified 108 people who had come in contact with Duncan, most of them health care workers. The team had already interviewed 90 of them and determined that 35 were not true contacts.

Not everyone was pleased that Lakey had decided to move to Dallas. State Emergency Management Chief Nim Kidd felt that plans were in place to assist Dallas without deploying the state health commissioner as a working member of the local EOC. "It put us in a position where our chief medical officer was taking care of one community instead of taking care of the entire state," says Kidd. DSHS Deputy Commissioner Mike Maples and DSHS Associate Commissioner Kirk Cole kept public health running in Austin, including communications, governmental affairs, and external affairs. Maples concurs that Lakey "kind of went offline of the state commissioner role."[39]

Kidd's preferred approach was to bring State Health Commissioner Lakey back to Austin, set up a local EOC according to existing county and state plans, and support it via health district disaster committees. He tried to warn Dallas County Judge Jenkins and Lakey that "we don't throw out the plan just because we haven't dealt with this particular instance before. We follow our organized structure." Kidd also objected to the control Judge Jenkins exercised over the release of information and access to the EOC. "Whatever the flavor of disaster, there has got to be a managed approach," he comments.

> We as cities, we as a state, we as a nation cannot have one-person shows.... We have to train together, exercise together and respond together, and we have to respond the way we have trained and exercised.... Instead, they tried to focus on it as a single event within the community, and no other resources were needed.

---

38. For a copy of the DCHHS press release, see: "Statement From Dallas County Judge Clay Jenkins," October 2, 2014, https://www.dallascounty.org/Assets/uploads/docs/judge-jenkins/press-releases/2014/100214_CJ_Statement.pdf.
39. DSHS Deputy Commissioner Mike Maples in phone interview with the author, March 3, 2015. All further quotes from Maples, unless otherwise attributed, are from this interview.

But such objections were set aside and Kidd made it his business to make sure Lakey—whose work he admired—was getting enough rest and the support he needed.

Some 15 state officials spent significant time in Dallas during the Ebola crisis. Quite a few DSHS officials were surprised by the roles they were asked to assume. DSHS Assistant Health Commissioner Gruber, for example, rather than representing the state in a locally driven effort, took over the operational details of waste disposal as well as patient transportation. "There's no reason for me ever to be in the position that I was in," he reports. "Much like State Health Commissioner Lakey should not have been as operationally involved as he was."

DECONTAMINATE

Thursday, October 2, and Friday, October 3, went to accomplishing the most urgent tasks. One was to calm the public. For example, parents fearing infection on Thursday pulled students from a classroom in the Richardson School District, and other schools experienced similar panic.[40] Another was to decontaminate the apartment where the Trohs were living. Both Dallas and Austin knew that special permits were required to remove the waste, but the process to obtain these permits was unclear, since even federal Department of Transportation permits had never been issued in the United States to allow transport of Ebola waste. EOC staff set to work finding out. It also wasn't clear which firm would be willing to take the job. "There has been a little bit of hesitancy for entities to want to do that," Lakey told a reporter.[41] Lakey had declared that, for the near term, costs were not to interfere with quick action. So even before the EOC opened formally, staff on Wednesday had contacted several hazardous-materials businesses—including Cleaning Guys in nearby Fort Worth, which had existing contracts with the city.

On Thursday, Cleaning Guys agreed to take the job. "A biological event is a biological event," owner Erick McCallum later told a reporter. "The type of gear, the decontamination, the protocols. All the same."[42] But the cleaners couldn't go in that day. As it turned out, the required US Department of Transportation permits to remove and dispose of Ebola waste had not yet arrived. The permits finally came on Friday morning and the crew—dressed in full hazmat suits—got to work.

Behind the scenes, the EOC dealt with countless details. For example, response leaders had resolved that the waste removal should be done quietly. However, on Friday DSHS Assistant Health Commissioner Gruber watched on TV as numerous fire engines

40. For other examples, see: Matthew Watkins, "Highland Park ISD Parents Told Jenkins Hasn't Created Risk," *Dallas News*, October 7, 2014, http://www.dallasnews.com/news/metro/20141007-highland-park-isd-parents-told-jenkins-hasnt-created-risk.ece. Also see: Christopher Hooks, "Breitbart Texas: Clay Jenkins Is Going to Give You Ebola," *Texas Observer*, October 8, 2014, http://www.texasobserver.org/breitbart-texas-clay-jenkins-is-going-to-give-you-ebola.

41. Tom Dart and Lauren Gambion, "Ebola Patient's Family Quarantined," *Guardian*, October 3, 2014, http://www.theguardian.com/world/2014/oct/02/ebola-patients-waste-remained-texas-apartment-two-days.

42. Bryan Burrough, "Trial by Ebola," *Vanity Fair*, February 2015, 95.

congregated at Ivy Apartments. He called Jenkins to say "if you're trying to make this quiet, this ain't the way to do it." Jenkins made some calls and the engines were withdrawn. By Monday, Cleaning Guys had finished the job and removed all contents—triple bagged inside industrial barrels—and burned them in an incinerator approved for hazardous waste.

But when Cleaning Guys started, the Trohs were still in the apartment. That was a problem. On Wednesday, global media had taken up stations outside the Ivy Apartments. The contrasting TV images of cleaners in hazmat suits versus the family in ordinary clothes was jarring. Many members of the public expressed outrage, both at the Trohs' living conditions and at lack of publicity in Ivy Apartments itself about Ebola. Something had to be done—and right away.

THE TROH FAMILY

On the morning of Thursday, October 2, Anderson Cooper, a CNN reporter, interviewed Troh, who said she knew of no plans to move her. A DCHHS spokesperson was quoted saying the family was responsible for obtaining its own clean linens, even though they couldn't leave the premises.[43] Although Lakey had arranged for public health agencies and charities to send the family groceries and other necessities, the news reports made the public health authorities look at best uncaring. The problem, as Lakey, Jenkins, and Rawlings were learning, was that no one—no motel, shelter, or apartment complex—would take the Trohs. Despite repeated reassurances from local, state, and national public health authorities, neighborhoods worried about contagion. Rawlings especially went to extraordinary lengths to find a willing landlord; at one point, the working solution was to use his son's recently renovated, empty bungalow.[44]

Visit

While the EOC researched residences, Jenkins on Thursday decided it was time to visit the Trohs. He recognized that of all the contacts likely to have contracted Ebola from Duncan, Troh led the list; she must be very anxious. As chief elected official of Dallas County and director of the Ebola response, Jenkins decided to go himself to Ivy Apartment 614. He checked with Lakey, CDC, and DCHHS that it was safe to enter the apartment in street clothing; all assured him that, so long as he remained 3 feet from any person and didn't touch anything, he was safe. The epidemiology teams had already conducted numerous home visits without PPE.

---

43. Dart and Gambion, "Ebola Patient's Family Quarantined." DCHHS Public Information Officer Erikka Neroes states: "The individuals, it's up to them … to care for the household."
44. Burrough, "Trial by Ebola."

Epidemiologists from CDC and DCHHS accompanied him to the doorway. He wanted to "let them [the family] know that we wanted to treat them the way we would treat our own families," recalls Jenkins. "I went out and met them, and apologized on behalf of the state and federal and local government that they weren't out of there." Like Thompson and Perkins on Wednesday, he found the apartment tidy but was disturbed that Troh was sleeping on a couch cushion on the floor. He notes:

> I thought if I were Thomas Eric Duncan and I were fighting for my life in a hospital bed, this certainly is not the way I would want my loved ones treated.

Jenkins's 15-minute visit stirred up a mini-storm of anger and fear. The Cleaning Guys were appalled that Jenkins would go in without head-to-toe protection. His own staff worried about contagion, as did his wife. As Jenkins later explained, "I think it was very important for Louise [Troh] and those three young men to be seen as human beings."

> There was a tremendous amount of fear, not based on science at that time, and I didn't want to ask the first responders to do anything that I myself wouldn't do. The main reason I did that was for Louise. I didn't want to unnecessarily dress up like a space man and de-humanize this person any further.[45]

Move

On the morning of Friday, October 3, Jenkins returned to the apartment to engineer the move itself. Mid-morning, the Catholic bishop of Dallas offered a church-owned house to the family. Again, the cleaning crew advised full hazmat gear for all. Jenkins vetoed that; they would all remain in their clothes.[46] But Jenkins did want a CDC medical professional onsite to witness the transfer. That never happened. As Jenkins learned in a phone call from the parking lot, CDC worried that if the move went awry, people in future might be afraid to come forward as contacts. CDC elected to remain uninvolved. So State Health Commissioner Lakey suggested asking DCHHS Chief Epidemiologist Chung, who readily agreed to be the medical representative onsite. That episode, says Jenkins, "does capture the chaotic nature of all this."

> In situations like this, it would be great if … you've got an exact plan and everything goes according to schedule and it looks like a sporting event, looks like a deal where everybody is working in unison and knows their parts and it's all well-rehearsed. But in reality, this never happened before in America. It hasn't been rehearsed at all and it's very chaotic and you're just doing the best you can.

---

45. NBC5, November 6, 2014.
46. Burrough, "Trial by Ebola." The epidemiologists differentiated between high-risk and some-risk contacts. None of the medical personnel who had worn PPE were on the high-risk list.

For example, it was not clear how exactly to move the family without a media carnival. News helicopters hovered over the apartment complex; news vans and cars were lined up outside. "In the midst of this media circus, how can you relocate them?" asks Lakey. "We were trying to figure out how do you move somebody, protect their dignity, give them a better condition, being as transparent as you can but understanding that some information doesn't necessarily have to be released to protect the public's health."

In the end, Rawlings advised Jenkins to call the intergovernmental affairs office at the White House and ask for help in clearing the air space above Ivy. Officially, the White House said that regrettably it could do nothing, but twice Friday afternoon (once before Chung arrived and once after), the helicopters vanished. In the second interlude, Jenkins loaded the Troh family into his Ford Explorer and spirited them away to the new location.[47] A few local news organizations that discovered the new address agreed to leave them alone.

TAKING STOCK

By the weekend of October 4, the EOC was functioning better. Some 24 epidemiologists had divided into two teams to track contacts—one followed health care workers, the other community contacts. The epis, as the epidemiologists were known, came 60% from CDC and the remainder from the county (DCHHS). They went in pairs to interview each contact. In addition, two epidemiologists from the state remained at the EOC to collect and coordinate numbers from the two teams.

The EOC had experienced early difficulties in reporting a consistent number of contacts because it was a moving target. Information on possible contacts was often incomplete, with no working phone numbers or e-mail addresses. Moreover, the electronic record-keeping software for contact monitoring that CDC brought had been designed for the Ebola outbreaks in Africa and could not be quickly configured for the situation in Dallas. Thus, a centralized database of contacts did not exist and the epidemiologists in the field at first could not enter and compile new contacts in real time.[48] Confusing to all, the press too easily conflated high- and low-risk contacts.

By the weekend, the EOC and CDC agreed to release one number, once a day—and everyone would refer to that number for the following 24 hours. The epis reported that, to date, those known to have been exposed to Duncan numbered 48 higher-risk community and health care contacts, plus a larger number of health care staff considered to have had "no known exposure" to Duncan because they wore PPE.[49] The 48 higher-risk

---

47. For a dramatic description of the transfer, see Burrough, "Trial by Ebola."
48. Later, CDC flew in a server to support multiple-user data entry and data access to resolve this issue.
49. Presbyterian had learned that taking care of an Ebola patient was labor-intensive, involving more than 30 individuals.

contacts were being monitored twice daily. On Saturday, Lakey published an op-ed intended, once again, to reassure the public. He wrote:

> Doctors and hospitals in Texas are well trained and have responded to numerous public health threats over the years. We have a history of successfully containing the spread of disease and protecting the public. I'm confident we'll do the same with Ebola.[50]

Criticism of Jenkins's visits to the Trohs continued, so the county in response published a statement Saturday that said, in part, "those that were not wearing protective gear were not doing clean-up or moving the potentially infectious materials."[51] On Tuesday, October 7, Lakey and CDC followed up with additional letters confirming that Jenkins had run no risk in dealing with the family unprotected. "Judge Jenkins was not at risk and posed no risk to others," Lakey wrote. "Judge Jenkins's action in moving them posed no danger of Ebola to himself or to anyone else and was consistent with good public health practice," wrote CDC Incident Manager Dr. Inger Damon.[52]

Daily routines had emerged. The EOC policy group met each morning at 8 a.m. in person or virtually to provide guidance to County Director Bass on what needed doing that day. Each member of the policy group played a distinct role. Rawlings, says Jenkins, "was very good at ascertaining what was going to be the next big thing that the public was going to be interested in." Lakey and Jenkins oversaw operations. At 11 a.m., there was a national CDC press call with Frieden speaking for the federal government, Lakey for the state, and Jenkins for Dallas. At noon was a call for all city emergency managers in north Texas. At 6 p.m. came a call of the principals: Jenkins, Lakey, Rawlings, and Dr. Lyle Peterson from CDC with, later, the White House Deputy Director of Intergovernmental Affairs Adrian Saenz and a representative from the Federal Emergency Management Agency.

The EOC had no shortage of tasks. It handled, for example, the decontamination of the police cruiser used to transport guards to or from the Trohs' apartment. The city and county police departments assisted Chung's teams to find a homeless man who had been in Duncan's ambulance after he used it and before he was diagnosed. The EOC handled relations with schools and publicized repeatedly the message that Ebola could be contracted only from direct contact with the bodily fluids of an infected person. It also managed a false alarm when a deputy who had been in the Troh apartment reported sick with an illness that proved unrelated to Ebola.

The EOC also worked through scenarios: What to do if Duncan died? What to do if an additional Ebola case arrived on US shores? What to do if a Duncan contact fell ill?

50. David Lakey, "Texas Health System Well Prepared to Deal with Ebola Threat," October 4, 2014, https://www.dshs.texas.gov/commissioner/op-ed-20141004.aspx.

51. Eric Aasen, "Dallas Ebola Patient Is in Critical Condition," *KERA News*, October 4, 2014, http://keranews.org/post/dallas-ebola-patient-critical-condition-hospital-says.

52. Ken Kalthoff, "Dallas County Judge Jenkins Not Ebola Risk: Health Officials," *NBCDFW*, October 7, 2014, http://www.nbcdfw.com/news/local/Dallas-County-Judge-Jenkins-Not-Ebola-Risk-Health-Officials-278461321.html.

"We were always planning for the next scenario that would present," recalls DSHS Deputy Commissioner Maples. They dealt with funding issues: who would pay for which aspects of the response? On the public health and medical front, DSHS Assistant Health Commissioner Gruber held regular calls with hospitals and health care delivery officials across Texas, sometimes as many as 2,000 people on a single call. "It was important to make sure that everybody knew what was going on, even if they weren't directly involved with it," says Gruber.

The EOC had also managed to regulate what messages went out to the public. To avoid rumors fueling panic, it was important to have a unified and authoritative daily account of the evolving situation. Early on, some EOC members had gone so far as to tweet photos and messages from the control center. "We had to take control of that," recalls Lakey. "It was a major challenge making sure that [the public wasn't] getting an updated message every 15 minutes or so by the next person that found themselves in front of a TV camera." Maples adds that "you needed to be judicious in doing press conferences…. If you didn't have anything to say, you opened yourself up for a lot of questions with no answers, and that wasn't helpful for anybody."

Jenkins recalls that clear communications among all responders were a challenge for the first week. "Everybody had a different boss," concurs Maples. "So we needed to say, you don't just report to your boss…. It had to be a much more coordinated chain of communication." To fill gaps, Lakey steadily added staff from Austin: a legislative liaison, legal counsel, a public information officer, and others. Moreover, CDC added personnel. "We didn't get good up- and down-stream communication going on this until we got a much larger CDC team in, probably the second week," says Jenkins.

Politics

Politics and politicians also played a role in the evolving situation. Duncan's case had drawn global attention and each release of any detail drew news reports, analysis, and criticism. On Monday, October 6, Governor Perry had issued an executive order for a task force on infectious diseases that would recommend improvements to the state's existing response plan. The task force, which included State Health Commissioner Lakey, set to work immediately. On Sunday, October 12, confident that the crisis was in good hands, Governor Perry departed on a long-scheduled trade promotion trip to Europe.

Meanwhile, public voices started to question why Duncan had been sent home after his first visit to Presbyterian on September 25. On Tuesday, October 7, National Civil Rights Leader Reverend Jesse Jackson held a press conference in Dallas to address the question. Jackson appeared with Duncan's mother, sister, and other family members and arranged for them to meet with Duncan's medical team. At the local level on Tuesday, Dallas County Commissioner John Wiley Price accused Presbyterian of using race and money in the decision to send Duncan away. "If a person who looks like me shows up without insurance, they don't get the same treatment," Price, who is black, told a local television station.[53]

The situation was generating state, national, and international anxiety. On Tuesday, the Texas Senate Health and Human Services Committee held a hearing on Ebola in Austin. Lakey was too busy working on the response to attend, but a deputy testified on his behalf. Later that day, CDC announced that the number of people under active observation for Ebola symptoms was 48, of whom only 10 had been in very close contact with Duncan. On Wednesday, CDC and the White House announced that Ebola screening for passengers arriving from West Africa would start at five national airports, beginning with John F. Kennedy International Airport in New York City on Saturday, October 11.

DUNCAN DIES

Meanwhile, Duncan had worsened. Lakey moved constantly between the EOC and the hospital; he kept track of the public health response, got regular updates on the patient for the daily conference call with CDC and the national press, and observed how hospital personnel were holding up. Over the weekend, doctors had started Duncan on an experimental regime of the drug brincidofovir. It was the only treatment option available (ZMapp supplies were exhausted) and required three sets of approval: from the federal Food and Drug Administration, the local institutional review board, and the company that made the drug.

Starting October 1, "we had people on the phones for literally hundreds of hours getting all this paperwork done, just tons of forms and e-mail," said the chief intensive care unit (ICU) doctor at Presbyterian.[54] In a related development, on Monday, October 6, a nurse in Spain who had tended the deceased missionary tested positive for Ebola. It was the first confirmed case of Ebola transmission outside Africa and provoked global alarm. The nurse was treated in a hospital; her dog was euthanized.

On Wednesday, October 8, at 7:51 a.m., Duncan died. His death was by then expected. The EOC had already laid detailed plans that answered such questions as who should notify the family, who should discuss with the family the need to cremate the body, and who would sign the cremation papers. The EOC, says Lakey, was worried about the potential for bioterrorism if the body was buried—that someone might deliberately obtain the Ebola virus from the corpse and use it to threaten society.

The EOC plan immediately went into effect. Dallas County Judge Jenkins and the family pastor told the Trohs in person that Duncan had passed away. Although Liberian

53. Kalthoff, "Dallas County Judge Jenkins Not Ebola Risk: Health Officials."
54. Burrough, "Trial by Ebola."

culture called for burial rather than cremation, the family accepted cremation given the public health concerns. As for legal approval, Duncan's 19-year-old son signed the papers. The body was removed for cremation on Wednesday afternoon, and the process completed on Thursday, October 9.

END IN SIGHT?

By Friday, October 10, cautious optimism infused the EOC. It had established a public education campaign that included schools, 2-1-1 and 3-1-1 emergency hotlines, and a coordinated message on all public Web sites. Contact monitoring was going well. A total of 142 barrels of waste from both the Troh apartment and the hospital had been successfully incinerated. There were no signs of illness among any of those getting twice daily temperature checks. Lakey and his DSHS team prepared to return home to Austin. During a 5 p.m. conference call with CDC and other key players, the tone was guardedly upbeat.

Late Friday, Lakey headed home. But on his way, he got a phone call: Presbyterian nurse Nina Pham, who had taken care of Duncan, did not feel well. Moreover, she had a fever. Lakey had decided that the CDC fever guideline of 101.5°F for an Ebola test was too high; he lowered that to 100.4°F—the fever threshold typically used by infectious disease doctors. When Pham's fever rose above that, she went to Presbyterian and they drew blood for an Ebola test. DSHS Assistant Health Commissioner Gruber, who returned to Austin Saturday, was asked to deliver Pham's blood sample to the state lab for testing; a second sample went to CDC.

Late Saturday night, the state lab confirmed that Pham had Ebola. That was a shock. Pham had treated Duncan, not when he was in the ED before his diagnosis, but after his transfer to the ICU. She had worn the PPE recommended by CDC. Lakey and the hastily reconstituted EOC team held a conference call with CDC at midnight. Judge Jenkins and Mayor Rawlings went straight to Presbyterian and remained there all night.

Back in Crisis

Lakey headed back to Dallas on Sunday, October 12, at 4 a.m. He took with him DSHS Assistant Health Commissioner Gruber, DSHS Communications Director Ricky Garcia, and DSHS Deputy Commissioner Maples; others followed later in the day. The Dallas County EOC returned to full operation. The conference calls were back: with CDC, with Judge Jenkins and Mayor Rawlings. Early Sunday, Jenkins and Rawlings made a public announcement of Pham's diagnosis based on the state lab results even before CDC had confirmed them. That day the hospital, in consultation with the EOC, decided to excuse from duty any Presbyterian doctors or nurses who had had any contact with Duncan. In addition, Presbyterian accepted no more ambulances; its ED business evaporated.

Pham named one potential contact she had had since displaying symptoms, and that person was placed under direct monitoring. Hazmat cleaning of her apartment started Sunday, with the Texas Commission on Environmental Quality in charge. Pham, like the nurse in Spain, had a dog. The decontamination crew gave the dog food and water inside the apartment until it was removed to quarantine. Pham's apartment and car were placed under protective order.

Then on Monday, October 13, a second nurse, Amber Vinson, complained of a fever. At nearly midnight Tuesday, she was confirmed positive. Vinson had recently flown twice on commercial airlines—once Friday and again Monday—headed to and from Ohio where she was planning her wedding. Vinson had obtained CDC permission to take the second flight after she developed a slightly elevated temperature of 99.5°F.

The consternation in Dallas was extreme. Mayor Rawlings reached Valerie Jarrett, senior advisor to President Barack Obama (who among other things was responsible for overseeing intergovernmental affairs at the White House), on Monday to say "I've got to assume this is going to get worse. You need to send somebody besides what we've got from the CDC, because we're not getting the help there," he recalls. Lakey remembers the many questions that beset him as he drove back to Dallas after Pham's diagnosis; they only doubled when Vinson was confirmed. "What's going on?" he and his colleagues asked themselves. He says:

> Obviously, this was a surprise. These individuals had been deemed by the protocols from the CDC to be at no risk. Now you have somebody that had been defined as no risk that's infected.... Who else could be exposed? How are we monitoring those individuals?... How big is "big" going to be?

The infection of the two nurses and the fact that Vinson had flown across state lines expanded exponentially the list of those potentially exposed to Ebola well beyond the Texas border. Who should now assume responsibility for tracing contacts? The new cases also opened for question what to do with the other nurses and doctors at Presbyterian who had treated Duncan. Did they all need to go into quarantine and, if so, where? What about Presbyterian? Could it continue to treat Pham, Vinson, and any other cases that might arise? Meanwhile, what should Presbyterian medical personnel tell their patients, and what should the EOC and DSHS tell the public? What exactly was the risk matrix? Did this mean an epidemic loomed?

Even before Vinson's case was confirmed, CDC Director Frieden in a press conference Tuesday expressed his regret that CDC had not responded more robustly at the start of Duncan's hospitalization. He declared CDC's intention going forward to send a larger Ebola response team anywhere a case arose. It would include not only epidemiologists but also experts in infection control, laboratory science, PPE, clinical management and experimental therapies, education and the environment, waste management, decontamination, and transportation. He said:

> I wish we had put a team like this on the ground the day the patient, the first patient, was diagnosed. That might have prevented this infection. But we will do that from today onward with any case anywhere in the US.[55]

Lakey welcomed the news of CDC's stepped-up involvement. But there remained pressing questions about Presbyterian, the two nurses, and Texas public health messages that he and the EOC team had to answer well before the expanded CDC team could come up to speed. Recalls Lakey: "We needed to get control of the situation, and to reassure the public."

55. CDC, "CDC Update on Ebola Response, 10-14-2014," October 14, 2014, http://www.cdc.gov/media/releases/2014/t1014-ebola-reponse-update.html.

Exhibit 2A-1. Interim Guidance for Monitoring and Movement of Persons With Ebola Virus Disease Exposure: Centers for Disease Control and Prevention; August 22, 2014

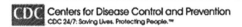 **Centers for Disease Control and Prevention**
CDC 24/7: Saving Lives. Protecting People.™

Interim Guidance for Monitoring and Movement of Persons with Ebola Virus Disease Exposure

Updated: August 22, 2014

The world is facing the biggest and most complex Ebola (http://www.cdc.gov/vhf/ebola/index.html) virus disease (EVD) outbreak in history. On August 8, 2014, the EVD outbreak in West Africa was declared by the World Health Organization (WHO) to be a Public Health Emergency of International Concern (PHEIC) (http://www.who.int/mediacentre/news/statements/2014/ebola-20140808/en/) because it was determined to be an 'extraordinary event' with public health risks to other States. The possible consequences of further international spread are particularly serious considering the following factors:

1. the virulence of the virus,
2. the intensive community and health facility transmission patterns, and
3. the strained health systems in the currently affected and most at-risk countries.

Coordinated public health actions are essential to stop and reverse the spread of Ebola virus. Due to the complex nature and seriousness of the outbreak, CDC has created guidance for monitoring people exposed to Ebola virus and for evaluating their travel, including the application of movement restrictions when indicated.

Definitions used in this document

For case and exposure level definitions, see: Case Definition for Ebola Virus Disease (EVD) (/vhf/ebola/hcp/case-definition.html).

Close contact

Close contact is defined as

a. being within approximately 3 feet (1 meter) of an EVD patient or within the patient's room or care area for a prolonged period of time (e.g., health care personnel, household members) while not wearing recommended personal protective equipment (i.e., standard, droplet, and contact precautions; see Infection Prevention and Control Recommendations (http://www.cdc.gov/vhf/ebola/hcp/infection-prevention-and-control-recommendations.html)); or
b. having direct brief contact (e.g., shaking hands) with an EVD case while not wearing recommended personal protective equipment.

Brief interactions, such as walking by a person or moving through a hospital, do not constitute close contact.

Conditional release

Conditional release means that people are monitored by a public health authority for 21 days after the last known potential Ebola virus exposure to ensure that immediate actions are taken if they develop symptoms consistent with EVD during this period. People conditionally released should self-monitor for fever twice daily and notify the public health authority if they develop fever or other symptoms (/vhf/ebola/hcp/case-definition.html).

Controlled movement

Controlled movement requires people to notify the public health authority about their intended travel for 21 days after their last known potential Ebola virus exposure. These individuals should not travel by commercial conveyances (e.g. airplane, ship, long-distance bus, or train). Local use of public transportation (e.g. taxi, bus) by asymptomatic individuals should be discussed with the public health authority. If travel is approved, the exposed person must have timely access to appropriate medical care if symptoms develop during travel. Approved long-distance travel should be by chartered flight or private vehicle; if local public transportation is used, the individual must be able to exit quickly.

Quarantine

Quarantine is used to separate and restrict the movement of persons exposed to a communicable disease who don't have symptoms of the disease for the purpose of monitoring.

Self-monitoring

Self-monitoring means that people check their own temperature twice daily and monitor themselves for other symptoms.

Early Recognition and Reporting of Suspected Ebola Virus Exposures

Early recognition is critical to controlling the spread of Ebola virus. Health care providers should be alert for and evaluate any patients with symptoms consistent with EVD and potential exposure history. Standard, contact, and droplet precautions (/vhf/ebola/hcp/infection-prevention-and-control-recommendations.html#table) should be immediately implemented if EVD is suspected. Guidance for clinicians evaluating patients from EVD outbreak-affected countries is available at http://www.cdc.gov/vhf/ebola/hcp/clinician-information-us-healthcare-settings.html (/vhf/ebola/hcp/clinician-information-us-healthcare-settings.html).

Health care professionals in the United States should immediately report to their state or local health department any person being evaluated for EVD if the medical evaluation suggests that diagnostic testing may be indicated. If there is a high index of suspicion, US health departments should immediately report any probable cases or persons under investigation (PUI) (/vhf/ebola/hcp/case-definition.html#PUI) to CDC's Emergency Operations Center (http://www.cdc.gov/phpr/eoc.htm) at 770-488-7100.

Important Evaluation Factors

Both clinical presentation and level of exposure should be taken into account when determining appropriate public health actions, including the need for medical evaluation or monitoring and the application of movement restrictions when indicated.

Recommendations for Evaluating Exposure Risk to Determine Appropriate Public Health Actions

This guidance provides public health authorities and other partners a framework for determining the appropriate public health actions based on risk factors and clinical presentation. It also includes criteria for monitoring exposed people and for when movement restrictions may be needed.

At this time, CDC is NOT recommending that asymptomatic contacts of EVD cases be quarantined, either in facilities or at home.

Exposure Level	Clinical Criteria	Public Health Actions
High Risk • Percutaneous (e.g., needle stick) or mucous membrane exposure to blood or body fluids of EVD patient • Direct skin contact with or exposure to blood or body fluids of an EVD patient without appropriate personal protective equipment (PPE) • Processing blood or body fluids of a confirmed EVD patient without appropriate PPE or standard biosafety precautions • Direct contact with a dead	Fever **OR** other symptoms (/vhf/ebola/hcp/case-definition.html) consistent with EVD without fever	• Consideration as a probable case (/vhf/ebola/hcp/case-definition.html#probable) • Medical evaluation using infection control precautions (/vhf/ebola/hcp/infection-prevention-and-control-recommendations.html) for suspected Ebola, consultation with public health authorities, and testing if indicated • If air transport is clinically appropriate and indicated, only air medical transport (/vhf/ebola/hcp/guidance-air-medical-transport-patients.html) (no travel on commercial conveyances permitted) • If infection control precautions (/vhf/ebola/hcp/infection-prevention-and-control-recommendations.html) are determined not to be indicated: conditional release and controlled movement until 21 days after last known potential exposure

body without appropriate PPE in a country where an EVD outbreak is occurring	Asymptomatic	• <u>Conditional release</u> and <u>controlled movement</u> until 21 days after last known potential exposure
Some Risk of Exposure • Household contact with an EVD patient • Other <u>close contact</u> with an EVD patient in health care facilities or community settings	<u>Fever **WITH OR WITHOUT** other symptoms</u> (/vhf/ebola/hcp/case-definition.html) consistent with EVD	• Consideration as <u>a probable case (/vhf/ebola/hcp/case-definition.html#probable)</u> • Medical evaluation using initial <u>infection control precautions (/vhf/ebola/hcp/infection-prevention-and-control-recommendations.html)</u> for suspected Ebola, consultation with public health authorities, and testing if indicated • If air transport is clinically appropriate and indicated, <u>air medical transport (/vhf/ebola/hcp/guidance-air-medical-transport-patients.html)</u> only (no travel on commercial conveyances permitted) • If <u>infection control precautions (/vhf/ebola/hcp/infection-prevention-and-control-recommendations.html)</u> are determined not to be indicated: <u>Conditional release</u> and <u>controlled movement</u> until 21 days after last known potential exposure
	Asymptomatic or clinical criteria not met	• <u>Conditional release</u> and <u>controlled movement</u> until 21 days after last known potential exposure
No Known Exposure • Having been in a country in which an EVD outbreak occurred within the past 21 days and having had no exposures	<u>Fever **WITH** other symptoms</u> (/vhf/ebola/hcp/case-definition.html) consistent with EVD	• Consideration as a <u>person under investigation (/vhf/ebola/hcp/case-definition.html#PUI)</u> (PUI) • Medical evaluation and optional consultation with public health authorities to determine if movement restrictions and <u>infection control precautions (/vhf/ebola/hcp/infection-prevention-and-control-recommendations.html)</u> are indicated • If movement restrictions and <u>infection control precautions (/vhf/ebola/hcp/infection-prevention-and-control-recommendations.html)</u> are determined not to be indicated: travel by commercial conveyance is allowed; <u>self-monitor</u> until 21 days after leaving country
	Asymptomatic or clinical criteria not met	• No movement restrictions • Travel by commercial conveyance allowed • <u>Self-monitor</u> until 21 days after leaving country

Page last reviewed: August 22, 2014

Page last updated: August 22, 2014

Content source: Centers for Disease Control and Prevention (/index.htm)

National Center for Emerging and Zoonotic Infectious Diseases (NCEZID) (/ncezid/index.html)

Division of High-Consequence Pathogens and Pathology (DHCPP) (/ncezid/dhcpp/index.html)

Viral Special Pathogens Branch (VSPB) (/ncezid/dhcpp/vspb/index.html)

Source: Reprinted from CDC, "Interim Guidance for Monitoring and Movement of Persons With Ebola Virus Disease Exposure," August 22, 2014.

Exhibit 2A-2. Sketch of Incident Command System Structure: Dallas County Emergency Operations Center Meeting; October 1, 2014

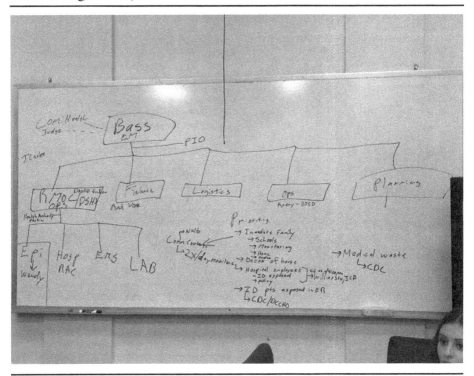

Source: Jenkins and others, White Board Organizational Chart, Dallas County EOC meeting, October 1, 2014. Used by permission of DSHS Assistant Health Commissioner David Gruber.

Fears and Realities: Managing Ebola in Dallas (Epilogue)

Kirsten Lundberg

Late Tuesday evening, October 14, 2014, the Centers for Disease Control and Prevention (CDC) doctors debated with the Dallas Emergency Operations Center (EOC) whether the country was on the verge of an Ebola epidemic. CDC officials wanted to designate a second Dallas hospital, Parkland, for future Ebola patients. But Dallas County Judge Clay Jenkins and Texas Department of State Health Services (DSHS) Health Commissioner Dr. David Lakey objected: that would take two of Dallas's hospitals out of general circulation, creating an impossible burden on the remaining three to treat all non-Ebola patients in the region.

Instead, Lakey and Jenkins decided to move the two nurses with Ebola out of Texas Health Presbyterian Hospital (Presbyterian). In Lakey's view, the Presbyterian staff was exhausted. In addition, many of them were themselves under medical observation after their colleagues contracted Ebola. So at midnight on Tuesday, October 14, they asked DSHS Assistant Commissioner for Regional and Local Health Services David Gruber to organize transport for the two patients.

Gruber spent much of the night on the phone with ambulance companies (the first one refused to provide transport); the State Department, which owned an airplane specially equipped for infectious disease patients; CDC; and the contractor who operated

---

This case was written by Kirsten Lundberg for Dr. Arnold M. Howitt, Executive Director of the Ash Center for Democratic Governance and Innovation at the John F. Kennedy School of Government, Harvard University. Funds for case development were provided by the Robert Wood Johnson Foundation for use at the Harvard Kennedy School as part of its State Health Leadership Initiative, sponsored in conjunction with the Association of State and Territorial Health Officials. HKS cases are developed solely as the basis for class discussion. Cases are not intended to serve as endorsements, sources of primary data, or illustrations of effective or ineffective management.

the aircraft.[1] Altogether, he dealt with 10 different organizations. Happily, a small group of people represented those organizations, and "every one of them pretty much had decision-making authority," recalls Gruber.[2]

Nurse Amber Vinson left first on Wednesday, October 15, bound for Emory University Hospital. It then took 15 hours to decontaminate the plane and return for Nurse Nina Pham, who was transferred Thursday to a National Institutes of Health clinical center in Bethesda, Maryland. The patients themselves, as well as the personnel who attended them, all wore personal protective equipment (PPE). On October 22, Vinson tested negative for Ebola and was moved out of isolation; she was discharged on October 28. Pham tested negative and was released on October 24.

Separately, 160 passengers who sat near Vinson on the flights she had taken just before diagnosis were contacted and monitored; none contracted Ebola, and monitoring concluded on November 7. By then, DSHS reported that it had monitored a total of 177 individuals, including health care workers, household members, or others who had been either in direct contact with Thomas Eric Duncan, Nina Pham, or Amber Vinson or who had handled medical specimens or waste.

Meanwhile, there were political consequences to the Ebola outbreak that percolated for weeks. On October 16, Texas Governor Rick Perry returned early from a trip to Europe in order to assert his oversight of the response effort. The Perry-appointed Texas Task Force on Infectious Disease Preparedness and Response on October 31 issued early recommendations for health care worker monitoring and passenger screening; it published a final report on December 1. At the federal level, Congress approved a $5.4 billion emergency Ebola-funding package. On October 17, President Obama appointed Ronald Klain as federal Ebola "czar" to coordinate the response nationwide.[3]

CDC made changes as well. On October 16, it changed the recommended fever protocol from 101.5°F to 100.4°F. It tightened its guidelines for PPE. CDC also acknowledged that not every hospital could handle Ebola. It asked hospitals to volunteer as Ebola centers; 35 that did so met CDC standards. Separately, many hospitals across the country ordered full-body hazmat suits and devoted hours to training staff in how to don and remove them. Some renovated in order to create isolation areas for suiting up. Ebola testing capacity expanded to 42 laboratories in 36 states.[4]

States and the federal government took a new look at quarantine for those arriving from Africa. Screening for Ebola was established at 12 US airports that received flights

---

1. The aircraft was specially equipped to carry an isolation pod.
2. DSHS Assistant Commissioner for Regional and Local Health Services David Gruber in phone interview with author, March 3, 2015. Gruber's division also had responsibility for health emergency preparedness.
3. Juliet Eilperin and David Nakamura, "Obama Taps Ron Klain as Ebola Czar," *Washington Post*, October 17, 2014, http://www.washingtonpost.com/blogs/post-politics/wp/2014/10/17/obama-taps-ron-klain-as-ebola-czar.
4. Felice J. Freyer, "Ebola Response Shows Flaws in System," *Boston Globe*, January 3, 2015, https://www.bostonglobe.com/metro/2015/01/03/ebola-exposed-flaws-nation-ability-respond-dangerous-new-germs/K26m73JZ5zn4tEXKKvLMZJ/story.html.

from Africa. On October 24, some governors—including from New York and New Jersey—adopted a mandatory 21-day quarantine for travelers who had had direct contact with Ebola patients. This strategy backfired and caused consternation as CDC, the federal government, and states sought to come to terms with public fears without violating civil liberties. On October 27, after fierce criticism from a nurse detained in Newark, New Jersey, Governor Chris Christie released her after three days and sent her home to Maine, where she remained in relative isolation and under observation for the remainder of the 21-day incubation period.[5] She did not contract Ebola.

Lakey remained in Dallas until late October. Looking back on the Ebola outbreak, he remarked: "As you approach [disaster] events, there will be surprises. Your plans are not going to be perfect and you need to accept that and be willing to change your plan in order to meet the challenge that you face on the ground."[6] As of February 6, 2015, Ebola had infected more than 22,000 people and killed more than 9,000, chiefly in Guinea, Liberia, and Sierra Leone.[7] The World Health Organization was much criticized for its failure to identify the epidemic early and respond swiftly. In the United States, 11 individuals—almost all flown in from Africa—were treated for Ebola. Only Pham and Vinson contracted the disease in the United States.

5. Sabrina Tavernise et al., "Seeking Unity, U.S. Revises Ebola Monitoring Rules," *New York Times*, October 27, 2014, http://www.nytimes.com/2014/10/28/nyregion/ebola-us.html?_r=0.

6. Krystina Martinez, "Texas' Top Health Official Reflects on Ebola Response in Dallas," *KERA News*, November 6, 2014, http://keranews.org/post/texas-top-health-official-reflects-ebola-response-dallas.

7. Editorial Board, "Reform After the Ebola Epidemic," *New York Times*, February 10, 2015, http://www.nytimes.com/2015/02/10/opinion/reform-after-the-ebola-debacle.html?nlid=28716017&src=recpb&_r=0.

Surviving the Surge: New York City Hospitals Respond to Superstorm Sandy

David W. Giles

EDITORS' INTRODUCTION

As Hurricane Sandy moved up the Atlantic Coast in late October 2012, forecasters warned of the storm's potential to inflict serious damage in and around New York City. Many area residents and institutions, however, wondered whether the storm would have much of an impact, given that a year earlier Hurricane Irene, despite dire predictions, had ultimately spared the city. In fact, Sandy proved to be far more devastating than many had anticipated, with its storm surge having severe consequences for parts of the city, including several prominent health care institutions.

This case study profiles how Sandy affected three Manhattan hospitals—the NYU Langone Medical Center (NYU Langone), Bellevue Hospital Center (Bellevue), and the Veterans Administration's NY Harbor Healthcare System/Manhattan campus (VA NY Harbor)—each of which is located in close proximity to the East River and is thus vulnerable to flooding. The case explores the actions each facility took prior to, during, and immediately following the storm, revealing how hospital administrators'

This case was written by David W. Giles, Associate Director, Program on Crisis Leadership, for Dr. Arnold M. Howitt, Executive Director of the Ash Center for Democratic Governance and Innovation at the John F. Kennedy School of Government, Harvard University. Funds for case development were provided by the Robert Wood Johnson Foundation for use at the Harvard Kennedy School as part of its State Health Leadership Initiative, sponsored in conjunction with the Association of State and Territorial Health Officials. HKS cases are developed solely as the basis for class discussion. Cases are not intended to serve as endorsements, sources of primary data, or illustrations of effective or ineffective management.

interpretations of storm-related risk, pre-event preparedness measures, and decisions made at the height of the storm had dramatic implications for the institutions and the safety of their patients.

State and local public health and emergency management officials initially refrained from ordering New York City hospitals and nursing homes to evacuate, recalling how the looming threat of Irene had prompted the relocation of thousands—a complex process that in hindsight appeared unnecessarily disruptive. Predictions worsened in the days immediately preceding Sandy's arrival, however, prompting the city to implement a sweeping set of measures. Authorities canceled school, shut down mass transit, and issued evacuation orders for residents of flood-prone areas. Although the city and state continued to refrain from issuing mandatory evacuation orders for most health care facilities, some hospitals—including VA NY Harbor—decided to evacuate voluntarily, having concluded that it was not worth risking their patients' safety no matter how Sandy played out. For their parts, NYU Langone and Bellevue released many of their patients, but not all, confident the investments they had made over the past year to safeguard their critical infrastructure, especially their emergency power systems, would enable them to withstand the storm.

In the early evening of October 29, Sandy's large storm surge swept over low-lying parts of the city, overwhelming neighborhoods and buildings, including both the NYU Langone and Bellevue medical complexes. At NYU, floodwaters quickly knocked out the hospital's back-up power supply, and as conditions deteriorated around them, hospital administrators decided they had no choice but to evacuate the remaining patients. The operation that unfolded would last 13 hours, with health care workers, hospital administrators, support staff, and city firefighters frantically working to move more than 300 people to more than a dozen host institutions during the very height of the storm.

Initially, Bellevue also thought that it had done enough to protect itself and its patients. And even as water began filling the hospital's basements, administrators there believed that they had escaped the very worst and could rely on emergency generators that continued to function. Still, a cascading series of systems failures eventually overwhelmed the hospital, and conditions at Bellevue soon mirrored those at NYU. By the next morning, it was all too clear that Bellevue's patients would also have to be evacuated. This effort would last several days, with National Guard troops and ambulance units from across the country pitching in to help move more than 700 people.

Not one patient died in the hospital evacuations conducted during and following Sandy. But the storm's toll on New York City's health care system was severe. As NYU Langone, Bellevue, and other storm-damaged institutions struggled to recover, the city's public health authorities and health care leaders were left to reflect on the severe challenges they had faced during Sandy. Despite their efforts at disaster preparedness and mitigation in advance of the storm, they had endured a serious crisis. To avoid a similar scenario in the future, they now had to consider what more they could do.

DISCUSSION QUESTIONS

1. Forecasting hurricanes is a science but not an exact one, as evidenced by New York City's experience with Hurricane Irene in 2011 and with Superstorm Sandy a year later. How do political leaders, emergency management professionals, and public health officials best communicate risk and appropriate preparedness strategies in advance of events like these, which have the potential for wreaking havoc (as was the case with Sandy), but often ultimately do not (as happened with Irene in New York City)?

2. Evacuating hospitals, nursing homes, and other health care facilities in the face of a major disaster can be a complex and disruptive endeavor, with serious implications for the well-being of the facilities' patients. But the alternative of sheltering-in-place runs the risk of exposing patients to a potentially devastating event in unsafe conditions. If you were in the shoes of local and state public health officials and hospital leadership as Sandy approached, how would you have weighed the costs and benefits of these two choices?

3. Would you characterize the hospitals featured in this case as having sufficiently planned and otherwise prepared for major emergencies, such as significant flooding? Why or why not?

4. NYU Langone and Bellevue took a number of important measures to prepare for a major storm but still experienced terrible damage from Sandy. Is it possible for them to be even better prepared for similar events in the future? How so? What is reasonable to expect, when also taking into account financial constraints and competing priorities?

* * *

By the late afternoon of Monday, October 29, 2012, millions of New Yorkers were hunkered down, awaiting the arrival of a late season hurricane. Although forecasters and public officials warned that the storm was imminent and potentially dangerous, many residents wondered whether it would actually do much harm. Indeed, a year earlier Hurricane Irene had prompted similar alarm but had ultimately caused little damage in and around the city. Within hours, however, it would become abundantly clear that this time around New Yorkers would not be so lucky.

Making landfall along the Jersey Shore the evening of the 29th, Superstorm Sandy[1] wreaked havoc across much of the Mid-Atlantic Coast, including the densely populated New York City area. (The largest metropolitan region in the country, greater New York, is home to more than 19.5 million people.)[2] There, fierce winds uprooted trees and spread fires that blazed through hundreds of homes and businesses.

In many parts of the city, however, it was Sandy's surge that proved the most devastating. Arriving at high tide and during a full moon (which elevated the tide about a half foot above usual levels), Sandy unleashed waves that reached approximately 14.5 feet in height and swept beyond the floodplain boundaries that the Federal Emergency Management Agency (FEMA) had established for the city.[3] Propelled by strong northwesterly winds, Sandy's surge pushed through New York Harbor and into the East River and Hudson River (which border Manhattan to the island's east and west, respectively), crashing ashore in low-lying coastal parts of the city's five boroughs. In a short period of time, the storm's surge had caused all kinds of damage, flooding key transportation routes and infrastructure (including major car and subway tunnels), overwhelming electrical facilities, swamping beaches and parks, and sweeping through New York's typically busy roadways. Sandy's toll, once all had been accounted for, was enormous: ranked as the second costliest natural disaster in US history (only surpassed by Hurricane Katrina),[4] the superstorm had destroyed numerous properties, caused thousands of injuries, and taken the lives of 43 New Yorkers.[5]

Reflecting on the extent of the damage, New York City Mayor Michael Bloomberg bluntly declared, "Hurricane Sandy was the worst natural disaster ever to hit New York City."[6] This was painfully true for far too many New Yorkers and city institutions; it was especially so for several of its most venerable hospitals. In addition to inflicting serious damage on several of the area's key health care facilities and causing significant

---

1. Although Sandy was of hurricane strength during much of its journey across the Atlantic, in the hours preceding Sandy's landfall the National Hurricane Center had reclassified the storm as a posttropical cyclone. This was due to several technical factors: Sandy's eye had disappeared, strong thunderstorm activity at its center had ceased, and it drew its energy from the jet stream—not from warm ocean waters. The term "superstorm" refers to Sandy's enormous size (at its height, the storm's wind field reached more than 1,000 miles across), to the extensive devastation it caused across the Northeastern United States, and to the particular climatic conditions that contributed to its intensity. As Sandy began moving up the Atlantic coast, a high pressure system blocked the storm's progress northward, while a low pressure system to the west provided it with energy, causing Sandy to make a sharp turn toward the New Jersey shore. See: Eric S. Blake and others, "Tropical Cyclone Report: Hurricane Sandy," National Hurricane Center, February 12, 2013, http://www.nhc.noaa.gov/data/tcr/AL182012_Sandy.pdf; City of New York, "A Stronger, More Resilient New York," June 11, 2013, http://www.nyc.gov/html/sirr/html/report/report.shtml.
2. US Census Bureau, "2010 Census and Census 2000, Population Change for Metropolitan and Micropolitan Statistical Areas in the United States and Puerto Rico (February 2013 Delineations): 2000 to 2010 (CPH-T-5)," March 2013, http://www.census.gov/population/www/cen2010/cph-t/cph-t-5.html.
3. City of New York, "A Stronger, More Resilient New York."
4. Blake and others, "Tropical Cyclone Report: Hurricane Sandy."
5. Amesh A. Adalja and others, "Absorbing Citywide Patient Surge During Hurricane Sandy: A Case Study in Accommodating Multiple Hospital Evacuations," *Annals of Emergency Medicine* 64, no. 1 (2014): 66–73; and City of New York, "A Stronger, More Resilient New York."
6. City of New York, "A Stronger, More Resilient New York."

disruptions to their operations, the storm triggered a massive and complex operation involving the evacuation of about 6,500 hospital patients and nursing home residents.[7]

Some hospitals, including the Manhattan campus of the VA NY Harbor Healthcare System, decided to organize full evacuations in advance of Sandy's landfall. But several others, including NYU Langone Medical Center and Bellevue Hospital Center, both of which were located just north of the VA complex, chose not to. They wagered that staying put would be less risky than moving hundreds of medically vulnerable patients. But as Sandy's surge pounded the city (and less than a decade after medical patients had endured horrendous and, for some, deadly conditions while stranded in New Orleans hospitals following Hurricane Katrina[8]), NYU Langone and Bellevue, along with several other health care facilities, were suddenly confronted with their own nightmares.

In response, hospital officials, along with their city and state public health and public safety counterparts, scrambled to safely relocate the remaining patients— most of whom required specialized care and medical support—during and in the immediate aftermath of the storm. As they did so, they were left to think back to the days and hours leading up to the evacuations. What lessons had they taken from Hurricane Irene and other past experiences? Had they prepared adequately for a coastal storm of Sandy's magnitude? And had they sufficiently weighed the benefits and costs of carrying out full-scale evacuations of their facilities?

For a map depicting the storm's track, see Exhibit 3-1. For a chronology of events, see Exhibit 3-2.

TRACKING SANDY, WEIGHING THE RISK

On Saturday, October 20, more than a week before Sandy would make landfall, New York City's Office of Emergency Management (OEM) began tracking the storm. At first, it appeared unlikely that Sandy would hit the United States' northeastern coast. In fact, as late as Wednesday, October 24, just one of the 20 models tracked by OEM showed Sandy doing so. But circumstances shifted considerably over the following two days, and by Friday an increasing number of forecasters were warning that Sandy would strike either late Monday, October 29, or early the following day, in or near southern New Jersey.[9]

---

7. Ibid.
8. For Harvard Kennedy School case studies exploring New Orleans' experience relocating hospital patients during Hurricane Katrina and subsequent storms, see: David Giles, *Moving People out of Danger (A): Special Needs Evacuations from Gulf Coast Hurricanes,* case no. 1943.0, (Cambridge, MA: President and Fellows of Harvard College, 2011); David Giles, *Moving People out of Danger (B): Special Needs Evacuations from Gulf Coast Hurricanes,* case no. 1961.0, (Cambridge, MA: President and Fellows of Harvard College, 2012).
9. Thomas A. Farley, "Testimony before the New York City Council Committee on Health, the Committee on Mental Health, Developmental Disabilities, Alcoholism, Drug Abuse, and Disability Services, and the Committee on Aging, Concerning Emergency Preparedness and the Response at the City's Healthcare Facilities," January 24, 2013.

Agencies and personnel across all levels of government accordingly accelerated their efforts to prepare for the storm. That Friday, New York Governor Andrew Cuomo declared a State of Emergency, while New York City's OEM activated its Emergency Operations Center. At the same time, both the city and the state also began implementing plans to support the possible evacuations of hospitals, nursing homes, and other health care institutions. As a first step, the State of New York's Department of Health and the city's Department of Health and Mental Hygiene jointly opened the Healthcare Facility Evacuation Center, which had first been utilized a year earlier during Hurricane Irene.[10] Charged with providing evacuation guidance to health care facilities in the lead-up to and during major emergencies, the center was also supposed to provide assistance to institutions unable to take action on their own.[11] Under the latter scenario, the center would coordinate the multiple organizations involved in transferring patients from an evacuating hospital or nursing home to one that could safely care for them. During Sandy, this effort would be led by the city's OEM and its Department of Health and Mental Hygiene, along with the Greater New York Hospital Association.[12]

Despite activating the center, NYC Health Commissioner Dr. Thomas Farley and his state counterpart, Health Commissioner Dr. Nirav Shah, refrained on Friday from issuing an evacuation order for health care facilities. This, Farley recollected, was largely shaped by their experience with Hurricane Irene. Then, in response to warnings that the storm would hit the city as a Category 1 (or even Category 2) hurricane, Farley and Shah had issued prestorm evacuation orders for hospitals and care facilities within Zone A (the parts of the city most prone to flooding). With the zone including 6 hospitals and more than 40 chronic care facilities,[13] Farley and Shah's evacuation order resulted in the eventual relocation of approximately 7,000 individuals. But in the end, Irene proved weaker than anticipated,[14] prompting leaders of many of the evacuated facilities to complain that the forced evacuation had unnecessarily endangered their patients. Farley sympathized with their concerns. As he observed,

> People in hospitals, nursing homes, and adult care facilities require round-the-clock care for their illnesses, and transporting them to other facilities is inherently risky. People in hospitals can die from an interruption in care during transport…. Therefore, in determining the best course of action before a tropical storm hits the area, City and State officials have to weigh the risks of evacuating these facilities against the risks of not evacuating.[15]

10. Ibid.
11. Ibid.
12. Adalja and others, "Absorbing Citywide Patient Surge During Hurricane Sandy."
13. Celeste Katz, "Mayor Bloomberg Update on Hurricane Sandy Storm Prep: Don't Be Complacent, NYC," NY Daily News, October 27, 2012, http://www.nydailynews.com/blogs/dailypolitics/mayor-bloomberg-update-hurricane-sandy-storm-prep-don-complacent-nyc-blog-entry-1.1692614.
14. Although not a devastating storm within the New York City metro area, Irene did have serious consequences for other parts of the Northeast, particularly inland New York and New England. In these areas, it caused extensive property loss, power disruptions, and heavy flooding. See Amit Uppal and others, "In Search of the Silver Lining: The Impact of Superstorm Sandy on Bellevue Hospital," Annals of the American Thoracic Society 10, no. 2 (2013): 135–142.
15. Farley, "Testimony," 3.

With forecasters predicting that Sandy's surge would be less than 4 feet (coupled with the knowledge that Irene's slightly larger surge had caused little damage in the city), Farley and Shah determined that the risks associated with organizing another large-scale evacuation were greater than the probability of patients being stranded and exposed to the effects of a destructive storm. That didn't mean, however, individual hospitals and nursing homes couldn't relocate their patients themselves. As Farley emphasized, "Health care facilities could have decided on their own to evacuate."[16]

But on Friday night, the forecast worsened; estimates of Sandy's anticipated surge now ran as high as 8 feet. Consequently, Farley and Shah began recommending more extensive preparedness measures. Although the storm was still believed to be, in Farley's words, "manageable," he and Shah directly reached out to hospitals and other health care facilities throughout the day Saturday, telling them to cancel elective admissions and surgeries and to discharge patients who were able to leave. They also learned that energy utility Con Edison planned to shut down Lower Manhattan's power supply as a precautionary measure, and as a result Dr. Shah subsequently ordered New York Downtown Hospital, situated just south of City Hall, to evacuate the next day. "We felt it was not wise for a hospital to enter a storm without grid power, even if it had an emergency generator," Farley explained.[17]

On Saturday evening, Mayor Bloomberg held a press conference to discuss the city's preparations. Among other things, he discussed the status of Zone A health care facilities. Bloomberg recognized Farley's and Shah's outreach efforts earlier in the day and assured reporters that in addition to cancelling admissions and discharging as many patients as they could,

> all of these health care facilities are taking additional precautions to prepare—including bringing in more staff. A lot of them do have backup generators and any outages are not expected to be more than hours or at most a day or so, so they'll be fine, they think. Every one of them has said that they're comfortable in going for a reasonable period of time dealing with a power outage if that should occur.[18]

Concern over Sandy's potential impact continued to mount, however, when on the following day forecasters once again revised storm surge estimates upward, warning that it could now reach as high as 11 feet. The latest predictions prompted President Barack Obama to take the unusual step of issuing prelandfall emergency declarations for several northeastern states, including New York, making a wide array of federal assets immediately available to protect lives, property, and public health.[19] For its part, the city

---

16. Ibid., 4.
17. Ibid., 5.
18. Katz, "Mayor Bloomberg Update on Hurricane Sandy Storm Prep."
19. FEMA, "Hurricane Sandy: Timeline," July 24, 2014; Sarah Parnass, "Sandy's Scope and Obama's Reaction Set Storm Apart Historically," *ABC News,* October 31, 2012, http://abcnews.go.com/Politics/sandy-scope-obama-reaction-set-storm-historically/story?id=17608888; Uppal and others, "In Search of the Silver Lining."

announced that it would implement additional emergency measures, including closing schools, shutting down public transportation, and ordering residents of Zone A to evacuate from their homes and apartments.[20]

All the same, said Farley, "It was [still] safer for the health care facilities to shelter in place than to try to accomplish an evacuation of a large number of facilities in the short time before the Zero Hour."[21] Zero Hour, he explained, was the moment when storm winds were predicted to be so strong that moving people was no longer safe. Because a full evacuation of health care facilities can last up to 72 hours, Farley continued, hospital officials typically must decide whether to conduct prestorm evacuations about three days before the projected Zero Hour. But on Sunday, as it became increasingly clear that Sandy would hit the region with substantial force, just 24 hours remained before its expected landfall. In other words, the window for safely organizing a large-scale evacuation of the city's hospitals had closed.

Neighboring Hospitals, Diverging Paths

The area in Manhattan bounded to the north and south by Manhattan's East 34th and East 23rd Streets and to the east and west by FDR Drive and 1st Avenue is home to three prominent medical institutions: NYU Langone Medical Center, Bellevue Hospital Center, and the Manhattan campus of the VA NY Harbor System. Their close proximity to Midtown and to the FDR, a major artery running the length of Manhattan's East Side, makes the hospitals easily accessible for emergency medical services and the populations they serve. But their location also has a potential downside: sitting just above sea level and with only the FDR separating them from the East River, all three facilities are vulnerable to severe coastal storms.

A year before Sandy, with Hurricane Irene bearing down on New York, both VA NY Harbor and NYU Langone had heeded evacuation orders and had closed their Manhattan facilities. This had entailed transferring or discharging hundreds of patients in the days leading up to the storm's anticipated arrival.[22] With Irene ultimately causing minimal damage (NYU Langone, for instance, experienced limited flooding of 2 to 3 feet of water in only one building), in hindsight some questioned whether it made sense to move so many individuals with serious medical conditions and needs.[23] But Martina

---

20. Farley, "Testimony"; Uppal and others, "In Search of the Silver Lining."

21. Farley, "Testimony," 5.

22. Kafi Drexel, "Veterans Affairs and NYU Langone Medical Centers Evacuate Ahead of Hurricane Irene's Arrival," *NY1*, August 26, 2011, http://www.ny1.com/archives/nyc/all-boroughs/2011/08/26/veterans-affairs-and-nyu-langone-medical-centers-evacuate-ahead-of-hurricane-irene-s-arrival-NYC_145885.old.html; Robert Kolker, "A Hospital Flatlined: Inside the NYU Langone Medical Center Evacuation," *New York Magazine*, November 3, 2012.

23. Elizabeth Cohen, "N.Y. Hospital Staff Carry Sick Babies Down 9 Flights of Stairs During Evacuation," *CNN*, October 30, 2012, http://www.cnn.com/2012/10/30/health/sandy-hospital.

Parauda, director of the VA NY Harbor Healthcare System, defended her own and her counterparts' decisions, which had been based on the prevailing forecasts, guidance provided by city and state officials, and—for her institution at least—memories of previous emergencies. "We had the 1992 nor'easter here at the Manhattan campus," she recalled. "We were flooded out, and we lost electrical power, and the generators could not accommodate us enough. That's why we realized, once we heard about Hurricane Irene, [we] could not safely keep the patients in place."[24]

A year later, even as frustrations over Irene lingered, VA NY Harbor decided to undertake a prestorm evacuation of its Manhattan campus yet again, transferring more than 100 patients to other facilities within its system, including hospitals in Brooklyn and the Bronx. "The safety of our patients is our top priority," Parauda declared over the weekend, while working out of VA NY Harbor's Incident Command Center. "With uncertainty about what the storm's impact will be, we feel that it is of critical importance to move our patients to care environments outside of the flood zone."[25]

Administrators at NYU Langone and Bellevue took a different course of action, however. At NYU Langone, the hospital's incident command team (ICT), comprising managers with crisis management responsibilities, spent several days assessing the threat posed by Sandy and determining the most appropriate response.[26] Aiming to strike a balance of sufficient precaution without overreaction, they decided to forgo a full-scale evacuation and to instead implement a separate set of emergency measures. Accordingly, hospital staff worked throughout the weekend to protect the complex from the physical effects of the storm and to discharge and transfer as many patients as possible.[27] (Prior to Sandy's arrival, staff members managed to reduce the number of NYU Langone's inpatients from about 575 to 325.)[28] Meanwhile, as late as Monday morning, with Sandy's winds strengthening by the hour and the storm advancing ever closer to the coast, officials continued to insist they had no plans to evacuate the entire facility.[29] As Dr. Bernard Birnbaum, head of the hospital's ICT, reitcrated, "There are significant risks to transferring patients.... It's the least desirable option."[30]

---

24. Drexel, "Veterans Affairs and NYU Langone Medical Centers Evacuate Ahead of Hurricane Irene's Arrival."

25. US Department of Veterans Affairs, "Goodbye, Sandy," November 1, 2012, http://www.nyharbor.va.gov/features/goodbyesandy.asp.

26. NYU Langone Medical Center, "All Hands on Deck," News & Views, November/December 2012, http://nyulangone.org/files/publication_issues/November_December_2012_N_and_V_Final.pdf.

27. NYU Langone Medical Center, "Annual Report," 2012, http://nyulangone.org/files/publication_issues/2012-annual-report.pdf.

28. Kolker, "A Hospital Flatlined: Inside the NYU Langone Medical Center Evacuation"; NYU Langone Medical Center, "All Hands on Deck"; David Remnick, "Leaving Langone: One Story," New Yorker, October 30, 2012.

29. Katie Moisse and Sydney Lupkin, "Superstorm Sandy Tests Hospital Preparedness: Generator Failure Prompted Patient Evacuation at NYU Medical Center," ABC News, October 30, 2012, http://abcnews.go.com/Health/superstorm-sandy-tests-hospital-preparedness/story?id=17597034.

30. NYU Langone Medical Center, "All Hands on Deck," 1.

THE SURGE HITS: NYU LANGONE AND BELLEVUE EVACUATE

Sandy made landfall at 7:30 p.m. on Monday, October 29, in Brigantine, New Jersey, 7 miles north of Atlantic City.[31] By then, the storm's winds were whipping across the Northeast and its deadly surge had begun smashing the coastline. In New York City, geological and meteorological conditions combined to make the surge particularly powerful, and among the places now facing its wrath were the three hospitals clustered along 1st Avenue in Manhattan. Fortunately, VA NY Harbor had by then completed its prestorm evacuation. But NYU Langone and Bellevue had only moved a portion of their patients, and over the following hours and days, a cascading series of events would overtake the two facilities, forcing administrators to make life-or-death decisions as the storm swirled around outside their hospitals' walls.

NYU Langone Evacuates

NYU Langone was the first of the two to face a full-blown crisis. There, between 7 p.m. and 7:45 p.m., a historically large surge of 14.5 feet propelled millions of gallons of water from the East River into the medical complex's basements and subbasements.[32] Quickly reaching 10 to 12 feet high, the floodwaters unleashed their fury, smashing doors, walls, and objects lying in their path. Soon, they had overwhelmed the hospital's backup power systems and infrastructure, plunging the hospital into darkness.[33]

In advance of the 2012 hurricane season, hospital administrators had made some significant investments in mitigating and preparing the facility for the effects of coastal storms. These included moving emergency generators to higher floors, placing the fuel tank that powered them in what was thought to be a watertight vault, and installing new fuel pumps in a secure pump house.[34] But both the fuel vault and pump house were still located in the basement, and although the latter survived Sandy's surge, floodwaters overtook the vault, triggering sensors that then abruptly took the generators offline.[35,36]

Soon, the situation became untenable. With the emergency generators no longer functioning, lights went out, water stopped running, and toilets no longer flushed.

---

31. City of New York, "A Stronger, More Resilient New York."
32. NYU Langone Medical Center, "Annual Report."
33. Cohen, "N.Y. Hospital Staff Carry Sick Babies Down 9 Flights of Stairs During Evacuation."
34. David B. Caruso, "The Big Story: Floods Render NYC Hospitals Powerless," *AP*, November 1, 2012.
35. Ibid.
36. According to NYU officials, the fuel vault was located in the basement because city code required it be placed in the lowest part of the building. See: Kolker, "A Hospital Flatlined: Inside the NYU Langone Medical Center Evacuation."

The hospital's communications systems, including its Web site, e-mail, and telephones, failed as well.[37] Reflecting on how quickly the surge upended NYU Langone's operations, Dr. Andrew Brotman, the hospital's senior vice-president and vice-dean for clinical affairs and strategy, observed, "Things went downhill very, very rapidly and very unexpectedly.... The flooding was just unprecedented."[38]

Although administrators had decided against organizing a full prestorm evacuation, the rapidly worsening conditions forced them to reassess their position. They now saw no other recourse but to move everyone off the premises.[39] Having made the decision, members of the ICT—which had formed an impromptu command center in the medical complex's main lobby—raced to launch the operation.[40] Among other things, they alerted the city's OEM, the New York Police Department, and the Fire Department of the City of New York (FDNY); notified on-duty doctors and nurses of their decision; and contacted other hospitals to begin arranging patient transfers.[41]

In total, about 1,000 people (including nurses, doctors, medical students, firefighters, and administrative and support staff) pitched in to carry out the evacuation.[42] Along with FDNY firefighters, who had quickly mobilized to assist with the effort, staff members organized themselves into teams of six or more to begin carrying patients on "Med Sleds" down the hospital's pitch black stairwells. Once patients made it to the ground floor, they were transferred to ambulances for transport to receiving institutions.

Many of these patients were highly vulnerable medically, and relocating them was by no means an easy process. One extreme case was a teenage girl suffering from epileptic seizures who had traveled from out of state to receive treatment from an NYU specialist. On Thursday, with Sandy's track still far from certain, she had undergone a craniotomy that involved the removal of skull tissue; afterwards, doctors had begun to induce seizures in order to identify the source of the problem. But now, as the evacuation swung into full gear, medical staff gave the patient Ativan to relieve the seizures. She was then placed on a sled and slowly carried down 12 flights of stairs.[43]

Transferring NYU's youngest patients also proved challenging. In advance of Sandy, the hospital had elected not to evacuate 20 newborns from its neonatal intensive care unit (NICU) due to their extremely fragile conditions. Now, as the storm's winds howled outside and its floodwaters swelled below, the process of moving the babies from the NICU, through the hospital, and then on to other medical facilities required exceptional care (this effort was believed to be the largest forced evacuation of a NICU

37. Moisse and Lupkin, "Superstorm Sandy Tests Hospital Preparedness."
38. Cohen, "N.Y. Hospital Staff Carry Sick Babies Down 9 Flights of Stairs During Evacuation."
39. NYU Langone Medical Center, "All Hands on Deck."
40. Jonathan Rockoff, "Among the Patients at Evacuated Hospital: A Benefactor," *Wall Street Journal*, October 30, 2012.
41. NYU Langone Medical Center, "All Hands on Deck."
42. Ibid.
43. Remnick, "Leaving Langone: One Story."

in US history). As medical students illuminated stairwells with flashlights, up to six people accompanied each baby down nine flights, vigilantly monitoring life-support systems and medications.[44] A medical student described the scene that played out in front of him as he watched one of the babies being moved:

> A nurse yelled, "NICU patient coming down! Silence!" The stairwell fell silent. No one moved. Flattened against a wall, I craned my head to see an orb of light. It was a phalanx of nurses guiding a doctor.... He held a baby in his arms and was manually ventilating the infant with one hand. The group moved forward silently, as one organism, down the steps into the darkness.[45]

Once they made it to the ground floor, the infants and the other evacuating patients were placed in ambulances and then driven, in the midst of the raging storm, to the 14 hospitals that had agreed to receive them.[46] (Although the Healthcare Facility Evacuation Center that the city and state had set up to help coordinate the evacuation process provided some overall guidance, a number of transfers were conducted directly by the two hospitals involved.)[47] Because many of the ambulances were driven by out-of-state volunteers, Sandy's winds and surge were not the only complicating factors during this final leg of the journey: limited knowledge of the local geography was also a problem. Remembered the mother of one evacuee, herself unfamiliar with the area, "None of us knew where we were going, so those guys [from Illinois] just switched on the GPS, and off we went.... I'm pretty sure we went uptown."[48]

Over the course of 13 hours—the last patient left the hospital by 11 a.m, on Tuesday—NYU Langone and its partners successfully transferred 322 individuals with highly complex medical conditions (in addition to the babies in the NICU and the teenager receiving treatment for epilepsy, they included adult critical care, pediatric cardiology, and transplant patients).[49,50] But even as hospital and emergency response personnel gave their all to sustain the operation, NYU Langone was already attracting public criticism. Speaking late Monday night, at the height of the storm and in the midst of NYU's evacuation,

44. Kolker, "A Hospital Flatlined: Inside the NYU Langone Medical Center Evacuation."
45. Samuel Penziner, "The Midnight Evacuation of NYU Medical Center," *Atlantic*, November 4, 2012, http://www.theatlantic.com/health/archive/2012/11/the-midnight-evacuation-of-nyu-medical-center/264504.
46. Among the hospitals agreeing to accept NYU's patients were Memorial Sloan-Kettering Cancer Center, North Shore-Long Island Jewish Health System, New York Presbyterian/Weill Cornell Medical Center, and Mount Sinai Medical Center. See: NYU Langone Medical Center, "All Hands on Deck"; Sumathi Reddy and Jonathan D. Rockoff, "Manhattan Hospital Transfers Patients after Losing Power," *Wall Street Journal*, October 30, 2012, http://www.wsj.com/articles/SB10001424052970204840504578087741520859014.
47. Adalja and others, "Absorbing Citywide Patient Surge During Hurricane Sandy."
48. Remnick, "Leaving Langone: One Story."
49. Mount Sinai Hospital, "The Mount Sinai Medical Center Accepts 64 Patients Evacuated From NYU Langone Medical Center and Is Preparing to Take Others," October 30, 2012, http://www.mountsinai.org/about-us/newsroom/press-releases/the-mount-sinai-medical-center-accepts-64-patients-evacuated-from-nyu-langone-medical-center-and-is-preparing-to-take-others.
50. NYU Langone Medical Center, "All Hands on Deck"; NYU Langone Medical Center, "Annual Report."

Mayor Bloomberg vented his frustration with the situation. "The one thing we had not counted on, New York University's hospital backup power—in spite of them making sure, assuring us that it's been tested—stopped working," he said.[51]

The hospital's top leaders pushed back. Among those who had been hospitalized at NYU Langone as the crisis unfolded was Kenneth Langone, the chairman of the hospital's board and a major benefactor for whom the medical center was named. Admitted the day before Sandy's landfall to receive treatment for pneumonia, he had watched from his hospital room as water swept across FDR Drive and then swamped the campus.[52] According to Langone, who was discharged early Tuesday morning, NYU Langone was adequately prepared for a significant storm. "We anticipated 12-foot surges, which we knew we could handle," he said. Among other things, he noted, the complex's emergency generators had routinely passed tests. But, he continued, Sandy's surge had exceeded the worst case scenarios for which the hospital had planned and trained.[53] Emphasizing his confidence in the hospital's administration and its decision to forgo a full evacuation in advance of the storm, he asked, "Do you think they'd have kept me in there if they thought I was going to be unsafe?"[54]

Bellevue Waits and Then Evacuates

Meanwhile, NYU Langone's neighbor to its immediate south, Bellevue—the oldest continuously operating hospital in the United States and a member of the New York City Health and Hospitals Corporation, the country's largest public hospital system[55]—had initially thought that it could weather the very worst of Sandy. Like their NYU Langone counterparts, Bellevue administrators were proud of the fact that they had taken steps, after the city's close call with Hurricane Irene, to protect the hospital's fuel pumps, placing them in a flood-resistant space (albeit still in the basement, but now sealed off by submarine doors). This, they believed, would safely protect the complex against a "100-year storm."[56] Despite these and other preparedness efforts, Bellevue was still forced to organize a poststorm evacuation—the first in its long history, during which it had endured blackouts, epidemics, and multiple natural disasters[57]—once it became clear that

---

51. Kolker, "A Hospital Flatlined: Inside the NYU Langone Medical Center Evacuation."

52. "Behind the Scenes of the NYU Hospital Evacuation," *CBS News*, November 1, 2012, http://www.cbsnews.com/news/behind-the-scenes-of-the-nyu-hospital-evacuation; Rockoff, "Among the Patients at Evacuated Hospital: A Benefactor."

53. Rockoff, "Among the Patients at Evacuated Hospital: A Benefactor."

54. Ibid.

55. City of New York, "About Bellevue," 2014, http://www.nyc.gov/html/hhc/bellevue/html/about/about.shtml.

56. Caruso, "The Big Story: Floods Render NYC Hospitals Powerless"; Uppal and others, "In Search of the Silver Lining," 142.

57. Uppal and others, "In Search of the Silver Lining."

its systems, too, had been compromised and that it would be too difficult to continue providing care.

As at NYU Langone, Bellevue's basement quickly filled with water late Monday evening. But for a while, Bellevue maintained an advantage over its neighbor: after losing its main power at around 9 p.m., the hospital's emergency generators kicked in, powering emergency lights and outlets. Still, the basement was completely flooded just an hour later; and at around 10:30 p.m., with the arrival of high tide, the view from hospital windows revealed a harrowing site: it was now entirely surrounded by water. With water pouring into the hospital, the fuel pumps that had been keeping the emergency generators functioning were compromised and ceased working. Doctors and nurses now worried that all power would be lost and anxiously began preparing for the very worst.[58]

But a valiant and improvised operation helped stave off immediate disaster, providing Bellevue a reprieve that NYU Langone had not enjoyed. In response to the failure of the fuel pumps, a brigade of Bellevue staff members and National Guardsmen lined 13 flights of stairs, passing buckets of fuel from one person to the next. Once at the top, each bucket was then carried up a small ladder and poured into the generator fuel tank. This labor-intensive effort succeeded in keeping the power going throughout the night and over the course of the next day.[59]

Conditions only worsened, however.[60] Because the generators could provide only about 30% of the hospital's usual level of electricity, equipment and systems lacked sufficient power to operate at full capacity. Meanwhile, the hospital was hit by several other challenges that emergency planners hadn't fully anticipated: all of Bellevue's elevators stopped working after water began cascading through their shafts; communications systems—including e-mail, landlines, and emergency phones—collapsed; food supplies dwindled; and water stopped running. More buckets, now filled with water, had to be carried up the stairs in order to flush toilets.[61] And with worries that oxygen supplies would run out, teams of National Guardsmen began lugging oxygen tanks, weighing about 180 pounds each, up 10 flights of stairs.[62]

Frustrated and exhausted, medical personnel pleaded with administrators to organize an evacuation. One of those on scene recalled the worsening conditions: "The phones didn't work.... We lost all communication between floors. We were in the dark all night. No water to wash hands—I mean, we're doctors!"[63] To the relief of many, as Tuesday dawned and the worst of Sandy ebbed, the decision to begin evacuating some of the

---

58. Ibid.
59. Ibid.
60. Ibid.
61. Caruso, "The Big Story: Floods Render NYC Hospitals Powerless"; Anemona Hartocollis and Nina Bernstein, "At Bellevue, a Desperate Fight to Ensure the Patients' Safety," *New York Times,* November 1, 2012; Uppal and others, "In Search of the Silver Lining."
62. Uppal and others, "In Search of the Silver Lining."
63. Hartocollis and Bernstein, "At Bellevue, a Desperate Fight to Ensure the Patients' Safety."

hospital's patients was finally made. But mirroring the operation that was now winding down at NYU Langone, moving patients out of Bellevue proved to be an incredibly complex and dangerous task. Several patients at Bellevue were extremely overweight, for instance, and they required teams of Guardsmen, working in shifts, to carry them down the stairs. Moving each one amounted to an hours-long effort.[64]

Meanwhile, other Guardsmen continued the arduous process of carrying fuel up and down flights of stairs, in support of a desperate attempt to keep the hospital going. By Wednesday, however, conditions had deteriorated considerably, and administrators decided that Bellevue had to be emptied entirely. "It was at that point that it was clear that it was just not tenable to keep patients for a longer term in the hospital," said Alan Aviles, who was president of the city's Health and Hospitals Corporation, which oversaw Bellevue.[65] By then, ambulance crews from across the country had flocked to assist with the evacuation, and with the continued aid of Guard troops, as many as 30 patients could now be evacuated every hour. By Thursday morning, more than 700 patients had been successfully evacuated, with just a few still remaining due to their conditions (such as several tuberculosis patients who could not easily be relocated).[66]

AFTER THE SURGE

On Wednesday morning, with the evacuation of NYU Langone completed and with Bellevue's own operation finally in full force, NYU Langone's leaders received a call. On the line was President Obama, who told them, "I want to thank you for the extraordinary work you and the whole Medical Center team did to safely evacuate patients.... I hope you know how much the whole country appreciates what you're doing."[67]

The president's words reflected what hospital administrators and government officials were most proud of: not one person had died in the hospital evacuations conducted during and immediately after the storm, despite the challenging weather conditions and the fragile medical state of many of the patients. "It's hard to imagine a worse case, but the worst case would have been if we had lost one patient. That would have been the worst case," reflected NYU Langone's medical dean and CEO, Robert Grossman.[68] New York City Health Commissioner Thomas Farley echoed that sentiment. "I can say that, while there was tragic loss of life from Hurricane Sandy, due to the heroic efforts of many people, no one lost their lives in health care facilities because of the storm."[69]

---

64. Uppal and others, "In Search of the Silver Lining."
65. Hartocollis and Bernstein, "At Bellevue, a Desperate Fight to Ensure the Patients' Safety."
66. Ibid.; Uppal and others, "In Search of the Silver Lining."
67. NYU Langone Medical Center, "All Hands on Deck," 7.
68. NYU Langone Medical Center, "Annual Report," 28.
69. Farley, "Testimony," 9.

All the same, Sandy had landed a powerful and devastating punch on healthcare facilities across the city. Although the hospitals had fortunately not lost a patient amidst the turmoil of the storm and the ad hoc evacuations, critics questioned NYU Langone's and Bellevue's decision not to follow VA NY Harbor's lead and evacuate before Sandy's arrival. Moreover, the storm's surge and subsequent power failures had damaged costly equipment and invaluable experiments and had taken the lives of thousands of lab animals.[70] For its part, NYU Langone lost a total of 7,660 cages of mice and 22 cages of rats that had been located in underground laboratories, which opened it up to further criticism. "This happens again and again and [research labs] never learn," Fran Sharples, director of the Board of Life Sciences at the National Academy of Sciences, said. "Anybody with half a brain knows you do a site-specific analysis … and it's really stupid to put your animals in the basement if you're in a flood zone."[71]

The damage caused by the surge was so devastating that it took months for Bellevue and NYU Langone to clean up and complete repair work. It was not until December 27 that NYU Langone had fully resumed services, and it took another five weeks after that until Bellevue was able to do so.[72] With other hospitals having to pick up the slack in the interim, Sandy's ripple effects would continue to tax the city's health care network well into the new year.

70. NYU Langone Medical Center, "Annual Report."
71. Sharon Begley, "New York University Faces Growing Criticism After Superstorm Sandy Kills Lab Mice at Medical Research Center," Reuters, November 7, 2012, http://www.reuters.com/article/2012/11/07/us-storm-sandy-animals-idUSBRE8A60L520121107.
72. Adalja and others, "Absorbing Citywide Patient Surge During Hurricane Sandy."

Exhibit 3-1. Best Track Positions for Hurricane Sandy: October 22–29, 2012

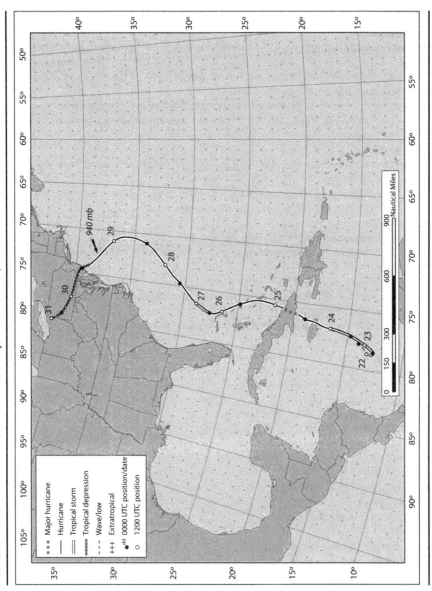

Source: Adapted from Blake and others, "Tropical Cyclone Report: Hurricane Sandy," National Hurricane Center, February 12, 2013, http://www.nhc.noaa.gov/data/tcr/AL182012_Sandy.pdf.

Exhibit 3-2. Chronology of Events: New York City Hospitals' Response to Superstorm Sandy, October 2012–February 2013

Saturday, October 20
- New York City's OEM began tracking Sandy.

Wednesday, October 24
- Just one of the 20 storm models tracked by the city projected that Sandy would hit the East Coast.

Friday, October 26
- Forecasters predicted that it was increasingly likely that Sandy would hit the East Coast by 2 a.m. the following Tuesday.
- New York Governor Andrew Cuomo declared a state of emergency.
- New York City's OEM activated its Emergency Operations Center.
- The New York State Department of Health and the New York City Department of Health and Mental Hygiene activated the Health care Facility Evacuation Center, while refraining from ordering health care facilities to evacuate their patients.

Saturday, October 27
- New York City and New York State public health officials reached out to vulnerable hospitals, instructing them to take precautionary measures.
- Mayor Michael Bloomberg gave a press conference in which he announced measures taken by the city in advance of the storm and reported that hospitals had assured officials that they were prepared.

Sunday, October 28
- Sandy's storm surge was now anticipated to be as high as 11 feet.
- The Manhattan campus of the Veteran Administration's New York Harbor Healthcare System voluntarily evacuated its patients.
- MTA suspended its subway, rail, and bus services.
- New York City Mayor Michael Bloomberg closed public schools and issued evacuation orders for Zone A (low-lying areas most vulnerable to flooding).
- President Barack Obama issued emergency declarations for several northeastern states, including New York.

Monday, October 29
- Superstorm Sandy made landfall at 7:30 p.m. in Brigantine, New Jersey, 7 miles north of Atlantic City.
- NYU Langone Medical Center began evacuating due to loss of power. The evacuation took about 13 hours to complete.
- Bellevue Hospital lost power but did not immediately evacuate. Instead, National Guard members maintained emergency power by carrying fuel up 13 flights of stairs.

Tuesday, October 30
- Bellevue Hospital began transferring select patients, due to loss of water pressure and extensive flooding.
- By 11 a.m., NYU Langone Medical Center had completed its evacuation.

Wednesday, October 31
- Bellevue Hospital continued evacuating its patients.

Thursday, November 1
- Bellevue Hospital completed its evacuation.

December 27
- NYU Langone Medical Center fully reopened.

February 7, 2013
- Bellevue Hospital fully reopened.

Source: Based on Amesh A. Adalja and others, "Absorbing Citywide Patient Surge During Hurricane Sandy: A Case Study in Accommodating Multiple Hospital Evacuations," *Annals of Emergency Medicine* 64, no. 1 (2014): 66–73; City of New York, "A Stronger, More Resilient New York," June 2013; FEMA, "Hurricane Sandy: Timeline."
Note: MTA = Metropolitan Transportation Authority; OEM = Office of Emergency Management.

II. EMERGENT INFECTIOUS DISEASE

The West Nile Virus Outbreak in New York City: On the Trail of a Killer Virus

Esther Scott

EDITORS' INTRODUCTION

This case study describes the difficult challenges that public health officials confronted in late 1999 in identifying and attacking an infectious disease previously unknown in this hemisphere. In many ways, New York City's experience with West Nile virus presaged issues that have intensified in the years since, as emergent infectious disease has become a vital concern not only in the United States but also worldwide.

Among the challenges described in Case 4A is the problem of enhanced disease surveillance—recognizing and tracking the incidence of infectious diseases in real time so that potential outbreaks might be averted or addressed with sufficient speed that they would not become epidemics. The surveillance systems in place in 1999 were heavily reliant on clinicians fulfilling their legal responsibility to bring incidents of specific, "reportable" diseases to the attention of public health authorities. But these systems were not well suited to detecting emergent infectious diseases that had not come under the surveillance regulatory regime. It applied mainly to already known diseases, reporting was spotty, and it was mostly post hoc—typically long after a case was discovered and treated.

This case was written by Esther Scott for Dr. Arnold M. Howitt, Executive Director, Taubman Center for State and Local Government, for use at the Executive Session on Domestic Preparedness, John F. Kennedy School of Government, Harvard University. Funding for the case was provided by the Robert Wood Johnson Foundation and the Office of Justice Programs, US Department of Justice. (0102)

Acute physicians, however, might note and promptly report anomalous clinical cases to public health authorities who in turn might initiate epidemiological investigations. That happened in the West Nile situation. However, although clinicians and public health authorities very quickly realized that something new was happening in New York City in 1999, the initial identification of the disease as St. Louis encephalitis proved faulty.

Case 4A thus highlights the importance of zoonotic diseases (i.e., those that pass between species). At about the time that human cases of West Nile were being recognized and misidentified, the metropolitan area was experiencing a large number of deaths of wild birds, especially crows. Similar infections soon spread to rare birds at the Bronx Zoo. An alert veterinary pathologist realized that there might be a connection between the bird deaths and the strange virus that had appeared in humans, but she also recognized that St. Louis encephalitis, the presumed cause of the human infections, did not kill birds. That insight ultimately led to the correct identification of West Nile.

The correct identification of West Nile depended importantly on robust organizational linkages and information sharing that stretched across broad networks of physicians, public health agencies, laboratories, and public agencies that normally had limited roles in public health matters. As Case 4B shows, similar interorganizational connections became crucial when a massive campaign of mosquito spraying became necessary to control the incipient epidemic. As NYC public health officials realized that the city was facing an outbreak of a new infectious disease, they reported through the organizational chain of the public health department and linked with the city's emergency management agency, the mayor's office, and eventually many other city agencies.

About two weeks after the first reports of the mysterious illness and shortly after the initial fatalities, New York Mayor Rudolph Giuliani called a press conference to explain the city's decision to initiate pesticide spraying, initially in one borough but eventually in all five. That was the beginning of an extensive communications campaign to explain the nature of the disease and ready the public for what might have been a deeply frightening pattern of events as spraying commenced. The city's strategy had to make use of multiple means of access to the public, and it had to be effective in dealing with special segments of the community, religious and ethnic minorities, and with dozens of linguistic minorities who received information imperfectly in English.

Case 4B also highlights the issue of implementation. New York City had not conducted mosquito spraying since early in the 20th century to control yellow fever outbreaks. Although the health department had the authority to initiate spraying, the capabilities of the city's Office of Emergency Management were critical in actually building the stakeholder support among elected officials and community groups; acquiring the necessary equipment; organizing complex, multidepartmental operations throughout the city; and effectively issuing information and reassurance so that the public would not be panicked by fear of the disease or by the spraying.

DISCUSSION QUESTIONS

1. To what extent would you characterize the recognition and belated identification of West Nile virus as a "success" or "failure" of the public health system?
2. How well did information and technical assistance flow among the health agencies involved in West Nile identification?
3. As New York City contemplated a massive mosquito spraying effort, what obstacles had to be overcome to implement its plans?
4. How important was the relationship between public health and emergency management in pushing forward with mosquito eradication? How did that connection develop?
5. How has disease surveillance improved to ensure early detection of new infectious threats?

* * *

In late August 1999, in the midst of a hot, dry summer, Dr. Marcelle Layton, assistant commissioner of the New York City Department of Health (NYC DOH), received a phone call from a hospital in Queens. The chief of infectious diseases at Flushing Hospital, Dr. Deborah Asnis, was calling to discuss two perplexing cases. Both involved elderly patients with symptoms of what looked like viral encephalitis: high fever, gastrointestinal distress, mental confusion. One of the two, however, also showed signs of profound muscle weakness—to the point of paralysis—an unusual symptom in cases of encephalitis. Concerned that she might not have gotten the diagnosis right, Asnis phoned the city health department for advice.

From Asnis's report, Layton thought that encephalitis was the likely culprit. On the face of it, this was no cause for immediate alarm. While not numerous, cases of viral encephalitis usually popped up in New York City every year, most often in summer. Still, as Layton recalls, "something bothered me" about Asnis's report, enough to prompt her to send a member of her staff to the hospital to review the two patients' charts. Less than a week later, Asnis was back on the phone to Layton to report a third case—again, an elderly patient with symptoms of encephalitis and, most disturbing, signs of muscle weakness; in the course of their conversation, a fourth case, in a different Queens hospital, was reported by another doctor. It was this second call "that got me more worried," Layton remembers. "I knew something unusual was going on," she would later say, "but I didn't know what it was, and the acid level in my stomach was skyrocketing astronomically as the phone call progressed."[1]

The phone call proved to be the opening act of a brief but intense drama that would involve several city, state, and federal agencies; an army research facility; a university laboratory; and a famous zoo. All would be on the trail of a virus whose precise identity

---

1. Interview with Marcelle Layton, *All Things Considered*, NPR, March 5, 2001.

proved elusive and controversial. When, less than four weeks later, the mystery of the virus was more or less solved, some observers believed its appearance constituted "one of the most important biological events to occur in the world of viruses in this century."[2] Many also felt that the unfolding drama offered a disturbing glimpse into the nation's capacity for quick detection of unknown disease agents, whether introduced by chance or by intention.

BACKGROUND: MARCELLE LAYTON AND THE COMMUNICABLE DISEASE PROGRAM

Marcelle Layton headed up the Communicable Disease Program in the NYC DOH, a venerable institution that traced its beginnings back to 1866. Essentially, the program was responsible for monitoring any infectious disease that did not fall into various categorical funding programs, the way that tuberculosis, HIV, or sexually transmitted diseases did. Of more than 70 "reportable" diseases (i.e., diseases that physicians were required to report to the city DOH under New York City's health code) about 54 fell under the purview of Layton's unit. In addition, new or emerging diseases were usually brought under the Communicable Disease Program's umbrella. Despite its wide range of responsibilities, the communicable disease unit was a small one: in 1999, its roughly 20-member staff was dwarfed by other NYC DOH infectious disease programs, such as HIV, which had a staff of several hundred. New diseases did not necessarily "come with more staff," Layton notes, "[so] you prioritize what you investigate." While reports of some illnesses were immediately investigated (i.e., field staff were sent out to review hospital charts and interview patients and their families) for others, Layton relied on a weekly data run to turn up signs of a disease cluster, indicating a possible outbreak.

Data on diseases, old and new, flowed into the Communicable Disease Program from the city's 72 hospitals and countless doctor's offices and clinics. Most reports were done on paper and arrived by mail or fax; in some instances—illnesses in which there was a "need for an acute intervention," Layton explains, such as bacterial meningitis— physicians were asked to phone in their reports. In all, Layton estimates, her program received anywhere from 50,000 to 60,000 reports a year.

Yet underreporting was a chronic problem in New York City, as in the entire nation. Busy doctors and understaffed hospitals and labs either failed to keep up with the paperwork or, in the case of many doctors, were simply unaware of reporting requirements.[3] In recent years, Layton had sought to raise the consciousness of the medical community

2. Richard Preston, "West Nile Mystery," *New Yorker*, October 18 & 25, 1999, 90.
3. According to NYC DOH Assistant Commissioner Dr. Marcelle Layton, hospitals were normally reliable in their reporting; "infection control" nurses routinely notified the city DOH of reportable disease cases. It was in office practices, Layton says, "where we start to lose reporting."

in regard to reportable diseases. Since 1996, her program had been responsible for working with the Mayor's Office of Emergency Management to prepare plans for dealing with potential bioterrorism incidents—the release of an anthrax "cloud" by terrorists, for example—as well as outbreaks of exotic new diseases that an international crossroads like New York City could unwittingly import. As part of this effort, Layton and other city DOH officials made the rounds of the city's hospitals, both to train physicians to recognize symptoms of rarely seen diseases, such as anthrax and smallpox, and to drive home the importance of reporting.

Despite the outreach campaign, however, there was evidence that underreporting persisted. When, later in 1999, the NYC DOH resorted to "active surveillance" of encephalitis (i.e., initiating contact with physicians and hospitals to gather data rather than waiting for reports to be sent in), it turned up 143 cases; this was in stark contrast to previous years, when the average number of reported cases of encephalitis was nine.

These figures pointed to a worrisome issue for an agency charged with monitoring the spread of diseases. In the case of some viral illnesses, like encephalitis and meningitis, the city DOH was particularly dependent on physician reporting. Because, as Layton notes, there were no quick and inexpensive tests for these diseases and because a specific diagnosis would not in most instances affect the treatment, suspected viral cases often went untested. This eliminated one important information source for the city DOH—laboratories—and left responsibility for both diagnosis and reporting almost solely in the hands of clinicians. The department's hopes of spotting early an outbreak of a disease with unusual manifestations in a city of more than 7.5 million people therefore rested on the sharp eyes and careful reporting of New York City's doctors.

THE CALL

When Dr. Deborah Asnis decided to phone the NYC DOH on Monday, August 23, 1999, it was not to report two cases of encephalitis at Flushing Hospital, a small community facility in northern Queens. "Most infectious disease doctors would not call the [NYC DOH] to report a case of encephalitis or meningitis," Asnis explains. "They would have the infection control nurse do it." But one of the two cases puzzled Asnis. The patients, both elderly, were being treated in the hospital's intensive care unit for encephalitis, but one of them had developed muscle paralysis, a symptom she did not associate with the disease.[4] "I could not understand why someone [with encephalitis] would be paralyzed,…" Asnis recalls, "and I wanted to make sure I wasn't overlooking" some other explanation for the symptoms she was observing. Neither patient was responding to the antibiotics and antiviral drugs being administered and, with both patients' families

---

4. Eventually, the other patient also became paralyzed. A third patient admitted at about the same time, ostensibly for cardiac arrest, was later found to have had encephalitis as well.

"very concerned about what's going on—why can't I give them an exact answer," Asnis turned to the Communicable Disease Program at the city DOH for help. "Fortunately," she says, "I didn't get a tape recording or a voicemail; I got a real live voice."

The voice belonged to Marcelle Layton who, after hearing Asnis's presentation of the cases, concluded that they did not fit the clinical picture of botulism, which Asnis had entertained as an alternative diagnosis, or of Guillain-Barré syndrome, which a consulting neurologist had proposed. She thought the original diagnosis of encephalitis was most likely correct and advised Asnis to send specimens of her patients' spinal fluid to the New York State DOH's laboratory in Albany, which had been funded and certified by the Centers for Disease Control and Prevention (CDC) to do viral testing.

Layton did not, however, feel totally at ease. She found herself wondering, as she recalls, "what type of encephalitis causes muscle weakness" and consulted her medical textbooks for an answer. "There are hundreds of viruses that cause encephalitis," Layton explains, and for almost all of these, her textbooks indicated that muscle weakness was an infrequent but not unknown complication, occurring in roughly 5% to 10% of cases. Still, she was not entirely reassured. Typically, when a case of encephalitis was reported, the Communicable Disease Program took no immediate action. "An individual report would just get entered," Layton explains, "and no investigation would be done … unless we got a clustering." In this instance, however, despite being shorthanded in the office—"August," says Layton, "is a bad time to have anything happen in New York"—she decided to send a member of her staff to Flushing Hospital to review the two patients' charts.

Just a few days later, on Friday, August 27, Asnis called Layton again. Another patient with symptoms of encephalitis and muscle weakness had been admitted to the hospital. While they were on the phone, a neurologist wandered into Asnis's office and, overhearing the conversation, said, as Layton remembers it, "This is very unusual. I'm seeing a very similar case at New York Hospital/Queens." It was at this point that Layton felt her stomach acid level shoot up. "All of a sudden," she says, "I went from one patient with what seemed to be viral encephalitis and another one that probably had it too, but with muscle weakness, to four. And they were clustered in this 16-square-mile area of town, when normally I only see nine in a year, citywide." Layton canceled her weekend plans and, along with Dr. Annie Fine, assistant medical director in the Communicable Disease Program, headed out to Queens to have a look for herself. "There's nothing like going out and reviewing a chart yourself," she says, "and actually examining the patients and talking to the families face to face."

A CLOSER LOOK

On the drive over to Flushing Hospital on Saturday, as Layton recalls, she and Fine speculated further on what might be causing the constellation of symptoms Asnis was reporting. A conference call with specialists from CDC on Friday had strengthened Layton's conviction that the patients were not suffering from botulism, although it was decided to test for it to be sure. Layton and her colleague briefly considered the possibility of polio, but, she says, "that didn't make sense" either. That left encephalitis as still the most likely candidate, though there were problems with this diagnosis as well. It was not unusual for viral encephalitis and its close kin, meningitis, to make an appearance in New York City in the summertime.[5] Almost without exception, these cases were caused by enteroviruses, which were transmitted by human contact. But the four Queens cases did not fit the pattern of an enteroviral outbreak, which usually sickened children and young adults, and typically was signaled by a rise in cases of meningitis. All of Asnis's patients were elderly, and there had been, to date, no clusters of meningitis reported in Queens or anywhere else in the city. Encephalitis could also be caused by arboviruses (i.e., viruses carried by mosquitoes and ticks) but this, too, seemed an unlikely source of the disease. While many parts of the United States, and of New York State, experienced periodic outbreaks of arboviral encephalitis, it was extremely rare in New York City: the last recorded arboviral outbreaks of any kind to occur there were the yellow fever epidemics of the 19th century.[6]

As Layton and Fine began interviewing patients' families—the patients themselves were too ill to talk—the mystery deepened. Although all of the families came from the same section of Queens, none of them knew each other or had recently participated in any community event that would have brought them into contact; this, plus the fact that other members of their families remained healthy, seemed to rule out an enteroviral outbreak. The one activity that all the patients had in common was spending time outdoors in the evening—to smoke, to socialize with neighbors, to garden—when mosquitoes typically came out in numbers to feed. This seemed to point to an arboviral source, but if it were so, it would appear to be an unusually isolated outbreak because, as Layton learned in a conversation with CDC officials, "there was no evidence of [arboviral] activity … anywhere on the East Coast, much less the Northeast." In fact, only a few weeks before Asnis's phone call, the *New York Times* reported that, due to an unusually dry summer, vacationers in the New York–New Jersey–Connecticut region were finding recreational areas remarkably free of mosquitoes.

Meanwhile, the number of cases, while still tiny, continued to inch up. On Saturday, August 28, while Layton was visiting Flushing Hospital, a fifth case "rolled in, in front of her eyes," Asnis recalls. By this time, Asnis herself had taken note of another unusually high statistic at the hospital: the number of spinal taps being administered. Asnis, who

---

5. Encephalitis and viral meningitis are both inflammations of the brain caused by viruses. Viral meningitis, the milder and more common of the two, refers to an inflammation of the lining of the brain, and encephalitis to an inflammation of the brain tissue itself. It is possible for patients to have elements of both diseases at the same time.

6. Annie Fine and Marcelle Layton, "Lessons from the West Nile Viral Encephalitis Outbreak in New York City, 1999: Implications for Bioterrorism Preparedness," *Clinical Infectious Diseases* 32 (2001): 278. In the mid-1990s, there was a small outbreak of malaria, a mosquito-borne illness, in Queens, but the disease agent in that case is a parasite, not a virus.

was consulted on every spinal tap done at the hospital, expected to see a small spike in the number of these procedures each summer, but typically they were requested for younger patients in cases where meningitis was suspected; this summer, however, "there were a lot of spinal taps being done on 70- and 80-year-old people,…" she says. "So I knew something strange was going on." Layton had come to the same conclusion. After calling around to other hospitals in Queens over the weekend, she had turned up a few more cases with similar clinical presentations. "By this point," she says, "I had eight cases, all adults, all relatively healthy before getting sick; seven of the eight had muscle weakness, half of them to the point of paralysis and being on ventilators.[7] This was something unusual." It was time, she decided, to ask for help.

GETTING THE WORD OUT

The first call Layton made, on Sunday morning, August 29, was to CDC, which, on request, provided assistance to state and local governments in investigating disease outbreaks.[8] Layton called the agency's emergency 800-number, which put her through to officials in both the enteroviral and arboviral branches of CDC. They, too, were perplexed by the unusual clinical picture presented by the cases, particularly the muscle weakness. "Everyone was impressed with the fact that that doesn't fit any known virus,…" Layton recalls. "Their advice was, you need a diagnosis." The following day, in what would be the first of many conference calls involving CDC and state and city health officials, it was agreed that the state health department lab, not CDC, would have first crack at analyzing the specimens taken from the Flushing Hospital patients, "because," Layton explains, "[CDC] was funding the state lab to do everything that they would do."

Efforts to get patient specimens to the state facility had stalled earlier when Flushing Hospital ran into problems preparing them for shipping; the hospital did not, it turned out, have the dry ice needed to preserve the samples while in transit. By Monday, August 30, the city health department had taken matters into its own hands, picking up the specimens at the hospital, bringing them back to its own lab, then packing and shipping them off to the state facility for testing.[9] Meanwhile, Layton began to widen the circle of officials who knew of the potential outbreak in Queens. She had already informally talked to her immediate boss, NYC DOH Deputy Commissioner Benjamin Mojica, before she visited Flushing Hospital; on Sunday night she e-mailed NYC DOH

---

7. Six of the eight patients ranged in age from 57 to 87 years; the other two were 29 and 49 years old.
8. US General Accounting Office (GAO), "West Nile Virus Outbreak: Lessons for Public Health Preparedness," HEHS-00-180 (September 11, 2000): 7.
9. The city sent spinal fluid specimens to the state virology lab and blood serum samples to the state serology lab; the two labs were 12 miles apart.

Commissioner Neal Cohen to apprise him of developments as well. In this, she was essentially following standard operating procedure at the agency. "We notify senior staff of all outbreaks," Layton explains, "both potential and confirmed." It was a practice that extended to the top of city government where appropriate. "We always err, and are encouraged to do so," Layton notes, "on early notification. We always clarify if the outbreak is confirmed or potential to put it in perspective. The leadership prefers to know what's brewing sooner [than] later."

At about the same time, Layton sent an e-mail alert to state health officials in New Jersey and Connecticut and to local health departments in counties bordering New York City. The purpose, she says, was both to ask, "are you aware of anything similar in [your] area, and to let them know about [the potential outbreak]." No other state or local organizations had any cases within their jurisdiction to report at that point, but Layton put them and others on a group e-mail list that she regularly updated over the following weeks. Also on Monday, August 30, Layton sent out a "broadcast fax"—the first of many—to all 72 New York City hospitals, alerting them to a "cluster of atypical viral encephalitis," and asking for specimens of any cases that fit the description to be shipped to the state lab for testing.

Getting to a Diagnosis

While NYC DOH officials awaited word from the state lab, which had received the first specimens from Flushing Hospital on Tuesday, August 31, the department, with help from epidemiologists on loan from CDC and an entomologist borrowed from the Museum of Natural History, launched a field investigation of the Queens neighborhood that was home to the patients. What they found strongly bolstered the theory that mosquitoes were the vectors that conveyed the encephalitis virus to humans. They observed, among other things, piles of old tires in a nearby park, bird baths in a garden, a swimming pool under construction, and buckets set out by a conscientious citizen to catch rainwater in that drought-stricken summer: all containers of water and, therefore, ideal breeding grounds for *Culex pipiens*, an urban mosquito whose larvae thrived in stagnant pools. Meanwhile, on Wednesday, September 1, Flushing Hospital reported the first death of a patient from the mystery virus.

The following day, city health officials received word of the first solid clue to the identity of the virus. State lab scientists, using a commercial antibody screening test,[10] had gotten positive results for a flavivirus, a family of about 70 different arboviruses; in particular, there was a strong reaction to the St. Louis encephalitis virus, the only

---

10. Simply put, these screening tests use antibodies, which are produced by the body to fight off foreign matter, to help identify a virus. The reaction of antibodies in patient serum samples to a virus indicates, to varying degrees of specificity, the type of virus that triggered the release of the antibodies in the first place.

flavivirus commonly found in the United States.[11] This was surprising news. While St. Louis encephalitis showed up periodically in outbreaks in the Midwest, Southeast, and West, it rarely turned up in the Northeast. It had made its last appearance in New York State in the 1970s, but there were no documented cases of St. Louis encephalitis in New York City itself.

The specter of an outbreak of a mosquito-borne encephalitis was a disturbing one, with serious public health implications, but city officials were counseled to hold off going public or taking any major action until the state lab's findings were confirmed by CDC. "There were many people at the lab level," Layton remembers, "who thought these [screening] tests [used in the state lab] are nonspecific; you can have false positives and false negatives.... Many people said, 'I wouldn't do anything until you know for sure this is positive.'" To NYC DOH Deputy Commissioner Ben Mojica, the advice made sense. "For us to really act on something in terms of controlling the vector—which was at that point [suspected to be] adult mosquitoes—without real proof that there is a disease transmitted by adult mosquitoes in the community, would be foolhardy." The city had, in fact, already had one unhappy experience with a false positive. The previous year, Layton explains, the state lab had reported positive test results for eastern equine encephalitis; the test results were made public, but later retracted when further testing by CDC did not confirm the original finding. Rather than unnecessarily alarm residents again, or launch a response that would prove pointless, NYC DOH officials decided to wait the extra 24 hours it would take for the specimens to be re-tested and the results confirmed.

The New York state lab had already shipped off specimens of blood and spinal fluid to the laboratory at CDC's Division of Vector-Borne Infectious Diseases in Fort Collins, Colorado, where they arrived on Thursday, September 2—the same day, city DOH officials were notified of the state's results.[12] There, scientists applied a more sophisticated and reliable antibody screening test, known by its acronym ELISA, to the samples, using what Dr. Duane Gubler, director of the Fort Collins facility, calls a "geographic panel of reagents"—that is, "a battery of antigens made up of viruses that we know occur in the region where these samples came from." These included viruses commonly found in the United States—the LaCrosse encephalitis virus, western and eastern equine encephalitis viruses, and St. Louis encephalitis virus; a few others from elsewhere in the western hemisphere—Central and South America—were added to the mix as well. The ELISA was a rapid test, but there would nonetheless be a day's wait. Results were not expected until sometime the following afternoon, Friday, September 3, the start of the Labor Day

11. US GAO, "West Nile Virus Outbreak," 44.

12. The facility in Fort Collins, Colorado, part of CDC's National Center for Infectious Diseases, acted as a "reference" laboratory, which meant that other labs could send it specimens for diagnosis, identification, and confirmation. See: "Expecting the Unexpected: The West Nile Virus Wake Up Call," Report of the Minority Staff, Senate Governmental Affairs Committee, to Senator Joseph Lieberman, July 24, 2000, http://concepts. gslsolutions.com/gov/senate/hsgac/public/_archive/wnvfinalreport.pdf.

weekend. Meanwhile, that Thursday, September 2, a second encephalitis patient at Flushing Hospital died.

Waiting

The roughly two-week period from Asnis's call to the arrival of the specimens in Fort Collins had been "tense," according to Mojica, but the final hours before the results came in from CDC were nail-biters. Still, the brief lull was useful in some ways, allowing city officials time to begin contingency planning. Members of the office of New York Mayor Rudolph Giuliani got their first inkling of an impending crisis on Thursday, September 2, when NYC DOH Commissioner Neal Cohen phoned Deputy Mayor Joseph Lhota to apprise him of the situation. "I said," Cohen recalls, "Joe, we have a problem." With "strong evidence [of] a mosquito-borne condition," Cohen says, and with CDC entomologists advising the NYC DOH that the city would need to attack the adult mosquito population with pesticides, he decided the time had come to involve city hall. Cohen also called Jerry Hauer, then-director of the Mayor's Office of Emergency Management, which would take the lead in handling the city's response. By that evening, Mayor Giuliani had been notified of the possible outbreak, and plans for managing it were percolating through the administration.[13]

As the time drew near for CDC to call, city officials grew increasingly tense. Mayor Giuliani "wanted to do something," Jerry Hauer remembers, "so we had decided that if in fact this came back positive, we would do a press conference between 2:00 and 2:30. We expected the results around 2:00." Two o'clock came and went, with no word from CDC. Giuliani "was on the phone about every 15 minutes asking about the results," Hauer says. "He was anxious. I was anxious. Neal [Cohen] was anxious." Finally, at around quarter of three, on Friday, September 3, the call came. The results of the ELISA test were reported to be, as Layton remembers it, "most consistent with St. Louis encephalitis." That is, the test was positive for St. Louis encephalitis but, because the ELISA was a "nonspecific serologic test," in Gubler's words, all that could be said at that point with certainty was that it was a flavivirus; any flavivirus—Japanese encephalitis, West Nile, Murray Valley encephalitis, for example—could be causing the positive results.[14] But, as Gubler notes, a number of factors seemed to point to St. Louis encephalitis in particular. The "serology was compatible with the St. Louis," he says, "the clinical information was compatible, the epidemiology was compatible." Although muscle weakness had not been associated with St. Louis encephalitis, it was known to cause more severe illness among the elderly—a

---

13. For an in-depth look at the city's handling of the outbreak, see Case 4B.
14. The viruses were customarily named after the area where they were discovered. Murray Valley encephalitis virus originated in Australia, West Nile in Uganda. See: Lawrence Altman, "Encephalitis Outbreak Teaches an Old Lesson," *New York Times*, September 28, 1999, 8F.

notable feature of the cases accumulating in Queens.[15] Moreover, while new to New York City, St. Louis encephalitis was a familiar virus; the other flaviviruses were virtually unknown in the United States. Additional, more time-consuming testing would have to be done to verify CDC's initial diagnosis, but in the meantime, the city would move forward on the assumption—which quickly translated into apparent certainty—that New Yorkers were dealing with their first-ever outbreak of St. Louis encephalitis.

Going Public

New York City residents got word of the outbreak, and of its first fatalities, at a news conference that Friday afternoon, held in the Whitestone section of Queens, near the "hot zone" for the virus. Within hours of Mayor Giuliani's announcement, the city commenced spraying sections of Queens with pesticides and handing out informational flyers and cans of insect repellent to area residents. Those who missed the coverage of the press conference on TV or radio woke the next morning to front-page news stories on the outbreak, perhaps most vividly depicted in the *Daily News*, which carried the banner headline, "Deadly Queens Mosquito."

While the Office of Emergency Management worked feverishly to exterminate the carriers of the encephalitis virus, and staff from the city health department fanned out across the city to determine how many the virus had sickened, others wondered about the possible connection between the St. Louis encephalitis outbreak and another odd happening in New York that summer. The question was raised at Giuliani's press conference, Layton notes. "Somebody came up to [Annie Fine, who was there along with Commissioner Cohen]," she recalls, "and mentioned the dead birds."

A BIRD DIE-OFF IN QUEENS

Precisely when birds started dying in the Queens area could not be pinpointed, but sometime in mid-June, residents began bringing in sick crows, which appeared to be suffering from a neurological disorder, to a veterinarian at a local clinic for treatment. By August, birds—almost exclusively crows—were dying in sufficient numbers to attract the notice of the local Queens press. Residents were reporting the disappearance of large flocks of crows from longtime roosts, and the discovery of crow carcasses in their backyards and in parks. Many of the dead birds were shipped off for examination to the New York State Department of Environmental Conservation (DEC), which

---

15. Lawrence Altman, "After a Phone Tip, Medical Detectives Track Down a Killer," *New York Times*, September 9, 1999, 1B.

had jurisdiction over wildlife, but the cause of the die-off proved elusive. Ward Stone, a pathologist with the agency who performed necropsies—the animal equivalent of a postmortem examination—on the birds, suspected that several unrelated factors were at work in the bird deaths; some, he hypothesized, were dying from pesticide poisoning, others from fungal pneumonia and metabolic bone disease. None of these, he told one reporter, posed a threat to area residents. "I don't see anything particularly hazardous to people," he said.[16]

At the Zoo

By mid-August, the crow deaths had also attracted the attention of Dr. Tracey McNamara, chief pathologist at the Bronx Zoo, a sprawling wildlife park that was home to more than 6,000 animals. McNamara had been hearing reports of dead birds for some weeks, but now she was observing the phenomenon firsthand. It began with one or two crows dying near or at the zoo, she recalls, "and then we started seeing them all over the place. You could literally be standing here, and you'd see a bird just take a nosedive into an exhibit." It looked, she later told a reporter, as if it were "raining crows."[17] These crows, like the ones in Queens, were sent to the DEC for examination, but McNamara grew increasingly skeptical of Ward Stone's proffered diagnoses, none of which, she believed, could cause bird deaths in the numbers she was seeing. Stone, who was, according to McNamara, not trained or certified as a veterinary pathologist, could not do the kinds of cell tissue analysis that she felt was crucial to understanding what was killing the birds. "When it became clear he was not doing histopathology," she recalls, "I [said], forget it. We're doing our own investigation."[18]

This was not, McNamara has pointed out, a matter of idle curiosity. Because of the vulnerability of its rare and exotic animals to infection from indigenous wildlife, a zoo was "always," she noted, "in a heightened state of surveillance, and very sensitized to unpredicted disease outbreaks."[19] Whatever sickened birds in the surrounding area could cross over and attack the zoo population; recently, two pheasants at the zoo had died, reinforcing her fear that the killer disease had begun to "spill over into our zoo birds." "You always have to be on the lookout for something new," McNamara observes; even a dead crow could be "a potential index case."

---

16. Brian Lockhart, "Queens Crow Death Cause Still Sought," *Times/Ledger* (Queens), September 2, 1999, 2.
17. Preston, "West Nile Mystery," 91.
18. In early September, Stone, who reportedly examined some 400 birds, began sending specimens to the National Wildlife Health Center laboratory in Madison, Wisconsin, part of the US Geological Survey, for testing and analysis; in a cover letter, he made note of the human encephalitis outbreak in New York City. Earlier, he had asked the New York State DOH lab to test the samples but was referred elsewhere because the state facility did not have the necessary reagents to test for bird viruses. See: US GAO, "West Nile Virus Outbreak," 43, 47.
19. Presentation at USDA satellite seminar broadcast, September 13, 2000.

What McNamara saw when she looked at cell tissue from the crows under the microscope was evidence, she believed, of something due to a "viral insult" that was "consistent with some kind of viral encephalitis." When news of the outbreak of St. Louis encephalitis in Queens began to surface over Labor Day weekend, she wondered whether there might be a link between the two. "The temporal and spatial relationships of people dying of encephalitis and birds dying of encephalitis in the same timeframe,…" she asks. "How could you ignore that?" But, as she knew, there was good reason to doubt the likelihood that the two outbreaks were linked. It was known that birds served as the "reservoir host" for St. Louis encephalitis virus (i.e., they carried the virus), which mosquitoes picked up when they bit birds and then transmitted to humans whom they subsequently bit; but it was also known that the St. Louis encephalitis virus did not kill the birds themselves. In fact, when McNamara consulted her textbooks over the Labor Day weekend, she discovered that flavivirus-related diseases like St. Louis encephalitis "had only been described in humans."

Mounting Losses

As McNamara had feared, whatever was killing crows in Queens began to attack birds at the Bronx Zoo as well. When she returned to work after the Labor Day weekend, on Tuesday, September 7, McNamara recalls, "all hell broke loose." On Tuesday, a flamingo, a longtime zoo inhabitant, died, as did a Guanay cormorant, both showing neurological symptoms before collapsing. The next day, McNamara recounts, "a bald eagle—our mascot—[developed] head tremors. Boom! Drops dead. Another pheasant. Boom! It ate breakfast; an hour later—dead on the ground." Over the next couple of days, the zoo lost a snowy owl and two Chilean flamingoes. "Something," McNamara says, was "sweeping through the zoo collection. The curators are going nuts, the veterinarians are going nuts, the keepers are going nuts…. It was emotionally a roller coaster here."

Again, McNamara turned to her textbooks for help but came away with more questions than answers. If St. Louis encephalitis virus did not kill birds, the viruses that did—chiefly the "alphaviruses," such as eastern and western equine encephalitis—seemed unlikely candidates in the current outbreak. If, for example, eastern equine encephalitis virus was at work, it would have devastated the zoo's emus, which were a "sentinel species" for the disease, being exquisitely sensitive, in McNamara's words, to the virus; but the emus at the Bronx Zoo were the picture of health. Similarly, Newcastle disease and avian influenza viruses, both of which caused encephalitis in birds, would have shown up among the domestic poultry—sentinel species for those diseases—in the children's zoo; but here, too, there was no evidence of ill health.

As birds continued to die at the zoo, McNamara and her staff "shifted into full emergency mode," conducting necropsies and preparing specimens for testing. They took extra precautions, donning disposable containment suits, visors, and three sets of gloves, "because," she explains, "I knew we were dealing with something I had never seen before." She was concerned that the unknown pathogen might be "zoonotic"—that is, a disease agent capable of sickening humans as well as animals or, as McNamara crisply puts it, "something that could kill us while we're working on it." Even so, a member of her staff accidentally stuck himself with a needle while euthanizing a dying flamingo—an unnerving moment, as McNamara recalls. "I was the only one who had seen how severe those lesions [in dead birds] were under the microscope," she says, "and I knew that whatever this was, he had just been inoculated with it, with a large-bore needle."

Looking for Answers

Concerned about the safety of workers at her lab, McNamara concluded that it was time to look outside the zoo for help with diagnostic testing. On Thursday, September 9, she placed a call to the National Veterinary Services Laboratory (NVSL) in Ames, Iowa, a veterinary reference laboratory run by the US Department of Agriculture. Normally, McNamara explains, protocol required her to talk first to the state agricultural veterinarian to get permission to send specimens to the NVSL; in this instance, however, although she did put in a call to the state, she spoke directly to Dr. Brundaban Panigrahy, director of the avian section of the NVSL and got his okay to ship the specimens to the lab immediately. "I was not going to wait," she says. "I knew we couldn't wait another day to get the samples out." By now, McNamara was convinced that there was a connection between the human and the bird deaths. In her conversation with Panigrahy, she remembers, "I told [him] I was certain that whatever it was, it was killing people and crows and now birds in the zoo. It was one and the same." She asked him to expedite efforts to isolate the virus, which would make possible a more conclusive identification than serological tests could provide. Panigrahy acceded to her request, and the samples were sent off to Ames that day.[20]

Her hunch about the link between the animal and human outbreaks in New York City also prompted McNamara to get in touch with CDC that same day. After being directed to the Division of Vector-Borne Infectious Diseases in Fort Collins, she called to ask if the lab would "check out these bird [specimens] to see if it's the same thing that the people have." If, as she suspected, a known "veterinary pathogen" was not at work in the animal outbreak, the NVSL might not be able to provide a definitive diagnosis, which to McNamara was the most urgent need of the moment. For this reason, she did not call the city DOH—its lab could not, she points out, "do the tests." The Fort Collins lab, on the

---

20. The day before, Ward Stone of the state DEC also sent bird samples to the NVSL, making note in a cover letter of the St. Louis encephalitis outbreak in New York. See: US GAO, "West Nile Virus Outbreak," 47.

other hand, could. "I had been told they were the only ones doing this [viral] diagnostic work," she explains, and it seemed a logical step to enlist its help in examining the bird specimens. In turning to CDC, "I thought I had gone to the top," she says. "If the CDC didn't want [the zoo samples], why would anyone else?"

As it turned out, however, the Fort Collins lab, which was already swamped with human specimens from New York needing immediate testing, was reluctant to accept McNamara's samples. The official she spoke to on September 9 "informed me," she recalls, "that there was no possible relationship [between the outbreaks] and he refused the samples." Irked but undeterred, McNamara called back, this time asking to speak to the secretary at the lab, who eventually agreed to fax her the appropriate forms for submitting samples. That day, she shipped out two flamingo specimens to Fort Collins by Federal Express. The day before, September 8, back in Queens, a third patient died of encephalitis.

Over the next couple of days and into the weekend, McNamara received a steady stream of serology test results from the NVSL, confirming her hypothesis that the familiar viruses were not implicated in the bird deaths in New York. But she heard "nothing from CDC," she recalls. "I'm calling them and leaving them messages on voicemail. Nobody talks."[21]

Then, on Wednesday, September 15, the NVSL called McNamara to report on its observation of the virus, which it had succeeded in isolating from one of her zoo specimens. Looking through an electron microscope, scientists at the lab saw a "flavi/toga-like virus, 40 nanometers in diameter."[22] According to McNamara, there was no mistaking the import of one key piece of data: the size of the virus made it too small to be an alphavirus, the group of viruses commonly known to cause encephalitis in birds. "I was like, 'Eureka,'" McNamara later told a reporter. "It's a flavivirus.... The group everyone thought it would be was the alphavirus, those are 60–65 nanometers.... No previous representative of that group of viruses [flaviviruses] had been known to ever kill birds. I knew we had something new."[23] For the NVSL, this was the end of the road in terms of virus identification. Because it was not a known veterinary pathogen, McNamara says, "they could take it no further.... No veterinary lab in the United States would be able to take the diagnosis the next step."[24]

Galvanized by the NVSL's findings, McNamara called the Fort Collins lab again. "I was leaving messages," she says, "and leaving messages, and finally I left a message to the effect of, 'Yo! ... Guess what? It is a flavivirus. It is in the brain of my flamingo. We've made

---

21. Bronx Zoo Chief Pathologist Dr. Tracey McNamara's and CDC's recollections of their communications differ. Officials at Fort Collins maintain that McNamara did not clearly convey to them her conviction that the virus that was killing birds was an unknown and likely connected to the human outbreak. They also note that they were in touch with McNamara by e-mail.

22. US GAO, "West Nile Virus Outbreak," 51.

23. Joyce Wadler, "Passionate Life in a Lab With Dead Animals," *New York Times*, October 1, 1999, 2B.

24. The NVSL did not have the "reagents"—the appropriate antibodies—that would allow it to identify specifically what kind of flavivirus it was observing through the electron microscope. The same was true for the National Wildlife Health Center in Wisconsin, which had, at about the same time, isolated a virus from bird samples sent to it by Ward Stone of the state DEC. See: US GAO, "West Nile Virus Outbreak," 50.

history. Will you look at my virus now?'" This time, her call was returned and, in the course of her conversation with a lab official, McNamara made a new discovery. She had hoped the CDC facility would compare the virus "isolate" taken from the zoo specimen with one taken from a human specimen. It was at this point that she learned that the lab did not in fact have a human virus isolate. This raised a new question in McNamara's mind: "How can you be so positive that people have St. Louis when you haven't isolated it?"

AT THE FORT COLLINS LABORATORY

As with all of the agencies and organizations involved in one way or another with the outbreak in New York, all hell could be said to have broken loose at the Division of Vector-Borne Infectious Diseases in the early weeks of September 1999. Once the lab had tendered its provisional diagnosis of St. Louis encephalitis on September 3, it found itself at the center of a massive screening and testing effort. The city DOH had launched an intensive campaign of active surveillance citywide, calling as many as nine different medical specialists at each of the city's 72 hospitals once a week and, in the process, turning up more than 650 suspected cases of viral encephalitis.[25] These cases, in turn, generated more than 1,000 serum and spinal fluid specimens, prepared by the city DOH lab and shipped off variously to state and CDC labs for testing. All of this severely taxed the limited resources of everyone involved, but in some ways the burden fell most heavily on the Fort Collins facility, as the final arbiter of diagnostic questions. "We were bombarding them with specimens," Marcelle Layton recalls. By her estimate, New York City alone sent between 1,000 and 1,500 samples to Fort Collins for testing at the height of the outbreak.

The diagnostic laboratory at Fort Collins was a small one. At the beginning of the outbreak, according to Duane Gubler, director of the Division of Vector-Borne Infectious Diseases, it had a staff of two to tackle the flood of samples pouring in. Although more staff members were brought in from elsewhere in the organization to help, "it takes a while to get people up to speed," he says. "We don't have the surge capacity that is necessary to deal with something like this on a minute's notice." It was in part for this reason, Gubler maintains, that the lab turned away Tracey McNamara when she asked for help in analyzing her zoo specimens. When she first called on September 9, he points out, "we were all of a sudden up to our ears in [the St. Louis encephalitis] outbreak.... We were just truly overwhelmed. So when her call came in, no question that my staff member was unnecessarily abrupt with her." But his staff's feeling was, he continues, that "these samples are coming in and we are dealing with a human epidemic of St. Louis encephalitis. Birds right now are not our high priority."

---

25. Fine and Layton, "Lessons from the West Nile Viral Encephalitis Outbreak in New York City, 1999," 280. The vast majority of these cases would test negative for encephalitis.

Moreover, Gubler notes, all the evidence to date indicated that the virus that was killing birds could not be the same one that was attacking humans. Members of the flavivirus family—not just St. Louis encephalitis, but other forms, such as Japanese encephalitis and Murray Valley encephalitis—"do not and have not in the past killed birds," he says. While there were reports of bird deaths from another flavivirus—West Nile—those had occurred in Egypt in the 1950s, when caged birds (hooded crows) were experimentally inoculated with the virus. "It just has not been in the nature of the [flavivirus]," Gubler maintains, "to kill [its] host." Accordingly, in Gubler's view, McNamara was following "the correct procedure" when she sent her specimens to a reference lab specializing in veterinary diagnostics; while the NVSL proceeded to test the zoo samples for "avian pathogens," the Fort Collins lab would be moving on a parallel track with the human specimens that were arriving in a steady stream from New York City.

Testing Issues

In the weeks immediately following its testing of the first specimens from Flushing Hospital, the Fort Collins lab faced a dual task: screening the new samples to see if they showed signs of St. Louis encephalitis, and confirming its initial diagnosis of St. Louis encephalitis. Neither would prove easy to do. Arboviral identification, wrote Dr. Charles Calisher, a professor of microbiology at Colorado State University and former head of the Fort Collins diagnostic laboratory, "can be [a tricky] business," particularly because members of a virus family could be extremely difficult to distinguish from one another.[26] Layers of testing were needed to pinpoint the true disease agent.

At Fort Collins, all of the specimens received were put through the ELISA antibody screening test, using the same geographical panel of viruses used on the first specimens. In view of the lab's limited resources, and the small quantities of patient serum or spinal fluid available, this panel, Gubler explains, provided an efficient first look that would "give us the most likely positive results." With hundreds of candidate viruses to choose from, "you have to set priorities," he maintains. "You look at the clinical [presentation], you look at the epi[demiology], and you look at the geographic region. You ask about [patients'] travel history. Where have they been? What could they have been exposed to? And then you select, based on those criteria, what tests—and with what agents—you will do."

But, as Gubler puts it, the ELISA was "a quick and dirty way to screen for large numbers of agents," and it was widely recognized that there was considerable "cross-reactivity" in such a test (i.e., a positive reaction could indicate the presence of a number of closely related flaviviruses in a patient's serum).[27] After the initial screening, Gubler says, the Fort Collins

---

26. ProMED post, September 25, 1999.
27. "Expecting the Unexpected," 9.

lab prepared to follow up with a lengthier, two-pronged analysis of the specimens to confirm its original diagnosis. One prong involved "virus neutralization tests"—the "Cadillac of all [serological] tests," according to Calisher; in this test, Gubler explains, "you actually try to specifically identify the antibody that is circulating in the [patient's] blood," and, by extension, the virus it originally reacted to. The other prong involved virus isolation—considered by many to be the "gold standard" of virus diagnosis[28]—which allowed for a more direct method of identification. Once isolated and put in tissue culture, a virus could be identified by testing it against a battery of known antibodies. But isolating an arbovirus from a human specimen was a notoriously difficult task, particularly in the case of St. Louis encephalitis. In fact, Gubler says, "in all of the history of St. Louis encephalitis in the United States, it has never been isolated from humans." The Fort Collins lab concentrated its efforts, therefore, on a more promising source of virus isolates—mosquitoes from the Queens area. "From our past experience, our best bet was to focus on mosquitoes," says Gubler. Although the lab did dispatch a vertebrate ecologist to New York City on September 11 to collect bird samples, he adds, "we were placing our priority on the mosquito isolates."

While the virus neutralization tests and the mosquito collection/virus isolation process would take the Fort Collins lab a couple of weeks to complete, there was one other, relatively new test that could produce quick results: polymerase chain reaction (PCR). Essentially, this technique enabled scientists to look for evidence of viral ribonucleic acid in specimens and map out the "genetic footprint" of a virus. PCR could, under the right circumstances, yield precise answers to questions of virus identity. "If you know what you're looking for, and you're sure you know what you're looking for," says Calisher, "… then PCR will not only tell you which one it is, but it will tell you how closely related [it is] to [other strains]." The New York State DOH lab had run PCR tests on the first patient samples it received, but it reported negative results for St. Louis encephalitis. When the Fort Collins lab ran its own PCR tests, it got the same negative reaction.[29] This was not, however, seen as a major cause for concern at the Fort Collins lab. "It's not uncommon to not have any positive evidence of virus in the serum or in the cerebrospinal fluid for St. Louis encephalitis," Gubler explains. Consequently, the negative results from PCR tests were "not unexpected" and hence not considered reason to question the initial diagnosis.

Questions

Elsewhere, however, questions about the validity of the St. Louis encephalitis diagnosis were beginning to surface. When, during a September 13 press conference, NYC DOH Commissioner Neal Cohen announced the latest tally of confirmed and suspected cases

---

28. Ibid., 10.
29. Fort Collins used an St. Louis encephalitis–specific "primer" in its PCR tests, which tested only for the presence of that flavivirus.

of St. Louis encephalitis, some observers were surprised to hear that a number of cases had been classified by CDC as "borderline." Commenting in an e-mail posting on ProMedmail—the Web site of the Program for Monitoring Emerging Diseases—Charles Calisher labeled the term "nonsensical," asserting that "[t]here is no such thing as a 'borderline' diagnosis.... [E]ither there is a significant rise or fall in antibody titer [i.e., concentration] or there is not." To Calisher, the use of "borderline" indicated poor communication or poor interpretation of test results, or both. Borderline, he remarks, "is a fine term if you're a psychiatrist"—as Cohen was—"but not a very good term if you're a serologist." The antibody "titer reactions" to St. Louis encephalitis, he argues, "ought to be dynamite," and the fact that they were not in some cases was reason enough, he believed, to prompt a rethinking of the diagnosis.

Meanwhile, questions had arisen as well in the New York State health department lab, which continued to get negative results from PCR tests on patients' spinal fluid specimens. In addition, notes Dale Morse, director of the Office of Science and Public Health at the state agency, the "serologic titers" (i.e., concentrations of antibodies) on "suspect patients were not especially high"—essentially the same "borderline" response that Calisher had questioned. Others, including Marcelle Layton and her colleague at the city DOH, Annie Fine, had also noted the borderline results in patients whose symptoms "were very consistent with the confirmed cases," says Layton. Concerns about the testing results were discussed in the course of conference calls involving city DOH officials, state health officials, and CDC that had been held on a regular basis since the beginning of the outbreak. As Layton recalls those conversations, however, state officials "did not once raise the issue that they doubted the St. Louis encephalitis diagnosis.... The comments were more about the ELISA test's accuracy [than] that it was the wrong virus."

Whatever the state's concerns, the question of the diagnosis was raised at the annual meeting of a working group studying encephalitis cases of unknown etiology[30]—part of a CDC project on unexplained deaths; coincidentally, the session was being held that year in Albany on September 14 and 15, less than two weeks after the announcement of the St. Louis encephalitis outbreak in New York City. The meeting was attended by, among others, officials from CDC in Atlanta, Georgia; representatives from the New York State DOH; and a number of academic researchers, including Dr. Ian Lipkin of the University of California at Irvine, a molecular biologist who had pioneered a PCR method of rapid virus identification. In the course of the meetings, according to Dale Morse, "we held several discussions about the potential cause of the cases and questions over St. Louis encephalitis as the diagnosis." As a result of these conversations, he continues, "specimens were shared with Dr. Lipkin."[31] On September 16, the New York State

---

30. US GAO, "West Nile Virus Outbreak," 50. According to a report in *Scientific American* in April 2000, two-thirds of all encephalitis cases each year are of unknown origin.
31. Layton, who did not attend the meeting, was told by some who did that doubts about the diagnosis were voiced by an academic infectious disease physician "in response to hearing about the negative PCR, and it was he that suggested submitting specimens to [Lipkin's] lab."

health department virology lab packed up samples of human brain tissue—taken from the three Queens patients who had by this point died of encephalitis—and shipped them to Lipkin's Emerging Diseases Laboratory in Irvine for analysis.

The state DOH did not, however, inform its city counterpart of its decision to send brain tissue specimens to Lipkin. Later, the *New York Times* attributed the state's silence to "age-old tensions" between the city and state health agencies,[32] but Marcelle Layton believed that a more innocent explanation could be found. It was a "lab-to-lab" arrangement, she maintains, which grew out of a "side conversation" at the encephalitis meeting. Other key players in the outbreak drama were not told either. Duane Gubler recalls that "we didn't even know that the New York [State] Health Department had shared the human brain tissues with [Lipkin]. They had given him brain tissue that we did not have."[33] Nor, Gubler says, was he apprised of the state's suspicions that the diagnosis of St. Louis encephalitis was problematic. "At the time," he reflects, "I don't know that there was any question that this was not St. Louis. If there was, then no one told us about it."

Reconsideration

Whatever doubts others might have been harboring about the St. Louis encephalitis diagnosis, by Thursday, September 16, the Fort Collins lab began to have its own. That was when it heard from the National Veterinary Services Laboratory that it had successfully isolated a flavivirus from McNamara's zoo specimens and from samples it had received from Ward Stone of the state Department of Environmental Conservation.[34] According to Gubler, the implications of NVSL's discovery were immediately apparent: since it was known that St. Louis encephalitis did not kill its bird hosts, some other flavivirus was apparently at work, and it could be the same one that was attacking humans. Simply put, the diagnosis of St. Louis encephalitis was possibly incorrect. "That's when you start saying," as Gubler puts it, "'Geez, if there's a flavivirus there [in bird specimens], then we need to start looking at other things.'" It was agreed that the NVSL would send its virus isolate to Fort Collins, waiting, at CDC's recommendation, until Monday, September 20, to ship it, in order to avoid having it in transit over the weekend.[35] When the isolate arrived the following day, the lab began analyzing it, this time expanding the panel of flaviviruses it was testing for.

---

32. Jennifer Steinhauer, "Battles Over Turf in Health Arena; Response to a Viral Outbreak Highlights City-State Tensions," *New York Times*, October 16, 1999, 1B.

33. According to Layton, the brain tissue specimens sent to Lipkin contained, by chance, the most viral material of any tissue samples, which as a result may have been easier to test. The brain tissue samples sent to Fort Collins, says Gubler, "were negative" for virus.

34. US GAO, "West Nile Virus Outbreak," 51.

35. Ibid.

By this time, however, others had gotten into the diagnostic act. In California, Ian Lipkin had begun genome-sequence studies on the brain tissue samples sent to him by the New York State DOH. Tracey McNamara, meanwhile, had enlisted the help of yet another organization—the US Army Medical Research Institute of Infectious Diseases (USAMRIID) in Fort Detrick, Maryland. Since learning from the NVSL that it was most likely a flavivirus that was killing birds, she had felt a keener sense of urgency about getting to the bottom of the mystery virus. Flaviviruses were dangerous to work with; only a "handful of laboratories" in the United States, according to McNamara, were equipped to handle them safely. Her Bronx Zoo lab was not one of them, and McNamara was uneasy about exposing herself and her staff to unnecessary risks.

Impatient with what she considered the unresponsiveness of the Fort Collins lab to her concerns and the slow pace of its investigation, McNamara decided to try USAMRIID. "I woke up in the middle of the night," she recalls, "and a little light bulb went off in my head: I'll call Fort Detrick. I'll call the Army." McNamara knew of USAMRIID through her work with the Armed Forces Institute of Pathology. "You can't just send samples to [USAMRIID]," she says, but a colleague from the pathology institute gave her the name and number of a virologist there. On September 21, she called the virologist and asked if USAMRIID would take a look at her specimens. "They were my choice to send something to," she explains, "because they're concerned about all these weird diseases that will kill soldiers in foreign countries, so they have the reagents [i.e., the antibodies to test unusual viruses]." USAMRIID agreed to take a look. "This was not their mission," McNamara points out, "but they got permission from the front office, essentially on a humanitarian basis and because this seemed to be such a unique situation, because the CDC was swamped with human samples, and because we suspected this might be something new."[36]

Zeroing In

By September 21, three different and widely separated facilities were closing in on the true identity of the virus. In Fort Collins, Colorado, scientists prepared to run PCR tests on bird specimens, using broader primers that would detect any flavivirus, not just St. Louis encephalitis, and to rerun the ELISA screening test on some of the human specimens, this time testing for Japanese encephalitis, West Nile, and several other viruses not found in the United States. In Irvine, Lipkin and his staff found evidence of a flavivirus in the brain tissue of the three New Yorkers who had died of encephalitis and began

---

36. At about the same time, on the advice of the medical officer at the Division of Vector-Borne Infectious Diseases, McNamara called the New York State DOH, which agreed to look at the NVSL virus isolates as well, and advised her on safety precautions in working with bird specimens. See: US GAO, "West Nile Virus Outbreak," 51–52.

comparing it with genome sequences of other flaviviruses. In Fort Detrick, Maryland, USAMRIID researchers began testing McNamara's bird samples and, by September 22, had ruled out alphavirus-related diseases.

From there, events moved very fast. On Thursday, September 23, the Fort Collins lab identified a "West Nile-like virus" in the isolate it had received from the NVSL. Also on the 23rd, USAMRIID came up with a preliminary identification of a flavivirus in the bird samples; according to McNamara's account, lab officials told her that it was "only weakly reactive" to the St. Louis encephalitis virus. The following day, after retesting showed high reactivity with West Nile virus, the Fort Collins lab began PCR testing for West Nile on human samples. That same day, the 24th, the New York State DOH got word from Lipkin that his analysis indicated that the virus in his specimens was not St. Louis encephalitis but was either the Kunjin virus (of Australian origin) or its almost identical flavivirus relative, West Nile.[37]

BACK IN NEW YORK CITY

Meanwhile, the NYC DOH had been largely in the dark about developments at the laboratory level. The possibility of a link between bird and human deaths had been raised early, during the first press conference on the outbreak back on September 3. "People in the community immediately connected [the two]," Marcelle Layton recalls, adding wryly that "in medicine you always hear, 'Listen to the patient.'" City health officials did check with CDC about a possible link on September 10 and were informed that the outbreaks were probably unrelated. Preoccupied with the task of sorting out hundreds of possible cases of St. Louis encephalitis and processing more than 1,000 specimens, the severely overtaxed city DOH let the matter drop.

It was not until September 22 that Layton by chance stumbled on an important fact about the bird die-off. She woke up that day to a news story on National Public Radio: scientists had determined that a virus isolated from a dead crow and from mosquitoes in Connecticut appeared to be identical. While the key point of the report was the potential link between the killer of birds and humans, for Layton it carried another revelation. "It was," she says, "the first that I heard that birds were dying of encephalitis." At that point, she adds, she knew nothing of Tracey McNamara and her pursuit of a possible connection between the human and animal encephalitis outbreaks. The city DOH was aware that dead birds from the Queens area were being sent to Ward Stone at the state DEC, but not of the magnitude of the die-off or of suspicions as to its cause. "We could have more actively called to find out," Layton acknowledges, "but they weren't calling us either."

---

37. US GAO, "West Nile Virus Outbreak," 52–54.

Breaking the News

On Friday, September 24, 1999, three weeks to the day after the Fort Collins lab had phoned in its provisional diagnosis of St. Louis encephalitis, the lab called to announce even more dramatic news. In a conference call that included city and state health department officials, Connecticut health officials, officials from CDC in Atlanta, and, at the invitation of CDC, Tracey McNamara of the Bronx Zoo, lab officials declared that the virus was not St. Louis encephalitis but West Nile. At that point, the lab was able to confirm the presence of West Nile virus in birds but wanted to postpone any public statement on the virus in humans until it had completed genome sequencing.[38] By this time, Layton and others in the city DOH had gotten word from the Fort Collins lab that a change in diagnosis might be forthcoming, but the news was stunning nonetheless. West Nile virus, which was indigenous to Africa and parts of Asia—it was first discovered in Uganda in 1937—and had surfaced periodically in Europe, had never been found before in the western hemisphere in either birds or people.[39] Its sudden appearance—from what source no one knew—was, Gubler would later tell the press, "a total surprise to us. There was no reason to suspect we'd find West Nile here."[40]

More surprises were in store for some. On the evening of the 24th, as Layton was working with colleagues on a press release announcing the discovery of West Nile in birds, she learned from an epidemiologist at the state health department about "this guy in California [who had] isolated West Nile from the human brain tissue. That was the first I heard of [Lipkin's work]." Duane Gubler was told of Lipkin's research the next day, Saturday, September 25, by the New York State DOH, and called Lipkin to discuss his results and those of the Fort Collins lab. As he recalls, Gubler "felt it was better to wait [to publish news of West Nile in humans] and make sure of our identification." That night, however, Gubler was awakened by a call from the *New York Times* inquiring about Lipkin's findings. The next day, the paper printed a story pinning the three deaths from encephalitis on the West Nile or the Kunjin virus.[41]

The arrival of an exotic new virus on American shores rang alarm bells throughout the city. "The press went nuts," McNamara later remembered. "They had a field day. We had helicopters circling the zoo. Unless you lived through this, you can't really capture the feeling of hysteria that went along with this."[42] the *New York Times* painted a similar picture. "In recent weeks," the paper wrote, "the region seemed close to hysteria over the virus: Phones lit up in record numbers at the health department, parents in

---

38. Ibid., 55.
39. Jennifer Steinhauer, "African Virus May Be Culprit in Mosquito-Borne Illness," *New York Times*, September 25, 1999, 1A. The worst modern outbreak of West Nile, the *Times* reported, occurred in Romania in 1996, when 90,000 cases, including 17 deaths, were confirmed.
40. Andrew Jacobs, "Exotic Virus Is Identified in 3 Deaths," *New York Times*, September 26, 1999, 43.
41. Later, in a September 30 press release, CDC clarified that a "West Nile-like virus" had been identified through "genomic analysis."
42. USDA presentation, September 13, 2000.

areas where there was not a single case kept their children indoors, TV reporters talked in stern tones about the plague among us."[43] Health officials hastened to reassure the public. There was no cause, Neal Cohen asserted, to fear that a virulent pathogen had been let loose in the city. "If anything," he told reporters, "the disease we are dealing with now is somewhat less severe than the one we were dealing with before."[44] More important, the change in diagnosis, both city hall and the NYC DOH stressed, would have no impact on the city's response. The discovery of the true identity of the virus was more a matter of scientific than public health "import," Layton points out. "If we had known about West Nile initially," she notes, "it would not have changed our response at all. We would have implemented the same active surveillance efforts, public education outreach, and most importantly the control measures of adulticiding [and] larviciding."

At the same time, however, officials acknowledged that there was some reassessment to do on the extent of the epidemic. On September 26, Cohen announced that blood and spinal fluid specimens from 77 patients who had tested negative for St. Louis encephalitis would be retested for West Nile. As expected, the new tests indicated higher numbers of cases connected with the outbreak than previously thought. In New York City, the number of confirmed cases rose from 18 to 25, and in adjacent Nassau County, from zero to four. By the time the first frost of autumn brought an end to any remaining adult *Culex pipiens*—and, with it, any further threat of infection—the final tally for New York City and its neighboring counties, Westchester and Nassau, stood at 62 confirmed cases, 7 of whom died.[45]

Postmortems

Even as the outbreak of West Nile encephalitis subsided, a flurry of concern over how the virus got to the United States arose in the press. Speculation had focused largely on an inadvertent importation: West Nile virus could have arrived, for example, in an infected bird brought, legally or not, from another country, or in an infected mosquito that made its way to the United States on a cargo ship or airplane. But in a *New Yorker* article published in mid-October 1999, author Richard Preston raised the chilling specter of a deliberate act of bioterrorism. "The mystery" of how the virus got to New York

---

43. Jennifer Steinhauer, "It's Infectious Fear That's Out of Proportion," *New York Times*, sec. 4, October 10, 1999, 16.
44. Jennifer Steinhauer, "Outbreak of Virus in New York Much Broader Than Expected," *New York Times*, September 28, 1999, 1A.
45. Fine and Layton, "Lessons from the West Nile Viral Encephalitis Outbreak in New York City, 1999," 277–278. All those who died were 65 or older. Later, after the city conducted a "serosurvey" of northern Queens residents, it was estimated that roughly 2.6% of the surveyed area population of about 46,000 had been infected by West Nile.

City, he wrote, "has been troubling the Central Intelligence Agency [CIA]." What troubled CIA analysts was an account by a defector from Iraq, published in a British tabloid newspaper the previous spring, which alleged that Iraqi leader Saddam Hussein was "developing a strain of the West Nile virus as a biological weapon and was preparing to release it."

Almost immediately, the CIA moved to squelch the story. "We have looked into that, and there's nothing that we've found that would support the notion [of a bioterrorist act]," one official told reporters. The agency had not done a formal investigation, he added, because that would lend the allegation "more credibility than it deserves."[46] Nonetheless, there was widespread agreement that the West Nile virus outbreak illustrated what terrorism expert Jessica Stern called "one of the most troubling aspects of biological warfare: it can be extremely difficult to distinguish germ warfare from a natural outbreak of disease."[47] As such, the West Nile epidemic was regarded by some as a "dress rehearsal" for a bioterrorist attack. Seen in that light, the response to the outbreak provided, in the words of one observer, "a sobering, not so reassuring, demonstration of the inadequacies of the US detection network for emerging diseases."[48]

The sharpest criticism fell on CDC for getting the diagnosis wrong. While some faulted the Fort Collins lab for initially testing the Flushing Hospital samples against a limited geographical panel of viral agents, others believed that was a reasonable first step in viral analysis. "You can't test against everything," notes Charles Calisher. It was subsequent lapses, in Calisher's view, that led to the lab's error. CDC, he maintains, had "blinders on" and failed to pay attention to other factors that did not necessarily fit the St. Louis encephalitis scenario: the huge numbers of dead birds being reported; the fact that there were no cases of St. Louis encephalitis anywhere else in the country; the presence of profound muscle weakness, which had never been seen in cases of St. Louis encephalitis; and, perhaps most important, the "squishy serologic results"—that is, the "borderline" reaction on some of the screening tests.

Calisher believed the misidentification was potentially a costly one for public health. "If somebody would have sat down and thought about all of this," he argues, "they'd have gotten to this point probably 10 days before [the correct diagnosis was made]. They might have lost the opportunity at that point of eradicating this virus rather than simply controlling the mosquitoes that carry it. Now we're going to have it forever." Gubler, however, strongly disputed this assertion. The delay in coming up with the right diagnosis, he maintains, did not compromise the response. The same mosquito transmitted both the St. Louis encephalitis and the West Nile virus, he notes, and, in either case, the method of attack would have been identical: vector control. "Clinical management of the two

---

46. Vernon Loeb, "CIA Finds No Sign Virus Was an Attack," *Washington Post*, October 12, 1999, A2.
47. Jessica Stern, "Is That an Epidemic—or a Terrorist Attack?" *New York Times*, October 16, 1999, 19.
48. Jennifer Steinhauer and Judith Miller, "In New York Outbreak, Glimpse of Gaps in Biological Defenses," *New York Times*, October 11, 1999, 1A.

viruses," he adds, "is also the same." Moreover, Layton argues, a diagnosis made just a couple of weeks earlier would "not have provided an opportunity" to eliminate the virus, because an epidemic curve graph later revealed that most humans had already been infected by mid- to late August—just as the first cases began surfacing in Flushing Hospital. "So by mid-September," she says, "the virus was well established."

Publicly, Gubler acknowledged the justice of some of the criticism leveled at his lab, in particular for the limited panel of viruses it used to screen samples. "We had tunnel vision on St. Louis virus," he remarked, "because all the clinical, epidemiological, laboratory, and geographic features pointed to St. Louis. We've learned a lesson here. We've got to be more open-minded."[49] Privately, however, he notes that open-mindedness, in the sense of greater inclusiveness in testing, "puts us in a real difficult spot, because we don't have the resources to do that." Along with highlighting the need to expand testing in an age of global trade and travel, Gubler says, the West Nile outbreak reinforced an old lesson about caution in diagnosis. "When you're working with flaviviruses," he says, "you better have a virus [isolate] in hand or neutralization test results in hand before you say anything definitive." Still, in Gubler's view, many of the lab's critics spoke from the vantage point of hindsight. At the time that "all of this was unfolding," he says, questions and doubts were not forcefully raised about CDC's handling of the virus testing.

Gubler did, however, recognize the key role played by animal health specialists in solving the mystery of the encephalitis outbreak in New York City. "CDC," he told the *New York Times* in late September, "would not have made the diagnosis of West Nile virus as quickly without Dr. McNamara's persistent sleuthing." Perhaps, he reflects, "the most important [lesson]" of the outbreak was the need for public health officials "to develop much closer working relationships and communications with non-traditional partners" in the animal health community.

While recognition of her role may have been welcome to McNamara, the frustration she experienced in the course of her sleuthing lingered on. The federal government spent "millions of dollars on bio-preparedness," she argues, but had little to show for it in the West Nile outbreak. "The people that cracked this diagnosis," she maintains—Lipkin, USAMRIID researchers, and herself, among others—"were not the people that are paid to do this work. They were people entirely outside of the public health community."[50]

---

49. Lawrence Altman, "Encephalitis Outbreak Teaches an Old Lesson," *New York Times*, September 28, 1999, 8F.

50. McNamara also noted that CDC's press release announcing West Nile virus in birds made no mention of NVSL, USAMRIID, Lipkin, or herself. The press release stated that "CDC, in collaboration with the New York City and New York State departments of health, has isolated and identified a West Nile-like virus from birds that died in New York City and were submitted for testing by the Bronx Zoo." Gubler explains that the original press release did include an acknowledgment of NVSL, but it was removed when "we could not get USDA clearance immediately, and it was important to get the story out." USAMRIID was not mentioned, Gubler adds, "because we didn't know of their involvement at that time." Later, in a ProMedmail posting, the NVSL "clarified" that it was the first to isolate the virus.

Gubler disagreed. The Fort Collins lab, he says, was also on the trail of the true identity of the virus. Using mosquito samples collected in New York City by CDC entomologists on September 12, the lab succeeded in isolating the West Nile virus on September 30, according to Gubler. "So," he concludes, "this case would have been cracked a week later if nothing else had happened."

Most frustrating to McNamara was what she viewed as the chronic indifference to wildlife in both the public health and the veterinary communities. "Four hundred crows [reported dead] in August," she points out. "It shouldn't have taken that long [to garner attention].… [But] until you have a significant death count in humans, it doesn't matter how many barrels of dead birds there are." Wildlife, McNamara maintains, fell between the cracks of the US public health system and a veterinary system interested either in "food animals" or domestic pets. "There is no funding for wildlife to speak of," she says—a state of affairs that the nation allowed to continue at its own peril. The lack of sophisticated "laboratory capabilities" to survey and diagnose wildlife diseases constituted a "big gap in the [US] biological defense system," she continues, and as long as it existed, "people will be the sentinels" for disease outbreaks.

Back at the city DOH, where the outbreak drama began, there was soul-searching as well. Despite weeks of regular, lengthy conference calls among city, state, and federal officials, significant gaps in communication—about bird deaths, about diagnostic question marks, about testing decisions—had opened up along the way. Layton expressed regret that neither the state DEC nor McNamara had informed the city DOH of the cause of mortality among crows, but she faulted the NYC DOH as well for failing to push the issue. In retrospect, Layton believed that the "true missed opportunity" in the West Nile virus saga was "the delay in diagnosing the avian deaths." Had the cause of the crow die-off been pursued "more aggressively," particularly within the veterinary community, she contends, the presence of West Nile virus might have been discovered as early as July, triggering control measures that could have prevented human cases and, conceivably, "the establishment of West Nile in the US."

At the same time, however, while acknowledging missed opportunities and communications gaps, Layton took issue with assertions that the handling of the West Nile virus outbreak revealed the sorry state of preparedness for bioterrorist attacks in the United States. Such critiques ignored the response of the city's public health system, which, she points out, acted rapidly and effectively along a number of fronts—sending out frequent alerts to the medical community, setting up a provider hotline to report suspected cases, managing the transport of clinical specimens to labs, and establishing a database for tracking the outbreak, among other things. "All of those steps," Layton says, "are key to outbreak detection and response, and worked well with West Nile due to the efforts of hundreds of [city] DOH staff who worked seven days a week and many 16-hour days." In doing this, she observes, the department had benefited from its participation in bioterrorism preparedness efforts. "Our ability to respond as quickly as we did—implementing active surveillance, rapid communication with the medical community and general public," Layton says, was enhanced by the bioterrorism training the department had done in recent years. "[I'm] not sure," Layton notes, "the [city] DOH could have mobilized overnight as we did if this had happened four or five years [earlier]."

Looking back, Neal Cohen, too, saw much to applaud in the story of the West Nile outbreak. He could point with "pride," he says, to his agency's handling of the early stages of the outbreak, "first in recognizing the significance of the call [from Deborah Asnis] and in Dr. Layton and Dr. Fine seeing the importance of going out into the field and doing the investigation almost immediately, taking their weekend to do that...." But, as she reflected on events, Layton believed the discovery of the outbreak had perhaps hung by the slenderest of threads. In a September 2000 account, written with Annie Fine, she noted that at the time they launched their active investigation, on August 28, there were already 19 patients hospitalized with what turned out to be West Nile encephalitis. Of these, 15—79% of the total—had not been reported to the health department. "Had the single infectious disease physician [Asnis] not reported the unusual cluster of neurological disease at her hospital," Layton and Fine wrote, "... it is not known when or if this outbreak would have been detected."

The West Nile Virus Outbreak in New York City: The City Responds

Esther Scott

O n a Thursday evening in early September 1999, just before the start of the Labor Day weekend, Jerry Hauer, director of the Mayor's Office of Emergency Management (OEM) in New York City, received a phone call from Neal Cohen, NYC Department of Health (NYC DOH) commissioner. "It was 6:30," Hauer recalls. "I was just getting ready to leave the office; I was literally walking out the door. The phone rang, and it was Neal. He said, 'We've got a problem, and we need your help.'"

The problem was a possible outbreak of an unusual form of encephalitis in northern Queens. Roughly eight people, most of them elderly, all of them from the same area of Queens, had been taken seriously ill over the past two weeks; two had died, and several others were on ventilators. After testing blood and spinal fluid samples taken from the Queens patients, the New York State DOH laboratory had come up with a tentative diagnosis of St. Louis encephalitis, a mosquito-borne viral disease never before seen in New York City. The city DOH was awaiting final word—due the next day—from the Centers for Disease Control and Prevention (CDC), but Cohen was calling for assistance in formulating a response in the event that the diagnosis of St. Louis encephalitis was confirmed. In essence, this would mean putting together, in very short order, two major initiatives: one to contain the outbreak, and the other to alert the public.

As director of the office responsible for emergency planning and response in the city, Hauer had handled numerous kinds of crises—snowstorms, building collapses, plane

This case was written by Esther Scott for Dr. Arnold M. Howitt, Executive Director, Taubman Center for State and Local Government, for use at the Executive Session on Domestic Preparedness, John F. Kennedy School of Government, Harvard University. Funding for the case was provided by the Robert Wood Johnson Foundation and the Office of Justice Programs, US Department of Justice. (0102)

crashes—and prepared contingency plans for many more, but nothing quite like this had ever confronted him or his staff. The city seemed ill-prepared to mount a rapid response to this rare event. New York City had not been visited by a mosquito-borne viral outbreak since the yellow fever epidemics of the 19th century; over the years, its mosquito control programs had steadily dwindled and, by the mid-1990s, largely disappeared. As a result, the city had neither the equipment nor the expertise on hand to track and destroy mosquito populations. Moreover, in the densely populated, polyglot neighborhoods of Queens, getting the word out quickly and clearly about St. Louis encephalitis would test OEM's skills at least as much in communications as in logistics. Hauer and his staff would be tackling these formidable challenges against a backdrop of deep uncertainty about what the city was up against. If, as expected, CDC confirmed the diagnosis, it would not be clear whether the outbreak would remain confined, as it currently appeared to be, to a 16-square-mile area of Queens, or whether it would spread out to engulf one of the most populous cities in the world. "The bottom line," says one OEM official, "is that the City of New York was dealing with a public health emergency the likes of which was unknown. We had no idea of what we were dealing with."

BACKGROUND: THE OFFICE OF EMERGENCY MANAGEMENT

OEM was a relatively recent addition to New York City government. It was the creation of Mayor Rudolph Giuliani, who was reportedly unhappy with the turf rivalries and lack of coordination that had plagued the city's handling of major emergencies and disasters in the past. Previously, responsibility for emergencies had been lodged in the police department, but, according to Hauer, "not much in the way of proactive emergency management" got done. "They did very little," he says. "[They] rarely coordinated, and had very little authority to do anything." Interagency squabbles over who was in command in emergency situations were not uncommon. "There have been well-documented incidents," says Deputy Mayor Joseph Lhota, "where [the police and fire departments] would literally argue with each other at the scene of something [over] who's in charge, and what happens."

In early 1996, Giuliani removed emergency management from the police department and established OEM in the mayor's office, with Jerry Hauer as its first head. By 1999, OEM had a staff of 65—a mix of civilians and uniformed services, detailed from other city agencies—and a large suite of offices at 7 World Trade Center in lower Manhattan. From the start, it was clear that the new agency bore the mayor's imprimatur. "We were in the mayor's office, and we had the power of the mayor," says Hauer. Other city agencies "knew I was very close to the mayor. I was one of the people that was on the phone with him eight times a day, and in his office all day long, so I got the cooperation I needed" from them. "Everybody knows OEM speaks for Rudy Giuliani," Lhota observes. "They are empowered."

The new agency was set up essentially to act as a coordinating body that would work with other city agencies in planning for and responding to emergencies of all types. It was given, according to OEM Deputy Director Calvin Drayton, a three-part mission: to prepare plans "to deal with emergencies" in New York City; to "make sure that once the plans were developed, that drills and exercises were done … to ensure that we were prepared"; and to act as the "on-scene coordinator" for emergencies that required a response across multiple city agencies. This latter duty included designating the incident commander, and providing the lead agency with the resources and personnel to manage the crisis.[1] Overall, says Lhota, OEM was "an oversight agency in a lot of ways. [It acted as] the catalyst for moving the ball forward [in emergency situations], making sure the whole thing is coordinated."

Over time, OEM officials had drawn up plans, in Hauer's words, for "pretty much all major types of incidents—hurricanes, heat waves, snowstorms, air crashes, civil unrest, power outages—you name it, we were working on or had plans for them." But, perhaps not surprisingly in view of its extreme rarity, there was no plan on paper for handling a mosquito-borne disease outbreak in New York City. Still, Hauer points out, OEM had been working for years on "bioterrorism" planning—that is, on preparing a response to a disease deliberately unleashed on the city by terrorists—and "whether it's [an] intentional or accidental [outbreak], the implications for the city can be very much the same." Perhaps more valuable than laying out any specific course of action, the bioterrorism preparedness effort had brought OEM into close contact with the city's DOH, which, at Hauer's urging, had been participating in planning and training exercises since 1996. "I do credit Jerry with involving public health a lot earlier than most other jurisdictions have," says Dr. Marcelle Layton, head of the NYC DOH's Communicable Disease Program and the department's chief liaison with OEM for bioterrorism planning. "I think public health has often been away from the table." The "biggest [advantage]," she continues, "is that we had a very collaborative and familiar relationship with [OEM] that we wouldn't have had without bioterrorism having brought us together.… I knew Jerry very well; he knew how to reach me 24 hours a day, and vice versa." It was a familiarity that would intensify as the NYC DOH and OEM joined forces to respond to the sudden appearance of a mysterious new disease in New York City.

An Outbreak in Queens

The outbreak first surfaced at Flushing Hospital, a small community facility in northern Queens, where a handful of elderly patients had been admitted with what appeared to be viral encephalitis. Along with the classic manifestations of the disease, however, was an unusual symptom shared by almost all of the patients: profound muscle weakness.

---

1. OEM constructed a matrix—called the "direction and control of incidents"—which identified the incident commander for an array of emergencies and disasters.

Since the first cases were reported on August 23, Layton and her staff at the NYC DOH had been working, with the assistance of the New York State DOH lab, to puzzle out the identity of the virus that was causing this atypical form of encephalitis.

By September 2, two patients had died and the number of cases of encephalitis in Queens had risen from four to eight. Meanwhile, the field of viruses had been narrowed to one likely candidate: St. Louis encephalitis, a virus typically found in other parts of the United States but never before in New York City.[2] Patient samples had been sent for further testing to CDC's Division of Vector-Borne Infectious Diseases in Fort Collins, Colorado, but it seemed probable that the city was facing an outbreak of a disease carried by mosquitoes—one that produced mild symptoms in most but could be deadly for young children and the elderly. Already, says NYC DOH Commissioner Neal Cohen, CDC officials were advising the NYC DOH that, in the event of positive results for St. Louis encephalitis, "we were likely going to need to spray with pesticides to contain the outbreak." It was the need to plan for this contingency that prompted Cohen to make two phone calls: one to Deputy Mayor Joseph Lhota and one to OEM Director Jerry Hauer.[3]

Cohen's call to OEM came on Thursday, September 2, normally a sleepy time of year in New York City, with much of the city—including many in city government—preparing to take off for the Labor Day weekend. Like others in OEM, "I was trying to get out of the office on that Thursday," Calvin Drayton remembers, "… when the call [from Cohen] came in. The next thing I know, we were pulling medical dictionaries off the bookshelf, trying to figure out what the hell is St. Louis encephalitis."

GEARING UP BIG-TIME

First Steps

After Cohen's call, Hauer pulled together a group of OEM deputy directors and staff members to consider what action to take while waiting for word from CDC, which, Cohen had told him, was expected the following day. "We started putting our [heads] together," recalls Edward Gabriel, OEM deputy director for health issues, "trying to figure out, first of all, very immediate goals. What do we do right now? And what do we do for the next 6 or 12 or 24 hours?"

For starters, it was agreed that, as Gabriel puts it, "we had to get out there [to the part of Queens where the cases had occurred] and have a look at it." Cohen had told Hauer

---

2. For an in-depth account of the discovery of the outbreak and its cause, see Case 4A.

3. According to Dr. Marcelle Layton, Hauer first learned of a potential outbreak on Tuesday, August 31, at a meeting to discuss a planned bioterrorism field exercise. Dr. Annie Fine of NYC DOH told him that public health officials were investigating an unusual cluster of encephalitis cases, possibly mosquito-borne. The September 9 field exercise was later cancelled when it became clear the city had a possible epidemic on its hands.

that the city DOH staff had spotted possible mosquito-breeding sites—piles of tires and rubbish in a park in Queens—which they thought would need to be removed. That night, after conferring with both Lhota and Giuliani, Hauer "sent some staff out" to inspect those sites and generally reconnoiter the area. They brought with them the OEM "command bus"—which Lhota describes as a "huge van" equipped with phones, computers, and a conference room—and stationed it in Powell's Cove, in the "hot zone" of the outbreak. Hauer also called several city departments—sanitation, parks, and environmental protection—and arranged for representatives of each to meet at the park in the morning to "evaluate the situation."

The next morning, Friday, September 3, after inspecting the sites himself, Hauer began "pulling more agencies in," he says, this time from the state and neighboring counties, to discuss the looming public health crisis and get their advice on how to respond to it.[4] In a nod to his bioterrorism training, Hauer also called the Federal Bureau of Investigation (FBI), which sent a representative from its joint terrorism task force to sit in on the early briefings on the outbreak. "I really wasn't [thinking this was bioterrorism]," he explains, "but I couldn't rule it out, so I felt it was important for him to be there and understand what was going on…." Officials from city, state, and county agencies, CDC, the FBI, plus Deputy Mayor Joe Lhota, hastily gathered in the OEM command bus to mull over the city's options and map out its first moves. Hauer was eager to get some response in place in advance of the call from CDC. "I just felt," he recalls, "that if this thing were going to be positive, we needed to react very quickly." CDC would not be in touch until sometime that afternoon, the start of a holiday weekend, Hauer notes, "and you don't want to be waiting [till] 5:00 to try and find people, because [by then], everyone's gone." It would be easier to dismantle the components of a response in leisure than to assemble them belatedly in haste. "If it came back negative," he points out, "you could always call things off." Accordingly, while city leaders waited nervously for CDC's call, "we were gearing up big-time."

Deciding to Spray

Essentially, the question before the group assembled in the command bus was what to do about the mosquitoes. The "vector" of St. Louis encephalitis—the *Culex pipiens*, an urban mosquito that breeds in stagnant pools of water—could be attacked in two ways: through "larviciding," which destroyed mosquitoes in their larval stage by eliminating their breeding sites where possible or by treating them with pesticides (in pellet, liquid, granular, or other forms); and through "adulticiding," which killed adult mosquitoes by spraying

---

4. These included representatives of the state health and environmental conservation departments, as well as officials from Suffolk and Nassau Counties, which had considerable experience in mosquito control.

pesticides in areas where, and when, they were flying. Larviciding was in a sense a more focused approach, aimed at eliminating specific larval habitats, but it required taking a fine-tooth comb to neighborhoods that might be harboring mosquito breeding sites. It meant, says Roger Nasci, a research entomologist with CDC's Division of Vector-Borne Infectious Diseases, "a yard-to-yard search," looking for the myriad havens that backyards afforded mosquito larvae—above-ground swimming pools, birdbaths, barrels, old tires. Adulticiding, by contrast, took a broader approach to mosquito control, but it required expensive machinery—specially equipped helicopters or planes for aerial spraying, and trucks for ground spraying—and trained personnel to operate it. In addition, pesticide sprays reached into human as well as mosquito habitats, leaving behind a whiff of chemicals and a host of anxieties as to their toxic potential.

There was one other, more defensive approach to dealing with mosquitoes: insect repellent. This had the virtue of confining the application of chemicals to individuals instead of covering huge swaths of the city indiscriminately with pesticides, but it also had its limitations. For one thing, residents could not be relied on to use it consistently. "There's times when it's going to wear off," says Jerry McCarty, a former deputy director of OEM. "There's times [people] forget; there's times somebody comes into the city who's not wearing repellent. And there's people who can't [use] repellent." For another, it would not get to the root cause of the outbreak. "Repellent provides the individual with protection," McCarty notes, "but that doesn't kill the insect."

In choosing a course of action, the city and its advisors were hampered in the early stages of the outbreak by an almost complete lack of information on the mosquitoes' whereabouts. The city had no mosquito surveillance program in place and, as a result, no way to know where the infected mosquito populations were to be found or what their rates of infection were (which would help determine the risk to humans). The CDC's Roger Nasci, who was based in Fort Collins, had begun packing up traps and other collecting equipment to send to New York City and was himself preparing to head for the city to help out with mosquito trapping; but in the meantime, a decision would have to be made for the short term without benefit of hard data.

Nonetheless, there was at least anecdotal evidence that the adult *Culex pipiens* population was booming in the city that summer. "We were looking at high urban *Culex* population densities late in the year," Roger Nasci says, "with a prospect of a rather prolonged late summer, early fall"—weather conditions, which favored an extended season for mosquitoes. Moreover, according to guidelines published by CDC, the disease cluster in Queens had reached the stage where more aggressive action than larviciding was warranted. Under these guidelines, New York City was experiencing at least a Category 3 outbreak ("probable") and appeared likely to reach the Category 4 stage: "outbreak in progress" (Exhibit 4B-1). "When you have infected adult mosquitoes flying around in an area, coupled with human cases," Nasci explains, "which verifies that you have levels of transmission activity that pose human risk, the appropriate action is to reduce mosquito density." All this seemed to point to one conclusion: while the city should work to eliminate larval habitats and encourage use of insect repellent, it should make its chief priority the control of adult mosquitoes. Joe Lhota recalls the strong consensus that emerged from the talks in the command bus. "I remember sitting around the table," he says, "and it became pretty obvious. Everyone agreed. Federal, state, and local officials involved said, 'We have to spray. We have to spray.'"

This was the recommendation that was brought to Mayor Giuliani. "He basically listened to CDC and the state," Hauer recalls, "... and he supported it, recognizing that ... we didn't know whether we were dealing with the tip of the iceberg or whether we were seeing the whole iceberg." If, Hauer adds, "we were in fact seeing the tip of the iceberg, we didn't want to have to look back and say, why didn't we get more aggressive in trying to deal with this?"

Preparing to Spray

Having made the decision to spray, New York City next faced the formidable task of figuring out how to go about doing it. There was virtually no internal capacity to build on. The city, according to the *New York Times*, had "one of the least aggressive mosquito control programs in the region." This in part reflected the fact that the city had largely been spared outbreaks of mosquito-borne diseases for more than a century, which made mosquitoes "more of a nuisance [than] a public health issue," in the words of one observer.[5] Some limited larviciding was done at wastewater treatment centers and in the Rockaway section of Queens; if the city sprayed with pesticides at all, it did so on a highly localized, "complaint-driven" basis. New York City "had not been spraying since about 1975 on a citywide basis," says Jerry McCarty. "So the institutional memory was not there." Neither was the equipment nor the personnel. As a result of belt-tightening measures in the early 1990s, the city's mosquito control program had a budget of $120,000 and a staff of two—meager by comparison to, for example, neighboring Suffolk County, which had a population one-fifth that of New York City's but a budget of $2 million and a staff of 33 devoted to mosquito control.[6]

Officially, pest control—mosquito and otherwise—was the responsibility of the city's DOH, but by 1999 its ability to mount a concerted attack on mosquitoes had all but atrophied. Aside from some backpack sprayers, says Hauer, "they had very limited resources to do any kind of spraying. I had to basically take over [the spraying]. The department of health did not have the money, the resources, the people.... And they also didn't have the

---

5. Jodi Wilgoren, "New York Mosquito Control Is Weak and Late, Experts Say," *New York Times*, September 8, 1999, 1B.

6. Ibid. In general, Marcelle Layton says, local governments were more likely to pay for mosquito control programs for "nuisance mosquitoes than disease—especially in tourist areas such as eastern Long Island."

coordination capability that my office did. They were not used to doing these kinds of projects." For its part, the city DOH welcomed what Neal Cohen calls Hauer's "take charge" style. Particularly in view of the "collegial relationship" the two agencies had developed in the course of their collaboration in bioterrorism planning, the city DOH was "comfortable," Cohen says, "with OEM's role in responding to a health emergency."

In this virtually unprecedented health emergency, there was no preordained incident commander. But, one OEM official reflects, "I think this is one of those situations where the mayor was in charge.... I think that because of our close working relationship with [Giuliani], he knew minute by minute what was going on, and he was able to guide our office as to how to guide the rest of the city." Generally, as the crisis played out, city hall took on the political side of the task—keeping the public and local politicians up to date on developments—while OEM, and particularly its director, shouldered responsibility for the operational side.[7] "Jerry," says Lhota, "took over."

Logistics

With the NYC DOH's sanction, Hauer and his staff set about readying the city's response in the event CDC confirmed the diagnosis of St. Louis encephalitis. To do so, they had to work on two tracks simultaneously: assembling the necessary equipment and personnel for aerial and ground spraying of selected Queens neighborhoods while assembling information on St. Louis encephalitis and the spraying schedule and devising a way to distribute it efficiently to area residents. In some regards, the spraying operation was easier to organize. For the aerial spraying, Hauer leased a helicopter from a private firm that specialized in such work. For the initial ground spraying, he started by borrowing a few trucks and their crews from Suffolk County. New York City and its neighboring counties had an informal mutual aid arrangement for providing assistance in emergency situations; normally, Hauer says, the aid was provided free of charge, but in this case, because county crews would be working overtime to help with the spraying in Queens, the city agreed to pick up the tab. OEM itself did not have budgetary funds to cover these and other costs it would incur in the pesticide spraying. The task of paying the bills, contracting for helicopter and, later, truck spraying services, and purchasing pesticides and insect repellent generally fell to the city's Department of Citywide Administrative Services. But when purchases had to be made on the spot, OEM's staff members put them on their own credit cards—the agency did not issue departmental ones—and were later reimbursed by the city.

Alerting residents to the outbreak and its consequences was a more complex affair. The focus of the spraying would be on three neighborhoods in the hot zone—where all

---

7. Lhota, for example, notified Queens Borough President Claire Shulman of the outbreak on the Friday of Labor Day weekend; he also spoke with key members of the New York City Council and state and federal legislators.

the known cases of St. Louis encephalitis had thus far originated—and then on immediately surrounding areas in northern Queens and in neighboring South Bronx. The total area earmarked for spraying included a sizable number of households that did not speak English. Hauer planned a leafletting campaign in which city workers would go door to door handing out information on St. Louis encephalitis and warning residents to stay indoors during the spraying. The leaflets themselves were composed by the city's DOH, which, according to NYC DOH Deputy Commissioner Benjamin Mojica, used census data to "help us in plotting out what the dominant languages were in those communities." Altogether, the leaflets would be published in eight languages (plus English)—including, among others, Korean, Russian, Hindi, and Urdu—but, Mojica says, this did not pose a severe challenge to the city DOH, which "purchases translation services routinely" to meet the needs of NYC residents who spoke, according to Lhota, "something like 180 different languages and dialects."

To distribute the leaflets, OEM initially rounded up a force of roughly 500 to 600 city workers, including police officers, to knock on residents' doors. Leaflets and cans of insect repellent, which residents were urged to use, would also be made available at neighborhood police and fire stations. Finally, in collaboration with the NYC DOH, a 24-hour emergency hotline, staffed by health department workers, was set up to answer questions about St. Louis encephalitis and the spraying, and to take residents' reports of possible mosquito breeding sites. "All this," says Hauer of the preparations, "had to happen, literally, in five or six hours," while the city waited for word from CDC.

When word finally came, it was almost 3 o'clock in the afternoon of Friday, September 3. Tests done in CDC's lab in Fort Collins, the city learned, had yielded results "most consistent" with a diagnosis of St. Louis encephalitis. A short time later, in "a hastily called news conference," the *New York Times* reported, Mayor Giuliani, flanked by Neal Cohen and other officials, announced the news, "as a group of bewildered-looking Whitestone [part of the hot zone in Queens] residents looked on." Later that day, city workers fanned out through neighborhoods in northern Queens to deliver the leaflets and answer questions, and that night, pesticide spraying began. The city's campaign to contain the outbreak of St. Louis encephalitis was on.

THE FIRST FIVE DAYS

Over the next several days, the city continued its aerial and ground spraying campaign, gradually enlarging it to include more of the Bronx, as "a preventive step," Giuliani told reporters.[8] OEM officials worked feverishly to keep one step ahead of the expanded

---

8. David Rohde, "Concerns Over Encephalitis Prompt Expansion of Spraying," *New York Times*, September 7, 1999, 1B. The city also did an aerial survey of the area to help identify mosquito breeding sites.

spraying schedule, making sure residents received advance warning. "We saturated the area with city employees," recalls McCarty, who was in charge of spraying operations. "Thousands of city employees would go door-to-door and announce [a scheduled spraying]." To get the job done, OEM mobilized "field people," McCarty explains, such as inspectors from the health and parks departments, "people who were already outside." The police out in the community—the "foot cops"—were also recruited to help get the word out to residents; in addition, police vehicles equipped with loudspeaker systems patrolled the streets, alerting residents to a spraying in their neighborhood. "We did everything we could possibly think of," says McCarty, "to notify [residents] that this specific area is going to be sprayed at this particular date at this particular time." Still, OEM worried about how well it was getting the message across. "We were hit-and-miss," McCarty notes. "We would go door to door and that was fine, but people who were passing through wouldn't be aware of it." In addition, there were concerns about the cost to the city of diverting a significant portion of its workforce to the door-to-door campaign. "We were taking people away from their primary function," McCarty says, "... and that wasn't good."

McCarty himself learned firsthand the drawbacks of leafletting as the primary means of communication. Keeping up with the demand for ever-increasing numbers of pamphlets had taxed the printing resources within city government to its limits; faced with the need for a huge printing, McCarty turned to the private sector. At 2 a.m., as he remembers it, he showed up at a Kinko's copy center on Queens Boulevard, unshaven and unkempt from working around the clock. "I come in, and I look like a homeless person," McCarty says. "I'm dirty and I'm tired and I must have a three-day beard on me.... And this poor kid [who was on duty] is looking [warily] at me, and I say, 'I need 100,000 of these.'" Eventually, after negotiations with the manager—awakened at his home in the middle of the night—Kinko's agreed to take on the job for 4 cents a page instead of the standard price of 10 cents. The total bill "comes out to a little over $4,000," McCarty continues. "I've got exactly $4,000 in my checking account ... to pay my mortgage and [monthly expenses]. So I give him my credit card, and he wipes me out." In a heroic effort by the Kinko's crew, the copies were made and delivered on time the next morning. "Jerry," says Hauer, "got the job done." But it was an experience that McCarty felt he could ill afford to repeat. "I couldn't do it anymore," he notes wryly, "because I had to pay my rent."

Meanwhile, other parts of the city's public outreach effort were also feeling some strain. The hotline set up by OEM and the city DOH was soon flooded with calls; by September 6—only three days into the city's mosquito control campaign—it had received more than 11,000 calls, breaking the city's record for calls to an emergency phone number.[9] The city DOH had increased the number of operators answering the lines from a

---

9. Ibid.

handful to about 20, according to Mojica, but they struggled to keep up with the growing volume of calls.

The calls to the hotline indicated that residents were as anxious about pesticide spraying as about St. Louis encephalitis. While city officials stressed that malathion (the primary pesticide used in aerial spraying) posed no health risks, they also cautioned residents to stay indoors during the spraying and instructed them to turn off their fans and air conditioners and to keep pets inside. Such pronouncements did little to allay the public's unease about the toxic effects of pesticide sprays. "It's kind of like germ warfare," one resident nervously told the New York Times.

Still, despite residents' concerns and the stresses of running the spraying operation, there was hope that the battle against St. Louis encephalitis and its vector, the *Culex pipiens* mosquito, would be a limited campaign. "We thought it would be very localized," Hauer recalls, "very focused." But on Wednesday, September 8, news of another case of St. Louis encephalitis shattered that assumption.[10]

A Case in Brooklyn

As Marcelle Layton remembers it, the news came during an internal meeting on the St. Louis encephalitis outbreak, held daily at the NYC DOH—with OEM representatives in attendance—and chaired by Ben Mojica. They were on the phone to CDC, reviewing new cases of St. Louis encephalitis, when the group realized that the latest patient to be diagnosed with the disease was from Brooklyn, "about 12 miles, as the crow flies," notes Roger Nasci, from the epicenter of the outbreak in Queens. At that moment, in the middle of the conference call, Layton says, "everyone stood up," and "started talking [on their two-way radios]." Moments later, the room emptied out. "I had to tell CDC," she recalls, "'I think we need to stop this conference call. I'm now the only one in the room.'" Officials were rushing to find out whether the Brooklyn patient had been in Queens in the last few weeks; when the answer came back in the negative and, the following day, reports of suspected cases in Manhattan began filtering in, the city was faced with an inescapable conclusion: St. Louis encephalitis had spread beyond Queens. It was now presumed to be at large in a huge and densely crowded metropolis, with an estimated 24,000 people per square mile.[11] The "fear factor" at this point "was overwhelming," recalls Lhota. "We didn't know what we were dealing with.... We didn't know [whether] we would have hundreds of people [coming down] with this illness."

---

10. As of September 8, according to a New York Times report, there were nine confirmed cases of St. Louis encephalitis, including three deaths, and 60 more suspected cases awaiting lab results.

11. Andrew Revkin, "Mosquito Virus Exposes a Hole in the Safety Net," New York Times, October 4, 1999, 1A.

Exhibit 4B-1. Definitions and Stepwise Response for Risk Categories for Mosquito-Borne Arboviral Disease Outbreaks in the United States

Category	Probability of Outbreak	Definition	Recommended Response
0	Negligible or none	Off-season; adult vectors inactive; climate unsuitable	None required; may pursue some reduction and public education activities
1	Remote	Spring, summer, or fall; adult vectors active but not abundant; ambient temperature not satisfactory for viral development in vectors	Source reduction; use larvicides at specific sources identified by entomologic survey; maintain vector and virus surveillance
2	Possible	Focal abundance of adult vectors; temperature adequate for extrinsic incubation; seroconversion in sentinel hosts	Response from Category 1 plus: Increase larvicide use in/near urban areas; initiate selective adulticide use; increase vector and virus surveillance
3	Probable	Abundant adult vectors in most areas; multiple virus isolations from enzootic hosts or a confirmed human or equine case; optimal conditions for extrinsic incubation and vector survival; these phenomena occur early in the "normal" season for viral activity	Implement emergency control contingency plan: Response in Category 2 plus: Adulticiding in high risk areas; expand public information program (use of repellents, personal protection, avoidance of high vector contact areas); initiate hospital surveillance for human cases
4	Outbreak in progress	Multiple confirmed cases in humans	Continue with emergency control contingency plan: Concentrate available resources on strong adulticiding efforts over areas at risk; hold daily public information briefings on status of epidemic; continue emphasis on personal protection measures; maintain surveillance of vector/virus activity, human cases

Source: Adapted from Centers for Disease Control and Prevention, "Guidelines for Arbovirus Surveillance Programs in the United States," April 1993.

Note: Risk categories are tentative and approximate. Local and regional characteristics may alter the risk level at which specific actions must be taken.

The West Nile Virus Outbreak in New York City: The City Responds (Sequel)

Esther Scott

After getting word, on September 8, 1999, that new cases of St. Louis encephalitis were cropping up beyond the original epicenter in Queens, officials from the Mayor's Office of Emergency Management (OEM) and the New York City Department of Health (NYC DOH) once again huddled with representatives from the Centers for Disease Control and Prevention (CDC) and the New York State DOH to consider their response to the widening outbreak. The advice they heard was unequivocal. "We made the recommendation," says CDC entomologist Roger Nasci, "along with the New York State and City health departments, that the mayor approve spraying citywide."

What information was available seemed to bolster the recommendation to spray. There was not enough time to do "a comprehensive surveillance program around the city," Nasci points out, "but we did have evidence of human case activity that needed to be addressed." Moreover, by that time, data from mosquito trapping around the city had begun to trickle in. It indicated, according to Nasci, "very high infection rates in mosquito populations," ranging from five to as high as 50 per thousand. "The literature about St. Louis encephalitis suggests that when you get infection rates in the *Culex* population of three per thousand or greater, you can expect widespread human cases," Nasci explains, "so we knew we were looking at a very high-risk situation for the human population. We were also looking at one of the densest human populations in the country.... So it was imperative that we take very aggressive action to reduce the number of infected biting mosquitoes that were on the wing."

This case was written by Esther Scott for Dr. Arnold M. Howitt, Executive Director, Taubman Center for State and Local Government, for use at the Executive Session on Domestic Preparedness, John F. Kennedy School of Government, Harvard University. Funding for the case was provided by the Robert Wood Johnson Foundation and the Office of Justice Programs, US Department of Justice. (0102)

After hearing out CDC and others, Mayor Rudolph Giuliani agreed. On Thursday, September 9, he held a press conference to announce the newest cases of St. Louis encephalitis and a "vastly expanded" pesticide spraying schedule, as the *New York Times* put it, that included virtually the entire city. Ground spraying was slated for Manhattan, because of the density of its buildings and the evening crowds that thronged its streets, but the rest of New York City would be sprayed by air. The "aerial assault," the *New York Times* reported, "would continue until the first frost, probably at least a month away."[1]

SPRAYING THE CITY

With the mayor's decision to expand the spraying, OEM's task was hugely multiplied. Instead of a relatively contained area where St. Louis encephalitis cases were closely clustered, the agency now faced the prospect of covering a vast city of roughly 800 square miles and 3 million households. It included large tracts of densely populated residential sections, long stretches of skyscrapers, acres of parklands and zoos, innumerable ballparks, and recreational areas. A finely tuned spraying operation, which focused on selected targets, would be almost impossible to do, in the hurried context of a health emergency. Lacking data from a comprehensive surveillance program, Nasci explains, "you do [not] have the luxury of anticipating where a virus is more active, where risk is higher, and targeting your program more precisely." Everything would have to be sprayed, equally.

Nor did OEM have the benefit of a plan on paper, or even comparable experience, to guide its work. "The planning we had done never [helped] us on this,..." says Jerry McCarty, who managed the spraying operation for OEM. "First of all, who would ever think [OEM] would be dealing with spraying?... It's something that a parks department or a health department does, certainly not emergency management." Without a plan, he continues, "a lot of it was myself and the folks working with me at three o'clock in the morning, on the hood of a vehicle, figuring out, okay, what do we do tomorrow?"

The improvisational nature of the spraying was reinforced by "the many variables involved," as McCarty puts it. During early morning strategy sessions, he and his staff asked themselves, "What's the weather forecast? Are there religious events? Are there street fairs anywhere in the city? We had a list of things to look at: baseball games, Little League games, soccer games in Staten Island or in Queens or in the Bronx." For each of these situations, OEM scrambled to devise a solution. The Jewish high holidays, for example, began on September 10, and orthodox religious leaders were concerned that worshippers would be leaving services and walking home just as the aerial spraying— which took place during the early evening hours—was getting underway. OEM Director Jerry Hauer "met with all the rabbis in Brooklyn," he recalls, and agreed to suspend aerial

---

1. Jodi Wilgoren, "Spraying Expands in New York Encephalitis Fight," *New York Times*, September 10, 1999, 1A. As it turned out, spraying stopped well before the first frost.

spraying near synagogues during the holidays.[2] Problems arose as well over outdoor sports events: the US Open tennis matches in Forest Hills, Queens, for instance, or Mets baseball games in Shea Stadium, also in Queens. In each case, officials tried to tailor the spraying to suit the particular demands of the occasion.[3] OEM even accommodated people who were allergic to malathion. "We had to move them," says McCarty. "We had to move them to New Jersey or move them to Connecticut."

Alerting the Public

With a hugely expanded spraying campaign on its hands, OEM could no longer rely on leaflets to notify residents of a spraying in their neighborhood. "It was good when the area was small," McCarty points out. But at this point, "you're talking acres instead of blocks, so it became impractical."[4] The city turned to the media to get the word out about the spraying. All of the city's major newspapers, many of its ethnic and foreign language papers, most local television and radio stations, and the city's Web site carried schedules and maps of each day's spraying and other pertinent information. It wasn't "a hit-or-miss type thing," as the leafletting effort had been, says McCarty. "We were just saturating the entire media."

But a well-informed public could turn irate when a spraying did not happen as planned. This was mostly due to bad weather. "We would tell a community we were going to spray them at night," Hauer explains, "and then the winds would kick up or it would rain, and we couldn't spray. And that got people upset." Other unforeseen events could disrupt the spraying schedule as well. McCarty recalls a bar fight that spilled out into the street in Brooklyn one night, just as a contingent of ground-sprayers was entering the area. "It stops our entire entourage of trucks," he says. "This whole street is full of [people] fighting, and we can't get around them." By the time the police had cleared the area, the sprayers were three hours behind schedule. It was not an uncommon experience for the ground crew, McCarty adds. "They'd come across muggings, they'd come across car accidents, they'd come across something, and it would [lead to] delay. This is one of the things you have to do when you deal with New York City."

Still, the job got done. In all, the city conducted two mass sprayings of the city—from September 3 to 13, and September 18 to 23.[5] "Every borough," says McCarty, "with the

---

2. According to McCarty, the city did ground spraying, which could take place late at night, but went back to these areas to do aerial spraying after the holidays were over; ground spraying was considered less effective because it did not penetrate into residents' backyards.
3. So, for example, OEM limited itself to "targeted spraying" in the wooded areas around Shea Stadium the day before a game, according to Nasci.
4. For example, OEM records indicate that 58,000 acres were sprayed by air between September 11 and 14; and 59,000 acres between September 15 and 22.
5. A third, smaller spraying, limited to Queens, was done between September 29 and October 3. See: Monica Schoch-Spana, "A West Nile Post-Mortem," *Biodefense Quarterly*, December 1999, 7. Six helicopters were leased for the aerial spraying, and a temporary airfield was built in Queens to provide a staging area for them.

exception of Manhattan, was sprayed twice," by air or by ground. New York City had "a few thousand miles of streets," he declares, "and I can [say] without fear of contradiction that every single street was covered, because I was there every single day.... For 29 days, I did nothing else but spray."

Other Measures

Although it was the chief focus, spraying was not the city's sole response to the suspected St. Louis encephalitis outbreak. Roger Nasci, who arrived in New York City on September 8 to help out with the mosquito surveillance effort, notes that "a very extensive larval control program was put in place" as well. This involved a door-to-door effort, largely by NYC DOH staff, to find and eliminate—by removal or application of larvicide—mosquito breeding sites in residents' backyards, as well as in parks and other public areas. It was labor-intensive work. The NYC DOH, says its Deputy Commissioner Ben Mojica, "mobilized our pest control people"—there were about 50 or 60 of them, he estimates—to do the job. Because they normally specialized in rodent control, "they needed a lot of training,..." he adds. "It's a very big shift in orientation from controlling rats to controlling mosquitoes."

Meanwhile, the city kept up its effort to get residents to use insect repellent when outdoors. OEM "distributed mosquito repellent all over the city," says Jerry Hauer. "I became the king of mosquito repellent." He and his staff scoured the country in search of stores of repellent, which, as the summer season wound down, were in short supply. Nasci recalls sitting in OEM's office at 7 World Trade Center, watching as Hauer "got his people on the phone with their credit cards, calling every warehouse that they could find in the country. I think they bought all the repellent east of the Mississippi. ... I have never seen so much repellent purchased so quickly and distributed so quickly in my life." In all, some 500,000 cans of repellent were bought and handed out to New York residents in the space of about a month.

PUBLIC RELATIONS

Since the early days of the outbreak, Deputy Mayor Joseph Lhota and OEM Director Hauer continued to keep local politicians up to date on developments. Lhota had phoned Claire Shulman, the borough president for Queens,[6] on the Friday that the St. Louis encephalitis diagnosis was confirmed; over Labor Day weekend, he also called the head of the health committee of the 51-member New York City Council, state legislators from

---

6. Each of New York City's five boroughs elects a president whose role, according to Deputy Mayor Lhota, is essentially that of an ombudsman for constituents.

the city, and the member of Congress whose district included Queens. Thereafter, he made sure that key city councilors were regularly briefed. "The worst thing you can ever do to a council member," Lhota observes, "is not inform them of what's going on." In addition, he recruited members to help hand out insect repellent in their districts and to appear in public service announcements in which they "were teaching little kids in the neighborhood how to spray [with repellent]." This outreach effort appeared to pay off handsomely. With minor exceptions, local politicians supported the city's spraying campaign. "We briefed the people we had to brief, that we felt were essential," says Hauer. "And the people that were briefed worked with us."

Among the general public, however, reaction was decidedly more mixed. The city had made a concerted effort to provide a steady stream of information not only on the spraying schedule but also on the status of the outbreak. The mayor held news conferences twice a day, according to Hauer, during which he briefed the press on the latest cases of St. Louis encephalitis and urged residents to take precautions to protect themselves against the disease and the pesticide spraying. But, as city officials acknowledged, the effort to inform and educate residents sometimes had the unintended effect of alarming them as well. "It is absolutely difficult," Health Commissioner Neal Cohen remarked, "to strike the balance between providing the public with all the information they need to know while at the same time not creating undue concern or panic."[7] The sense of crisis was enhanced, the New York Times noted, by the sights and sounds of the spraying campaign, with helicopters that "clattered ominously above the city" and vans with bullhorns that "crawled down city streets bellowing public health warnings."

Giuliani chided the press for "botching the facts," the New York Times reported, and "spreading alarm and fear," but sometimes the anxiety was inadvertently triggered. Hauer remembers a phone call from an irate council member who insisted that his community had been sprayed by helicopter during the Jewish high holidays despite the city's promise to refrain. Using flight records of the helicopter fleet, Hauer ascertained that no helicopter had been spraying in the area. The council member insisted, however, that he had seen the spraying, because he had observed a helicopter overhead. It was, Hauer realized, a "media helicopter," not a city-leased one, that the council member had spotted. "So every time a media helicopter was overhead," he says, "people thought we were spraying."

Concern about the spraying and its effects spiked each time a new round of spraying was announced. Residents called the emergency hotline in record numbers; at one point, it was reported to have received 500 calls an hour.[8] To meet the demand, the city DOH added new phone lines and beefed up the number of operators; at its peak, some 75 people were handling phone calls on a single shift.[9] As September wore on, and the number of fatalities in

---

7. Jennifer Steinhauer, "Giuliani's Challenge in Outbreak: To Warn But Not to Panic Public," New York Times, September 11, 1999, 1A.
8. Maggie Haberman, "Swarms of Callers Tie up Hot Line," New York Post, September 11, 1999, 7.
9. This further strained the overburdened city DOH, which had to train the new operators, who were often borrowed from other city agencies.

New York City from St. Louis encephalitis did not increase appreciably, concern in some places turned to anger; environmentalists began to speak out against the spraying campaign, and there were protests in Brooklyn and Queens against the wide use of pesticides.[10] Hauer dismissed many of the opponents as "environmental nutcases." "There are legitimate concerns that people have," he says, "and we tried to address those. And then there's the nuts." The city, Hauer says, consulted widely on its choice and use of pesticides. "We were using good science," he maintains. "[Opponents] were using emotion."

The "emotion" did, however, cause problems for the city, particularly the mayor who took considerable heat for adhering to a hard line on pesticide spraying. "The more dead mosquitoes," he declared to reporters, "the better." There was, he insisted, "no point in not spraying, because there's no harm in spraying. So even if we're overdoing it, there's no risk to anyone in overdoing it."[11] But residents were not convinced that the remedy for St. Louis encephalitis was less risky than the disease itself. On radio talk shows, the *New York Times* reported, questions about "the spraying operation were far more prevalent than questions about the encephalitis itself." Residents, said one radio producer, did not "feel they were being told the truth of long-term effects of malathion."[12] The spraying, McCarty reflects, was "a political nightmare" for Giuliani, who nonetheless did not waver in his conviction that an aggressive response was needed.

Some of New York City's neighbors were less resolute, however, and this created occasional tensions. It could be a touchy issue, notes Perry Smith, an epidemiologist with the New York State DOH, "when one jurisdiction would decide to spray, and the other wouldn't." Smith recalls conversations in which officials from both Westchester and Nassau counties, where suspected cases of St. Louis encephalitis began to crop up in mid-September, were "agonizing" over the "appropriate response." They did have "a few human cases," Smith notes, but "they were not as focused geographically and [were not] as numerous" as in New York City. "There was so much uncertainty," Smith points out. When Westchester County began to get positive test results for St. Louis encephalitis, he says, "I think we didn't know how to put that in context—whether spraying would be like taking a sledgehammer to a fly, or whether not spraying would be seen as public health neglect of a clear warning." But Hauer saw political cowardice at work. Westchester County officials, he maintains, "saw the political grief we were getting, so they opted not to spray for a very long time." In his view, this was a "really irresponsible" course of action. "It showed a county," Hauer argues, "that instead of focusing on the public health issue, chose to go the political route."[13]

10. Schoch-Spana, "A West Nile Post-Mortem," 7. The following year, when the city resumed spraying, environmentalists went to court in an effort to block it.
11. Wilgoren, "Spraying Expands in New York Encephalitis Fight," *New York Times*, September 10, 1999.
12. Andrew Revkin, "As Mosquito Spraying Continues, Officials Stress Its Safety," *New York Times*, September 14, 1999, 1B.
13. By September 23, however, after three confirmed cases were reported, Westchester began to spray. See: Mike Allen, "Scientists Detect Encephalitis at 2 Connecticut Sites," *New York Times*, September 22, 1999, 1B.

A Surprise

In late September, arguments about the wisdom of spraying took a backseat to a stunning piece of news. During a conference call with city officials on Friday, September 24, CDC announced that it was changing its diagnosis: the virus that New York City had been battling for three weeks was not St. Louis encephalitis after all. The discovery of the true identity of the virus was a saga in itself, involving agencies and laboratories across the country. At its heart lay the belated realization that the mystery killer responsible for the deaths of hundreds of birds—chiefly crows—in recent months in Queens and neighboring boroughs was the same agent that had been causing encephalitis symptoms among humans. The connection had been made in large part as a result of the efforts of Tracey McNamara, chief pathologist at the Bronx Zoo, who entered the diagnostic fray after several rare birds at the zoo had begun dying over Labor Day weekend. After weeks in which many specimens—bird and human—changed hands and many diagnostic tests were performed, CDC confirmed what McNamara had already suspected: the virus in birds and humans was one and the same. Moreover, it was not St. Louis encephalitis but West Nile virus. West Nile belonged to the same family of viruses as St. Louis encephalitis, but it was new to American shores. In fact, not only had it never been seen in the United States; it had never been reported anywhere in the western hemisphere before.

The news of the discovery of West Nile virus created a stir within the scientific community, where the appearance of a virus in a new setting was considered "exciting" and "interesting," in the words of a CDC official,[14] and among the general public who viewed the virus chiefly as an unsettling and unwanted presence. When the story broke in newspapers on September 25, city officials hastened to calm residents' fears about an exotic and potentially virulent new disease agent at loose in the city. West Nile virus, NYC DOH Commissioner Neal Cohen pointed out, was in fact "somewhat less severe" in its effects than St. Louis encephalitis. Moreover, city officials stressed, the new diagnosis would not necessitate a different approach to combating the outbreak. Mosquitoes were still the vector of the virus—although other species, in addition to *Culex pipiens*, were known to be carriers—and would continue to be attacked with pesticide sprays.

But by then, the city had finished its second mass spraying and, except for a brief round in Queens at the very end of September, its spraying campaign came to a close. With that, and the coming of autumn, the uproar over West Nile subsided, at least until the next summer would bring a new hatching of mosquitoes and, with them, renewed anxieties about an outbreak of encephalitis.

---

14. Jennifer Steinhauer, "African Virus May Be Culprit in Mosquito-Borne Illnesses," *New York Times*, September 25, 1999, 1A.

Reflections

Looking back, Lhota sees the misdiagnosis as something of a "blessing in disguise." "It would have probably scared us a lot more if it was [known to be] West Nile upfront," he muses, "because while St. Louis encephalitis is something that [occurs] in North America, West Nile had never been in North America [before]." Still, he acknowledges, it did create "a credibility issue … in some ways" for the city. The misidentification was "only a problem," Cohen explains, "in relation to public confidence" in the city's response to the outbreak. After the West Nile story broke, he says, "we did see some perception that maybe we didn't know what we were doing." Critics of the city's spraying policy "exaggerated the significance of [the misdiagnosis]," Cohen maintains, "to make the case that we might not have made an informed decision when we chose to use pesticides in the first place."

In defense of its response, the city could point to figures from CDC indicating that no new encephalitis cases "had onset" in New York City once citywide "control measures" began on September 11 (Exhibit 4C-1). Whether this was the result of the spraying, or an indication that the disease had run its course, was not clear. When the first frost of the fall brought an end to the mosquito season and officials could tally the figures, what was clear was that the West Nile outbreak had not been as devastating as some had feared. A total of 62 cases of West Nile encephalitis were confirmed in 1999: 46 in New York City, the remainder in Westchester and Nassau counties; of the seven who died from the disease, four lived in New York City.

The pricetag for New York City's 1999 campaign to contain the encephalitis outbreak came to an estimated $10 million,[15] but city officials were not inclined to second-guess the cost, either in monetary or political terms. "We were luckily in a situation of a surplus," Lhota says. "We were in good [fiscal] shape." Moreover, he notes, out of a total city budget of about $36.5 billion, $10 million was "infinitesimal." From an operational point of view, Jerry Hauer saw little he would do differently, except to fashion "a more aggressive public communications program…. Our biggest frustration was in working with the public and getting accurate information out quickly…," he says. "We needed to keep the public informed. I think we did, but I think we could have done it better." But the relatively modest number of people who contracted West Nile encephalitis did not shake his conviction that New York City had made the right choices in attacking the outbreak aggressively. "I wouldn't have changed anything we did," Hauer maintains. "Hindsight is perfect. You don't have that luxury during an outbreak." Lhota agreed. "We didn't know how many people were going to die at first," he points out. The city had to spray "based on the information we had at the time…. I do not believe spraying killed anybody, but it did kill thousands, if not millions, of mosquitoes, which could have infected other people."

---

15. Schoch-Spana, "A West Nile Post-Mortem," 1.

Exhibit 4C-1. Seropositive Cases of West Nile–like Virus by Week of Onset: New York, 1999

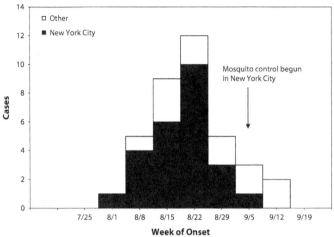

Source: Reprinted from Centers for Disease Control and Prevention, "Update: West Nile-Like Viral Encephalitis–New York, 1999," *MMWR Weekly* 48 (1999): 890–892.

5A

Emergency Response System Under Duress: The Public Health Fight to Contain SARS in Toronto

Pamela Varley

EDITORS' INTRODUCTION

In late February 2003, China was only gradually becoming aware of the epidemic of severe acute respiratory syndrome (SARS) that had originated there and in coming months would grip it tightly. But SARS had already traveled halfway around the globe, carried by an elderly woman from Hong Kong to her home in Toronto, Canada, where she unknowingly set off a public health crisis.

This case study raises a number of issues about public health readiness and performance in an emergency. The first concerns the difficulty of detecting a gradually emerging threat that at the beginning looks very much like a routine problem—in this instance, an uptick in influenza or pneumonia cases. But ordinary infection controls in hospital emergency departments, while functional for such illness, proved grossly inadequate for controlling the spread of the SARS contagion to other patients and clinical staff.

In SARS as in any emergent crisis, it is extremely challenging for emergency responders—not only clinicians, but also public health workers, firefighters, or law enforcement officers—to see and realize that they face something new and must respond with significantly different measures. Human cognitive processing can easily miss the signs of

This case was written by Pamela Varley, case writer at the John F. Kennedy School of Government, Harvard University, for Dr. Arnold M. Howitt, Executive Director, Taubman Center for State and Local Government, Harvard University. It was funded by Harvard's National Preparedness Leadership Initiative, a project of the Centers for Disease Control and Prevention, US Department of Health and Human Services, and by a grant from the Robert Wood Johnson Foundation. (0505)

novelty, and it is particularly difficult to spot a gradually emerging "break" in normal operating experience. Teams that have practiced and refined their abilities to handle ordinary challenges deploy and work on the problem from the perspective of the routine. Experienced practitioners may ignore or simply not perceive information that disconfirms their expectations, and they may resist adapting or abandoning tried-and-true methods. So the recognition of novelty may be delayed or denied.

This case also shows the additional difficulties of establishing situational awareness when scientific understanding of the challenge is evolving rapidly. While clinicians were struggling with the burgeoning number of cases presenting in hospitals and public health officials were trying to track the epidemic and develop preventive measures, medical researchers worldwide were discovering more about how to diagnose the disease, how SARS behaved, and how clinicians should treat it and protect themselves. In order to integrate that emerging knowledge into professional practice, it had to be captured and transmitted from researchers to world and national public health officials, then to networks of regional and local treatment centers, and finally down to individual practitioners. Technical documents and treatment guidelines changed frequently, initially outpacing the systems in place in Toronto to communicate within the health care and public health communities and to reach the general public in language that nonmedical people could understand.

How to organize the response at the provincial and metropolitan levels was also a major challenge. The national and provincial public health agencies were not hierarchically organized, and public health and emergency management agencies did not closely interconnect. Health care institutions, moreover, were not under the direct control of government agencies. Thus, because public health and health care networks are what organizational theorists call "loosely coupled" systems, leaders of the Toronto emergency response were challenged to establish a decision-making structure and communicate and implement preventive and treatment methods to frontline practitioners. As a result, they had to develop means of collaboration and mesh different organizational cultures under the intense pressure of a raging epidemic.

The SARS crisis also challenged and strained the operational capacities of even the world-class health care system of Toronto. Institutions had to scale up their activities in many ways, including managing high caseloads of highly contagious, hospitalized individuals; ramping up epidemiological systems to find and keep track of people exposed to SARS; finding supplies of protective equipment; and making sure that those who self-quarantined after exposure were adequately monitored for symptoms and had access to meals and other necessities.

As the crisis peaked, therefore, the response was not simply the domain of health care and public health professionals but required the engagement, cooperation, and compliance of the general public. People had to be educated about how to minimize the risk of exposure, what symptoms to be alert for, and how to self-quarantine.

DISCUSSION QUESTIONS

1. For the region's public health and hospital systems, what were the major obstacles to recognizing and responding to the developing SARS crisis?
2. How did the SARS crisis impact the emergency management agencies of the region?
3. What factors hindered the collaboration between public health, health care, and emergency management that proved necessary to fight SARS? How were these obstacles overcome?
4. What should jurisdictions outside the Toronto area have been doing as Toronto's SARS crisis deepened?
5. What implications does Toronto's experience with SARS have for jurisdictions preparing for future incidents of emergent infectious disease or contagious agents loosed by bioterrorists?

* * *

On February 23, 2003, the severe acute respiratory syndrome (SARS) virus slipped, undetected, into Toronto's Pearson International Airport aboard a commercial flight from Hong Kong. At the time, the illness—so new that it had not even been named—was known only as a mysterious and virulent pneumonia[1] spreading in mainland China's Guangdong Province. The person who unwittingly brought the disease to Toronto—setting off an outbreak that would infect 375 and kill 44[2]—was a 78-year-old Toronto grandmother, Kwan Sui-chu, returning home from a 10-day trip to Hong Kong with her husband.[3] Two days after their return, Kwan began to feel sick. On February 28, she went to a doctor. But public health officials did not learn that the mystery pneumonia had entered their city until March 13. By that time, five other members of Kwan's family were visibly sick. Unbeknownst to public health or hospital staff, the virus had also spread to a group of patients and health care workers at one of Toronto's community hospitals. By the time this group fell sick, the virus had moved on, silently infecting a new set of victims.

For a chronology of events and a cast of characters, see Exhibits 5A-1 and 5A-2.

---

1. Pneumonia is not a single disease but a category of diseases. These diseases share symptoms—inflammation of the lungs and the collection of fluid in air passages—but these symptoms have a variety of causes.

2. Because there was no definitive test to diagnose SARS, public health physicians labeled cases as "probable" SARS or "suspect" SARS (and in Ontario, there was a third category: "persons under investigation") based on clinical, laboratory, and epidemiological evidence. The convention, internationally, was to count only the "probable" cases for official record-keeping purposes. Thus, there were 375 "probable" SARS cases in the Toronto area between February and June 2003. Within the Toronto city limits, there were 199 probable SARS cases and 38 deaths.

3. Official government documents about the SARS outbreak keep the names of all SARS patients and their relatives confidential. Local reporters were able to find some of the names, however. In this case study, names are used, for the sake of clarity, if they have already been made public by the press.

THE EMERGENCE OF SARS

SARS made its quiet arrival in Toronto—Canada's largest city and its thriving, cosmopolitan economic center—three weeks before the World Health Organization (WHO) had officially identified the disease as something new and distinct from other known types of pneumonia. Before that, it seemed just as likely that the virulent disease spreading in China was the resurgence of a previously identified illness. Public health experts later observed that it was Toronto's bad luck to be part of the first small cluster of SARS cases exported from China. While SARS would travel, via passenger jets, to many cities around the world in the course of the outbreak, its arrival came days or weeks later to most of these places, which gave them time to prepare. By contrast, SARS had killed two people and—though no one knew it at the time—infected between 12 and 20 others[4] in Toronto before WHO issued its first global alert about the disease on March 12.

The Chinese-Canadian Community

This is not to say that no one in Canada had been aware of the mystery illness before WHO's March 12 alert. As early as January 2003, Chinese enclaves in Vancouver and Toronto had been hearing about the deadly new disease from panicky relatives in Mainland China.[5] That month, surgical masks began disappearing from local pharmacy shelves in Vancouver as Chinese patrons bought them up to send back to China. In a prescient early February news story, Toronto's *Sing Tao Daily*, a Chinese language newspaper, anxiously predicted that an infected person from Asia might bring the disease to Canada. After all, tens of thousands of people traveled from Asia to Toronto's Pearson airport every month. But Health Canada, the country's massive federal health agency, assured *Sing Tao* that the agency was on top of the situation and was "closely monitoring the spread of pneumonia" diseases globally.[6]

WHO, for its part, had been receiving unofficial reports of the virulent disease for a number of weeks. One e-mail message from an undisclosed source, which WHO

---

4. Figures assume that SARS patients who had become symptomatic by March 16 or March 17 had been infected March 12 or earlier. The incubation period for the virus ranged from 1 to 12 days in Toronto, but the statistical average was 4.7 days. Jim Young, Ontario's public safety commissioner and, later, the co-chair of the province's emergency response to SARS, suspects the number of people infected by March 12 was greater than 20, but there is no way to know for certain.

5. The first known case of SARS—thought to have crossed the species line from an animal—occurred in Guangdong Province in November of 2002. Many of the world's new infectious diseases originate in this part of China.

6. The information in this paragraph was drawn from "Behind the Mask," *CBC News*, November 19, 2003, http://www.cbc.ca/news2/background/sars/behindthemask.html.

received February 10, 2003, said that more than 100 people had died of the illness in Guangdong Province in a single week, that panic was widespread, and that there was a run on pharmacies as people bought up "any medicine they think may protect them." Until this point, the Chinese Ministry of Health had refused to acknowledge the existence of the mystery disease. But on February 11, 2003, the Ministry did notify WHO that an acute respiratory syndrome of unknown origin had struck Guangdong Province. The official statistics were far less dire than the rumors, however. The disease had killed five people, according to the Ministry, and infected another 300. Later, Chinese authorities would acknowledge that these figures represented a significant undercount.

SARS ENTERS THE HOSPITAL SYSTEM

By their nature, stories about the early spread of SARS are personal and in retrospect full of odd and tragic happenstance. Perhaps the most frequently repeated of these stories is how SARS traveled, in rapid succession, from Guangdong Province to Hong Kong, and from Hong Kong to Toronto, Singapore, and Hanoi.

The tale began on February 21, the day Dr. Liu Jianlun, a 64-year-old respiratory specialist, who had been treating severely ill pneumonia patients in Guangdong Province, traveled to Hong Kong with his wife to attend his nephew's wedding. The pair checked into Room 911 at the Metropole Hotel.[7] Liu had been bothered by respiratory symptoms for five days before his trip to Hong Kong but had paid them little heed. He did not want to miss the wedding, for one thing, and, for another, he hoped to get the chance to talk to colleagues at the University of Hong Kong about the devastating pneumonia that was spreading through his hospital in Guangzhou. That evening, however, his condition took a dramatic turn for the worse and the following day, he checked himself into a nearby hospital. He died 10 days later, on March 4. But during his few hours in the Metropole, Liu infected at least seven other hotel guests. According to one account, he exposed most of them when, formally dressed for a wedding party, he was seized with a bout of sneezing and coughing in a hotel elevator lobby.[8]

Meanwhile, on February 25, two days after Kwan and her husband returned to the Toronto apartment they shared with their two grown sons, daughter-in-law, and five-year-old grandson, Kwan developed a fever, sore throat, cough, and aches. On February 28, she went to see her primary care physician, who diagnosed flu, prescribed antibiotics,

---

7. After the fact, the Metropole reportedly renumbered the ninth floor rooms so as to eliminate number 911.
8. Carolyn Abraham, "How a Deadly Disease Made Its Way to Canada," *The Globe and Mail*, March 29, 2003, A1; Jan Wong, "How China Failed the World," *The Globe and Mail*, April 5, 2003, F6; WHO, "Update 95—SARS: Chronology of a Serial Killer," http://www.who.int/csr/don/2003_07_04/en.

and sent her home. On March 2, she began to have trouble breathing, and three days later, on March 5, Kwan died at home, tended by family. Because she had a history of heart disease, the local coroner identified her cause of death as a heart attack.

On March 7, two days after her mother's death, Kwan's 38-year-old daughter, Cora, who was feeling unwell herself, became urgently concerned about the deteriorating health of her 43-year-old brother, Tse Chi Kwai, who had been Kwan's primary caretaker during her illness. For several days, Tse had struggled with fever, cough, and respiratory symptoms. By this point, he had gone twice to see a doctor and was taking antibiotics but was getting rapidly worse. Tse's sister persuaded him to go immediately to seek medical care at a nearby community hospital, Scarborough-Grace.

The young triage nurse at the Scarborough-Grace Emergency Department (ED) took one look at Tse—feverish, shaky, gasping for breath, and frightened—and immediately escorted him into the emergency room, which was, per usual, overwhelmed and under-staffed.[9] The ED doctor recommended that Tse be hospitalized, but there were at the moment no beds available in the inpatient hospital wards—also a commonplace circumstance. In the meantime, the ED staff moved Tse to the observation unit of the ED, where he spent the night on a gurney a few feet from those of other patients, some of them elderly. The gurneys were separated from one another by sliding cloth curtains. To ease his difficulty breathing, the ED staff placed a noninvasive bilevel positive airway pressure (BiPAP) ventilator over Tse's face. The BiPAP's forced air helped Tse to breathe but also probably aerosolized his virus-laden respiratory droplets, thereby dispersing them across a wider area.

Emergency Department Infection Controls

Later, these actions would face scrutiny. Even if no one on the ED staff suspected that Tse had acquired a deadly infectious disease never before seen in Toronto, critics asked why had *any* seriously ill pneumonia patient been placed so close to other patients? "What on earth was this patient, who had trouble breathing, doing next to an elderly man?" demanded Natalie Mehra, director of the Ontario Health Coalition, a public health advocacy group. "Why was anybody left lying in emergency for 12 hours?"[10] And among respiratory specialists came the question—why had BiPAP been used on an infectious patient while he was lying chock-a-block with other patients in a confined area?

But the way the Scarborough-Grace ED handled Tse's case was characteristic of ED practices citywide, according to a number of hospital-based physicians. In many a hospital, the ED had become the densely populated holding area for patients who were

9. Daffyd Roderick, Cindy Waxer, and Leigh Anne Williams, "Canada," *Time*, May 5, 2003.
10. Linda Diebel, "10 Questions for a SARS Inquiry," *Toronto Star*, June 8, 2003, A01.

awaiting an available hospital bed. In some hospitals, at busy times, a patient might have to spend as many as three or four days on a gurney in the ED hallway before a bed was available. There was generally very little space in the ED for isolating infectious patients. What's more, hospitals did not, as a rule, isolate pneumonia patients. Pneumonia was extremely common and, for the most part, easily treated and not terribly contagious. Hospital workers were therefore not required to use special precautions or barrier infection controls (masks, goggles, gowns, gloves) when treating pneumonia patients. Putting on and taking off such items was time-consuming. Wearing them was thought to be alienating to patients and, for staff, cumbersome and uncomfortable. Masks, in particular, caused breathing difficulties, dizziness, and rashes for many wearers. Even the most basic precautions against spreading infection, such as frequent handwashing, tended to be a low priority in the hectic ED atmosphere.

Dr. Brian Schwartz, director of prehospital care at Toronto's Sunnybrook and Women's College Health Sciences Centre, who would later play a key role in the response to the SARS outbreak, believes doctors, nurses, and other health care workers should always wear masks when delivering care to patients with febrile respiratory illness. He argues that in contemporary times, medical workers have grown dangerously blasé about infection control in general—an attitude that may date to the eradication of smallpox in the Western hemisphere in 1971.[11] After that, infectious diseases suddenly seemed an old fashioned concern. In fact, in 1970, US Surgeon General William Stewart famously told the US Congress that the nation was "ready to close the book on infectious disease as a major health threat."[12] In the new era, a doctor's coat spattered with blood and gore began to carry a certain cachet, as the mark of the unflappable veteran, Schwartz says, and anyone who seemed overly concerned about infection control risked eye-rolling from colleagues. In the case of blood, that attitude changed with the advent of AIDS in the 1980s, but "I think as an international medical community, we became very complacent with respect to respiratory illnesses, except in pockets where you might have TB [tuberculosis]," he says. "We [developed] an air of invincibility that is unwarranted."

The ramifications of this new attitude have been far-reaching, according to infection control experts. For one, a generation of hospital EDs was designed and maintained with little regard for infection control. Allison McGeer, director of infection control at Toronto's Mt. Sinai Hospital, told a reporter that this state of affairs gave the SARS virus its first real opening in Toronto. "We could have gotten away without the full outbreak," she said. "If we had EDs that had higher air speeds of ventilation and negative air pressure,[13] if we had single rooms in our [ED] observation areas, if we had

---

11. Credited to the vaccination campaign of WHO, begun in 1956.
12. Commission to Investigate the Introduction and Spread of SARS in Ontario, *First Interim Report: SARS and Public Health in Ontario* (Toronto, 2004).
13. Negative air pressure refers to a system by which the air in a room is sucked out—and fresh air pumped in—at a rapid rate.

adequate hand washing facilities and training—and *time* for people to wash their hands—that transmission might not have happened."[14]

PUBLIC HEALTH IN TORONTO AND ONTARIO

Toronto Public Health

Across Canada, the primary responsibility for controlling infectious diseases belonged to local government and, in Ontario, that meant 37 local public health units, each governed by a medical officer of health[15] and local health board. Toronto Public Health (TPH) was Canada's largest public health unit and was known across the country for its strong advocacy, community participation, and wide array of programs. As in the public health field generally, the mission of TPH had broadened over time. Communicable disease control—once the centerpiece—had now moved over to make room for health promotion, health protection, and the prevention of chronic diseases.

TPH's Communicable Disease Control division employed 300 of TPH's 1700 employees and was still the agency's largest single division. It received 40,000 communicable disease reports each year and oversaw 300 minor disease outbreaks annually, each generally controlled in two or three days. But the division did not have the legal responsibility, the legal authority, or the staff resources to promote compliance with Ontario's minimum mandatory infection control requirements in institutional settings such as hospitals, long-term care facilities, nursing homes, and day care centers, according to Dr. Barbara Yaffe, then-director of TPH Communicable Disease Control.[16] Provincial law did require TPH to assign a staff member to each hospital's internal infection control committee, which TPH did. In addition, TPH oversaw the handling of any cases of reportable diseases within the hospitals. (Reportable diseases were those communicable diseases identified under law as posing a potential threat to public health.) But because TPH did not oversee infection control broadly within the hospitals, there had historically been few well-developed relationships between TPH and the hospitals' infection control staffs. This had just begun to change in late 2002, when TPH established a Pandemic Influenza Steering Committee that included representatives from the hospital infection control field. These burgeoning new relationships, in fact, would prove valuable during the SARS outbreak, according to Yaffe.

---

14. *Toronto Observer*, October 22, 2003.
15. In the United States, the administrators who lead local, state, or federal public health agencies typically have a master's-level professional degree but need not be medical doctors. In Canada, by contrast, public health—like neurology or pediatrics—is a medical specialty. Thus, the leaders of Canada's public health agencies at all levels of government are generally public health doctors.
16. In fact, Toronto's largest teaching hospitals were relatively well resourced and had more infection control expertise than TPH, itself, did.

Ontario Public Health Department

Even in theory, it was not clear what role the Ontario Public Health Department—a division of the provincial Ministry for Health and Long-Term Care—was supposed to play in the event of a communicable disease emergency. Some public health experts were under the impression that if an outbreak overwhelmed the resources of the local public health unit or if it spread beyond the boundaries of a single local jurisdiction, the provincial Public Health Department was supposed to step in and take charge. But in reality, Ontario Public Health was small (TPH had 15 times more staff) and was, by reputation, weak—in terms of its statutory authority, its resources, and the skill level of its staff. The province's chief medical officer of health, who directed Ontario Public Health, rarely reversed the decisions of local medical officers of health. Provincial law did give the chief medical officer the authority to do so in certain circumstances, but local medical officers were "not ordinarily subject to the review or influence, of the chief medical officer of health," according to a provincially sponsored report written after the SARS outbreak. The report also described the "machinery … under which the province might ultimately bring to heel a rogue board of health" as "cumbersome." This lack of centralized authority had terrible implications for emergency management, the report continued. For example, two adjacent communities might have inconsistent quarantine policies or inconsistent diagnostic practices.

Not everyone in the Ontario public health field agreed with this assessment. Some argued that provincial law did, in fact, provide the chief medical officer of health sufficient discretion to override local authorities, but the provincial government had not traditionally made use of this discretion. Whether a product of limited authority, limited resources, or limited leadership skill over some 15 to 20 years, Ontario Public Health was not widely viewed as a helpful or galvanizing force in Ontario by the local medical officers of health, nor was it held in high esteem outside Ontario in the public health field. Several of Ontario's medical officers of health later reported that they had long found the agency resistant to sharing information with the field and to approaching issues in an open, collegial fashion. As a result, relations between Ontario Public Health and the public health units were generally wary and strained at the point that Tse walked into the Scarborough-Grace ED on that fateful Friday, March 7.

TUBERCULOSIS?

On Saturday March 8, after 12 hours on an ED gurney, Tse's condition was visibly declining and he was placed in the Scarborough-Grace Intensive Care Unit (ICU). ICU Director Sandy Finkelstein examined the patient later that day, noting that Tse was dangerously ill and that his mother, who had also been sick with respiratory symptoms, had just died. Finkelstein was puzzled by Tse's condition, but his first instinct was to check for the possibility of TB, an illness common in Tse's Toronto neighborhood of Scarborough, home to many immigrants. The doctor ordered TB tests and immediately moved Tse to an isolation room in the ICU.[17]

By this point, Kwan's husband, Tse's wife, and Tse's two siblings all had a fever, cough, and labored breathing.[18] Finkelstein ordered x-rays for the four, checking for TB. As a matter of protocol, the Scarborough-Grace Hospital notified TPH of a possible TB cluster within a family on March 9, a Sunday. This raised no special alarm, as some 400 TB cases were reported in Toronto each year. TPH referred the case to its TB unit for investigation and follow-up—the usual procedure.

Afterward, infectious disease experts would note that, even though Finkelstein's TB concern proved wrong, it had been a lucky instinct to pursue it. Even a remote chance of tuberculosis—unlike pneumonia—required the isolation of the patient and the use of special infection control precautions by health care workers and visitors. As a result, hospital staff, other patients, and visitors were all much better protected from SARS once Finkelstein made his tentative diagnosis and moved Tse into an isolated room. Meanwhile, members of the TPH staff asked the rest of Tse's extended family to stay home until the tentative TB diagnosis was either confirmed or ruled out, to avoid spreading it to others.

OR IS IT BIRD FLU?

On Monday, March 10, Agnes Wong, a nurse and patient care manager in the Scarborough-Grace ICU, returned to work after an off-duty weekend. During her days off, she had enjoyed a favorite pastime—reading Chinese language newspapers. One story, in particular, had haunted her—the story of a young family in Hong Kong. The 33-year-old father had traveled with his nine-year-old son and eight-year-old daughter to Fujian Province on Mainland China in January 2003. While there, the girl had died of unknown causes. Back in Hong Kong, the father died on February 17, and his son—also sick—was hospitalized. On February 19, father and son were diagnosed with bird flu. (Bird, or "avian," flu, once a disease found only in chickens and ducks, was diagnosed in 18 humans in Hong Kong in 1997, but the outbreak was quickly halted. Between the 1997 outbreak and the two cases diagnosed in February 2003, no other cases of bird flu had been reported.) In late February, TPH had learned of the bird flu cases in Hong Kong and had sent an alert about bird flu to infectious disease specialists, hospital EDs, and infection control practitioners in Toronto.

---

17. Tanya Talaga and Kevin Donovan, "Why SARS Alert Was Late," *Toronto Star*, September 22, 2003, A1; Roderick et al., "Canada."

18. Not everyone in the extended family was sick, however. Tse's brother-in-law and the three children in the family—aged 5 months, 9 years, and 17 years—were free of symptoms.

When Wong returned to work at the ICU on March 10, she learned about the worrisome new patient, Tse, who was extremely sick, with a tentative diagnosis of TB. His story was a compelling one. He had just lost his mother—perhaps also to TB. And he had recently married a 24-year-old woman from China. The couple now had a five-month-old baby boy. "Somehow I connected this event with the other event I'd read about in Hong Kong," Wong later told a *Toronto Sun* reporter. "He was such a young man—in his forties—he shouldn't be so sick. I asked the nurse to check their traveling history." When Wong learned that Tse's mother had, in fact, recently returned from Hong Kong, she became more and more persuaded that Tse's illness might be bird flu. "I said, 'Something very unusual is going on. Two members of a family getting so sick? And one already dying?' Somehow I knew something was wrong." Wong took her hunch to Finkelstein and the hospital's infection control division. "I didn't have any proof except what I read in the Chinese newspaper—but they took it very seriously," she later told the *Toronto Sun*.[19]

As Tse's condition worsened, Finkelstein considered what other disease he and his family might have contracted. Bird flu was a possibility. Certainly from a clinical perspective, Tse's illness appeared to be progressing far too quickly to be TB. What's more, the Vancouver Public Health Department was now reporting a mysterious respiratory case, too. Vancouver's patient had also stayed at the Metropole Hotel in Hong Kong. He had then traveled on to Bali, where he developed fever and respiratory symptoms. He was sick enough by the time of his return flight to Vancouver on March 7 that local city authorities were notified and met the patient at the plane with an ambulance. He was quickly taken to an isolation room at the Vancouver General Hospital.[20]

THE WORLD HEALTH ORGANIZATION ALERT

On Wednesday, March 12, WHO issued a global alert about outbreaks of atypical pneumonia[21] in Viet Nam, Hong Kong, and Guangdong Province. Very little was known about the disease at this point. It appeared that the same disease had broken out in all three locations, but even this much was uncertain. Only sketchy information was available from public health authorities in Mainland China, but in Hanoi and Hong Kong, there had been significant outbreaks of the respiratory syndrome among health care workers in hospitals treating patients with the disease. In Hanoi, 20 hospital staff had become sick, and in Hong Kong, 26 had developed fever and respiratory symptoms. It had still not been determined whether this new disease was bird flu or something else.

---

19. Michele Mandel, "Our Christmas Angels: Grace ICU Doc Isolated First SARS Case," *Toronto Sun*, December 21, 2003.
20. The patient recovered, and the disease did not spread to anyone else.
21. Atypical pneumonia refers to a subset of pneumonia diseases marked by particularly rapid onset and severity of symptoms.

ProMED

There were several ways that local physicians generally learned that WHO had issued an alert. The most traditional was the chain of communication through the government. That is, WHO would notify the national government, which would notify state or provincial governments, which would notify local governments, which would notify local hospitals and doctors. In addition, some local officials and doctors might see word of the WHO alert on television or in the newspaper. But some Toronto doctors say they first learned of the WHO alert from Programs for Monitoring Emerging Diseases (ProMED), an Internet service sponsored by the International Society for Infectious Diseases. Indeed, this was a harbinger of the critical role ProMED was to play throughout the SARS outbreak.

ProMED had been designed as a clearinghouse, receiving infectious disease information from experts around the world and disseminating it within hours to an international network of subscribers. The ProMED subscribers received word of the WHO alert the evening of March 12. This was faster than the traditional news media could manage and much faster than the traditional government chain of communication. All across the world, doctors and other health experts on the front lines of the SARS battle would come to rely on ProMED to learn the most current information about the disease and the outbreak. "This outbreak was to ProMED what the first Gulf War was to CNN," observes Dr. Donald Low, microbiologist-in-chief at Toronto's Mt. Sinai Hospital. "It put ProMED on the map."

TORONTO GOES PUBLIC

On Thursday, March 13, the day after the WHO alert, Tse died at Scarborough-Grace of respiratory failure. When Tse's younger brother and sister arrived to view his body, hospital staff members were appalled at how sick they both appeared, and sent them directly to the Scarborough-Grace ED. An ED physician placed a call to Andrew Simor, microbiologist-in-chief at Sunnybrook and Women's College Health Sciences Centre, and asked whether Sunnybrook had an isolation room free and could take one of the Tse siblings. Simor agreed, and—mindful of the WHO alert—stipulated that the patient go straight into an isolation room upon arrival rather than entering via the ED.[22]

In the meantime, Finkelstein's TB tests for Tse and his family came back—as predicted—negative. At this point, Finkelstein phoned McGeer, Mt. Sinai's infection control director. Mt. Sinai's Infectious Disease Department was the largest in the area, and its laboratory served 11 area hospitals. In addition, the department had forged a cooperative relationship with many local hospitals: The hospitals cooperated in Mt. Sinai research

---

22. Carolyn Abraham, "How a Deadly Disease Made Its Way to Canada," *The Globe and Mail*, March 29, 2003, A1.

projects, and Mt. Sinai served as a resource for the hospitals' trickiest infectious disease cases. McGeer agreed to admit Tse's sister, as well as his young widow and baby,[23] to Mt. Sinai. Kwan's husband, too, was sick by this point, and he was soon admitted to Mt. Sinai as well.

Late Thursday afternoon, Simor, McGeer, and Irving Salit, director of the Infectious Disease Division of the University Health Network, held a teleconference to discuss treatment for the new patients. The first two Toronto residents to contract this virulent pneumonia had both died. Now there were four more cases, three of them critical. They decided on an aggressive course of treatment—a complement of three broad-spectrum antibiotics and two antivirals.

After a teleconference with McGeer Thursday night, the Toronto and Ontario public health departments decided to hold a press conference on Friday night, March 14, to inform the public about the cluster of cases and to urge anyone who had been in contact with the family or had suspicious symptoms to call a TPH hotline, which TPH hastily established Saturday morning. McGeer also notified Health Canada, the Centers for Disease Control and Prevention (CDC) in the United States, and WHO of the cluster of cases. "So by Thursday night, everything was buzzing," recalls Low, who was out of town until the following day but was keeping abreast of events through e-mails from McGeer. McGeer told a reporter, "I knew we were dealing with something that was very serious," but even so, she added, "I never, in my wildest dreams, could have imagined what we were in for."[24]

THE RACE TO UNDERSTAND SARS

In Hong Kong, meanwhile, medical laboratories had run tests to determine whether the new outbreak of atypical pneumonia was actually an incarnation of the old bird flu virus, and those tests had come back negative. Tests for several other recognized types of atypical pneumonia came back negative as well. That meant the disease was new, and its cause, unknown. Health officials knew it was crucial to identify it as quickly as possible. Without knowing the cause, it was not possible to make a definitive diagnosis, to develop vaccines to fend off the disease, or to design better medicines to treat it.

WHO moved quickly on several fronts. On Saturday, March 15, the organization named the new disease SARS—for severe acute respiratory syndrome—and declared it "a worldwide threat." WHO also announced criteria for identifying a "probable" or

---

23. The baby was not sick, which created a dilemma: what to do with the child, since there were at the moment no healthy adults in the family to take care of him. As a stopgap measure, Mt. Sinai admitted the child "for observation."

24. *Toronto Star*, May 25, 2003.

"suspect" SARS case and sent them to the national health agency of every country.[25] In addition, over the course of the next three days, WHO set up a network of 11 leading laboratories in nine countries to expedite discovery of the SARS causative agent and, if possible, to develop an accurate diagnostic test. In parallel, an international network was set up to pool clinical knowledge of the symptoms, diagnosis, and management of SARS. And a third network was established to study SARS epidemiology—empirical data about how the disease was being spread.

In Toronto, Mt. Sinai's Low—who had just arrived home from his trip—made it his personal mission to make sure Tse was given an autopsy and then to gather and send as many disease specimens as possible from the autopsy and from Tse's ill relatives to the Ontario provincial laboratory, the National Microbiology Laboratory in Winnipeg, and the CDC laboratory in the United States. Mt. Sinai's infectious disease research group collected detailed clinical information about the signs and symptoms of the disease in Toronto's six cases. On Sunday night, March 16, Mt. Sinai sent these clinical data to ProMED and sent a copy to CDC in the United States. "So as of Sunday night, we had the feeling we were doing a pretty good job," says Low. "We had gotten all this information. We were sharing it around. Things were going along tickety-boo."

THE LULL BEFORE THE STORM

As of Saturday, March 15, there was still no discussion within Toronto's infectious disease and public health circles that SARS might sweep through Toronto's hospital workers, the way it was sweeping through hospital workers in Hong Kong and Hanoi. Through the infectious disease grapevine, Low had learned a little about one of the largest outbreaks, at Hong Kong's Prince of Wales Hospital, where a local man had been diagnosed with pneumonia and hospitalized on March 4. (Later, when it was clear that he had SARS, epidemiologists pieced together the information that he had been infected by Dr. Liu at the Metropole Hotel.) Over the next week, this patient transmitted SARS to 47 health care workers, including 16 medical students. Hearing the story from afar, Low was sure there had been an egregious breach of safety precautions at Prince of Wales. "I'm thinking, 'Obviously, they're screwing up somehow,'" Low recalls. "They're letting their health care workers get sick. It must just be *terrible* infection control, for gosh sakes. It's not going to happen to us."

Over the next few days, this confident mood mostly held steady, but there were a few worrisome developments. First, a primary care physician who had seen Tse and his wife for about 15 minutes in an outpatient clinic was now home sick with pneumonia. She was

---

25. If WHO was to keep track of a disease worldwide, it was important that everyone use the same definitions. While WHO did not have the authority to require other countries to use the WHO definitions, most countries used these or close variations.

quickly diagnosed with SARS and hospitalized. "So she was the first example that this had gone outside the family—and after a relatively minor degree [of contact]," says Low.

On the evening of Sunday, March 16, there was a second worrisome development. Joseph Pollack, 76, came to the Scarborough-Grace Hospital ED for the third time in 10 days. On March 7, he had come to the ED with heart arrhythmia. A few days later, he returned with a fever and pneumonia but was not deemed sick enough for hospitalization and was sent home. On March 16, he arrived by ambulance, very sick and gasping for breath. This time, he was immediately placed in an isolation room in the ICU. The ED staff checked his recent history and ascertained that on March 7, Pollack had spent 12 hours in the ED observation room, lying on a gurney next to Tse. "So now we've got another case that's outside the family, and evidence of transmission in the hospital setting, which is a bit more disconcerting," says Low. After all, he adds, "We were trying to wrap this thing *up*."

IN RETROSPECT, A CRUCIAL JUNCTURE

After-the-fact, some critics remarked that if the Scarborough-Grace Hospital had temporarily isolated itself at this point—that is, if the hospital had halted all transfers of patients to other hospitals; if it had closed its doors to new patients, outpatients, and visitors—the magnitude of the SARS outbreak in Toronto would have been vastly reduced. Richard Schabas, chief of staff at York Central Hospital and Ontario's former chief medical officer of health, put it this way:

> One of the things you would think you would do in a situation like that—where you've got an outbreak of a new infectious disease about which you know little or nothing, in a hospital—is you would put a wall around that hospital. At the very least, you'd stop transferring patients from that hospital to other hospitals.

A sharply critical *Toronto Star* article, written several months after the SARS outbreak, echoed this sentiment, noting that in a similar situation, a hospital in Hanoi had, in fact, closed immediately. Hanoi's outbreak was limited to 63 cases and five deaths, compared to the Toronto area's 375 cases and 44 dead.[26]

Hindsight is always 20/20, counter the decision-makers who were on the scene at the time but did not advocate closing Scarborough-Grace to new in-patients and day-patients—at least not for a few more days. All that had apparently happened at Scarborough-Grace, by that point, was that SARS had passed, in the ED, from Tse to an elderly and susceptible man lying right next to him. It wasn't a good thing, but it didn't indicate a virus running amok, either. "I was out at Scarborough-Grace in the middle of

---

26. Kevin Donovan, "Crucial SARS Experts Fail to Testify," *Toronto Star*, October 5, 2003, A1.

this thing, and nobody was thinking about closing the hospital on March 18 and 19. Nobody had even a clue about it," says Low.

To close a hospital was tantamount to declaring that the hospital was too overwhelmed to continue its normal functions. "You're basically saying something is out of control, and you have to go into shut-down mode," says Ontario Health Minister Tony Clement. In addition to the stigma, it was very expensive for a hospital to curtail its revenues in this way, and Ontario hospitals, as a group, were already running significantly in the red.[27] A hospital shutdown also cut off an avenue of medical care to many patients. Emergency patients would have to go to another hospital. Patients already in the hospital could no longer enjoy the visits of family members and friends. Patients who required specialized care could no longer be transferred to the appropriate facility. And, already, outpatients complained that they had to wait far too long to receive many kinds of treatment. In other words, a hospital shutdown was disruptive and inconvenient to staff, doctors, patients, and family. "To close any hospital—the consequences are tremendous. It's not something that you do lightly," says Low.

HEALTH CARE WORKERS IN TROUBLE

By Thursday, March 20, things took an abrupt turn for the worse, however. One by one, Scarborough-Grace nurses and hospital workers began to straggle into the Scarborough-Grace ED complaining of high fevers. The following day, March 21, Pollack died—the city's third SARS fatality. With Scarborough-Grace workers continuing to turn up at the hospital ED, there was an active discussion in Toronto about whether Scarborough-Grace should close. The hospital management resisted closing completely but did shut down its ED and ICU to new patients. By evening, hospital staff began appearing at the EDs of other Toronto hospitals and in the hospitals of neighboring York, Durham, Peel, and Simcoe jurisdictions, where many health care workers lived. By Sunday, March 23, 12 members of the Scarborough-Grace staff had been diagnosed with probable-SARS.

That Sunday, under growing pressure from the Ontario Health Ministry, Scarborough-Grace closed altogether. At the same time, Toronto Medical Officer of Health Sheela Basrur and her executive team decided they needed to take a rather drastic step: they issued a public appeal to all hospital staff and all other persons who had visited Scarborough-Grace Hospital, for any reason whatsoever, on or after March 16 to (1) contact the TPH and (2) put themselves in self-quarantine for a period of 10 days from the date of their most recent exposure to the hospital. "We recognized that was a pretty broad sweep, a big extension of quarantine—that it might affect thousands of people," says Basrur. "But I think at the outset, given the tremendous number of unknowns we were facing, it was the only reasonable thing to do."

---

27. Karen Palmer, "Hospital Crisis Feared," *Toronto Star*, June 21, 2003, B2.

Meanwhile, within Toronto's hospitals, another worry was building. Citywide, there were very few hospital isolation rooms available. In general, Toronto's hospitals ran very close to full capacity, which allowed for almost no "surge capacity" in an emergency, and the need for isolation rooms made the problem that much harder. No one knew what the magnitude of the SARS outbreak would be at its peak. Hospital-based infectious disease doctors McGeer and Simor began to discuss the dramatic possibility of calling in the military to set up a mobile hospital where all the SARS patients in the city could be treated. On Sunday, a rehabilitation and long-term care facility called West Park, in northwest Toronto, offered at least a temporary solution: it would revive its 25-bed tuberculosis hospital, long shut down, to create a SARS facility. With help from staff at Scarborough-Grace and Mt. Sinai hospitals, West Park readied the facility in fewer than six hours—a feat likened to a miracle.

But there was a catch. Collective bargaining agreements precluded hospital workers from being transferred to the facility against their will. By this time, doctors, nurses, and other hospital workers were very frightened of catching SARS, and West Park was able to find staff enough to care for only 14 patients. Mt. Sinai's Low himself volunteered to serve as the doctor-in-charge of the facility.

COULD WE HAVE SEEN THIS COMING?

In retrospect, physicians realized that there had been some intimations of coming trouble earlier in the week, but no one had picked up on them. Low, for instance, recalls that on Tuesday, March 18, while at Scarborough-Grace to collect clinical samples to send to laboratories for assessment, a nurse remarked to him that Pollack's 73-year-old wife, Rose, was running a fever. "I remember thinking 'Well, that's not good,'" Low says, but, on the other hand, many things could explain a fever. Rose Pollack was not suffering any respiratory symptoms—the sine qua non of the SARS illness. The following day, back at Scarborough again, Low recalls a nurse casually remarking that she herself, who rarely fell sick, had run a fever the night before—but it had broken, and now she felt fine. This remark, too, made him vaguely uneasy—but, after all, hadn't the nurse said she was fine? "These things just didn't gel at that time. It was still early," he says, then adds, "In outbreaks, there's quite a denial component. The psychology is really to try to minimize it. You're trying to say, 'We've got this under control.'"

RESURRECTING AN AGE-OLD STRATEGY: QUARANTINE

Before the illness that had killed Kwan and Tse had been identified as probable-SARS, TPH had informally tried to halt the spread of the disease—whatever it might be—by asking family members to stay home and avoid exposing others. But once the disease was tentatively identified as SARS, TPH and, in particular, its Communicable Disease Control Division had to face an uncomfortable fact. For the first time in decades, Toronto was confronting a disease of unknown biological cause—potentially fatal and perhaps highly contagious—against which there was no immunization available and for which there was no cure. This meant that contemporary approaches to preventing the spread of contagious illness—immunizing against the flu, for example, or, in the case of AIDS, providing condoms, clean needles, and public education—would not be sufficient. Instead, TPH leaders, in line with recommendations from WHO, decided they must resort to the old-fashioned techniques of isolating those with probable- or suspect-SARS in the hospital (as the hospitals were already doing) and quarantining those who had been exposed to the disease.

It was daunting to think about cranking up the machinery of quarantine, which had not been used in Toronto in at least 50 years—that is, not in the working life of anyone presently working for TPH. The TPH leadership had to come up to speed quickly on how to run a quarantine program, train staff, and educate the public about why quarantine was necessary and what it entailed.

What Quarantine Entailed

The idea behind quarantine was deceptively simple. When a person was diagnosed as a possible SARS case, the first task for TPH was to determine how long the person had been infectious, and then to review this infectious period with the patient (and sometimes with close family or friends).[28] The goal was to get the patient to remember every place he or she had gone while infectious and every person with whom he or she had had sufficient contact to transmit the disease.[29] Then each of these exposed persons was contacted and placed under quarantine for the "incubation" period of the disease—the length of time between infection and the first sign of symptoms. The incubation period was thought to last between 2 and 10 days for SARS. If no symptoms appeared after 10 days, the person was considered safe from contracting the disease at that point. If SARS symptoms did appear, the person was hospitalized in an isolation room. If indeterminate symptoms appeared—just a cough, for instance—the person remained in quarantine until the symptoms expanded to meet the criteria of SARS, disappeared, or took the shape of a recognizably different ailment. While under quarantine, the person had to remain home and avoid

28. In the case of most infectious respiratory diseases, a person was infectious as soon as he or she felt the onset of symptoms. The assumption was that this was true of SARS, although in some diseases a person could be infectious before feeling sick.
29. It was not clear what level of contact was, in fact, sufficient. Overall, the disease behaved like a droplet-spread illness that needed quite close contact to spread, but in some anecdotal situations, it seemed to have spread with more remote contact, and scientists were not sure why.

all contact with other household members. That meant abiding by such unpopular requirements as eating alone and sleeping alone. If contact was unavoidable, the person was to wear a surgical mask. The person was also required to closely monitor his or her health and, in particular, to check for fever every day. TPH's job was to call each person under quarantine daily to check on his or her health status and to ensure that the person was complying with quarantine rules. Hospital workers who were considered contacts—but not close contacts—of a SARS patient were to be placed on work quarantine. This meant that they observed quarantine procedures at home, traveled alone to and from work, and followed full infection control procedures at work.

A SNOWBALLING CRISIS

Between Sunday, March 23, and Wednesday morning, March 26, the number of SARS cases rose, though not dramatically, from 12 to 18. Between morning and evening on March 26, however, the number suddenly shot up—from 18 to 49. By Wednesday evening, every isolation room in the city was occupied, 10 Scarborough-Grace staff members were awaiting hospital admission, and other sick hospital workers were at home, waiting to be seen.

That same day, Mt. Sinai Hospital doctors concluded that one of their intensive care patients, a liver transplant recipient who had been transferred a day and a half earlier from Scarborough-Grace, almost certainly had SARS as well. For 31 hours, he had been treated at Mt. Sinai without infection control precautions. As a consequence, Mt. Sinai announced that it would transfer the patient to Toronto General and close its ED and ICU for 10 days. All hospital workers who had been exposed to the patient were instructed to quarantine themselves. During Mt. Sinai's shutdown, the patient's doctor, seven health care workers from the Mt. Sinai ICU, and six members of the patient's own family would develop SARS symptoms.

The Mt. Sinai experience was a blow to the Toronto medical community, given its leading role in infectious disease work and the desperate need in the city for SARS hospital beds. Sunnybrook stepped into the breach and announced that it would convert 40 standard hospital rooms to isolation rooms over the next 48 hours.

By this point, says Low, no one was denying that Toronto was in trouble. "It was sort of the realization that we had lost control of this thing," he says. In fact, he and others now feared that SARS was not only a virulent disease but also a highly contagious one. "I thought that it was only going to be a matter of time before it would spread out into the community in Toronto. Then it would be Ottawa, Hamilton—other communities. Because you couldn't contain everybody," he says. "I thought that at the end of the day, we'd be recognized as the epicenter for SARS in North America."

Exhibit 5A-1. Chronology of Events: 2003 Toronto SARS Outbreak

February 21
- Kwan Sui-chu is infected with the SARS virus in Hong Kong's Metropole Hotel.

February 23
- Kwan returns home to Toronto.

February 25
- Kwan begins to feel ill.

February 28
- Kwan goes to see her primary care physician and is prescribed antibiotics.

March 5
- Kwan dies at home.

March 7
- Kwan's son, Tse Chi Kwai, goes to the Scarborough-Grace Hospital Emergency Department with a severe case of pneumonia.
- A Vancouver citizen, who had also stayed at the Metropole Hotel, returns home from Bali very sick and is rushed directly from the plane to isolated care at Vancouver General Hospital.

March 8
- Tse is tentatively diagnosed with tuberculosis and placed in an isolated room in the intensive care unit.

March 9
- Scarborough-Grace Hospital notifies Toronto Public Health of a possible cluster of tuberculosis cases in an extended Scarborough family.

March 10
- Scarborough-Grace Patient Care Manager Agnes Wong raises the possibility that Tse might have bird flu—at the time, considered a possible cause of the mystery pneumonia in China's Guangdong Province.

March 12
- The World Health Organization issues a global alert about outbreaks of atypical pneumonia in Viet Nam, Hong Kong, and Guangdong Province.

March 13
- Tse dies at Scarborough-Grace Hospital.

March 14
- Toronto and Ontario public health officials hold a joint press conference to alert the public to the fact that two members of a Toronto family have died and another four are sick as a result of contracting a mysterious, virulent pneumonia—perhaps the same one circulating in China and Viet Nam.

March 15
- The World Health Organization names the new disease SARS, for severe acute respiratory syndrome, declares it a "worldwide threat," and releases diagnostic criteria for it.
- Primary care physician who saw Tse and his wife in her outpatient clinic is diagnosed with SARS.

March 16
- Joseph Pollack, 76, cardiac patient who spent 12 hours on a gurney next to Tse's in the Scarborough-Grace Emergency Department on March 7, is rushed to the Scarborough-Grace Emergency Department and swiftly diagnosed with SARS.

March 20
- Scarborough-Grace health care workers begin to appear at the hospital's Emergency Department with high fevers.

March 21
- Pollack dies at Scarborough-Grace.
- Scarborough-Grace shuts down its Emergency Department and intensive care unit.

March 23
- Scarborough-Grace closes to all new hospital admissions, places sharp restrictions on day patients and visitors.

March 25
- Ontario Health Minister Tony Clement declares SARS a "reportable" disease under provincial law.

March 26
- SARS caseload in greater Toronto rises from 18 to 49 during this single day.
- Mt. Sinai Hospital discovers that an undetected SARS patient spent 31 hours in its intensive care unit without being isolated. Hospital closes its Emergency Department and intensive care unit for 10 days and orders all exposed hospital workers to quarantine themselves.

Exhibit 5A-2. Cast of Characters: 2003 Toronto SARS Outbreak

Public Officials in Spring 2003
- Sheela Basrur, MD, Toronto Medical Officer of Health
- Tony Clement, Ontario Minister of Health and Long-Term Care
- Ernie Eves, Ontario Premier
- Barbara Yaffe, MD, Toronto Public Health Communicable Disease Control Director

Medical Experts
- Sandy Finkelstein, MD, Scarborough-Grace Intensive Care Unit Director
- Donald Low, MD, Mt. Sinai Microbiologist-in-Chief
- Allison McGeer, MD, Mt. Sinai Infection Control Director
- Irving Salit, MD, University Health Network Infectious Disease Division Director
- Richard Schabas, MD, former Ontario Chief Medical Officer of Health and York Central Hospital Chief of Staff
- Brian Schwartz, MD, Sunnybrook Pre-Care Director
- Andrew Simor, MD, Sunnybrook Microbiologist-in-Chief
- Agnes Wong, Scarborough-Grace Intensive Care Unit Patient Care Manager

SARS Patients
- Kwan Sui-chu, 78
- Liu Jian Lun, 64
- Tse Chi Kwai, 43
- Joseph Pollack, 76
- Rose Pollack, 73
- James Dougherty, 77
- Adela Catalon, 46
- Eulialo Samson, 82
- Nestor Yanga, 54
- Maurice Buckner, 57
- Kitty Chan, 66
- Hubert Chan, 44
- Lewis Huppert, 99

Others
- Natalie Mehra, Ontario Health Coalition Director

Emergency Response System Under Duress: The Public Health Fight to Contain SARS in Toronto

Pamela Varley

INTRODUCTION

On March 26, 2003, Ontario Premier Ernie Eves declared the severe acute respiratory syndrome (SARS) outbreak an emergency under the province's Emergency Management Act. Emergency responders launched an intensive effort to isolate everyone with the disease, to quarantine everyone who had been exposed to it, and to protect hospital workers from contracting it. After the month-long battle that followed, culminating in a tense Easter-week vigil, the public health community heaved a collective sigh of relief, convinced that the worst was over—that SARS was all but extinguished in Toronto. Unfortunately, they were wrong. There was to be another chapter to the story.

For a chronology of events and a cast of characters, see Exhibits 5B-1 and 5B-2.

ONTARIO'S ROLE

Between March 13 and March 26, Ontario Public Health and the larger Ontario Ministry of Health and Long-Term Care, both headquartered in Toronto, were well aware of the SARS outbreak but had played a backstage role in it. The Ministry had

This case was written by Pamela Varley, case writer at the John F. Kennedy School of Government, Harvard University, for Dr. Arnold M. Howitt, Executive Director, Taubman Center for State and Local Government, Harvard University. It was funded by Harvard's National Preparedness Leadership Initiative, a project of the Centers for Disease Control and Prevention, US Department of Health and Human Services, and by a grant from the Robert Wood Johnson Foundation. (0505)

leaned on the Scarborough-Grace Hospital to close on March 23 and had declared SARS a "reportable" illness under the province's Health Protection and Promotion Act on March 25. (This required hospitals and health care providers to report any and all cases of SARS to their local public health department. It also allowed public health units to track infected people and issue isolation and quarantine orders to prevent the spread of the disease.) The Ministry had also collected SARS data from Toronto Public Health (TPH) and public health units from several adjoining communities and had passed it on to Health Canada, which in turn passed it on to the World Health Organization (WHO).

Once hospital workers began to come down with SARS, Colin D'Cunha, Ontario's chief medical officer of health and public health commissioner, had participated in a daily telephone conference with decision-makers in the affected public health units and infectious disease experts at the hospitals to share information about the latest developments and to try to figure out what to do next. On March 25, Ontario Public Safety Commissioner Jim Young, who believed he should be playing a role in the outbreak—both as safety commissioner and as the province's chief coroner—asked D'Cunha if he might join these teleconferences and D'Cunha readily agreed. Young had, in the past, managed such provincial emergencies as plane crashes, ice storms, and power failures. From this vantage point, what Young heard in the March 25 conference call made him nervous. The group was intelligent, well informed, well intentioned, and everybody was doing his or her best to think constructively about the problem, he says, but in his view, the group was neither bold enough nor quick enough in its decision making:

> What you have to do in an emergency is—you have to have structure enough to make decisions quickly. You can't sit there and ponder decisions all day. You have to have a meeting, make decisions, let everybody go out and do them, and then have another meeting.

"It seemed to me the situation was getting a whole lot worse, not better," he continues. Not only was the number of people visibly sick with SARS growing, but also there was an unknown number of people infected but not yet symptomatic. After sitting through a second group conference call the following day, Young says, "I hung up the phone and went and saw Colin [D'Cunha], and said, 'Colin, I think this is growing too fast. This is an *emergency*, and it should be treated and managed as an emergency.'" That meant the province needed formally to declare the SARS outbreak an emergency, under the terms of the Emergency Management Act, he argued. Doing so would give the province the flexibility to take swift and decisive action if necessary—confining individuals who refused to abide by quarantine orders, for instance; closing down borders; commandeering buildings; and handing down orders to doctors and to hospitals. He suggested that he and D'Cunha each urge their respective ministers—the solicitor general in Young's case, and the health minister in D'Cunha's—to advise Ontario Premier Ernie Eves to make the declaration, posthaste. D'Cunha was quick to agree.

In fact, it did not prove difficult to persuade the solicitor general, the health minister, or Premier Eves to take this action. They were elected officials—laymen, without expertise in infectious diseases. Faced with the spread of a mysterious, often fatal illness—and faced with the observable alarm of public health and infectious disease experts who had been grappling with the outbreak thus far—no one wanted to underreact. Health Minister Tony Clement recalls thinking, "If they're going to accuse me of anything after this is over, it's better to say, 'He did too much' rather than 'He did too little.' So I was very quick with my recommendation to the Premier that we declare the state of emergency. He got a full briefing from myself and Colin at the time, and it was decided within an hour."

AND YET ... WHO'S IN CHARGE?

On March 26, Health Minister Clement announced that Premier Eves had formally declared the SARS outbreak an emergency. This automatically activated the Provincial Operations Centre (POC)—a well-equipped central gathering area that facilitated information exchange and cooperative decision making among the 12 Ontario ministries deemed pertinent to the emergency at hand. But who was to manage the emergency day by day and moment by moment? All things equal, this responsibility would have fallen to the Health and Long-Term Care Ministry. The ministry did have—on paper—a plan for addressing emergencies. In the aftermath of the September 11, 2001, terrorist attacks in the United States, each major division of the Health and Long-Term Care Ministry had been directed to write up its own plan, describing what it would do in an emergency; but the result, says Allison Stuart, then-director of the ministry's Hospitals Division, was "a patchwork quilt, with no overall sense of strategy." Like every other Ontario ministry, the Health and Long-Term Care Ministry had also created an internal Ministry Action Group (MAG), which was supposed to take action on behalf of the ministry in a crisis. Each of the ministry's major divisions was represented at the MAG. The group had met about four times a year to participate in tabletop exercises that postulated the occurrence of a province-wide emergency—for example, an overturned train—and asked each MAG to come up with a response plan.

In reality, however, the MAG had never been a priority within the ministry, says Stuart. It was not, for the most part, made up of senior administrators but of a rapidly changing stable of junior staff members, reluctantly pressed into service and uncertain what they were supposed to do. In addition, the MAG's meeting space—while adequate for a tabletop exercise—was not adequate for a real emergency. It was small, ill equipped, and located in a building about a half-hour subway ride from Queens Park, the seat of provincial government in downtown Toronto. "Their MAG was smaller than [my office]," says Young, "with one table, one phone, and nobody who knew how to run an emergency."

Young had managed many kinds of emergencies in the past, but he had never managed a public health emergency. Although he was a medical doctor by training, he was not expert in infectious diseases or public health matters. Premier Eves therefore decided to make Young and D'Cunha cochairs of the emergency response, in charge of developing a workable decision-making system under the mantle of POC. In terms of the chain of command, they would report to Health Minister Clement, who would report to Eves. This kind of joint management approach "can work," Young muses, "or *cannot* work. The major problem with it is—what if your approaches are different and you've got different personalities? And how do you break ties [in the event of a disagreement]?" He adds, "It wasn't a problem initially. We each had areas we looked after." Over time, though, conflicts would emerge.

OPENING SALVOS IN THE WAR ON SARS

As soon as Eves had declared a provincial emergency on March 26, Young called a 7 p.m. meeting of the frontline decision makers in the SARS outbreak—doctors and administrators from TPH and the Mt. Sinai Infectious Disease Department along with D'Cunha and Stuart from the Health and Long-Term Care Ministry. Young asked the group to explain to him where the outbreak stood. "Initially," recalls Toronto Medical Officer of Health Sheela Basrur, "there had been an assumption by those who were relatively new to the situation—in other words the provincial folks—that we could establish a planning structure, get some advice, consider what the best approach would be, and then issue something as guidance to local hospitals." The reaction from the local public health and hospital personnel was fast and adamant, she continues: this would not be sufficient.

> Something had to be done *tonight* for *tomorrow*, because we did not know how far this had spread, and the fish were already swimming away from the net. Waiting another day to see how big the net should be was going to miss more fish than it caught.

So the group sat together until 4 a.m., hammering out a set of emergency operating instructions—the first of many—for Toronto-area hospitals.

One of the group's first decisions was to make these mandatory directives rather than advisory guidelines. "If you sent out 'guidelines' to 100 hospitals and 100 hospital administrators and then 100 doctors got ahold of them, there'd be 400 ways of doing it by the end of the day—if they did it at all," Young says. "The administration would think they were doing one thing, and the doctors would think another, and the nurses would get on with the job and do it their way."

Whether the province actually had the legal authority to issue mandates to the hospitals was somewhat blurry under provincial law. "The hospitals aren't owned by municipalities, they aren't owned by private industry. They're stand-alone nonprofits," says Young. But this did not deter him:

> The funding for them, almost entirely, comes from the province. And so we had the ability to turn around in an emergency and say, "Well, we're going to take some of your independence away." … You assume you have the legal responsibility and ability to do it, but if it's hazy, you err on the side of doing what you have to do anyway, and then you let the courts sort it out afterward. Did we have the authority? I'd like to think we did.

The group agreed to impose a rather draconian set of restrictions on all the hospitals in the Greater Toronto Area (which included York, Durham, and Peel Counties) plus Simcoe County, just north of the Greater Toronto Area (GTA). The directives were faxed or e-mailed to the 44 hospitals in these affected areas on the morning of March 27.

The First Set of Directives

Under the directives, each hospital was required to invoke its Code Orange emergency plan—that is, to activate a preexisting blueprint for closing down the hospital to all but essential care. The hospital could continue to receive patients needing urgent medical care (unless, for its own specific reasons, a hospital had closed its emergency department [ED] and intensive care unit [ICU]). But many elective services would be either suspended or limited to the most serious medical conditions.

In addition, there were a number of additional directives aimed at infection control. Among the most important:

- Tightly restricted access to the hospital—limited to staff with identification and patients needing emergency care. Visitors would not be permitted to enter except in certain specific cases—for instance, parents of an admitted child, close relatives of a terminal patient, the partner of a woman giving birth.
- Everyone entering the hospital was to be screened—that is, staff would be posted to take their temperatures and ask about recent health symptoms and possible contacts with people at high risk of having SARS.
- Every hospital was to create a SARS unit. That meant emptying an existing ward by discharging or moving patients and ensuring that each room had a negative pressure ventilation system or the equivalent.
- All hospital personnel—whether or not they were directly involved in patient care—were to wear an N95 mask, isolation gown, gloves, and protective eyewear or face shield. (N95 masks were designed to filter out smaller particles than, for instance, standard surgical masks. Thus, they were said to be 95% effective in screening out airborne viruses. The masks had not often been used in the health

care field, although they were used when caring for tuberculosis patients. The masks originally had been created for construction workers—for instance, people who did plasterwork, or spray-painted cars.)

- Part-time staff who had worked at Scarborough-Grace after March 16 were prohibited from working their scheduled shifts in other hospitals.
- Patient transfers from outside the area into Toronto-area hospitals were stopped, and transfers from one hospital to another in Greater Toronto/Simcoe were limited to urgent cases.

Four days later, on March 31, the provincial decision-makers decided to extend the screening and other infection precautions to all 160 hospitals in the province. Only the hospitals in the GTA and Simcoe County were instructed to implement the more extreme Code Orange provisions, however.

A JURY-RIGGED MANAGEMENT GROUP

The Provincial Operations Centre Executive Committee

Because the Health Ministry MAG was deemed incapable of serving as an executive decision-making body in the provincial emergency response to SARS, Young and D'Cunha created and cochaired a group they called the POC Executive Committee, initially made up of key provincial and municipal decision-makers in the response effort (or their designees). The Executive Committee began as a group of about eight people—the hospital doctors treating SARS patients, infectious disease and emergency medicine experts, and representatives from TPH. Over time, however, more and more officials petitioned to join the committee, and its membership swelled to two dozen. The newcomers included infection control nurses, broader representation from local public health agencies, assorted academic experts, occupational health doctors, and family physicians. Because many of its members were also managing the outbreak response, the POC Executive Committee quickly developed a modus operandi that allowed its members to participate but also attend to other pressing duties. The committee met each morning at 10 a.m.[1] to review the events of the last 24 hours, raise concerns, and, when necessary, make a major decision about the course of the emergency response.

Early on, for example, the committee debated the question of whether the province should try to contain the SARS disease in a single designated hospital and to transfer all present and future SARS cases there. Proponents of the idea argued that it would be easier to bring the disease under control in a single hospital, where it would be possible to enforce the strictest infection controls. But opponents of the plan noted that it would

---

1. The meeting time was later changed to 1 p.m.

expose SARS health care workers to a concentrated risk that was, at present, dispersed more democratically among a number of city hospitals. In the current anxious climate, there was an excellent chance that the health care staff would refuse to work there; the West Park experience had given a pretty good indication of that. It also raised the specter of inciting a union battle in the midst of a health care emergency—a thing no one wanted to contemplate. In addition, some argued that creating a designated SARS hospital would give the other non-SARS hospitals a false sense of security. If a SARS patient were mistakenly admitted to a hospital that was not on guard against SARS, the undetected spread of the disease would begin all over again. In the end, these latter arguments won the day.

INFORMATION AND ADVICE

In organizational terms, the Ontario Health Ministry's Public Health Department might have been the logical choice to provide staff back up to the POC Executive Committee, in the form of information, analysis, and recommendations. But Ontario Public Health possessed neither expertise in the infectious disease field nor in-house capacity for epidemiological analysis, two areas of major importance in the SARS outbreak. So Young and D'Cunha set out to fill these gaps as best they could, on the fly.

The Science Advisory Committee

Young created the ad hoc Science Advisory Committee (SAC), by asking Mt. Sinai's well-respected and well-connected infectious disease expert, Dr. Donald Low, to send out an SOS to his infectious disease colleagues around the province and the country, asking them to come to Toronto to help the province turn the daily arrival of new bits and pieces of information into practical advice about how to stop SARS from spreading, especially within Toronto's hospitals. Over time, it would become clear that other areas of expertise were needed as well, so the group was gradually broadened to include experts in public health, emergency medicine, and family medicine. The SAC met daily in a conference room provided by the Public Safety Ministry and reported to Young.

The Epi Unit

D'Cunha, meanwhile, created within Ontario Public Health a temporary Epi Unit, which reported to him. He recruited Bill Mindell from the York Region Public Health agency to set up and administer the unit, and Mindell recruited Dr. Ian Johnson, a professor at the University of Toronto, to direct the epidemiological work itself. Johnson's staff consisted primarily of a rotating group of epidemiologists volunteered by municipal public health units in communities not (or not yet) affected by SARS and four federal field epidemiologists.

The SARS Operations Centre

Young also created a temporary SARS Operations Centre within the Hospitals Division of the Ontario Health and Long-Term Care Ministry. This center, headed by Hospitals Division Director Stuart, had responsibility for writing and disseminating special emergency infection control directives to hospitals and other health care facilities based on recommendations handed down from the SAC. It was also responsible for managing the logistics of the outbreak—for example, providing help in rounding up N95 masks for hospitals and doctors.

A Word About the Incident Command System

Students of emergency management may note that the organization of the SARS response effort did, in a few respects, borrow concepts from the Incident Command System (ICS), a widely embraced though somewhat controversial organizational template for managing a broad array of emergencies.[2] For example, ICS called for a clearly identified incident commander, or for multiple commanders working closely in a "unified command" structure. Young and D'Cunha arguably fit this description, at least in theory—two commissioners managing the emergency response together. As done in ICS, they brought in outside experts to advise them in making decisions, via SAC and the Ontario Public Health Epi Unit. Young says he used ICS principles "as was practical," but notes that the ICS model was not familiar to many in the health care system, nor was

2. ICS featured a preestablished organizational template that had the advantage of being simple, consistent, and flexible. A basic structure was prescribed, but the pieces of the structure could be expanded, contracted, or eliminated to adapt to emergencies of varying sizes and types. Critics charged, however, that Incident Command, which was originally created to eliminate chaotic management in the case of large fires that cut across two or more jurisdictions, was not a good one-size-fits-all solution for all emergencies. Under the system, the emergency response was managed by either a single Incident Commander or a joint Unified Command Team. This commander or team oversaw four major sections that could be subdivided into assorted branches, divisions, groups, and units, depending on the demands of the incident: The Operations Section managed all tactical activities; the Planning Section gathered and evaluated current and forecasted information so that the command group could create and update the Incident Action Plan; the Logistics Section provided ongoing supports for the responders—ordering new equipment and replacing supplies; arranging for facilities, transportation, equipment maintenance, and fuel; and providing food, counseling, rest/sleeping arrangements, medical care, etc.; the Finance/Administration Section kept track of the money and time spent on the emergency response by any agency that did not have the in-house capacity to track such information.

the health care system organized to operate in line with the model. For example, ICS called for a single, clear chain of command linking every frontline responder straight up to the Incident Commander(s). This chain of command—absolutely crucial to ICS— was absent from the response organization in Ontario and, in fact, would have been impossible to establish under provincial law and practice. The frontline activities of the responders—to identify and isolate those with SARS, to identify and quarantine those exposed to SARS, to provide information to the public about avoiding exposure to SARS, and to gather and report data about SARS cases and SARS contacts—were all carried out by a combination of doctors, hospital personnel, and staff members of the local public health units. Doctors—though ultimately accountable to their own professional and accreditation organizations—were not, in a day-to-day way, accountable to anyone. Hospitals had their own internal hierarchies, and each hospital was ultimately governed by an independent private board of directors. Local public health units, likewise, had their own internal hierarchies, and were ultimately accountable to their local medical officers of health and boards of health. However, proponents of ICS would note that, especially under unified command, participation in ICS was voluntary. As a result, inclusion in the ICS structure was often based on willing participation rather than hierarchical accountability.

In this case, although Young created the SARS Operations Centre to carry out the writing of the emergency directives for hospitals and other medical institutions and clinics, the hospitals and other recipients of these directives were left to their own devices to figure out how to comply. In addition, there was no mechanism to ensure that they did, in fact, comply, beyond their own self-interest in remaining on the safe side of the law with respect to medical malpractice. In the absence of any legal authority (or organizational capacity) to proceed differently, the SARS emergency response relied on the existing and highly decentralized medical and public health systems to carry out the outbreak response.

THE COST OF MISSED CASES

On March 28, two days after Eves had declared a provincial emergency, the staff at York Central Hospital made a dismaying discovery. James Dougherty, a 77-year-old heart-attack patient, had been transferred from the Scarborough-Grace Hospital to York Central on March 16 for dialysis treatment. He had arrived with a low fever and respiratory trouble—symptoms that, at the time, doctors assumed were byproducts of the heart attack. But by March 28, Dougherty was near death with a virulent pneumonia, and York Central doctors concluded that he had SARS. Further investigation revealed that a week before his heart attack—on March 7—Dougherty had come to the Scarborough-Grace ED with congestive heart failure and had spent the night on a gurney in the observation unit—across from Tse Chi Kwai and Joseph Pollack. After his March 14 heart attack, Dougherty had spent two days in the Scarborough-Grace cardiology ward without infection precautions, followed by 12 days at York Central, also without infection precautions.

This news was a terrible blow to those trying to contain the outbreak. It meant that the Scarborough-Grace Infection Control Unit and TPH had not, in fact, tracked down every hospital patient that had been exposed to Tse; at least one had slipped through the cracks. In addition, it wasn't until 14 days into his second hospitalization that Dougherty's SARS case was finally recognized. Once the diagnosis was made, York Central immediately closed down its ED and ICU and more than 3,000 staff members, patients, and visitors were placed under quarantine.

Over the next days and weeks, public health officials would tally the effects of the Dougherty case. At Scarborough-Grace, Dougherty spread SARS to an estimated 21 health care workers, patients, and visitors (including the liver transplant recipient who was transferred from Scarborough-Grace to Mt. Sinai on March 25, forcing the 10-day shutdown of the Mt. Sinai ED and ICU). At York Central, he infected an estimated 15 people. "In hindsight," says Dr. Allison McGeer, Mt. Sinai Hospital's director of infection control, the Dougherty case "was the worst miss of the early days of the investigation."[3]

Another early "miss" also proved consequential for many weeks to come. When Joseph Pollack had been rushed to the Scarborough-Grace ED on March 16 with an advanced case of pneumonia, his wife, Rose Pollack, had accompanied him. Though Joseph was quickly identified as a probable-SARS patient and isolated, no one had thought to worry about Rose, who was feverish herself that evening but not otherwise symptomatic. She too had been infected with SARS, however, and was highly infectious. She checked her husband in at the registration desk—and while there, she infected three ward clerks. She sat in the waiting room for about two-and-a-half hours—during which time she infected five other people seated in the waiting room, along with a security guard, three nurses, and a housekeeper. In the end, public health workers calculated that Rose Pollack infected a total of 24 people. She and Dougherty became the first SARS patients identified as super-spreaders.[4]

The Dougherty and Pollack cases revealed a frustrating truth about SARS: It was a hard disease to diagnose, especially in its early stages, before all symptoms were manifest. The early SARS symptoms were extremely general.

---

3. Daffyd Roderick, Cindy Waxer, and Leigh Anne Williams, "Canada," *Time*, May 5, 2003.
4. The term "super-spreader," akin to yesteryear's term "Typhoid Mary," was imprecise but referred to SARS patients who were thought to excrete the virus in unusually large quantity, thus infecting an unusually large number of people. After the fact, some epidemiologists questioned whether the notion of the super-spreader might not be entirely myth. The explanation, instead, might be that the hospital environment—where large numbers of people were infected—was especially conducive to the spread of SARS for a number of reasons: warm, humid air in a relatively contained environment; close contact between health care workers and SARS patients at their sickest; high risk procedures that put health care workers in direct contact with respiratory secretions; SARS patients in proximity to susceptible fellow patients.

THE DIAGNOSIS DILEMMA

Researchers would not isolate the SARS virus until April 16. Even though this discovery paved the way for the rapid development of a laboratory test for SARS, the test was not reliable for patients in the early stages of the disease. Thus, doctors were forced to rely on a combination of the patient's clinical symptoms and the epi link—the moment of contact with a person or place that could have exposed the patient to SARS.

The World Health Organization's Diagnostic Criteria

As soon as WHO identified SARS as a new infectious disease and global threat, the organization had identified diagnostic criteria for making both a probable- and suspect-SARS diagnosis. WHO's criteria for a suspect-SARS diagnosis were as follows:

- The patient must have had SARS symptoms after February 1, 2003.
- S/he must have had a fever of 100.4°F or higher and one or more respiratory symptoms (e.g., cough, shortness of breath, difficulty breathing).
- In addition, the patient must have had either close personal contact with a diagnosed SARS patient or a recent history of travel to an area reporting SARS cases.

A probable-SARS case included all the suspect criteria *plus:*

- a chest x-ray finding of pneumonia or respiratory distress syndrome[5] *or*
- a death owing to an unexplained respiratory illness, with an autopsy examination demonstrating the pathology of respiratory distress syndrome without an identifiable cause.

Other symptoms sometimes associated with SARS included headache, muscular stiffness, loss of appetite, malaise, confusion, rash, and diarrhea, WHO added. For purposes of developing an official disease count, WHO used only the probable-SARS numbers from each country.[6]

Health Canada's Diagnostic Criteria

The official definition in Canada, developed by the federal health care agency, Health Canada, was the same as WHO's except that instead of a chest x-ray finding of pneumonia or respiratory distress syndrome, Health Canada required a clinical finding of severe,

---

5. Refers to a syndrome of life-threatening progressive pulmonary insufficiency in the absence of a known pulmonary disease.
6. Over time, a number of suspect cases evolved into probable cases.

progressive pneumonia. Later in the outbreak, this disparity would prove consequential, but in the early days, it had little effect.

The Possibility of Asymptomatic Carriers

The problem with both the WHO and the Health Canada definitions, says Ian Johnson, who managed the epidemiological work of the province's emergency Epi Unit, was that they assumed that everyone who was infected with SARS would be symptomatic. But what if some of the people infected with the virus never became sick themselves but did spread the disease to others? Most infectious diseases included such asymptomatic carriers. In the case of hepatitis B, for example, a full 60% of the people who spread the disease did not get sick themselves. If this were true of SARS, then it would not be possible to find the epi link in every case; a person might catch SARS from someone who appeared perfectly healthy. Thus, public health personnel were loathe to rule out a SARS diagnosis on the basis of the epi link alone. "So then we had to try to start monitoring for other kinds of SARS-like illnesses that did not have an epidemiological link," says Johnson. "Otherwise the thing could be spreading way beyond our control and we would just be happily looking at this one little area—because we could *link* it all."

On the other hand, to consider every pneumonia patient a possible SARS case would overwhelm the hospital system and confuse efforts to distinguish SARS from other kinds of pneumonia. Ontario therefore created a third category called persons under investigation (PUI), which primarily consisted of people with all the clinical symptoms of SARS but no apparent epi link. In addition, a person with an epi link and just one SARS symptom—for example, a Scarborough-Grace health care worker with a fever but no respiratory symptoms—was often categorized as a PUI.

Likely Alternatives

Despite the failsafe PUI category, it was still easy to miss SARS cases, doctors noted. One of the most confounding situations arose if a doctor believed a pneumonia patient not only had no epi link to SARS but that his or her pneumonia symptoms had a very likely alternative cause. This, in fact, had happened with Dougherty, whose respiratory symptoms were assumed part of his congestive heart condition until they became extremely virulent.

Finding the Epi Link

In addition, it was often very difficult to find the epi link—a job that belonged to the local public health department. There were several reasons for the difficulty. For one, the primary source of information was necessarily the patient's own memory, perhaps supplemented by the recollections of close family or friends. Public health staff had to question patients—who were often woozy with fever and struggling to breathe—to recall everything they had done, every place they had gone, every person they had been near, for the 10 days preceding the first onset of symptoms. "Think of yourself—how hard it is to remember what you were doing in the last 10 days," says Barbara Yaffe, then-director of TPH's Communicable Disease Control Division. "Now think if you were *sick* and trying to remember."

What's more, the links could be Byzantine, and public health staff had practically to become gumshoe detectives to uncover them. For example, in mid-April, health authorities in Manila, the Philippines, would announce that a 46-year-old Toronto woman, Adela Catalon, had brought SARS to the country when she arrived from Canada to visit her ill father and attend a wedding. During her stay, her symptoms worsened, leading to diarrhea and labored breathing. She finally went to a hospital where she was diagnosed with SARS. She died 10 hours later, on April 14. According to an article in the *Toronto Star*, the case set off a panic in the Philippines. Catalon had potentially exposed many people before her hospitalization. She had, for example, attended an April 7 wedding with 500 guests. Armed troops forcibly quarantined three towns in the Philippines, and members of Catalon's extended family were reportedly shunned and lost jobs.[7]

Ontario public health authorities at first disputed the Philippines' claim: they could find no epi link to Catalon from the known pool of SARS cases. But eventually, TPH did find a link. Just before Catalon's departure, she reportedly helped care for the ill 69-year-old mother of her roommate. That 69-year-old woman was later diagnosed with SARS and died on April 25—11 days after Catalon, herself, had died in the Philippines. Published reports indicate that the roommate's mother may have contracted SARS at the Lapsley Family Clinic in late March from a member of the Samson family. Some 17 members of this family reportedly contracted SARS from the family patriarch, 82-year-old Eulialio Samson, who was not diagnosed with SARS until a few days after his April 1 death. Samson and his son contracted SARS on March 16 in the Scarborough-Grace ED from Rose Pollack, who was seated near them in the waiting room.

A Shifting Approach to Diagnosing SARS

Through the month of April, the number of probable, suspect, and PUI cases mushroomed. While public health officials continued to believe that it was disastrous for a SARS case to go undiagnosed, they also saw the downside to casting too wide a net for SARS. If the child of a health care worker on quarantine came down with the flu, for example, and—erring on the side of caution—public health doctors decided to consider

---

7. "Adela Catalon," *Toronto Star*, September 27, 2003, H3.

it a possible SARS case, the diagnosis could close down an entire school for days. If a hospital patient acquired pneumonia and, again on the side of caution, doctors diagnosed possible SARS, it could close the hospital ward and send hundreds of health care workers into quarantine. A SARS diagnosis, in other words, could prove extremely disruptive. If it was crucial not to miss cases, it was almost as important not to bend over backward to diagnose the disease when the chances were remote. "Overcalling of cases causes huge resource problems, public panic, and potentially discredits the operation," says Young.

In mid-April, hoping to reduce overdiagnosis of SARS, D'Cunha began to stress the need to pay strict attention to the SARS criteria listed in the Health Canada SARS definition. In addition, with the support of the POC Executive Committee, he created a provincial adjudication program, in which questionable or conflicting local diagnoses were subject to the review of one of several provincially designated experts, who would look at the patient's case file and make a final judgment call.[8]

THE MONTH OF APRIL: LONG HOURS, CAMARADERIE, AND A LARGE DOSE OF EXASPERATION

During the month of April, the emergency response to SARS settled into a basic modus operandi, buoyed by a high level of expertise, professionalism, and earnest good will among the participants and hobbled by limited information, inadequate staff resources, and unworkable systems for the exchange of vital incoming information about the behavior of the disease. Within this basic context, each of the major organizational players in the response—Toronto Public Health, the Epi Unit, the Science Advisory Committee, and the Greater Toronto Area hospitals—faced a distinctive set of challenges and frustrations.

TORONTO PUBLIC HEALTH AND THE PROBLEM OF "OVERWHELM"

The tasks that fell to the local public health units during the outbreak were all extremely labor-intensive, especially for TPH, as most of the SARS caseload was in Toronto. For example, a TPH staff member had to investigate every potential SARS case in an effort to find the epi link. In some cases, the link was obvious, but in others it took a full-blown investigation to track it down—and that might take days. The average epi-link

---

8. Some public health units objected to this move, which they regarded as an unlawful usurpation of their authority.

investigation took nine hours to complete. In the course of the outbreak, TPH investigated 2,000 potential cases.

Once a patient had been identified as a possible SARS case, TPH had to come up with a list of every person who might have been exposed to the patient since the onset of his or her symptoms. In the course of the outbreak, more than 26,000 people were identified as contacts. If the contact had no SARS symptoms but had been exposed to the SARS patient less than 10 days before, the virus might be incubating in the body of the contact person. Thus the contact had to go into quarantine for the remainder of the 10-day period. That meant getting the person a mask and thermometer and calling once or twice a day to make sure the person was complying with quarantine and to check on his or her health status.

As a practical matter, TPH caseworkers would find that they had to help people under quarantine in a number of other respects as well. If the person became severely anxious or depressed, for instance, the caseworker had to arrange psychological support by phone. If the parent of young children was quarantined, the caseworker might have to help him or her find childcare. If the person had no way to get food, TPH had to find him or her a free food delivery service. Or if an employer refused to allow an employee to comply with quarantine, TPH had to call the employer to advocate on the employee's behalf.

In addition to the casework itself, TPH leaders had to figure out a way to keep track of assorted details of every possible SARS case and every possible contact of every possible SARS case. The existing software for reporting infectious diseases in Ontario was unworkable as it was limited to a set of specific, known diseases. They then tried to develop a system using Excel spreadsheets, but even the Excel template was too limited for the task at hand. TPH asked its internal computer experts to devise a viable tracking system—which they did, but they were not able to complete it until late April. As Toronto's Medical Officer of Health Basrur put it, this "was like designing the bucket when you're fighting the fire."[9] In the meantime, TPH resorted to old-fashioned paper files. As Basrur has explained:

> We had flip charts and color-coded Post-Its as one of the key ways in which we shared information and passed it on between shifts. It [was] absolutely manual—highly visual. Expeditious, but not efficient, if you know what I mean, when it comes to such things as reporting to the Ministry or to the media what was our total number of cases, how many were in hospital, how many were in ICU, how many were on ventilators. At one point, it was practically a matter of counting stick men every single time they called us up to ask for more recent numbers, and that's no way to run a public health unit.[10]

Given the amount of work involved and given the burden to those under quarantine, there were questions, early on, about what categories of people to place under quarantine. Everyone at TPH agreed on the need to track down the contacts of all the probable- and

---

9. "Behind the Mask," *CBC News*, November 19, 2003, http://www.cbc.ca/news2/background/sars/behindthemask.html.
10. Ibid.

suspect-SARS cases. But what about the PUIs? Did all their contacts have to be quarantined as well? "That was the dilemma," says Yaffe, director of the TPH Communicable Disease Control Division. "We decided to err on the side of caution. So if there was any doubt that the person was a case, we kept investigating very carefully to figure out if they were or they weren't. In the meantime, we had to deal with them as if they were, and deal with their contacts as if they were the contacts of a case."

Similar questions arose with respect to the degree of exposure to SARS. It seemed clear that the virus was at least primarily spread by droplets; an airborne virus would have spread the disease far more widely and quickly. Droplets were heavy enough that they could only travel about 3 feet before falling to the ground. They could also land on flat surfaces and be spread by the hands. That meant that close contact between people was generally necessary to spread the disease. But there were also examples of disease transmission that seemed to have occurred from a more remote level of contact. In terms of identifying people who should be quarantined, this uncertainty posed a dilemma. The members of a SARS patient's household were a clear-cut case: they should be quarantined. But what about someone who had walked through a hospital at a time when SARS was spreading, unchecked, among health care workers? Early on, TPH decided to quarantine anyone with a plausible level of contact—again, erring on the side of caution—but later the agency adopted a position in the middle ground: "active surveillance" instead of quarantine for a low-likelihood contact. That meant allowing the person to go about his or her regular life but monitoring closely for SARS-type symptoms. There were 13,374 people under quarantine in Toronto over the course of the outbreak—as many as 8,000 at once during the outbreak peak.

While TPH received wide praise for the long hours and unstinting efforts of its leadership and staff, there were, in the final analysis, not enough trained people to carry out all this work, even when an additional 400 people were redeployed to the Communicable Disease Control Division from other parts of TPH, and even when a few nearby communities volunteered public health workers to help out. Nor was the old fashioned paper information system really viable. As a result there were many mistakes of various types reported by a frustrated public. There were hours spent on hold when trying to call TPH for information. There were people under quarantine who were never called—and then those who were called repeatedly. There were people who had to repeat their entire story over and over to a string of TPH staff members, as the information given before could not be located. There were deceased SARS patients whose grieving relatives received calls asking about the patient's condition. There were SARS-exposed individuals who were not contacted soon enough to prevent the possibility of further spread of the disease.

In fact, a number of Toronto residents figured out they had been exposed to SARS and placed themselves under quarantine—not at the request of TPH, but because they had heard about the protocols from TV news reports and decided to do the responsible thing.

The impression of widespread cooperation and compliance with quarantine in Toronto would later be a topic of some wonder to officials at both WHO and at the Centers for Disease Control and Prevention (CDC), according to Health Minister Clement, although there was no way to calculate the actual compliance rate, and estimates ranged from 50% to 90%. There were also a few infamous examples of noncompliance—in particular, a Hewlett-Packard employee who scoffed at the idea that he might be infected and went to work, persuading his wife to cover for him on the phone when public health workers called. Not only did he have a fatal case of SARS, but he also infected a coworker who also died.

Although it created an overwhelming workload, most people in the public health field agreed that, given what was known at the time, there had been little choice but to use quarantine in Toronto. There was one prominent exception to this viewpoint, however. Dr. Richard Schabas, chief of staff at the York Central Hospital and Ontario's former chief medical officer of health, believed that quarantine was ineffective and a waste of resources. "Quarantine was abandoned by public health a hundred years ago because it doesn't work," he argues.

> When it comes to quarantine diseases, there are two categories. There are those diseases where quarantine is ineffective because the disease is too infectious—like measles or influenza. And then there are diseases where quarantine is unnecessary because the disease isn't sufficiently infectious—your standard garden-variety pneumonias. Why would you put immense effort into a control measure which doesn't work for any other infectious disease? You might as well bring out the leeches.

What's more, Schabas says, epidemiologists should have been able to see that the outbreak was almost entirely hospital-based and focused resources there, not exhausted themselves trying to halt the small amount of community spread. Even after the fact, Schabas's view was well out of the mainstream, however, and certainly at the time, the TPH leadership did not doubt the need to use quarantine, however arduous and imperfect.

THE EPI UNIT AND THE BAD INFORMATION REPORTING SYSTEM

One of the greatest difficulties in arresting the spread of SARS was to come up with infection control protocols in the absence of clear information. For example, there was an operating assumption that everyone infected by the virus got sick—but was that really true? Might there not be people who were infected but asymptomatic, and might they not still spread the disease? Was SARS spread only by droplets—and did the virus transmit only through respiratory secretions or also through fecal matter? Was the maximum incubation period 10 days, or was it really 12? Were some SARS patients "super-spreaders"—people who were highly infectious because their secretions contained an unusually large volume of the virus—and, if so, did they have identifiable characteristics?

The job of the Epi Unit was to provide the answers to these kinds of questions by analyzing statistical data about the behavior of the disease. In addition, the Epi Unit was to provide authoritative data about all SARS cases in Ontario. It was information and analysis that many agencies and interest groups desperately wanted, including Health Canada, WHO, SAC, the scientific researchers, provincial politicians, and the media.

This would have been challenge enough to an established epidemiology office working with the latest and most flexible computer software. In Ontario, the Epi Unit had to be created from scratch by people outside government in the midst of the outbreak. "This fact, in and of itself, is stunning," according to the interim report of the province's post-hoc analysis of the SARS response effort.[11] "[Y]ou cannot, in the event of an outbreak, suddenly hire your whole work force, implement your computer system, and then implement the processes and the legislative frameworks in which to produce a coherent surveillance system," says an anonymous observer, quoted in the report.

As the Epi Unit began work, its staff consisted of Johnson, the professor seconded from the University of Toronto, four field epidemiologists loaned by Health Canada, and a revolving pool of epidemiologists loaned from the local public health units. This latter situation necessitated constant training of incoming epidemiologists and created some problems with consistency in the work product.[12] But the biggest problem for the Epi Unit leaders concerned the hopelessly antiquated and inappropriate system for reporting data from the province's 37 public health units to the Epi Unit. This Reportable Disease Information System was an outdated computer system that dated from the late 1980s and only worked for specific, known diseases.[13] By the time the Epi Unit was up and running, each public health unit affected by SARS had come up with its own means of recording patient data, using Excel spreadsheets, which they e-mailed to the Epi Unit. There were several problems with this, from the point of view of the Epi Unit. For one, the data were inconsistent from one public health unit to another. Also, the information the unit was trying to record often did not fit the design of the Excel template. For example, a public health unit might list a date of death in a field intended for yes/no information, which made it impossible even to do a simple calculation like a fatality rate without having to count the fatalities manually. In addition, the sheets did not track changes in a

11. *SARS & Public Health in Ontario*, Interim Report, (Problem 13: No Provincial Epidemiology Unit), 2004.

12. Early on, the managers of the Epi Unit tried to get the Ontario Public Health Branch staff to assist the Epi Unit but were turned down on the grounds that the staff was too busy working on other projects. According to the province's later analysis, there was an odd dynamic in play, in which the Epi Unit volunteers were working long hours at a frantic pace, while the Public Health Branch staff worked their usual 8:30 a.m. to 4:30 p.m. schedule at a deliberate and unhurried pace on non-SARS matters.

13. The inadequacy of this system was no secret to the Public Health Branch or to the local public health units. D'Cunha had tried and failed to obtain provincial funding to upgrade it in 2000. A 2003 provincial report had also noted the inadequacy of the system in reporting information about the West Nile virus (2003 Annual Report, Provincial Auditor of Ontario).

patient's condition. Thus, the only way to see, for example, whether the diagnosis of a particular patient had changed from suspect to probable SARS was to rifle through past spreadsheets. Even worse, the sheets did not record enough detail about patients to allow epidemiologists to do the kind of analysis urgently required by SAC and Health Canada. For example, to calculate the incubation period of the disease, the Epi Unit needed to know the date of the patient's exposure and the date of the onset of fever or other symptoms. In some communities, however, the spreadsheets had been set up to give only a yes or a no for a list of symptoms (e.g., fever-yes, cough-no).

In collaboration with Health Canada, therefore, the Epi Unit devoted a great deal of energy, early on, to bringing in the more state-of-the-art Integrated Public Health Information System (iPHIS). The iPHIS system was ready to use in mid-April just when TPH, York, and other public health units were at their busiest, however, and did not feel able to make the switch. What's more, while the iPHIS system would have allowed for better analysis of SARS, it did not have the capacity to track quarantine contacts—an important need for the local public health units. Further, TPH was well along in developing its own system, which TPH leaders insisted would be superior to iPHIS.

In the end, the Epi Unit could not persuade the public health units to switch to iPHIS. Instead, the Epi Unit quietly hired a group of caseworkers to go back out to the community and re-research every SARS case, in order to capture the data the Epi Unit needed—a time-consuming process and one that raised hackles among hospitals and public health units.[14]

THE SCIENCE ADVISORY COMMITTEE AND THE LACK OF DATA

SAC was created out of Young's conviction that Ontario should take advantage of any new discoveries about SARS—gleaned from research scientists or from the behavior of the disease in the outbreak itself. And who better to interpret the new information than a group of infectious disease experts? They would be able to extrapolate from small discoveries to recommend the best possible outbreak policies, Young reasoned.

When Low and others put out a call to infectious disease experts around the country to come and help Ontario, many responded—in some cases, spending weeks away from work and home. After the fact, the provincial analysis of the outbreak would praise the group's good will, camaraderie, and civic-mindedness, but argue that—because SAC was created without the advantage of emergency planning ahead of time—it was created

---

14. The information in this section was largely drawn from the following: *SARS & Public Health in Ontario*, Interim Report (Problem 13: No Provincial Epidemiology Unit; Problem 14: Inadequate Infectious Disease Information Systems), 2004.

without thought to important topics: Should other areas of expertise be represented on the committee, and if so, what areas? Who, exactly, should the committee report to? What kinds of questions should the committee take up—and what kinds not?

Over time, the membership of SAC did broaden to include, in particular, public health doctors and—after some campaigning—primary care physicians, but not without first incurring bad feeling among those left out. One committee member later commented that disease surveillance and epidemiology experts were never well enough represented on the committee. Committee members also expressed confusion over whether they were reporting to Young or D'Cunha, both of whom were members of the committee.

There was additionally some doubt about the purview of SAC and how it should prioritize its tasks. As the post-hoc provincial analysis would later put it, "[T]he Science Committee not only had to answer the questions but had to identify the issues at the outset, prioritize them, and determine who best could help answer the question. [In addition,] the Science Committee quickly became inundated with requests for guidance and information." Thus, for example, in addition to recommending directives to hospitals, the committee was lobbied to send out guidance to long-term care facilities and primary care physicians. A handicap in this regard was the fact that—because the province had never gotten very far with emergency planning for pandemic influenza—SAC did not have the advantage of starting with a set of prototype directives for hospitals and other medical settings that could be tailored for the particulars of the SARS outbreak. They had to start entirely from scratch.

The committee also received questions from hospital administrators, confused about aspects of the directives that had been sent out. Sometimes, the committee was also asked to address questions that were coming in from the media. It was nearly impossible to do everything, and definitely impossible to do everything all at once, though committee members reportedly often put in 14- and 16-hour days.

In addition, except for three or four core members, the SAC members could not serve on the committee for more than a week or so, as they had work and personal demands elsewhere. The turnover meant the continual need to bring new people up to speed, says Sunnybrook's Dr. Brian Schwartz, director of prehospital care, who cochaired SAC from beginning to end. "There was a learning curve—and in an outbreak, you don't have time for that. It might take them two days to figure out what was going on and start contributing—especially if they were from out of the area."

> People would come in from other provinces saying, "Oh, why can't you do it this way?" Which, in a normal environment, is great, but [in this situation] you needed people to just leave that stuff at the door and say, "OK, we'll take it from here."

In addition, Schwartz says, many of the experts had a tendency to offer information in all its complexity but were reluctant to make hard-and-fast recommendations. Schwartz, with his background in emergency medicine, was the person who pushed them to do so. "I was the guy that had to bring closure on a lot of things," he says, "and I was the guy who had to stand up and sometimes take responsibility for things that were less than perfect." It would have been better, he suggests, to establish ahead of time a roster of experts who had agreed to help out in an emergency, and who had received training in the particular nature of decision making in an emergency, and the role of scientific experts in that process.

To the committee members, themselves, the great frustration was the lack of daily-breaking epidemiological data and analysis on which to base their recommendations. "Put yourself in the position we were in, in the second week of April," says Schwartz. "We do not yet know the results of the protection measures [in the hospitals] and the quarantine measures and all the other things we were doing. We don't know whether it's working or not. We still aren't sure whether [SARS transmission] is *airborne*." It was crucial to know, yea or nay, in order to know whether to stay the course or take a new, more draconian approach.

After-the-fact analyses have cited several reasons for the information problem. One was, simply, that the Epi Unit was struggling with insufficiently detailed information in unwieldy form and, thus, the data were often not available or not available in timely fashion. But a further problem was the fact that D'Cunha insisted that he receive all data from the Epi Unit so that he could ensure its accuracy before passing it on. Reportedly, this became quite a bottleneck, though D'Cunha steadfastly denied that it caused any significant delays. He was, however, adamant that his department not release flawed data. At one point, for instance, he explained to the SAC that patients were sometimes double-counted—once in the city or region in which they lived and once in the city or region in which they were hospitalized—and he insisted that such errors be corrected. "One of the things we said was, we'd rather have flawed data than no data," says SAC Cochair Schwartz. "At least we'd have *something* to work with, even if some patients were counted twice. And Dr. D'Cunha's retort was, 'Well, no, we can't do that.'"

When the SAC was able to have direct contact with the Epi Unit, Schwartz added, the exchange was generally very useful. On several occasions, however, D'Cunha directed the Epi Unit leaders to cancel scheduled presentations to the SAC. Such episodes were enraging to the SAC. In mid-April, the SAC wrote an official letter of complaint and, at one point, even threatened to disband. Young and a high-level Health Ministry official tried to intervene to speed up the flow of data to SAC, with mixed results. Says Young, "You see, the problem we ran into is—how do I fix that? They're my committee, but he's got the information. How do I fix that? We tended to find ways to fix it by going around the edges and developing side pathways—stuff that you shouldn't do in an emergency."

In Fact, Many Resort to Side Pathways

The frustration, from many quarters, at not having the newest and best data led to assorted efforts to circumvent the official reporting structure and recreate the data from scratch, leading to some of the most unpleasant tensions in the outbreak response.

One example was the decision of the Epi Unit, frustrated at not getting the detailed information it needed through regular channels, to hire caseworkers to go out and collect all the information they could on the SARS cases again, one at a time. But the Epi Unit was not alone. At various times, D'Cunha's staff, SAC, Health Canada, and POC all ended up calling hospitals, public health units, and even patients or their relatives to get data. Not only did this result in assorted discrepancies in the data, but already overloaded hospitals and public health units were flooded with calls for information on specific cases. Many times, the hospital or public health person who received the calls had never heard of the person who was calling and was reluctant to give out confidential patient information over the phone. But, under increasing pressure from WHO, Health Canada pressured D'Cunha, and D'Cunha, in turn, pressured the Epi Unit staff and his own staff. Sometimes five different people would be asked to get the same information—and all would call the public health unit, insisting that the matter was extremely urgent, and—if the call was not returned within 5 minutes—calling again. Civility was reportedly a casualty of this dogged fight for data. "I had people coming into my office *crying* about being harassed," says TPH's Yaffe.

THE HOSPITALS AND THE PROBLEMATIC DIRECTIVES

According to an article in the *Toronto Star*, the Ontario Health Ministry sent out more than 50 bulletins and directives to hospitals and other medical settings in the course of the outbreak response.[15] The system for developing the directives began with deliberations by SAC. SAC then made a recommendation and passed it to Young, who passed it on to the SARS Operations Centre, which was supposed to take the SAC advice and—in rapid order—write it up as a clear, workable directive. Any big changes were sent to Schwartz or his SAC cochair for approval—then on to Young and D'Cunha for their signatures—up to Health Minister Clement for final approval—then back to the SARS Operations Centre for dissemination.

From the perspective of the hospitals, these directives were cumbersome, confusing, overly long, and overly complicated—not at all what was needed in an emergency—and some members of SAC and the Health Ministry concede the point but say they were

---

15. Karen Palmer, "SARS Bureaucracy Inundates Doctors," *Toronto Star*, June 21, 2003, B01.

doing their best. "As a personal comment, we didn't have the time or the strength to be able to simplify it more than we did," says Schwartz. "The science advisory group was made up of individuals who each had expertise in an area, but had never met as that kind of a group before, and had zero time to be able to exchange knowledge enough so that we could translate the infectious disease expertise into emergency response expertise—and so it came out cumbersome." Even more exasperating to the hospitals was the fact that, based on new information and complaints from the field, SAC and the SARS Operations Centre would reissue directives. The new version would be sent out without summaries of what changes had been made, so hospital personnel had to spend hours wading through them all over again, hunting out the new bits and pieces. The problem, says Stuart, was that there were many changes, scattered all through the documents. In retrospect, Young notes, a simple expedient might have been to highlight the changes, but he adds that in the press of the moment, no one thought to do this. Stuart acknowledges that this made the directives difficult for hospitals to deal with. "But it wasn't done out of malice," she says. "It was a huge amount of work to send out a directive—a *huge* amount of work."

Hospital administrators additionally complained that some of the directives were simply impossible to fulfill. The most obvious example, perhaps, was the decision— included in the province's first batch of directives—to require all hospital personnel to use N95 masks, which offered much better protection against airborne viral particles than did standard surgical masks. The preponderance of evidence suggested that SARS was droplet-spread, but there were enough anecdotal exceptions to this that the group decided to err on the side of caution by mandating the more protective masks.

Unbeknownst to SAC or the Health Ministry, however, there were not enough N95 masks available for all Greater Toronto Area hospital workers to use them. "Once we decided we needed the N95 masks, the reality is, we couldn't get [them]. So the complaints that the hospitals didn't get what they needed—they were legitimate, but there was no way around it," says Schwartz. "It just took some time to get the supply chain revved up to be able to get people the equipment they needed."

Eventually—cleaning out the supply of stored N95 masks all across North America— the hospitals were able to get the masks. But then there was a second problem. The Ontario Labor Ministry required that these particular masks be "fit-tested," an elaborate procedure requiring trained personnel and special testing equipment. SAC and the Health Ministry had not known about this occupational safety requirement when they adopted the directive.

"There was a recognition that, operationally, you just couldn't do this," says Schwartz. But despite these difficulties, he stands by the N95 requirement. "My feeling as a frontliner was—get the damn masks out there. Even if you're not exactly sure how to use it, even if it's not perfectly fit-tested, it will provide you a level of protection. Better than nothing—and better than the surgical masks." Was it fair to require hospitals to do something that was—at least immediately—undoable? Says Schwartz:

> I think it was the idea that people need to be pushed to do what they need to do—and I don't think that anybody was particularly punished for not following the directives—but there had to be a fire lit under them to understand the seriousness of the problem. And, ultimately, people were able to procure the masks, and I think there was some leeway given in terms of fit testing from Labor.

But the fact that, for a time, the provincially required masks were not available to them made some health care workers extremely uneasy, especially as they watched their colleagues with SARS growing sicker and sicker. Some filed union grievances about having to work without the N95 masks.

Former Ontario Chief Medical Officer of Health Schabas argues that the whole notion of sending out detailed directives during the outbreak was benighted from the beginning. "Hospitals are large and complex and, for the most part, very sophisticated organizations," he says.

> [The provincial leaders of the response] were dealing with institutions that in many cases had far more expertise than they did at the [Health] Ministry. Basically, the Ministry's approach was to deal with the hospitals like they were small children: "Here are Our Rules, written down." Of course, it's enormously difficult to write a coherent policy in black and white, yet that's what they tried to do. And of course as a result, they had to change their policies every few *hours* because people found flaws in them.
>
> They should have issued general guidelines and left it to the hospitals how they implemented them—and they should have had the capacity to respond to questions and to troubleshoot. That's not what they did—and so there was tremendous wasted effort, tremendous ill will created between the hospitals and the Ministry.

THE WEEKEND FROM HELL

In the week before Easter Sunday, April 20, the emergency responders endured the two most dispiriting and frightening developments in the outbreak. The first was the discovery of an undetected cluster of SARS cases—not in a hospital, but at large in Toronto.

The Cluster in the Bukas-Loob Sa Diyos Covenant Community

On Friday, April 11, TPH discovered that SARS had been spreading, just outside the radar of the public health surveillance system, within a 500-member, mostly Filipino, charismatic Catholic group called Bukas-Loob Sa Diyos Covenant Community

(BLD). As of April 11, TPH reported, there were 10 probable- and 19 suspect-SARS cases in the BLD. In addition, two community-based doctors who had treated some of these patients had also acquired SARS. Although TPH had been following most of these cases individually, it had taken some time to see the connections among them.

The two cases that began the cluster were those of Eulialo Samson, the man who had, fatefully, gone to the Scarborough-Grace ED on March 16 with a knee injury, and his son, who had accompanied him. There, they had contracted SARS from Rose Pollack, who was sitting nearby in the waiting room. The 82-year-old Samson, who was the patriarch of a large family, had 10 children and dozens of grandchildren. He was not diagnosed with SARS until after his April 1 death, but in the meantime he had infected 17 members of his extended family.

At least one of those family members had attended two large BLD events—a March 28 religious service with 500 people and a March 29 religious retreat with 225. In addition, an April 3 funeral visitation service for Samson had been attended by a combination of BLD members and family members who had been infected with SARS.

At first, TPH authorities tried to identify which BLD members in particular had been exposed to SARS, but they found this impossible to reconstruct, given the large numbers of people at each gathering. By April 13, TPH reluctantly decided it had to quarantine the entire BLD community.[16] But TPH leaders were not confident that they could get the word of the quarantine out to everyone in the BLD fast enough and persuasively enough to avoid a major spread of the disease during Easter weekend, April 18 to 20. All things equal, many BLD members would either visit or host out-of-town family members over Easter. Such visits had the potential to disperse the disease widely. In addition, officials worried that some BLD members might be unwilling to miss services for Easter, the holiest religious holiday in the Catholic faith. They also worried that some of the rites of Easter in Catholic and Protestant churches might facilitate the spread of the disease—for instance, drinking wine from a common cup, giving communion wafers in the mouth, conducting confession in a small confessional stall, kissing the crucifix on Good Friday, widespread shaking of hands in the Salute of Peace.

Health Minister Clement appealed to the local Catholic archbishop for help in encouraging BLD members to observe the quarantine. He also asked the archbishop (and some Protestant church leaders) to substitute bows and other noncontact rituals for the traditional rites. Church leaders pledged their help, but the leaders of the outbreak response were still on tenterhooks. They worried that this could be the moment they had fought hard to avoid—the moment when a disease that was still traceable, and therefore still controllable, spilled out of control. "We were on the precipice," says Clement. "We were on the razor's edge."

---

16. Public health officials and BLD leaders worried that BLD, in particular, and Filipinos, in general, might be stigmatized as a result of the quarantine. Already, Toronto's Chinese community was suffering from a mistaken impression that SARS was widespread among Chinese-Canadians. Chinese restaurants were experiencing a pronounced drop in business, although in mid-April political leaders began to make a show of eating in them in an effort to persuade citizens of their safety.

The Sunnybrook Intubation Fiasco

In the midst of the BLD anxiety, the leaders of the emergency response learned, to their horror, that at the Sunnybrook hospital, 11 health care workers—who had taken pains to follow infection control precautions carefully—had all contracted SARS during a particularly difficult intubation procedure. Intubation in this context refers to the insertion of a tube down a patient's trachea to clear the airway.

On April 8, Nestor Yanga, a 54-year-old family doctor who contracted SARS from one of his patients at the Lapsley Family Clinic, had been admitted to Sunnybrook. By April 12, his condition had deteriorated, and he was having extreme difficulty breathing. Hospital staff moved him to the ICU and placed a bilevel positive airway pressure (BiPAP) mask over his face, but he kept pulling it off to cough. They therefore tried to intubate Yanga, but secretions rose up from his lungs, blocking the tube. The tube had to be removed and drained, then reinserted—all in the rushed atmosphere of a respiratory emergency. Doctors speculate that the combination of the techniques and the circumstances led to the aerosolization of the patient's secretions, which increased the virus's ability to spread. In addition, the procedure took place in crowded quarters and lasted 4 hours in all.

Still, the doctors, nurses, respiratory technicians, and other health care workers present had worn the requisite N95 masks, goggles, gloves, and gowns. Three days later, they began to get sick and by the end of the Easter weekend, four were diagnosed with probable SARS and another eight with suspect SARS. On April 20, Sunnybrook closed its ED and ICU for 10 days. This was a blow to morale in the medical community, as Sunnybrook was a flagship hospital with the largest trauma center in Canada. It had played a leadership role in the outbreak and had treated about half of the area's SARS patients.

To the SAC advisors, the episode was especially devastating. They had banked on the idea that these precautions were—if anything—cautious to a fault and that they would be utterly reliable at protecting health care workers. At this point, they began to fear that there might be *nothing* that health care workers could do to keep safe. "We thought we'd see health care workers walk out of the hospitals—because we weren't protecting them," says Low. "They were getting SARS even though we were using precautions. That was a dark time."

BRACING FOR THE WORST-CASE SCENARIO

At the least, the BLD outbreak demonstrated that Toronto's contact tracing and quarantine efforts were not foolproof. And the Sunnybrook episode demonstrated that the new hospital safeguards were not foolproof either. Were these cases aberrations, or was the emergency response, more broadly, failing to stop SARS? The data that would answer that question were not yet available. Thus, on April 22, Health Minister Clement called a meeting with SAC to ask the scientific experts a distressing question: If their best efforts failed, if SARS continued to spread, what was the worst-case scenario? What dire and extreme choices might he and Premier Eves be forced to face? "I wanted to know how bad this could get," he says. "You hope for the best, but plan for the worst—that was my motto during this whole thing."

SAC laid out a shocking picture. Under the worst-case scenario, SARS would turn out to be a highly contagious disease, impossible to contain, that would begin spreading uncontrolled in the community. The very worst-case scenario—it would eventually infect everyone. Given the projections at the time of a 10% mortality rate, that would mean one million people dead in Ontario and three million dead in Canada before the virus burned itself out.

In terms of the government response—if the disease began spreading out of control in the Toronto area, the government might have to close down all nonessential venues for public mixing, by shutting movie theaters, for instance, or canceling ball games. Worst-case scenario—the province might have to quarantine the entire Greater Toronto Area in an effort to save the rest of Ontario and Canada.

A SIGH OF RELIEF

Once Toronto had gotten past the Easter weekend, however, the situation brightened considerably. In fact, the BLD community did comply with the city's quarantine order; the outbreak did not, after all, slip out of control.

Nor did health care workers walk out en masse. SAC members and provincial authorities candidly expressed their distress and bewilderment at the fact that health care workers were still getting SARS and vowed to redouble their efforts to understand why. In support of that effort, Health Canada requested assistance from CDC.[17]

At SAC's recommendation, the province issued new protective regulations—for example, the use of face shields in place of goggles and double gloves, double gowns, and double masks when caring for SARS patients, so that the top layer could be shed as the worker left the patient's room. They stopped short of mandating Stryker "space" suits for high-risk procedures such as intubation, suctioning, bronchoscopy, or the use of BiPAP masks. These suits, which resembled the suits worn by astronauts, entirely enclosed the worker and provided him or her with a special protective air filter. But they were hot, unwieldy, and reportedly took about 3 minutes to put on—far too long in a respiratory emergency, some experts argued. In the wake of its own intubation disaster, however, Sunnybrook did require its own staff to use the Stryker suits for high-risk procedures on SARS patients.

The best news, though, was that data were now available that indicated that in the past two weeks, there had been only one new case identified as probable or suspect SARS

---

17. Nothing conclusive came out of the CDC consultation, but CDC did heighten SAC's consciousness about the importance of removing protective clothing correctly to avoid becoming infected from the protective gear itself. CDC recommended removing the gear in a strict order, interspersed with frequent handwashing.

in the Greater Toronto Area. The outbreak seemed to be dying out; the end was in sight. The emergency response group heaved a collective sigh of relief. But not for long.

BLINDSIDED: THE WORLD HEALTH ORGANIZATION CAUTIONS AGAINST TRAVEL TO TORONTO

On Wednesday, April 23, WHO issued a global advisory against all nonessential travel to the City of Toronto. Although WHO officials insisted that Canada's federal leaders should have seen this coming, local and provincial health officials were dumbfounded. *Why*—when SARS had been almost entirely confined to Toronto-area hospitals? And why *now*—when the outbreak was nearly over? "The day they called it, we knew we had it under control," says Young.

WHO had issued SARS travel advisories to only four other cities or regions—Hong Kong, Beijing, and two provinces in Mainland China—Guangdong and Shanxi. Although the purpose of the alerts was pragmatic—to minimize the spread of SARS to other regions and to other nations—any city or region named in such an alert regarded it as a tremendous blow, sure to exact a heavy penalty in lost revenue from foreign visitors.

What's more, for a wealthy industrial nation like Canada, inclusion in a WHO travel advisory was a significant embarrassment. The government of such a nation was expected to have the public health sophistication to rein in infectious diseases expeditiously. After all, Canada was on a short-list of countries that, by many widely accepted measures, offered the best quality health care in the world. Canada was accustomed to *advising* WHO, not receiving its injunctions. And within Canada, Toronto was no Podunk outpost; it was the nation's largest city—its lively, thriving, cosmopolitan economic center. How, officials wondered, could Toronto be placed in the same category as the province of Guangdong in China?

COMPLAINTS ABOUT POLITICAL LEADERSHIP

The fury and indignation of the health authorities upon learning of the WHO travel advisory were immediately joined by the fury and indignation of local, provincial, and federal politicians of every stripe. "I've never been so angry in all my life," said Toronto Mayor Mel Lastman. "Let me be clear: It's safe to live in Toronto.... It's safe to visit this city.... This isn't a city in the grips of fear and panic."[18] Federal Health Minister Anne McLellan telephoned WHO Director General Gro Harlem Brundtland to argue that the advisory was unwarranted and should be rescinded immediately. Brundtland refused to do that but did agree to listen to Canada's arguments at a WHO review of the decision

---

18. Nicolaas van Rijn, "Britain Warns Its Citizens Not to Travel to Toronto," *Toronto Star*, April 24, 2003, A1.

the following week.[19] The next day, Canadian Prime Minister Jean Chretien called Brundtland, personally, to reiterate McLellan's call for an immediate end to the advisory. He also put in a similar call to the Deputy Secretary-General of the United Nations, Louise Frechette.[20] (WHO and the United Nations stuck to their guns, however, and WHO Communicable Disease Director David Heymann would later call Canada's April lobbying effort "very inappropriate."[21])

But the sudden visibility of political leaders seemed to remind local reporters of their prior invisibility. Except for Ontario Health Minister Tony Clement, elected leaders had played almost no role during the first month of SARS. Chretien, followed by other federal officials and later by Ontario Premier Eves, did troop, one by one, into Toronto's Chinatown in the second and third weeks of April to eat in local restaurants and assure a jittery public that these establishments were perfectly safe. But reporters observed pointedly that during the darkest hours of the SARS outbreak—when the leaders of the emergency response had been sick with worry at the thought of an uncontrolled community outbreak and/or an angry walk-out by health care workers, and when the Ontario Health Minister had been facing the frightening implications of a SARS "worst-case scenario"— the top political leaders of the city, the province, and the country were nowhere to be found. Where had they *been*? the reporters asked.

The answer, it turned out, was that, during Easter week, Prime Minister Chretien had been in the Dominican Republic on a golfing holiday. The parliament was likewise in vacation mode, enjoying the Easter recess. Ontario Premier Ernie Eves was golfing in Arizona and had, since the start of the outbreak, not deemed SARS the kind of emergency that required the interruption of the Ontario legislature's four-month recess. Toronto Mayor Mel Lastman had been receiving arduous medical treatment for hepatitis C, which made him a more sympathetic figure, but in the course of excoriating the WHO travel advisory, Lastman mortified partisans and enemies alike by appearing frankly befuddled on international news broadcasts. For example, ABC News aired the following exchange with reporters:

> Mayor Lastman: What I'm doing right here, right now, is sending out a message to this CDC group, whoever the hell they are.
> Reporters: The WHO.
> Lastman: Who?
> Reporters: The WHO.
> Lastman: The WHO. Sorry. Well, who's the CDC?
> Reporters: The Centers for Disease Control.
> Lastman: Okay, the WHO.

19. Tim Naumetz and Joan Bryden, "WHO Won't Back Down on Warning," *Ottawa Citizen*, April 25, 2003, A1.
20. Valerie Lawton and Les Whittington, "Chretien Wants to Show Toronto Is Safe," *Toronto Star*, April 26, 2003, A14.
21. Martin Regg Cohn, "WHO Rebukes Canada for SARS Lobby," *Toronto Star*, June 17, 2003, A1.

Though later briefed by his staff, Lastman made another gaffe on a subsequent and more widely disseminated CNN broadcast. Apparently trying to diminish the stature of WHO, the mayor remarked, "I don't know who this group is. I've never heard of them before." The tactic, if such it was, backfired. "There's a vastly greater chance of dying from embarrassment in this city over the performance of our political leaders than there is from succumbing to SARS," wrote *Toronto Star* columnist Jim Coyle on April 26, 2003. With respect to Lastman, in particular, Coyle continued, "To admit, as he has, to not even knowing what WHO is demonstrated a degree of ignorance inconceivable in any newspaper-reading adult. For that admission to come from the leader of a cosmopolitan metropolis is mind-boggling. To have gone on CNN and admitted as much is just plain stupid—a credibility-destroyer that was total."

On April 30, another *Star* columnist, James Royson, described the prime minister, premier, and mayor, collectively, as "lame," "lax," and "lethargic." "The SARS outbreak is a classic case of How Not to Handle a Crisis."

For their part, the politicians insisted that they had been taking the high road by stepping back and letting the professionals handle the situation—that they did not want to exploit SARS for political capital, nor did they want to increase public alarm. In fact, their biggest role would come later, with a partisan federal versus provincial (and Liberal versus Tory, respectively) tussle over who was going to foot the bill for the SARS emergency response and how much of the economic loss suffered by individual citizens, businesses, and hospitals in the Greater Toronto Area would be offset by government spending in some form or other.

THE CAVALRY RIDES TO GENEVA

After receiving Canada's enraged response to its Toronto travel advisory, WHO did agree to hear an appeal of its decision on April 30, and Canada sent a delegation to Geneva, headed by Ontario Health Minister Clement. In addition to Clement, the delegation included Ontario Public Health Commissioner D'Cunha, Toronto Communicable Disease Control Director Yaffe, and two federal officials—a political assistant to the federal health minister and the ambassador to WHO and the World Trade Organization.

The delegation came armed with facts and figures and suggested that WHO had probably not seen the best and most current data from Toronto and thus did not understand that SARS was well in-hand in the city; there had been no new transmissions of the disease in the last 10 days. Clement recalls, "When we gave them the numbers on the decline in new cases, and when we gave them the information on how we were handling the cases in the hospitals, what they said to us was, 'OK, what about the border issue?'"

The Border Issue

Clement says that it rapidly became clear to the delegation that WHO's primary concern with respect to SARS was to prevent the disease from traveling to developing countries that had little public health infrastructure. WHO's sudden focus on Toronto, in fact, may have resulted from the claim of the Philippine government that Adela Catalon had brought SARS to Manila from Toronto, setting off a panic reaction in the areas she visited. (Whether Catalon really had SARS was in sharp dispute at that time, and the question was never completely resolved, though TPH did eventually find a clinical link between Catalon and other SARS patients in Toronto.)

On March 27, well before the Catalon incident, WHO had called upon the federal government in Canada to institute health screening of all passengers aboard international flights out of Toronto's Pearson International Airport. Ontario officials had urged their federal counterparts to comply, but federal officials were reportedly not convinced of the efficacy of airport screening. Instead, they arranged for the distribution of information cards at the airport, asking passengers with SARS symptoms to put off traveling and see a physician. To WHO—which favored the use of questionnaires to identify potential SARS carriers along with infrared scanners to detect passengers traveling with a fever—the Canadian information cards were anemic indeed. "They said, 'Why are Singapore and Taiwan doing x, y, and z, including infrared scanning, and why are you doing nothing?'" Clement recalls. "'Why are we getting better compliance on border control from Asia than we are from North America?'"

From Geneva, Clement and his delegation colleagues were able to broker a deal. Health Canada committed itself to carrying out a set of specific, robust airport screening measures, including infrared scanning, and WHO rescinded its advisory on April 30—one week after issuing it. The advisory would otherwise have lasted three weeks.

IT'S OVER!

Back in Toronto, meanwhile, leaders of the emergency response to SARS were worn out, dispirited by the WHO advisory, and eager to put this difficult chapter behind them. Luckily, the prospects of doing so appeared promising: There had been 10 consecutive days without a new probable-SARS case. Once the city had gone 20 consecutive days without a case—two incubation periods—the epidemiologists believed it would be safe to declare the outbreak at an end.

They waited, impatiently, for the next 10 days to tick by without event. On May 9, Toronto's Basrur jubilantly told the press that the outbreak was over. On May 14, WHO removed Toronto from its list of areas with recent local transmission. On May 17, Ontario Premier Eves formally ended the province's declared emergency and dismantled the

Provincial Operations Centre. That same day, the Ontario Health Ministry ended Code Orange for Greater Toronto hospitals, so they could return to their full complement of health care services. But the post-SARS celebration was to be brief.

FALLING APART BEFORE OUR EYES

On Friday, May 18, Maurice Buckner, a 57-year-old double-lung transplant recipient at St. John's Rehabilitation Hospital, went home for the Victoria Day long weekend. Almost immediately, he became feverish and exhausted. In alarm, his wife took him to the ED of the Toronto General Hospital. Doctors there stabilized him and sent him back to St. John's, where he developed pneumonia symptoms. But one Toronto General doctor, fearing SARS, ordered a bronchoscopy and tested Buckner's respiratory secretions for signs of the SARS virus. On May 22, that test came back positive. When TPH received this grim report, it sent an envoy to St. John's posthaste. In dismay, the TPH doctors discovered a cluster of four patients with probable SARS.

At 9 p.m. that night, according to the Canada Press, "a clutch of ashen-faced public health officials" gathered at the headquarters of TPH to report this dispiriting piece of news to the public.[22] They did not yet have the answer to the crucial public health question: where had this cluster come from?

At first, public health workers held out the hope that the St. John's outbreak would turn out to be a small and isolated incident, easily contained. They learned that Kitty Chan, the mother of St. John's leg surgery patient Hubert Chan, had recently returned with her husband from a trip to Hong Kong, where the couple spent part of each year. Both Kitty Chan and Hubert Chan were now sick with probable SARS. Had Kitty brought SARS back from Hong Kong and infected her son, who had, in turn, passed the disease to others at St. John's? TPH wondered. But the answer was no. Kitty Chan and her husband had returned from Hong Kong on April 22 and had immediately placed themselves in a 10-day self-quarantine, just to be on the safe side. After that, they went to visit their son who was at the time at North York General Hospital. On May 9, he was transferred to St. John's. On Mother's Day, May 11, Kitty Chan visited him there. Over the next two or three days, both Kitty and Hubert became feverish and weak with respiratory symptoms. Kitty Chan was admitted to Centennial Hospital soon thereafter.

Another of the St. John's SARS cluster had also been a patient in North York's orthopedic ward. On May 23, two TPH doctors and Low headed to North York General and asked to look at the medical charts of all the pneumonia patients. They soon discovered that there were a large number of pneumonia cases—perhaps 20—clustered in the orthopedic ward. Even as they sat in North York General, poring over the charts, they learned that members of the hospital staff had just turned up in the ED with suspicious symptoms. It was all too

---

22. Canadian Press, "Strange Twists During SARS Four-Month Outbreak," July 6, 2003.

familiar. "The day we sat in that conference room, I remember, it was really quite surreal, because things were falling apart before our eyes," Low recalls. That night, at TPH's instigation, North York General closed down. TPH announced that anyone who had visited St. John's between May 9 and May 20, or North York between May 13 and May 23 must go into quarantine. The outbreak was back.

SARS II

Call it SARS II or call it the moment when Toronto realized that SARS I had never actually ended—either way, the second go-round of the outbreak had a very different character from the first. "Phase One was sort of a rah-rah kind of outbreak," says Low. "And Phase Two—everybody was sick of it. They didn't want it. It was a mistake. People were fed up with SARS. It was a failure. It was a very different atmosphere than the first wave."

For all that, the actual containment of the second outbreak was smoother and more efficient than the first, public health experts agree. Working with better information about SARS and having learned from the experience of SARS I, hospitals and their workers had clearer protocols from the start—and so did public health departments. In fact, once the second outbreak was detected, it took only one week to halt nearly all transmission of the disease. WHO removed Toronto from its list of active SARS outbreak areas on July 2. But 118 people became sick during SARS II and 13 of them died. Thus, the city was much occupied with figuring out what had gone wrong—what had allowed the resurgence of SARS when it had been all but extinguished in late April.

By mid-June, with the help of epidemiologists from CDC, Toronto Public Health doctors believed they had worked out the basics of the link between SARS I and SARS II, though some of the particulars remained a mystery. According to the CDC report, the chain of infection went all the way back to Tse, who had passed the disease to James Dougherty, the cardiology patient who had spent the night of March 7 on a gurney near Tse's in the Scarborough-Grace ED. When Dougherty was readmitted to Scarborough-Grace on March 14 with a heart attack, he spent two days in the Scarborough-Grace cardiac unit, without being recognized as a SARS patient and without being isolated. There he is believed to have passed SARS to a female heart patient, who returned home on March 17, where she developed respiratory symptoms but was never diagnosed with SARS. She passed the virus to her daughter who was a nurse at North York General. The nurse began to feel sick on March 30 but did not immediately stop working. CDC is not sure how she could have come into contact with Lewis Huppert, a 99-year-old North York patient with a fractured pelvis, as she was not assigned to his ward. But epidemiologists believe that, somehow, she did pass the disease to him.

Huppert developed pneumonia symptoms on April 2, but doctors assumed he had aspiration pneumonia—common to elderly, bedridden patients. Especially confusing,

Huppert's symptoms seemed to abate when he was given a round of antibiotics.[23] By April 19, however, he was worse again, with a fever and diarrhea. On May 1, Huppert died. Meanwhile, other patients in the orthopedic ward began to develop pneumonia symptoms. So, too, did Huppert's wife, daughter, son-in-law, and granddaughter—all of whom came, at some point, to the North York ED as patients. None of the four was diagnosed with SARS, and none was hospitalized.

A junior doctor at North York and a number of nurses were convinced that the family had SARS, however. They finally insisted on a meeting with hospital management on May 20 to press the issue. North York's management team reportedly tried to calm the group and repeated the common wisdom that the SARS outbreak was over.

Political Pressure?

Once the news of the missed SARS cluster became public, there was much public speculation about whether the WHO travel advisory had led to direct or understood political pressure on doctors, hospitals, and public health personnel not to "find" any more SARS cases. For one thing, the WHO's travel advisory had resulted in an abrupt shift in public rhetoric about SARS. Before the advisory, the rhetoric had consisted of (some said alarmist) warnings to the public and exhortations to stay home if suffering from flu-type symptoms. Afterward, the rhetoric was reassuring and stressed that the outbreak was well in hand and the city safe. Some remarked wryly that the city and province had gone directly from panic to denial with no stop in between.

What's more, a late May dustup over Health Canada's diagnostic criteria for SARS enhanced the picture of a nation trying to minimize its SARS profile through a bit of fancy footwork. The issue erupted when Low and TPH doctors were deciding how to diagnose the cluster of cases at North York General in late May. The dilemma was whether they should be labeled probable SARS or suspect SARS. In terms of stopping the spread of the disease, this distinction did not matter, as all the cases would be isolated and handled with the same barrier infection precautions. But only the probable-SARS tally was reported to WHO. Infectious disease and public health doctors had actually paid little attention to the Health Canada definition until mid-April, when D'Cunha had begun pushing for a more exacting diagnosis of SARS, in an effort to cut down on the false-positive diagnoses of the disease. But the Health Canada definition of probable SARS was stricter than the WHO definition and, in Low's opinion, stricter in a way that made no sense.[24]

---

23. Antibiotics should have no effect on a viral disease like SARS.
24. The Health Canada definition required a clinical finding of severe progressive pneumonia, while the WHO definition required only an x-ray finding of pneumonia or respiratory distress syndrome.

When asked by a radio journalist to characterize the scope of the North York outbreak, on May 28, Low publicly criticized the Health Canada definition, arguing that it led to a significant undercount of probable-SARS cases. "There was no question what was going on—yet when you went through the Health Canada definition, nobody fit the definition," he says. "They were all 'suspect.' In the first wave, we would have called them all [probable] cases." He had spoken out of frustration but was stunned when his comments set off an international media uproar. WHO expressed indignation at being given a deceptively low SARS "count" from Canada. Health Canada expressed indignation at Low, saying that this was the first the agency had heard of the problem. "By the end of the day, I was ready to leave town," Low recalls. "But within 24 hours, Health Canada had changed the definition," he adds, bringing it in line with the WHO language. Under the new definition, there were not just a handful but 43 probable-SARS cases in Greater Toronto.

Infectious disease experts and public health doctors at all levels of government resolutely insist that there was no political pressure not to find SARS cases after the WHO advisory. "It is an urban myth. It did not occur," says Young. Yaffe says that, for its part, TPH "remained vigilant for any new cases of SARS and did not let down our guard." In the case of hospital physicians, the pressure not to find SARS cases—to the extent that it existed—was subtle and internal, according to Low. "I don't think anybody tried to hide a case they thought in their hearts was SARS," he says. But, for all kinds of reasons, doctors ardently wanted to believe that SARS had gone for good. And, given the general nature of SARS symptoms and the prevalence of pneumonia among hospital patients, it was not difficult to find ample evidence for an alternate diagnosis. There was a climate, he explains, in which "subconsciously, people were more apt to say no as opposed to yes."

Exit Strategy

None of that would have mattered though if Ontario had consciously developed an outbreak exit strategy back in April, Low continues, voicing the common wisdom of the emergency responders. On May 14, the day WHO removed Toronto from the list of areas with local SARS transmission, "everybody should have gone into their hospitals and identified everybody over the next week that had febrile respiratory illness with pneumonia. [You then assume] that person has SARS until proven otherwise, and therefore you don't allow [any further] transmission to occur."

This was, more or less, what happened at the end of SARS II, though Low says that the second time around, the province and the hospitals erred on the side of extreme caution. Many precautions remained in place long after the threat of SARS had passed. "We just kept everything in place until there was absolutely no possible way in the world that we could ever have missed a case. And then," he adds, "we added a buffer of two to three months."

Exhibit 5B-1. Chronology of Events: 2003 Toronto SARS Outbreak

March 26
- Ontario Premier Ernie Eves declares a provincial emergency.

March 27
- On the recommendation of an ad hoc group of frontline public health and infectious disease experts, the Ontario Health Ministry requires all Greater Toronto hospitals to invoke their Code Orange emergency plans, closing down the hospitals to all but essential care. The Ministry also issues a set of directives to the hospitals for improving infection controls.
- Public Safety Commissioner Jim Young creates a SARS Operations Centre within the Health Ministry to translate the hospital policy recommendations of the Science Advisory Committee into hospital directives.
- Young asks Donald Low, microbiologist-in-chief at Mt. Sinai Hospital, and others to recruit infectious disease experts from across Canada to form a Science Advisory Committee.
- WHO calls on Health Canada to institute health screening of all passengers aboard international flights out of Toronto's Pearson International Airport.

March 28
- York Central Hospital discovers that James Dougherty, an undetected SARS patient, spent 12 days in its hospital without being isolated. York Central closes its emergency department and intensive care unit and sends 3,000 staff, patients, and visitors into quarantine.n
- A person with undiagnosed SARS attends a religious service of the Bukas-Loob Sa Diyos Covenant Community, a mostly Filipino religious group, where 500 people had gathered.

March 29
- A person with undiagnosed SARS attends a Bukas-Loob Sa Diyos Covenant Community religious retreat attended by 225 people.

March 31
- Ontario extends infection control directives (but not Code Orange) to all Ontario acute care hospitals.
- Colin D'Cunha, Ontario Chief Medical Officer of Health, asks Bill Mindell, Medical Officer of Health in the York Region, to create a temporary Epi Unit in the Ontario Public Health Branch.

April 2
- Experts believe Lewis Huppert, 99, a patient at North York Hospital, had SARS and not aspiration pneumonia, as doctors had initially believed.

April 11
- Toronto Public Health discovers SARS spreading within the Bukas-Loob Sa Diyos Covenant Community.

April 12
- Eleven health care workers at Sunnybrook and Women's Health Care Centre are infected with SARS during a difficult intubation procedure. They begin to show symptoms on April 15.

April 13
- Toronto Public Health quarantines the entire Bukas-Loob Sa Diyos Covenant Community.

April 20
- Sunnybrook Hospital closes its emergency department and intensive care unit for 10 days.

April 23
- WHO issues a worldwide advisory warning against nonessential travel to Toronto.

April 30
- A delegation of health officials from Toronto, Ontario, and Canada meets with WHO officials in Geneva to try to persuade them to rescind the travel advisory. Canada agrees to put in place rigorous airport screening of passengers traveling internationally and WHO agrees to lift the advisory.

May 9
- Toronto Public Health declares the SARS outbreak over.

May 14
- WHO removes Toronto from its list of areas with active SARS transmission.

(Continued)

Exhibit 5B-1. (Continued)

May 17
- Ontario Premier Eves ends the province's formal emergency.

May 20
- A group of North York General nurses and other health care workers holds a meeting with hospital management expressing concern over a possible SARS cluster in the hospital.

May 22
- Maurice Buckner, 57, a patient at St. John's Rehabilitation Hospital, tests positive for the SARS virus. Toronto Public Health doctors diagnose three other St. John's patients with probable SARS. Toronto and Ontario public health officials announce the cluster of four cases.

May 23
- Toronto Public Health and Mt. Sinai's Low discover a large cluster of patients with suspect or probable SARS at North York General.

May 28
- Low publicly criticizes the Health Canada definition of probable SARS, saying it leads to a pronounced undercount vis-à-vis the WHO definition.

May 29
- Health Canada brings its definition of probable SARS in line with the WHO definition.

July 2
- WHO once again removes Toronto from the list of areas with active SARS transmission.

Exhibit 5B-2. Cast of Characters: 2003 Toronto SARS Outbreak

Public Officials in Spring 2003

- Sheela Basrur, MD, Toronto Medical Officer of Health
- Tony Clement, Ontario Minister of Health and Long-Term Care
- Colin D'Cunha, MD, Ontario Chief Medical Officer of Health and Public Health Commissioner
- Ernie Eves, Ontario Premier
- Bill Mindell, MD, York Region Medical Officer of Health
- Allison Stuart, Ontario Health and Long-Term Care Ministry's Hospitals Division Director
- Barbara Yaffe, MD, Toronto Public Health Communicable Disease Control Director
- Jim Young, MD, Ontario Public Safety Commissioner

Medical Experts

- David Heymann, MD, World Health Organization Communicable Disease Director
- Ian Johnson, MD, University of Toronto Professor of Public Health and the Epi Unit's Epidemiology Director
- Donald Low, MD, Mt. Sinai Microbiologist-in-Chief
- Allison McGeer, MD, Mt. Sinai Infection Control Director
- Richard Schabas, MD, former Ontario Chief Medical Officer of Health and York Central Hospital Chief of Staff
- Brian Schwartz, MD, Science Advisory Committee Cochair and Sunnybrook Prehospital Care Director

SARS Patients

- Kwan Sui-chu, 78
- Liu Jian Lun, 64
- Tse Chi Kwai, 43
- Joseph Pollack, 76
- Rose Pollack, 73
- James Dougherty, 77
- Adela Catalon, 46
- Eulialo Samson, 82
- Nestor Yanga, 54
- Maurice Buckner, 57
- Kitty Chan, 66
- Hubert Chan, 44
- Lewis Huppert, 99

Emergency Response System Under Duress: The Public Health Fight to Contain SARS in Toronto (Epilogue)

Pamela Varley

INTRODUCTION

Severe acute respiratory syndrome (SARS) infected and killed more people in Toronto than it did anywhere else in the western industrialized world. The disease was brought to heel in Toronto later than in any other country in the world but Taiwan. However, there are mixed views about whether the emergency response mounted by Ontario and the Greater Toronto Area was fundamentally a success, or fundamentally a failure, and why. "You would have thought that of all the cities that were hit by SARS, that Toronto was the one that should have handled it the best," says Dr. Richard Schabas, the former provincial chief medical officer of health and prominent critic of the government's response to the SARS outbreak. "In fact, you can make the argument that maybe we handled it the worst." The heart of Toronto's problem, he claims, was a series of wrongheaded decisions and judgments by the leaders of the outbreak response.

Federal and provincial postmortem analyses of the Toronto SARS outbreak painted a different picture—one of a system under significant duress because of a 20-year

This case was written by Pamela Varley, case writer at the John F. Kennedy School of Government, Harvard University, for Dr. Arnold M. Howitt, Executive Director, Taubman Center for State and Local Government, Harvard University. It was funded by Harvard's National Preparedness Leadership Initiative, a project of the Centers for Disease Control and Prevention, US Department of Health and Human Services, and by a grant from the Robert Wood Johnson Foundation. (0505)

erosion of investment in the public health system and because, as a consequence, many building blocks of an effective emergency response were not in place when SARS hit the city. These reports praised the Herculean efforts of the city, provincial, and medical community but called for extensive improvements in the country's public health infrastructure.

No matter what the ultimate assessment, it was unnerving for observers of the outbreak response to realize that, at the end of the day, SARS was only moderately contagious compared to other communicable diseases. If the local, provincial, and federal governments had struggled this hard to control a moderately infectious disease in Toronto, how would they fare in the face of something more deadly and more infectious—a true pandemic, say, or bioterror attack?

OPPOSING ASSESSMENTS

Even granting that Toronto had a heavy dose of bad luck in facing the SARS virus before the world was on-guard against the disease, almost everyone involved in the SARS outbreak in Toronto, Ontario, and Canada acknowledges that aspects of the emergency response went awry. Learning the right lessons from the Toronto SARS outbreak, however, was tricky. Mistakes and lapses were made at every level—due in part to poor or partial information. Doctors missed SARS cases when they mistook them for different kinds of pneumonia. People who had been exposed to SARS were sometimes contacted too late to keep them from spreading the disease. Doctors, bureaucrats, and politicians wanted to believe the SARS outbreak was over before it was. Were these errors at the heart of what went wrong—or were systemic problems with preparedness at the heart?

The Schabas Critique

For his part, Schabas believes that common-sense leadership judgments, rather than—for example—a lack of sophisticated epidemiological systems, was at the heart of the difficulty. His has been a sometimes-abrasive and sometimes-lonely voice of criticism in Toronto, and some have questioned his credibility, as he has a track record of criticizing the Progressive Conservative Party, which was in control of Ontario government during the SARS outbreak. But even his detractors have admitted that he has made some good points. For example, there is general agreement with Schabas's argument that at the apparent "end" of SARS I, all Toronto-area hospitals should have instituted a "pneumonia surveillance protocol," observing strict infection controls and closely watching every pneumonia case to be sure there was no stealth case of SARS in the system that could rise up to continue the outbreak. In other respects, though, Schabas's views were controversial and some dismiss them out of hand. They do, however, make a provocative counterpoint to the conventional wisdom.

To Schabas, the emergency response lacked a certain steady-minded common sense. At first, he says, there was an underreaction in the failure to follow the common-sense precaution of halting all patient transfers out of Scarborough-Grace Hospital as soon as it was clear that a patient with an unknown, virulent disease was being treated there. Then, he says, there was a wild overreaction in the decision to close down the hospital system and institute mass quarantine, setting off "public panic." Both those initiatives were so draconian and exhausting that people did not have the energy or clarity to focus in on the few things that were really most important, he says. "All you need to stop SARS is to identify cases, put them in private rooms, and nurse them with a mask," he says.

Schabas's critics say that his arguments are willfully simplistic, on the one hand, and reflect the advantage of 20/20 hindsight, on the other. At the time, they did not know how contagious SARS was, or the circumstances under which it would spread. Yes, in retrospect, it turned out that it was not very contagious and that it was mostly droplet-spread by people in hospitals. True that, ultimately, there was little community spread. *But there might have been.* And the responders say they had to act on that possibility. Says Ontario Public Safety Commissioner Jim Young, codirector of the provincial response to the SARS outbreak, "Intuitively, he may have been right, but I don't make any apologies. Richard was on one side saying, 'This isn't the pandemic.' There were others coming to me and saying, 'It is.' When you're in the middle of something like this, you're getting contrary advice from different people. I didn't feel that we could take the chance."

Schabas counters, though, that simply by graphing the incidence of new cases—creating an epi curve—the responders should have been able to see pretty quickly that SARS was not terribly contagious. "The fundamental problem, in my view, was that people jumped to conclusions about SARS," he says.

> From the very beginning, there was this perception that this was a highly infectious pandemic disease that was going to spread like wildfire around the world. All efforts were put into, quote, "controlling this disease"—forgetting the fact that if it *was* a highly infectious disease, we didn't have a hope in hell of controlling it. But they did not put sufficient effort into understanding what was going on—into challenging their basic assumptions about this disease and collecting and analyzing the data. They were just too busy.

Basically, he says, there were just two critically important pieces of data: the date that each diagnosed probable SARS patient got sick and the likely route of transmission. "There were about 150 SARS patients in SARS I—maybe 200 if you count the suspect cases," he says. With two pieces of data for each case—that's a total of 300 pieces of data, he continues. "You need a piece of graph paper and four colored pencils—I'm not kidding. You don't need an information system. Infectious disease epidemiology is not rocket science. It's really not." By about April 10, he says, the pattern was clear enough to

Schabas himself that he sat down and wrote an editorial arguing that the reaction to SARS was overblown—that the disease was not terribly infectious, after all. As a confirming piece of evidence, he adds, Hanoi brought its outbreak under control quickly, and its epi curve was "up on the WHO Web site by the end of March."

> Hanoi had a nice curve that went up and came down, and it was over. And I said to people, "If you can control an infectious disease in Hanoi, I mean, how hard can it be?" And I'm not being disparaging to the Vietnamese. It's true.

The Government-Sponsored Reports

Meanwhile, both the federal government of Canada and the provincial government of Ontario commissioned after-the-fact studies of the emergency response to SARS in order to learn for the future and, in the case of the Ontario study, to identify the things that went wrong and led to SARS II.

Federal Health Minister Anne McLellan established the National Advisory Committee on SARS and Public Health under the leadership of David Naylor, dean of medicine at the University of Toronto, in May 2003. The report of that committee, titled "Learning From SARS,"[1] summarized the committee's viewpoint as follows:

> The SARS story as it unfolded in Canada had both tragic and heroic elements. Although the toll of the epidemic was substantial, thousands in the health field rose to the occasion and ultimately contained the SARS outbreak in this country, notwithstanding systems and resources that were manifestly sub optimal. The challenge now is to ensure not only that we are better prepared for the next epidemic, but that public health in Canada is broadly renewed, so as to protect and promote the health of all our present and future citizens.

The committee made 75 recommendations in all. The biggest was to call for the creation of a Canadian Agency for Public Health—a sort of "CDC North"—that would be led by a chief public health officer. It also recommended the infusion of $700 million of new federal spending in public health by the year 2007. The committee called on federal and provincial/territorial governments to work jointly to address the country's shortage of public health nurses, public health doctors, microbiologists, and infection control experts. It also called on Canada to take a lead role in advocating international standards for issuing travel advisories and warnings.

Ontario Premier Ernie Eves commissioned an inquiry into Ontario's handling of the SARS emergency response, conducted by Ontario Superior Court Justice Archie Campbell. The interim version of this report, "SARS and Public Health in Ontario,"

---

1. National Advisory Committee on SARS and Public Health, "Learning From SARS: Renewal of Public Health in Canada" (Ottawa: Health Canada, 2003): 12, http://www.phac-aspc.gc.ca/publicat/sars-sras/naylor/index-eng.php.

was more detailed than the federal report in its analysis of what went wrong during the emergency response to SARS and more passionate in tone. While the federal report characterized systems and resources as "manifestly sub optimal," the provincial report stated, "SARS showed Ontario's central public health system to be unprepared, fragmented, poorly led, uncoordinated, inadequately resourced, professionally impoverished, and generally incapable of discharging its mandate." Like the federal report, however, Campbell's report praised the heroic efforts of frontline health care and public health workers and their medical advisers.

The Ontario report endorsed the recommendations of the federal report and made its own set of recommendations with respect to Ontario's public health system. It called for the creation of a provincial Centre for Disease Control, independent of the Ministry of Health, and established to support the Chief Medical Officer of Health. This Ontario Centre for Disease Control should have "a critical mass of public health expertise, strong academic links and central lab capacity," Campbell wrote.

"The SARS crisis exposed deep fault lines in the structure and capacity of Ontario's public health system," the report said and, in its aftermath, the province faces "a clear choice":

> If it has the necessary political will, it can make the financial investment and the long-term commitment to reform that is required to bring our public health protection against infectious disease up to a reasonable standard. If it lacks the necessary political will, it can tinker with the system, make a token investment, and then wait for the death, sickness, suffering and economic disaster that will come with the next outbreak of disease.

6

X-Treme Planning: Ohio Prepares for Pandemic Flu

Pamela Varley

EDITORS' INTRODUCTION

The severe acute respiratory syndrome (SARS) epidemic of 2003 sounded a shrill alarm for public health officials and government leaders alike: a future pandemic of a virulent infectious disease—most likely a deadly strain of influenza—could spread rapidly across national borders and continents and potentially sicken hundreds of millions and kill tens of millions of people worldwide.

One possible source of a pandemic was already known. The H5N1 variety of avian flu, spread from chickens to humans, had caused a localized outbreak in Hong Kong in 1997. Although it infected just 18 people, 6 died, and the outbreak was brought under control only by slaughtering all of Hong Kong's 1.5 million chickens. Since then, there had been sporadic occurrences of H5N1 in humans, but it had been widely detected in bird populations in Asia, not just chickens, and increasingly elsewhere in the world.

In 2005, President George W. Bush and the Centers for Disease Control and Prevention launched a national effort to strengthen the country's preparedness should an influenza pandemic occur, whether caused by H5N1 or another viral strain. This case study describes how one state thought through the issues of pandemic readiness and developed its plan—mobilizing the Ohio Department of Health (ODH) to complete its preliminary plan in just four months.

This case was written by Pamela Varley, a senior case writer at the John F. Kennedy School of Government, Harvard University. It was sponsored by Dr. Arnold M. Howitt, Executive Director of HKS's Taubman Center for State and Local Government and faculty co-director of HKS's Program on Crisis Leadership. It was funded by The Robert Wood Johnson Foundation. The Kennedy School takes sole responsibility for the content of this case. (0507)

There was great uncertainty about the timing and extent of such a pandemic. The planners knew that a pandemic would spread rapidly given the density of human settlements, modern transportation means, and the complex interaction patterns of urban life. It would effectively strike everywhere in the world in a short period of time, meaning that state/local public health and health care institutions could expect only limited help from outside.

The challenges of developing a workable plan were enormous. The elements of flu defense were well known: recognize the outbreak of a new influenza strain as fast as possible; rapidly develop and manufacture an effective vaccine; provide antiviral medications to people exposed to the virus but who had not yet manifested symptoms; implement social distancing measures to reduce opportunities for the spread of the disease; and educate the public on how to reduce exposure. But actually implementing these strategies was immensely challenging. Numbers alone were daunting. The World Health Organization urged that planners assume a 25% infection rate, which would mean 2.8 million cases in Ohio, a caseload that could swiftly overwhelm the health system. It would therefore be necessary to find unconventional ways of providing health care to affected Ohioans, probably using some methods of care that would not be acceptable under ordinary conditions. Since health care staff would be among the people who contracted the flu, keeping health facilities operating while demand for care soared could prove extremely difficult. Fatality management was yet another serious problem: tens of thousands of Ohio residents might succumb—in hospitals, public places, their homes—requiring vastly more capacity to transport and store bodies, certify deaths, maintain death records, obtain permits for burial, and interact with grieving families who might themselves be critically ill.

Although ODH was the institution doing the planning, it was far from the only entity that would have to engage with an influenza pandemic. ODH would be the interface between the federal government, other state agencies and officials, local public health agencies and governments, and a complex web of hospitals, clinics, pharmacies, and independent practitioners. It therefore had to determine how it would relate to each of these stakeholders—communicating, educating, coordinating—all the while under the immense pressure of the pandemic's impact on ODH's own personnel.

DISCUSSION QUESTIONS

1. Are there weak links in the planning process that Ohio has devised? What are the major pitfalls that it needs to avoid as the planning process concludes?
2. How should ODH sell its finished plan to the Governor's office, the state legislature, and other state agencies? What commitments and support are needed once a plan is written?

3. What methods should be employed in advance of a pandemic to reach out to the wider public health and health care system of Ohio in order to enlist other institutions in their own planning and in efforts to link and coordinate these entities in readiness for a pandemic?

4. In what ways is it important to engage the general public in pandemic planning? How should public health officials try to get citizens to recognize and prepare for a potential pandemic?

5. Since the timing of a pandemic cannot be known in advance, how should ODH seek to sustain preparedness over the long term? What are the main needs for and obstacles to sustainable preparedness?

*　*　*

In the fall of 2005, President George W. Bush unveiled a federal initiative to ready the country for a looming danger: the possibility of a severe worldwide influenza pandemic. The plan emphasized the positive, promising to use "all instruments of national power to address the pandemic threat." President Bush called on state and local governments, private industry, and private citizens to prepare together, in advance, to meet that threat. Between the lines of the President's call to arms was a stark truth, however—and a warning. If the flu pandemic were to come, it would quickly sweep the entire country. The federal government could provide information, advice, technical assistance, and probably—a few months into the crisis—a cache of vaccines tailored to protect against the pandemic flu virus. But short of sending in the military to quell riots and enforce quarantines, the federal government would not be able to help with the crisis on the ground. As one Ohio public health official put it, "the cavalry isn't coming."

In many states—Ohio among them—top political and government officials took the warning to heart, especially as it came just weeks after the painful spectacle of Hurricane Katrina, the flooding of New Orleans, and the slow, poorly coordinated government response. In October 2005, Ohio Governor Bob Taft announced the launch of a statewide pandemic influenza preparedness effort. His health director, Nick Baird, followed up with a bold promise: the Ohio Department of Health (ODH), which would lead Ohio's emergency response in event of a flu pandemic, would develop an operational pandemic flu plan in 120 days.

PANDEMIC FLU

For two years, and with gathering urgency, virologists had been warning that conditions were ripe for a worldwide influenza pandemic. A flu pandemic was, by definition, the product of a new virus—one for which the human population had little immunity.

The danger of a flu pandemic was ever-present; in the 20th century, there had been three—in 1918, 1957, and 1968. But the severity of any given pandemic depended on the ease with which the virus spread and the virulence of the disease it caused—and both could vary dramatically. Thus, for instance, the 1918 flu had been devastating, but the two most recent pandemics had been relatively mild.[1] In a world full of dangers, concern about pandemic flu had receded until 2003, when virologists and influenza experts grew worried about the sudden proliferation of an exceptionally pathogenic and deadly new strain of the bird flu virus, H5N1.

Human flu pandemics are often a manifestation of a zoonotic disease, one that can be passed between animals and humans.[2] An animal virus—from birds or pigs, for example—is mutated or reassorted[3] into a subtype that could infect humans (sometimes by way of an intermediary species) and spread easily from person to person. H5N1 had first been detected in humans in 1997, when, in the midst of an H5N1 poultry epidemic in Hong Kong, 18 people were diagnosed with the virus. Authorities acted quickly to kill 1.5 million domestic birds and no further H5N1 outbreaks were detected for several years. In February 2003, two more human cases of H5N1 were diagnosed in Hong Kong—a man and his son, who had just returned from a trip to China. This was a worrisome development as it indicated that H5N1 was still circulating under the radar in China. In the March–April 2003 issue of *American Scientist*, renowned virologist Robert Webster warned that the world had dodged a bullet in 1997 but was nonetheless "teetering on the edge of a pandemic that could kill a large fraction of the population." Later that year, H5N1 was diagnosed in zoo animals in Thailand and several Korean poultry farms. Within a few weeks, the virus had appeared in poultry farms in Viet Nam, Japan, Thailand, Cambodia, Lao PDR, Indonesia, and China. It had also infected two human clusters of 23 and 12, respectively, in Viet Nam and Thailand.

Over the next two years, H5N1 continued to spread quickly, infecting new bird and mammal species, and appearing in new geographic areas—all typical precursors of a human pandemic. By the end of 2005, H5N1 had infected fewer than 200 people and, crucially, there was still no sign of efficient human-to-human transmission. But bird flu viruses were famously mutable, and H5N1 might gain the capacity to spread from person to person at any time. In the process of becoming a transmissible human virus, H5N1 would lose virulence; but in present form, it was extraordinarily deadly, killing more than half of its human victims. Many flu experts feared that even a weakened H5N1 could easily kill five million people worldwide and, in the worst case, might kill an unimaginable 150 million.

---

1. According to CDC, the 1918 pandemic killed more than 50 million people worldwide and more than 675,000 in the United States. The 1957 pandemic killed between 1 and 2 million worldwide and more than 70,000 in the United States. The 1968 pandemic killed more than 700,000 worldwide and more than 34,000 in the United States.

2. CDC, "Zoonotic Diseases," http://www.cdc.gov/onehealth/zoonotic-diseases.html.

3. This refers to the exchange of genetic material between flu viruses.

PANDEMIC PLANNING ON THE FAST TRACK

Within ODH, the Division of Prevention, one of the agency's three programmatic divisions, had traditionally managed public health emergencies and taken charge of emergency planning. The Division of Family and Community Health Services was primarily focused on the delivery of maternal and child health services, and the Division of Quality Assurance on regulation, training, and technical assistance. At the staff level, the three divisions had historically had little interaction. But some of Ohio's recent disease outbreaks had been large enough to strain the staff resources of the Division of Prevention, and a bad pandemic flu would dwarf any public health emergency in living memory, both in scope and duration. In the event of such a pandemic, Ohio Health Director Baird believed that employees throughout the agency would be needed in the emergency response. Therefore, Baird suggested that staff from all three divisions and ODH's central administrative offices participate in the development of the plan, under the leadership of the Division of Prevention. Staff from the other divisions and offices would bring fresh resources and perspectives to a large and fast-paced planning effort, he argued, and, in the process, a range of staff people throughout the agency would learn about pandemic flu and about emergency response work.

Faced with the task of writing a major plan in short order and involving colleagues in other divisions, Deborah Arms, chief of the Division of Prevention, and her leadership team made two requests. One, they would like Baird's personal backing to persuade staff in the other divisions to participate. And two, they would like to use the Incident Command System (ICS) to manage the process of developing the pandemic flu plan.

The flexible ICS system—developed to provide a consistent, integrated framework for managing any emergency—had become the standard approach for emergency responders across the country.[4] But the idea of using ICS for a planning process—even an intensive one—was a little unorthodox. The Division of Prevention had used ICS with relative success, however, to create a state emergency plan for a smallpox outbreak.

---

4. The system was defined by several key concepts: (1) *Modular organization*—a scalable template for organizing response activity. Key components included an incident commander (or two or more commanders working jointly) overseeing four sections: operations (actions on the ground to carry out the incident action plan), planning (collecting/sharing information related to the incident and developing and revising the incident action plan), logistics (providing resources, services, supplies, support needed to carry out the response), and finance/administration (tracking costs, personnel records, requisitions, etc.). (2) *Incident action plan*—designed to make sure the response to an event was guided by a single consolidated plan, prepared by the Planning Section. (3) *Span of control*—designed to keep the responsibilities of any one individual manageable in an emergency. No ICS manager was to have more than seven direct reports. (4) *Unity of command*—designed to avoid confusion by ensuring that each individual in the response reported to one, and only one, supervisor. (5) *Common set of facilities* to carry out defined tasks in the response, such as the incident command post, staging areas, bases, and camps. (6) *Common terminology*—to ensure that people from disparate organizations shared an understanding of the response structure and their own role in it. (7) *Integrated communications*—to make sure responders from different organizations could readily communicate with each other during the emergency.

Arms's chief strategist, Steve Wagner, had proposed ICS for pandemic flu planning for several reasons. First, it would signal the importance of the pandemic flu planning project within the agency. It would offer a practical way to organize a cross-agency planning group quickly, by task, without having to invent a structure from scratch or tiptoe around the existing ODH hierarchy. It would familiarize ODH staff outside the Division of Prevention with ICS. After all, if the entire agency was expected to participate in the emergency response to pandemic flu, the entire agency would have to learn about ICS. In 2005, few ODH staff outside the Division of Prevention had had much exposure to it.

Baird approved the use of ICS, and Arms chose Mary DiOrio, a public health physician and medical epidemiologist in the Division of Prevention's Immunization Program, to serve as Incident Commander for the planning process. DiOrio had written ODH's existing pandemic flu response plan, completed in September 2005. She described the plan as "strategic" rather than "operational," as it identified the key functions ODH would carry out in a pandemic but did not lay out a detailed blueprint for action. DiOrio had also participated in developing operational plans for bioterror threats, such as anthrax and smallpox, but she had long argued that the state should place a higher priority on planning for pandemic flu. For one, unlike a bioterror attack, a flu pandemic was not a maybe. It was sure to come at some point and even a moderate pandemic would overwhelm Ohio's medical and public health resources. In addition, she believed that if the state were prepared to cope with a crisis as large as an influenza pandemic, it would be well positioned to cope with any other imaginable health crisis.

At an October 2005 meeting of some 40 members of the ODH leadership team, Arms and Wagner introduced the pandemic flu planning effort. ODH's assistant directors told the group that this planning effort was to span the agency—that they all were expected to participate personally and to free up time for their staff members to participate.

OVERWHELMING MAGNITUDE AND GREAT UNCERTAINTY

Under the ICS model, the heart of the action—whether it was to put out a fire or to write a plan—was carried out by task-driven teams. At a practical level, therefore, the architects of the pandemic flu planning project decided to identify a list of planning tasks and assign a team to address each one. Before doing so, however, the project leaders had to take stock of several issues.

Pandemic influenza posed the twin challenges of immensity and uncertainty. Unlike a bomb or a hurricane, a flu pandemic would not be bounded geographically; it would hit everywhere. It would not affect a limited group of people; everyone would be vulnerable to it. The precipitating crisis would not end quickly; most likely it would come in waves of six to eight weeks, separated by a few weeks or months. And the severity of a pandemic could vary widely. A mild pandemic, like the 1968 Hong Kong flu, had only been slightly worse than a seasonal flu. On average, seasonal flu infected between 5% and 20% of the population in the United States, sending 200,000 to the hospital, and killing 36,000. By contrast, a severe flu could infect up to 35% of the population and kill millions.

The World Health Organization (WHO) recommended that emergency planners assume an infection rate of 25%. In Ohio, with a population of 11.5 million, that meant 2.8 million people. In a June 2005 report, the health care advocacy group Trust for America's Health estimated the number of people in each state that would (1) need hospitalization and (2) die in a flu pandemic. The organization assumed a 25% infection rate and, using a formula developed by the Centers for Disease Control and Prevention (CDC), provided estimates for pandemics that were mild (akin to 1968), virulent (akin to 1918), and moderate (midway between the two). In Ohio, Trust for America's Health estimated that the number of people requiring hospitalization would range from 46,000 to 200,000; the number to die, from 8,000 to 33,000.

Level of Severity	Ohio Cases, Assuming 25% Infection Rate	Ohio Cases Needing Hospitalization	Ohio Cases Ending in Death
Mild (akin to 1968 pandemic)	2.8 million	46,393	7,732
Moderate (midway between mild and severe)	2.8 million	99,979	23,197
Severe (akin to 1918 pandemic)	2.8 million	199,956	33,326

Source: "A Killer Flu?" Trust for America's Health, Special Report, June 2005.

This range of possibility was enormous, but even a mild pandemic flu would badly strain Ohio's resources. In 2005, the state had 163 acute care and community hospitals with a total of 32,981 beds that were, on average, 75% to 85% full. Some hospitals had to activate parts of their emergency plans—freeing up beds by releasing patients early, limiting elective procedures, etc.—just to get through the annual seasonal flu.

PANDEMIC FLU PLANNING 101

The basic formula for a pandemic flu response plan was not a mystery. Infectious disease experts knew a lot about the behavior of influenza viruses. And, in a number of respects, an outbreak of a virulent influenza required the same response as many other infectious disease outbreaks.

1. See It Coming

As with any disease outbreak, the first order of business was to identify it at the earliest possible moment. That required a good surveillance and laboratory testing system—one especially attuned to early signs of a novel flu virus and one that could quickly ratchet up if a new flu virus began to spread elsewhere in the world. Though in theory, a flu pandemic could begin anywhere, including Ohio, in the likeliest scenario, it would begin in Asia.

2. Limit the Spread

The next order of business was to try to limit the spread. In the case of pandemic influenza, however, there were limited options, and some of those options would be disruptive and unpopular.

Immunization

In general, the best tool against influenza was vaccination. By definition, however, a pandemic flu virus was new to the world and to the human immune system. That meant, at best, it would take several months to develop an effective vaccine.[5] Even then, it would take several months more before there was enough of it for universal immunization, which meant it would be necessary at first to ration. Any rationing scheme for a life-saving vaccine was guaranteed to be controversial. CDC had completed a priority list in June 2005, which the states would be free to use or modify.[6] ODH had made a tentative decision to use the CDC list. The federal government would take responsibility for acquiring the new vaccine and distributing it to the states. Thus a crucial aspect of preparedness at the state level was the logistical task of receiving vaccines from the CDC's Strategic National Stockpile and distributing them to local distribution spots. The local health districts would

---

5. The seasonal flu vaccine might offer partial protection—for instance, a 30% reduction in the chance of becoming infected—and, if so, then mass vaccination would be encouraged.

6. This list created seven categories of people who would, in priority order, be eligible to receive the vaccine in advance of the general public. In the top category were the manufacturers of the vaccine and health care workers. In the second, the people whose health conditions placed them most at risk from complications of the flu. In the third, pregnant women and people living in a household with babies or severely immunocompromised people. In the fourth, key public health emergency response workers and key political leaders. In the fifth, people 65 and older and others at greater risk from the flu than the general public. In the sixth, five groups of essential workers including first responders and some utility, transportation, and telecommunications workers. In the seventh, others in government important to managing the response and funeral directors/embalmers. This list was likely to undergo changes, however. Some argued for adding groups to the essential workers category and moving them up in the queue. Some argued for prioritizing the vaccination of children on the grounds that they spread the virus more quickly than adults. Also, if children were vaccinated, it might be possible to keep schools open or reopen them sooner.

need the capacity to get the vaccines into the right hands in the case of rationing and later to conduct a mass-vaccination effort when vaccines were available for the general public.

Antiviral prophylaxis

Another possibility was antiviral prophylaxis—that is, giving a person who had been exposed to the illness but had not yet become sick antiviral medicine in hope of staving it off. In early 2006, however, there was not enough antiviral medicine stockpiled for treatment, let alone for prophylaxis.[7] CDC policy at the time called for using antivirals only for treatment, but the question of whether to stockpile the huge quantities necessary for prophylaxis was a matter of active debate within CDC and in the larger public health world. On the one hand, all measures that reduced the number of people who became sick would lessen the burden and expense of the pandemic response. On the other hand, a person would need to take prophylactic antivirals for months, not just for a one- to two-week course as in treatment. That would require a far greater supply. Also, there was evidence that some people suffered serious side effects when they took these medications over a protracted period. In addition, there was no guarantee that the available antiviral medicines would be effective; the pandemic flu virus might be resistant to them. And, finally, the proven shelf life of antivirals was only five years; that meant stockpiling them would be a frequently recurring expense.[8] The bottom line was that, at the moment, ODH needed to develop a system to receive and distribute antivirals only for treatment. But CDC's policy might change, and thus some ODH planners advocated developing a plan to distribute them for prophylaxis as well—a more involved project, as it meant distributing a far larger volume to the local health districts which would, in turn, have to find a way to get them into the hands of the general public.

Social distancing

Another strategy was to limit the opportunity for the virus to spread by restricting exposure. There were a number of possible ways to do this, nearly all of them difficult and disruptive. For instance, authorities could restrict travel into, or out of, an area. Also, if physicians caught the first case or two in any area, before it spread further, it might be

---

7. Antivirals represented the only means of attacking the virus in a person ill with the pandemic flu. WHO recommended that every country/jurisdiction stockpile enough antiviral medication to treat 25% of its population. In the United States, the federal government was stockpiling enough to cover 15% to be divided among the states based on population. Each state would make its own decision about whether to buy and store enough antivirals to make up the difference—that is, enough to treat another 10% of its own population. The federal government encouraged the states to do so and offered to defray 25% of the cost. In 2006, the Ohio General Assembly appropriated $17 million to purchase Ohio's share of this antiviral supply.

8. It was possible that future testing would show that the antivirals remained safe and effective for a longer period, in which case their shelf life would increase.

possible to isolate the patients and quarantine the people they had exposed in order to try to halt the disease in its tracks. Ultimately, however, influenza experts doubted that this strategy would succeed given (1) the short, 1- to 4-day incubation period (the time between exposure and symptoms) of flu illnesses, (2) the fact that many flus were contagious even before the host became symptomatic, and (3) the likelihood that the earliest flu symptoms would be general enough to cause a delay in diagnosis, increasing the amount of time before a pandemic flu patient was isolated.

Once the virus was in circulation, authorities could recommend that everyone stay home as much as possible. They could close gathering places—for instance, theaters, bars, churches, universities, malls, and, of course, schools and day care centers. Children were infamous viral shedders and thus spread the virus more quickly than did adults. But the ramifications of closing schools were extensive. How would such a thing be implemented? Where would the children go instead? What would they do with their time? Would the teachers be paid? Would education of children continue in some form? How would schools cope with the legal requirement to keep children in school a set number of days in the school year? All these matters would have to be resolved in advance.

Health education

Finally, the general public would be in a state of heightened anxiety, and there would be a need for an immediate, consistent public education campaign to explain the nature of the flu, the measures government and health care providers had taken in response, and the best general methods of protecting against exposure.

3. Cope With the Illness and Its Repercussions

It was in the interest of any community to contain the pandemic to the fullest possible extent, but experts were not sanguine that these efforts would spare many places from having to cope with a large number of seriously ill people, a large number of deaths, and a host of related problems. Thus, to prepare for a pandemic meant facing these difficult circumstances. Among the biggest issues in emergency preparedness parlance were "medical surge," "fatality management," "continuity of operations," and "mass care."

Medical surge

One certainty about an influenza pandemic was that the hospitals would not have enough beds, ventilators, or health care workers to serve all the sick. Clinics, too, would quickly be overwhelmed. Preparing for pandemic flu therefore meant coming up with a system to triage patients and devising a way to care for the sick either at home or in some sort of alternative care setting. It meant changing standards of care—the rules mandating minimum staff-to-patient ratios, for instance, and those dictating which types of personnel could perform which procedures. It meant making decisions about who would and would not receive scarce resources, such as intensive care beds and ventilators. It meant mobilizing additional health professionals—people with professional training who were not in the active workforce because they were still in school, retired, or had made a career change.

Fatality management

In a lethal flu, tens of thousands of Ohio residents might die in short order. To keep the management of dead bodies from spiraling out of control, it would be crucial to remove the bodies from homes, health care facilities, and public places and to manage them in a manner protective of public health and the water supply. That meant arranging methods of transport and identifying additional sources of refrigerated storage. It also meant streamlining the process of certifying deaths, obtaining burial permits, and maintaining official death records. It might also mean lining up emergency burial grounds in advance.

Continuity of operations

One of the dangers in a pandemic, with staff outages as high as 30% (perhaps 40% among health care workers), was a general breakdown of essential services. Such breakdowns—for example, a power company that failed to supply power—would further impair the operations of other agencies, businesses, and organizations. Therefore, it was important that government agencies and other entities that supplied essential services create continuity of operations plans, identifying their most essential functions and training reserve staff (several deep, if possible) to keep them going if the regular staff members were out ill. In addition, they would need to provide protective equipment (for example, disinfecting hand gels) and institute protective procedures (for example, frequent disinfectant cleaning) to protect staff from exposure to influenza in the workplace. All businesses were advised to do the same.

Mass care

In a severe pandemic, there would be all kinds of secondary effects as well. Dependents would need day-to-day care if their caregivers became sick or died. Traditional supply chains might break down, leading to shortages of food, water, and medicines. State and local governments, in coordination with state relief organizations, would have to be prepared to detect and respond quickly to such problems.

THE DILEMMA OF LIMITED AUTHORITY

In addition to the difficulty of planning for the sheer magnitude of a severe pandemic flu, ODH faced another dilemma: its own limited purview. ODH would be the lead agency to manage Ohio's emergency response to the flu pandemic, yet it lacked the authority to make and implement some of the most crucial decisions in that response. To some degree, this was true for every state in the country. Authority in the health care sector was shared, in complex fashion, among a vast variety of actors—local, state, and federal agencies; private hospitals; clinics; health management organizations; professional organizations; insurance companies; accreditation agencies. But as a home rule state, Ohio state government had even less authority vis-à-vis local government than most states. It was the state's 135 local health districts, not ODH, that bore primary responsibility for protecting the health of citizens in their respective jurisdictions. What's more, Ohio stood alone among the 50 states in neither licensing nor regulating any of the state's nationally accredited hospitals.[9] In addition, an influenza pandemic would require action from a number of agencies and entities outside the public health and medical care sectors, such as school departments and social service providers.

ODH's operational responsibilities in a pandemic emergency response were primarily to serve as an interface between the federal government and local communities and to provide the clearest possible information and guidance to all affected parties in the state in timely fashion. Among ODH's specific tasks:

- Conduct surveillance, receive disease reports from the field, provide fast laboratory tests so as to detect the first cases of pandemic flu in Ohio as soon as possible, in an effort to contain the disease early.
- Activate ODH's Emergency Operations Center and ICS to manage the response. (Another state-level Emergency Operations Center and ICS system would also be activated, to provide support to the ODH effort and to address issues outside the purview of public health.)
- Serve as a central information source, receiving and analyzing information from local health districts to provide a statewide view of the pandemic, and passing the latest CDC information and guidance to the local health districts and other relevant partners.
- Mobilize a major communications initiative to provide specifically tailored materials about coping with pandemic influenza to the general public and an array of audiences with more specific concerns.
- Recommend (or, if necessary, mandate) actions to contain the community spread of the disease by limiting the movements of people into and out of certain areas;

---

9. This included most of the state's 163 acute care and community hospitals. ODH did regulate the maternity wards in accredited hospitals, however. The department also regulated nonaccredited specialty facilities—for example, long-term care facilities, rehabilitation centers, dialysis centers, and rural hospitals.

closing schools and other public venues; and encouraging people to stay home as much as possible.

- Receive all available flu supplies from state and federal stockpiles (vaccines, antivirals, face masks, ventilators, etc.) and distribute them according to an established plan, along with guidance on how to ration items in short supply.

In addition, as the lead state agency for addressing pandemic flu, ODH did bear a responsibility to make sure the state as a whole was prepared to face down a pandemic. ODH did not interpret this responsibility to mean that the agency could or should write a plan that told other agencies what to do in a pandemic. Every local health district, every community, every hospital, every health care provider, every school district would have to prepare itself for pandemic flu. There were, however, important aspects of a statewide strategy that necessitated close collaboration among independent government agencies. For example, ODH had the authority to order one or more public schools to close for health reasons.[10] But for ODH to exercise such authority, in the absence of a local plan to implement it, might actually worsen the spread of the pandemic. Says DiOrio, "It doesn't help anything to close the schools and then have a mom down the street with 100 kids in her house—or [to have the kids congregate] at the mall."

In addition, some decisions exceeded the jurisdiction of any single agency or entity. A single hospital, for example, could implement an emergency plan but could not on its own create a system of triage or change standard patient care requirements without the risk of substantial liability. In addition, there was general agreement that, with hospitals overwhelmed, there would be a need for some kind of alternative care centers to take care of the thousands of patients the hospitals could not accommodate. There was no general agreement, however, about what agency or organization, in either the public health or health care systems, should establish, manage, and operate such centers.

Public health agencies—ODH and the local health districts—tended to argue, with reason, that they had no authority, resources, or capacity to address issues of health care delivery, observes ODH Prevention Chief Arms. But she notes that, in the midst of a pandemic, the general public was guaranteed to see things differently:

> When people need care and can't get into emergency rooms and can't get into their primary care provider, they're going to come to public health. I don't think the constituents or legislators are going to look at the hospitals and say, "This is *your* fault." They're going to look at the state health department and say, "How did you not plan for this?"

The reality is, Arms says, "it's going to fall in our laps."

---

10. In fact, the decision to close a school could be made by any one of five government entities: the school itself, the school district, the local board of health, the state Department of Education, or ODH.

Thus, the Division of Prevention leadership agreed that a part of ODH's job was to understand the role that all participants in the response must play and to keep well informed about how well or ill prepared they actually were. In addition, ODH would have to do what it could to guide, assist, support, inform, facilitate, persuade, and, perhaps, pressure them to become better prepared.

In this effort, ODH did have several important advantages:

- good political support from Governor Taft;
- three years of work as a participant with other organizations in the state in developing a regional approach to mass casualty emergencies; and
- four years of experience in distributing and overseeing various federal emergency preparedness grants to local areas, which had created a foundation upon which the state could now build—both in improved capacity to respond to health emergencies and in a general familiarity with the emergency planning process.

Support from the Governor

Ohio Governor Taft had made emergency preparedness, in general, a top priority of his administration. He also encouraged state agencies to conduct frequent workshops and exercises as they were developing and refining their emergency plans, and committed himself and his office to participating in a number of them.

In October 2001, Taft created a cabinet-level group called the State of Ohio Security Task Force (SOSTF). This task force organized working groups, or committees, to develop a state-level strategy for various complex emergency management issues that might arise in Ohio. Even before the state began its initiative to prepare for pandemic flu, multiagency committees were already beginning to address certain issues that would be important in a pandemic flu response—for example, the creation of a voluntary medical reserve corps.

In December 2005, Taft also created a Pandemic Preparedness Coordinating Committee under the SOSTF, led by ODH Director Baird. This committee, with representatives from the Department of Agriculture, the Department of Natural Resources, the Department of Public Safety, and the Department of Public Safety's Emergency Management Agency, would address issues of coordination among these state agencies that would be specific to a flu pandemic. Taft and his administration also put their weight behind a successful request to the state legislature to budget a major sum—$17 million—for the purchase of an antiviral drug stockpile for Ohio.[11]

---

11. See footnote 7.

The Basics of a Regional Structure

Beginning in 1996, the US Department of Health and Human Services (HHS) funded development of a Metropolitan Medical Response System, intended to enhance the capacity and coordination of local and regional responders in major metropolitan areas during terrorist attacks. Under the leadership of ODH, this program evolved over time into a regional system to cope with any large, mass casualty emergency. On a voluntary basis, first responders, hospitals, health care providers, and others within each of eight state regions had been working together since 2002 to develop emergency response plans for various scenarios and to exercise those plans together.

Building on a Foundation

Over a period of seven years, ODH had overseen the management of a number of federal emergency medical preparedness grants. For the most part, grants from HHS were aimed at improving the preparedness of the local health districts, and grants from the US Health Resources and Services Administration, the hospital system. These grants came with federal requirements but also gave ODH some latitude to improve its own preparedness and to influence the preparedness approach taken by the local health districts and hospitals. For example, federal grants had been used to fund a group of regional coordinators who worked out of the local health districts and facilitated regional planning. Federal grants had also enabled ODH to develop an advanced Web-based disease reporting system, create a system for real-time reporting of emergency department admissions in 110 hospitals, develop and drill mass prophylaxis plans, and devise a Web-based system for collaboration and information sharing among state and local public health agencies. Ohio was due to receive an additional $11 million in HHS grants specific to developing preparedness for the flu pandemic.

CREATING THE PLAN

In late 2005, when ODH was beginning its intensive 120-day project to create a pandemic influenza response plan, CDC had not yet developed detailed guidance to offer the states. But the US Department of Homeland Security had published a 600-page target capabilities list—an effort at compiling a comprehensive list of all capabilities that might be needed at the state and local level in any conceivable emergency response. Attached to each of the 36 broad capabilities—for example, providing mass prophylaxis medications to the public—was a more detailed description of the critical tasks necessary to accomplish this end.

Many of the capabilities on this master list would not apply to pandemic flu. For example, unless the pandemic coincided with an earthquake or an explosion, there would be no need to mobilize urban search and rescue teams. But Arms and Wagner reasoned that, if they started with the master list, they could select the relevant capabilities, leave out the rest, and feel secure that "we hadn't missed anything," Wagner says.

In November, DiOrio and the other leaders of the pandemic flu planning group used the target capabilities list to structure the planning project, creating 21 teams, clustered in four major subgroups, to address the target capabilities relevant to a pandemic influenza response. Each team was assigned responsibility for analyzing one or more target capabilities and reporting back up the chain of command with a list of capacities that would be necessary to meet the target and a summary of other issues or dilemmas that would need to be addressed. The leadership of the planning group would then take these reports and translate them into a plan.

In all, about 200 ODH staff, at all levels, participated in the planning project. Those in top command positions in the ICS structure worked full time–plus over the four month period. Those in midlevel positions—leading the target capability teams—were expected to devote about 20 hours a week to the effort. And rank-and-file team members were expected to spend about eight hours per week.

The pandemic flu planning process proved controversial within ODH for a number of reasons. Staff in the Division of Family and Community Health Services, the Division of Quality Assurance, and the ODH administrative offices had little familiarity, in general, with emergency preparedness work. Many argued that they had no expertise in the topics they were supposed to address and thus had little to offer. In addition, they protested that their time had already been obligated to other grant-funded projects. Thus, despite assurances from ODH leadership that they would be given time to work on the pandemic flu plan, they felt that, in reality, they had to do the pandemic planning work on top of their regular workload. In addition, frustrations ran high as they did not, in some cases, ever entirely understand what an emergency plan should (and should not) include. Many did not understand ICS or the DHS target capabilities. Some had a poor grasp of pandemic flu.

By hook or by crook, however, the ODH pandemic flu group did produce a plan by March 15, 2006. "People were good soldiers," says Arms. Despite their frustrations, "they tried to do the best job they could, because this was something that the health department had committed to, and the director wanted us to do."

Within the Division of Prevention, there were mixed views about the product, however. Some regarded it as a good start and others, as a disappointment. All acknowledged, however, that it was a draft and that many things remained still to do before Ohio would be prepared for a pandemic.

In general, the project leaders believed the plan succeeded best at detailing ODH's own operational role in the pandemic response. The planners had identified the specific set of tasks that the agency was authorized and responsible to perform in a pandemic flu emergency, and the steps ODH must take beforehand to develop the capacity to perform them. For example, in the heat of the emergency, it would be crucial to have a quick, reliable means of sharing information back and forth with the local health districts and other frontline partners in the response. But the time to develop such an information-sharing system—to work out the kinks—was in the present. The plan thus included several components:

1. The list of specific capacities that ODH would need to fulfill its role.
2. If such capacity was lacking, the division or office responsible for developing it, and the anticipated completion date (if relevant—some were ongoing).
3. The operational plan for what ODH would actually do, step by step, in the emergency.
4. A year-long schedule of workshops and exercises to train staff, practice the plan, and—based on feedback from these sessions—refine it.

ADDRESSING OVERALL STATE STRATEGY

The plan was less sure-footed in mapping out ODH's role in shaping the overall state strategy. But even if these projects were not clearly set down in the plan, they were either underway already or were identified in the course of the planning effort. Thus, once the 120-day plan was complete, ODH continued to participate in a number of collaborative projects aimed at developing pandemic preparedness.

Guiding the Local Health Districts

For four years, ODH had been distributing federal emergency preparedness grants to the local health districts and, through this oversight role, steering the local preparedness efforts to some degree. In addition, ODH was often in the position of go-between, trying to clarify current CDC thinking and policies to the local health districts. To a large degree, therefore, developing the flu pandemic plan was a continuation of an existing relationship. The 135 local health districts ranged widely in size and sophistication. Some were ahead of the curve and had developed aspects of a local pandemic flu plan well before the nationwide initiative began.

ODH tried to help the local health districts with their pandemic flu plans in a number of ways. In February 2006, the agency hosted a statewide pandemic influenza summit, attended by state officials, community leaders, and industry representatives who participated in a panel discussion about cooperative approaches to pandemic flu planning. A speakers bureau sent out ODH representatives to address local pandemic planners. Barbara Bradley, director of the Bureau of Infectious Disease Control in the Division of Prevention, held a weekly teleconference with local health district administrators, to discuss a wide array of issues, including pandemic influenza. ODH created a pandemic influenza information and planning Web site that included quarterly pandemic planning newsletters tailored to the local health districts and descriptions of best practices by local governments. ODH provided information and planning advice to all the local health districts about a wide array of populations that would have special needs during a pandemic. In January 2006, ODH created a planning checklist for the local health districts, based on a list prepared by CDC.

For local governments, there were a number of issues that made pandemic flu preparedness especially difficult. For example, there were yet-unresolved questions about whether the local health districts should take responsibility for planning and operating alternative care centers when hospital capacity was overwhelmed—a topic under discussion by the Medical Surge Committee. In addition, the question of how a school department would handle a lengthy school closing was complicated and required considerable discussion.

And sometimes things that, on their face, appeared straightforward proved more complicated in fact. One example was the stockpiling of masks to protect emergency response workers and others from exposure. Should a community buy any masks and, if so, should they buy simple surgical masks, or N95 face masks designed to protect against airborne matter? The underlying question had to do with flu transmissibility. For many years, CDC had taken the position that flu viruses were overwhelmingly droplet-spread rather than airborne. The agency did advise that hospital workers wear the N95 masks, as some hospital procedures were known to aerosolize flu virus. But CDC recommended that emergency medical technicians and others with passing contact with flu patients should wear surgical masks, which were less expensive and less complicated to use. This position had been controversial; several other professional organizations had advised far more widespread use of N95s. But ODH had agreed with CDC and strongly advised the local health districts to stockpile surgical masks. (In fact, ODH would not allow a local health district to use its federal grant funds to buy N95 masks unless the local agency described their scope of use and created a plan for fit-testing the wearers and providing them with medical assessment.) "We said, 'We're going with the CDC recommendation—this is *science-based*,'" says Arms. "Well, wouldn't you know, a year later, CDC changed its mind," recommending a wider use of N95 masks. "We look like idiots!" Arms adds.

In general, however, DiOrio says the local health districts were doing well with their planning efforts. Many had held community-wide pandemic flu summits. And some had come up with creative approaches to difficult problems. For example,

Clark County decided to set up a drive-through clinic for mass immunization—a popular idea that other communities decided to try as well.

Anticipating the Problems of Groups With Special Needs

ODH also decided to take a lead role in identifying, up front, the problems that special needs populations, from dialysis patients to migrant farm workers, were likely to face. Thus, ODH drafted a model plan for the local health districts to consider in addressing the needs of special populations. ODH also identified alternatives and resources for people in need of dialysis, prescription medicines, and home care supplies. ODH wrote a plan for addressing the particular needs of those whose illnesses or treatments left them immunocompromised. Together with the Ohio Department of Jobs and Family Services, ODH wrote a plan for migrant populations. ODH also cooperated in a project of the Ohio Legal Rights Council to create an "Emergency Management Be Prepared Kit" designed for developmentally disabled, elderly, HIV-positive, and medically fragile populations.

Developing a Host of Educational Materials to Assist in Pandemic Flu Planning

ODH created a Web site with information about pandemic flu; published quarterly planning newsletters for businesses, schools, local government, and faith-based and community organizations; took out print and broadcast ads advising residents how to prepare for pandemic flu and other emergencies; and created an informational DVD and informational fact sheets and guides for distribution at state fairs and other public venues.

Helping to Create the Volunteer Medical Reserve Corps

In 2002, President Bush launched the national Medical Reserve Corps program to encourage doctors and other health care workers—including those not in the active medical workforce because they were still in training, retired, or had dropped out—to volunteer their medical services in an emergency. To operate smoothly, volunteers in the program would have to register, establish their credentials, and attend special training sessions. In Ohio, ODH worked on this initiative in collaboration with the Ohio

Community Service Council. One of their goals was to create a medical reserve corps in each of the state's 88 counties. ODH and the Council were also working together on the management of nonmedical volunteers, donations, and volunteer relief efforts to deliver mass care.

Assisting State Agencies With Continuity of Operations Plans

ODH worked with the other state agencies to help them plan for continuity of operations, working on the assumption that as much as a third of the staff—including key leaders and subject matter experts—might be out sick or caring for sick children or other relatives.

Participating in Fatality Management Planning

The Ohio Emergency Management Agency was Ohio's lead agency for managing mass fatalities (though ODH's Vital Statistics office was the keeper of official death records). Under the Governor's State of Ohio Security Task Force, the Ohio Emergency Management Agency organized a committee that included coroners, funeral home directors, health commissioners, hospitals, pathologists, the American Red Cross, and several state agencies—the Ohio Environmental Protection Agency, the Department of Administrative Services, the Department of Alcohol and Drug Addiction Services, the Department of Mental Health, the Department of Transportation, the State Highway Patrol, and ODH—with the goal of planning how to cope if the state were faced with thousands of fatalities in a few weeks' time. This included questions about how to store bodies safely until they could be processed, how to process the bodies during the height of the emergency, whether to acquire land for burials, and how to streamline the registration of deaths.

THE TOUGH PROBLEM OF MEDICAL SURGE

By the spring of 2007, many of these multiagency preparedness activities were still not complete, but Arms said that if a pandemic flu were to strike the next day, she believed Ohio's emergency response would be good enough in most categories. "My biggest concern would be medical surge," she says. Under the auspices of the Governor's State of Ohio Security Task Force, ODH organized a statewide Medical Surge Committee in April 2006 to sort through this challenging set of issues.

Well before the pandemic influenza planning effort, Ohio hospitals had, as a require-ment of accreditation, each developed an emergency plan to cope with a sudden surge of patients at its facility, from any cause. What counted as a patient surge varied by the hospital. For small hospitals, a single highway accident with several casualties might con-stitute a surge. For large hospitals, a toxic spill with 100 casualties might constitute a surge. Most hospitals in Ohio had adopted a flexible, three-tiered approach to scaling up capacity, according to Carol Jacobson, director of emergency preparedness for the Ohio Hospital Association:

- In the event of a minor patient surge, hospitals implemented Tier 1—freeing up hospital beds by halting elective procedures, transferring less sick patients to less acute facilities, and getting permission from the federal Center for Medicare and Medicaid Services to temporarily lift required set-asides of beds for patients with particular needs, such as rehabilitation or mental health treatment.
- If still more beds were needed, a hospital would move to Tier 2, converting hospital gyms, offices, and outbuildings to patient rooms.
- Tier 3 involved a cooperative arrangement among hospitals in a given region (one of the state's seven emergency response regions) to share information about bed availability. If certain hospitals were experiencing a surge, other hos-pitals and long-term care facilities in the region would take on some of the patient load.

These measures would allow hospitals, individually and regionally, to handle many small- to medium-sized emergencies, but they would not be sufficient for a large med-ical surge—and certainly not sufficient for the kind of surge anticipated from an influ-enza pandemic. In April 2006—just after completion of the 120-day plan—ODH created a statewide Medical Surge Committee to come up with a plan for large-scale emergencies. The group included hospitals, long-term care facilities, primary care pro-viders and clinics, emergency medical ambulance services, home care organizations, health professional boards, and several state agencies including the Emergency Management Agency, the Department of Mental Health, the Department of Youth Services, the Department of Corrections, and the Ohio National Guard. The commit-tee was to design a general plan to address medical surge issues, but ODH Prevention Chief Arms recalls:

When we got the Medical Surge Committee together, we struggled with, "Okay, what disaster are we talking about here?" Because every disease is different in terms of what resources we're going to need, how we're going to do things. And what we decided to do was go with the disaster-of-all-disasters, which would be pandemic flu.

The group began with the assumption that even if every hospital in a given region activated its Tier 1, 2, and 3 emergency plans, the existing medical care system would not be able to meet the region's needs. When hospitals and other medical care providers in any region were too overwhelmed to continue with business-as-usual operations, they could collectively decide to activate the state's medical surge plan in their region, provided the decision was approved by the director of the Ohio Department of Health.[12] This would set in motion a more centralized system of patient triage, rationed medical care, altered standards of care, and alternative care options. There would be some regional variations in implementation, but the basics of the plan would be the same, wherever it was implemented.

Individual hospitals and other medical care providers would not be legally obligated to comply with the scheme, but they would have two powerful incentives for doing so: (1) state legislation (still to be written and enacted) to provide liability protection to those who followed the medical surge plan and (2) eligibility for government funding to help defray the costs of providing care during the emergency.

The committee began with a basic concept of operations, developed by the US Department of Defense, called the Modular Emergency Medical System (MEMS). Under this system, anyone needing medical attention would go to a triage center, where s/he would be examined quickly and sent to a hospital, an alternative care center, or back home with medication and instructions for care.

Triage

One of the tasks for the Medical Surge Committee was to come up with decisions about which patients belonged in which of the four triage categories:

1. Red for urgent cases that would receive the most intensive resources. These patients would be sent to the hospital and would receive priority for scarce resources such as ventilators and antiviral medications. Typically, these patients were judged healthy enough to survive their current illness if they received intensive medical care but were in danger of dying without it.
2. Yellow for less urgent cases. If there was room for them in the hospitals, they too would be sent there. If not, they would be sent to alternative care centers or home with home health care providers or relatives.
3. Green for minor cases. These patients would be treated in alternative care centers or at home with home health care providers or relatives.

---

12. The mechanism for making this decision was still a work in progress. There was a regional hospital board in each region, but hospitals were not the only organizations that would have to implement the medical surge plan. Wagner advocated the creation of a board with broader representation in each region—for example, from hospitals, local health districts, and other medical providers.

4. Black/blue[13] for patients that, however urgent, were deemed too sick to survive, and were therefore eligible only for palliative care in an alternative care center or at home. Typically, these were people who were already suffering progressive, systemic, irreversible organ failure. In some triage systems, anyone over the age of 85 was also placed in this category. In some triage systems, children were never placed in this category.

In addition to deciding on triage categories, the Medical Surge Committee would have to make a string of other important decisions:

- Hospitals would be operating with as many additional patients as they could handle under their emergency plans and might be operating with a staff outage as high as 40%. Therefore, they would need to adopt altered standards of care. For example, it would be necessary to accept higher-than-usual patient-to-staff ratios and place fewer restrictions on which procedures various categories of health care workers were permitted to perform. The Medical Surge Committee would have to delineate these altered standards.
- Even if hospitals only treated "red" patients under the triage system, there would likely be shortages within the hospitals of certain kinds of facilities, equipment, and medications. Thus, the plan must include a system for prioritizing which "red" patients would receive beds in the intensive care unit, ventilators, antiviral drugs, etc.
- The MEMS plan called for the creation of alternative care centers. Many health care planners believed it was the responsibility of the local health districts to make arrangements to use certain buildings for this purpose, to stockpile equipment, to develop a set of operating rules and procedures and, in the emergency response itself, to set up the centers, to staff them, and to manage them. Many local health districts, however, argued that they had no resources or capacity to do so. The Medical Surge Committee had to figure out a plan—one that would likely vary by region and community.
- The MEMS plan called for the creation of triage centers. The committee would also have to decide where such centers would be located, and who would manage and staff them.
- The MEMS plan called for providing palliative care to patients in the "black/blue" triage category. It would be necessary to organize the delivery of such care.
- The MEMS plan called for caring for patients at home via home health care providers or relatives who received quick training. The plan would have to come up with a way to expand available home health care and an efficient means of training patients' relatives in the basics of caring for pandemic flu patients.

---

13. In traditional triage nomenclature, "black" was used for the category that would not receive active medical care. For reasons of cultural sensitivity and to avoid confusion, some systems elected to call this category "blue."

- The Medical Surge Committee would also have to draft language for inclusion in the Ohio Revised Code to create immunity or assume liability for health care providers practicing under altered standards of care in an authorized medical emergency.
- The Medical Surge Committee would have to ensure that private health insurance companies would pay for care to patients regardless of where they were treated and regardless of the altered standards of care.

Beginning in April 2006, the Medical Surge Committee met monthly to hear the reports and proposals of various subcommittees working on specific aspects of the medical surge plan. By the spring of 2007, the Medical Surge Committee was reportedly making headway, with proposals on the table in a number of areas, but there was a great deal of work still to do before the plan would be complete.

7

On the Front Lines of a Pandemic: Texas Responds to 2009 Novel H1N1 Influenza A

David W. Giles

EDITORS' INTRODUCTION

By the mid-2000s, following the 2003 severe acute respiratory syndrome (SARS) outbreak and in the face of isolated cases of H5N1 avian influenza (commonly known as "bird flu") in Asia, public health officials in the United States and beyond had begun paying increasing amounts of attention to the threat of pandemic influenza. Many in the public health and medical communities focused on the potential of the highly lethal bird flu to trigger the anticipated pandemic, which was predicted to strike in the near future based on historical patterns of occurrence. But because it continued to be difficult to transmit from one human to another, outbreaks of H5N1 remained relatively contained. Instead, in 2009, a different strain of influenza (novel H1N1, widely referred to as "swine flu") began spreading rapidly among humans in North America and then across multiple continents. By June of that year, based on the global spread of H1N1, the World Health Organization had declared the first flu pandemic in more than 40 years.

This case study explores how state health officials in Texas, one of the first places to experience the disease, confronted H1N1 in its earliest stages. The case opens

This case was written by David W. Giles, Assistant Director, Program on Crisis Leadership, for Dr. Arnold M. Howitt, Executive Director of the Ash Center for Democratic Governance and Innovation at the John F. Kennedy School of Government, Harvard University. Funds for case development were provided by the Robert Wood Johnson Foundation as part of its State Health Leadership Initiative. HKS cases are developed solely as the basis for class discussion. Cases are not intended to serve as endorsements, sources of primary data, or illustrations of effective or ineffective management.

with a brief review of the state of pandemic planning in the United States leading up to the emergence of H1N1, before recounting how reports of early cases of an unknown respiratory disease in Mexico (eventually identified as H1N1) triggered intense international media coverage and an extensive set of public health interventions across that country. Revealing the challenges of obtaining adequate situational awareness about what was soon to become a full-blown pandemic, the case explores how authorities in Texas learned about the appearance of the disease in both Mexico and in their own state and how they subsequently sought to design and implement a response, even as significant questions about H1N1 remained, including ones related to its contagiousness, lethality, and the populations it most seriously affected.

Told largely from the point of view of senior state health officials in Texas, the case details the key actions they took to get a handle on the rapidly escalating outbreak. To improve their situational awareness, this included launching extensive and time-consuming epidemiological investigations, which required close coordination with other state agencies, localities, and the federal government. They also had to think expansively about how best to fight H1N1. Because this was a new strain of the flu, it would take several months to produce and then distribute an effective vaccine, meaning that in the short term, they would be without one of the most effective tools for curtailing the spread of H1N1. In the hope that limiting person-to-person contact could minimize transmission, they thus considered, and in several instances implemented, several social distancing measures, such as the closure of schools where confirmed or probable cases of H1N1 had been identified. But social distancing has its own drawbacks (for instance, closing schools means that parents might have to miss work—and forgo much needed income—in order to care for their children), and health officials simultaneously pursued additional strategies to combat the disease. Among other things, they improvised ways to distribute antiviral medications, which seemed to help mitigate the effects of H1N1, to as many people as possible. All the while, they also sought to communicate effectively across multiple sectors and jurisdictions and to a wide array of stakeholders—no easy challenge in a state as large and diverse as Texas and with strategies and guidance rapidly evolving from one day to the next.

Fortunately, the situation in Texas stabilized considerably during the summer of 2009. But with the annual North American flu season looming on the horizon, health authorities realized that the threat was far from over. Anticipating another wave of H1N1 outbreaks in the fall, they spent the summer reviewing and revising their response plans. By building off of the key lessons they had learned from their frontline experiences that spring, they hoped to be as prepared as possible for a resurgence of the disease.

DISCUSSION QUESTIONS

1. Would you characterize the 2009 H1N1 pandemic as truly novel? And if so, how did the unique aspects of the outbreak affect early response efforts in Texas?
2. How useful were Texas's past experiences and its pre-outbreak planning and preparedness efforts for helping the state respond to H1N1?
3. In hindsight, how appropriate and necessary were the various strategies (e.g., social distancing, antiviral distributions, methods of risk communication) employed by the state of Texas in responding to H1N1? If you were a state health official and also had a limited amount of data about the disease (and limited options for fighting it), would you have done anything differently? How so?
4. What similarities, if any, do you see in the early response to H1N1 in Texas and the responses to Ebola in Dallas and SARS in Toronto, as discussed earlier in this book?

* * *

The public health response here and in the United States has been quick and aggressive. It had to be. H1N1 was a new virus, unpredictable, and spreading widely to people who had little or no immunity. There was no public health track record to label who was at risk, how severe the outbreak would be, or how lethal the virus could be.

–Texas Commissioner of Health Dr. David Lakey[1]

In early 2009, the world's first influenza pandemic in more than 40 years emerged not in Asia but, surprisingly, in North America. Sparked not by the highly lethal H5N1 strain (also known as avian or bird flu) to which the public health community had paid considerable attention over the past decade, the pandemic appeared to have originated in pigs before jumping to humans. Designated 2009 novel H1N1 influenza A, or H1N1 for short, the virus was originally termed "swine flu," although subsequent laboratory analysis determined that it contained genetic properties of avian, human, and swine strains. Early reports from Mexico, which seemed to indicate high case–fatality ratios, raised alarm worldwide. Fortunately, this new form of influenza eventually proved to be generally mild for most of those it affected.[2]

---

1. David Lakey, "Commissioner's Commentary: A Pandemic by Definition," June 18, 2009, http://www.dshs. state.tx.us/commissioner/commentary/commentary-20090618.shtm.
2. Institute of Medicine (IOM), *The Domestic and International Impacts of the 2009-H1N1 Influenza A Pandemic: Global Challenges, Global Solutions* (Washington, DC: The National Academies Press, 2010); Marc Lacey and Donald G. McNeil, "Fighting Deadly Flu Outbreak, Mexico Shuts Schools for Millions," *New York Times*, April 25, 2009, A4.

All the same, the disease spread quickly, and on June 11, 2009, the World Health Organization (WHO) declared a full-blown pandemic. By then, public health officials in several places, including the state of Texas, had been battling multiple outbreaks of the disease for well over a month. As an ever-increasing number of states and countries confronted H1N1, Texas's experiences on the front lines of the pandemic offered many valuable lessons. Among them: How had the pandemic response plans put in place in the face of bird flu stood up in the earliest days and weeks of H1N1? How had rapidly evolving conditions and a high degree of uncertainty and unpredictability affected the initial response? And what, exactly, was the severity of this disease? As H1N1 continued to circulate throughout the summer and into the fall, understanding what had taken place in Texas earlier that spring would be vital for authorities hoping to keep the pandemic's ill effects in check.[3]

For a chronology of events and a cast of characters, see Exhibits 7-1 and 7-2.

A PANDEMIC EMERGES

In the late 1990s and early 2000s, several outbreaks of emergent infectious disease, coupled with the rising threat of bioterrorism, spurred public officials in the United States to bolster public health preparedness across all levels of government. At around the same time, concerns over the threat to human health posed by highly virulent H5N1 avian flu intensified dramatically, and by the mid-2000s, the Bush administration had begun paying particular attention to the United States' capacity to prepare for and respond to future influenza pandemics. In short order, the federal government was investing in the expansion of surveillance and testing systems, funding pandemic modeling initiatives, and developing guidance on key issues that would likely arise during a pandemic, such as the distribution of scarce resources (e.g., limited supplies of vaccine or facemasks) and the implementation of social distancing measures.[4]

In November 2005, the US Department of Health and Human Services (HHS) released its *Pandemic Influenza Plan,* which addressed the federal government's role in preparing for and responding to a pandemic. It also offered guidance to state and local health departments as they set about designing their own response frameworks.[5] Although the public health community by and large recognized the tremendous amount of uncertainty regarding the shape and scale of any future pandemic, worries about H5N1 significantly influenced the planning process. The focus on H5N1 led many to assume that the next pandemic would likely originate overseas, which would provide at least some advance

---

3. Case 9 explores Tennessee's own experience in confronting H1N1, with a particular emphasis on issues relating to vaccine distribution in fall 2009.
4. IOM, *Domestic and International Impacts*; HHS, *HHS Pandemic Influenza Plan* (Washington, DC: HHS, 2005).
5. HHS, *Pandemic Influenza Plan.*

warning, and that it would be extremely deadly, given the high case–fatality ratio among the limited number of humans who had contracted H5N1 to date.[6]

Beginning in March 2009, an unusually large number of people exhibiting symptoms of flu-like illness began appearing in hospitals and health clinics across Mexico. Initial reports indicated that an abnormally high proportion of ill individuals were developing serious forms of pneumonia and, ultimately, dying.[7] At first, Mexican health authorities believed that they were dealing with an outbreak of severe acute respiratory syndrome, which in 2002 and 2003 had taken hundreds of lives in Asia and dozens more in Canada. But an investigation of cases in Mexico City soon ruled out that theory. Instead, laboratory testing conducted by the US Centers for Disease Control and Prevention (CDC) and Health Canada (the Canadian national public health agency) determined that a formerly unidentified strain of influenza had triggered the outbreaks.[8]

With the number of confirmed cases of this new strain (subsequently termed novel H1N1) growing rapidly, senior government officials convened in late April in Mexico City to formulate a response.[9] On Friday, April 24, Mexico's Health Secretary, Dr. Jose Angel Cordova, briefed reporters who had assembled from around the world. "We're dealing with a new flu virus that constitutes a respiratory epidemic that so far is controllable," he told them.[10] But, he warned, "This is highly contagious, it can be fatal and it has pandemic properties."[11] Cordova acknowledged that hundreds, if not thousands, of Mexicans were likely suffering from H1N1 and that at least 68 people had died of "respiratory problems" since the onset of the outbreak.[12] Perhaps most worrisome, many of the ill and dead were young and previously healthy adults, populations generally less vulnerable to influenza.[13]

As news of these deaths spread, residents in and around Mexico City—a massive metropolis of approximately 20 million people—sought to protect themselves as best they could. They flooded hospitals in search of vaccine, depleted stocks of facemasks, and followed a series of sweeping social distancing measures instituted by the government.[14]

---

6. HHS, *Pandemic Influenza Plan*; IOM, *Domestic and International Impacts*; David Lakey, *Novel H1N1: Lessons Learned, Pandemic Planning, and Preparations*, Legislative Briefing (Austin, TX: September 16, 2009).
7. IOM, *Domestic and International Impacts*; Center for Infectious Disease Research and Policy, "H1N1 2009 Pandemic Influenza," 2010, http://www.cidrap.umn.edu/cidrap/content/influenza/swineflu/biofacts/ swinefluoverview.html; Alexandra Minna Stern and Howard Markel, "What Mexico Taught the World about Pandemic Influenza Preparedness and Community Mitigation Strategies," *JAMA* 302 (2009): 1221–1222; CDC, "Outbreak of Swine-Origin Influenza A (H1N1) Virus Infection—Mexico, March–April 2009," *Morbidity and Mortality Weekly Report* 58 (2009): 1–3.
8. IOM, *Domestic and International Impacts*; CDC, "Update: Swine Influenza A (H1N1) Infections—California and Texas, April 2009," *Morbidity and Mortality Weekly Report* 58 (2009): 435–437.
9. Lacey and McNeil, "Fighting Deadly Flu Outbreak."
10. Ibid.
11. Ioan Grillo, "Swine Flu Outbreak Stirs Alarm," *Houston Chronicle*, April 25, 2009, A1.
12. Ibid.
13. Lacey and McNeil, "Fighting Deadly Flu Outbreak."
14. Grillo, "Swine Flu Outbreak." Mexico initially tried inoculating people with existing supplies of seasonal flu vaccine, but it soon became clear that the vaccine was ineffective against this new strain of flu.

Beginning April 24, all schools and colleges in the Mexico City area closed indefinitely, as did museums, public cinemas, and sports facilities. A few days later, the federal government extended the measures nationwide. [15]

Poor disease surveillance and reporting systems limited situational awareness, however, contributing to an initial distortion of case–fatality ratios, which, in turn, heightened fears over H1N1's lethality.[16] To help Mexican authorities gain a better understanding of the extent of the outbreak and the disease's actual severity, the US federal government provided assistance with testing specimens and conducting epidemiological investigations.[17] The United States also made available antiviral medications to help alleviate symptoms and to minimize infections. "Flu viruses don't stop at the border and it is imperative we do whatever we can to slow the spread of the virus and help stop this outbreak," US Secretary of Health and Human Services Kathleen Sebelius said as she explained the Obama administration's rationale for providing aid.[18]

In fact, by the time Sebelius spoke, H1N1 had quietly found its way into the southwestern United States, with CDC confirming first on April 15 and then on April 17 that a 10-year-old Californian and a 9-year-old, also of California, had contracted this new strain of flu.[19] With the situation in Mexico continuing to intensify, the news from California prompted the United States to begin conducting an epidemiological investigation on its own soil. The investigation would expand, when just a week later, on Thursday, April 23, Texas health officials learned that laboratory testing had confirmed H1N1 in two students attending Byron P. Steele High School, located in Guadalupe County, not far from San Antonio. [20] (For a map of Texas and its counties, see Exhibit 7-3.)

Seeking to establish an epidemiological, or epi, link (an identifiable line of contacts connecting infected individuals) between the California and Texas cases, investigators pursued several early leads. For one thing, three of the four cases had initially been flagged by military surveillance systems.[21] Was the virus primarily circulating among military populations? But investigators also learned that one of the two Californians had recently traveled to Dallas, and epidemiologists from California and Texas teamed

15. Grillo, "Swine Flu Outbreak"; Stern and Markel, "What Mexico Taught the World."

16. Stern and Markel, "What Mexico Taught the World."

17. CDC, "Update: Swine Influenza A."

18. HHS, *Secretary Sebelius Takes Two Key Actions on Strategic National Stockpile* (Washington, DC: HHS, 2009).

19. Novel Swine-Origin Influenza A (H1N1) Virus Investigation Team, "Emergence of a Novel Swine-Origin Influenza A (H1N1) Virus in Humans," *New England Journal of Medicine* 360 (2009): 2605–2615; CDC, "Swine Influenza A (H1N1) Infection in Two Children-Southern California, March-April 2009," *Morbidity and Mortality Weekly Report* 58 (2009): 1–3.

20. CDC, "Update: Swine Influenza A"; David Lakey, *Panel 1: Vaccine Distribution,* Testimony to the Senate Committee on Health and Human Services (Austin, TX: February 24, 2010); Belinda Pustka, *Lessons Learned from a School Closure in Response to H1N1,* Presentation at the Texas Pandemic Influenza Summit (Austin, TX: August 10, 2009).

21. Don Finley, "Flu Strain Matches Mexico's," *San Antonio Express-News,* April 25, 2009, A1; CDC, "Swine Influenza A (H1N1) Infection in Two Children."

up to follow that trail as well.[22] In the end, however, the investigations failed to connect the four cases.[23]

Unable to identify an epi link, US health officials concluded that H1N1 had established itself in the American Southwest. They also determined that since none of the individuals infected with H1N1 had any known contact with pigs, this novel strain of the flu was now spreading through human-to-human contact.[24] As laboratory tests confirmed several more cases of the new virus within a matter of days in Texas and, with intense media attention now focused on the state, public officials at all levels of government moved to respond to the rapidly unfolding health crisis.

TEXAS LAUNCHES ITS RESPONSE

Despite collaborating regularly with Mexican health officials, Dr. David Lakey, Commissioner of the Texas Department of State Health Services (DSHS), did not learn about the extensive H1N1 outbreaks occurring south of Texas's border from his Mexican counterparts or from federal health officials in the United States.[25] Instead, he said, he first heard of the respiratory illnesses in Mexico just as CDC confirmed the two Guadalupe County cases and even then, through a much less formal channel. Upon returning home one evening, Lakey had sat down at his computer to scan health updates online. An alert about the mounting cases in Mexico, posted by the University of Minnesota's Center for Infectious Disease Research and Policy, caught his eye. It was then that he realized that the few cases of H1N1 so far identified in Texas and California were likely part of a much larger event. "There's something going on just south of our border, and we had this very unusual swine flu in two different parts of the United States. You start putting two and two together that this could indeed be a pandemic—the first pandemic in 40 years," Lakey recollected.[26]

---

22. DSHS, *Two Human Cases of Swine Flu Confirmed in Texas* (Austin, TX: DSHS, 2009).

23. DSHS, *Two Human Cases*; Novel Swine-Origin Influenza A (H1N1) Virus Investigation Team, "Emergence of a Novel Swine Origin Influenza A."

24. CDC, "Update: Swine Influenza A;" Lacey and McNeil, "Fighting Deadly Flu Outbreak."

25. A number of mechanisms exist to coordinate and facilitate crossborder activities and communication, including the United States–Mexico Border Health Commission (USMBHC), which seeks to address health problems across the border area through binational action. USMBHC's membership consists of both the US and Mexican secretaries of health, as well as the chief health officers of the 10 states on either side of the border. The commission covers a region with a total population of almost 12 million people, a large number of whom live in poverty with limited access to important health resources and inadequate or no health insurance. The annual average income for US residents living in the area is around $14,500, while 25% to 30% of the US border population is uninsured. See: United States–México Border Health Commission, 2010, http://www.borderhealth.org.

26. All statements and quotations attributed to state and local officials are from interviews conducted by the author in February and April 2010, unless otherwise noted.

Texas Department of State Health Services Stands Up Its Multiagency Coordination Center

After learning of the first two cases of H1N1 in California, senior DSHS staff had convened quietly at the department's headquarters in Austin to begin discussing possible response options. But with the confirmation of the two cases in Guadalupe County and growing awareness of the situation in Mexico, state health leaders quickly realized that they faced a potentially serious health threat, requiring a more formal response apparatus. Consequently, on Friday, April 24, DSHS activated its multiagency coordination center (MACC) at its sprawling Austin campus.[27] The MACC would serve as the center of the public health response to the emerging disease in Texas. At the same time, Lakey directed his border health team to gather any information they could about the respiratory illnesses occurring in Mexico. But getting a clear picture of events to the south proved challenging amidst the escalating crisis. "It just wasn't as clean a communication as it could have been," said Dr. Adolfo Valadez, Assistant Commissioner for Prevention and Preparedness Services at DSHS.

Meanwhile, the interagency State Operations Center (SOC), also in Austin, ratcheted up its own activities. Although the outbreak clearly qualified as a public health emergency, with DSHS taking the lead in the overall response, the effort would require the direct involvement of a host of other state agencies, chief among them the Governor's Division of Emergency Management (GDEM), the Texas Education Agency (TEA), and the Texas Department of Agriculture. To coordinate their activities, department heads and key partners from the private and nonprofit sectors convened at the SOC over the course of the weekend of April 24 to 26. Both Commissioner Lakey and Jack Colley, director of GDEM and the governor's point man for disaster response, said that the decision-making process at the SOC proceeded relatively smoothly, due in large part to the trust they had in each other. This trust, they elaborated, came from working closely in response to one high-stakes disaster after another, including not only Hurricanes Gustav and Ike but a series of smaller emergencies as well—an unfortunate reality in a state as large as Texas.

Gathered together at the SOC, state officials realized that their response to H1N1 would require regular communication with a large number of key stakeholders and decision-makers outside of government, such as hospitals, professional associations, school districts, and businesses, as well as with local and regional officials from across the state. (A massive home-rule state, Texas consists of 254 counties and more than 1,000 municipalities, to which it delegates a considerable amount of governmental responsibility.) Thus, on Sunday, April 26, DSHS joined with GDEM in initiating the first of what became daily, statewide conference calls. State officials conducted the calls at the SOC, which offered a teleconferencing system that supported 3,000 dedicated phone lines.

---

27. Lakey, *Panel 1: Vaccine Distribution.*

Valadez described the nature of the calls:

> Our commissioner, or myself, when he couldn't do it, would give an update of what we knew at the time, what we didn't know, and then what our plans were, what we were doing in terms of disease surveillance, laboratory surveillance, vaccine, antivirals. And then literally we would just answer any questions that people had. We'd be there for about two hours answering hundreds of questions.

With these calls, which on some days included up to 10,000 participants, state officials aimed to help local leaders communicate directly with their communities and the local media, instead of trying to control all communication in a centralized manner. "If there was a big event, I would be out there, but if we could equip the locals so they could be effective, we thought that would be a better strategy," Lakey explained, noting that conditions varied tremendously from one part of the state to another, necessitating a locally based approach.

DSHS officials acknowledged that some in the public health community eventually found the process tedious, as the calls often covered the same ground. All the same, they say, it was one of the few ways they and other state leaders could speak directly to their partners from across Texas all at once.

Grappling With Unknowns

As they set up their command structure and communication systems, state health officials, with assistance from their federal counterparts, scrambled to overcome a number of significant unknowns. Realizing that H1N1 was moving rapidly, they understood that they would have to make some important decisions fast. But to do so, they needed to know what, exactly, they faced. Had the disease remained confined to Guadalupe County, or was it now widespread across the state? Reports emerging from Mexico indicated that H1N1 was extremely virulent. But had Mexican authorities captured the complete picture? As Adolfo Valadez put it, "Yes, there are 100 people dying, but remember, there's 24 million people in Mexico City. So is it just a bad outbreak? … We didn't know, and that was a problem."

To gain a better understanding, DSHS dispatched teams of epidemiologists to investigate suspected cases and to collect specimens from ill individuals. DSHS also tapped into the Texas Medical Association's communication network, asking the group to encourage member physicians to report cases of influenza-like-illness and submit samples for testing. Meanwhile, in Austin, state and CDC epidemiologists huddled together at DSHS's MACC to analyze collected data and determine the nature of the disease and the extent of its spread.

Senior DSHS officials also kept in constant communication with CDC and other federal health authorities, discussing a range of possible interventions that might stem, or at least mitigate, the spread of the new disease. Although the federal health bureaucracy was experiencing significant transition (the outbreak occurred just 3 months into the Obama administration), Lakey said that he and his team had little trouble communicating with CDC's leadership. Dr. Richard Besser, the agency's acting director, had previously headed CDC's public health preparedness programs and had played a large role in the pandemic planning process. In addition, Lakey had worked closely with Besser during Hurricanes Gustav and Ike in 2008, personally giving him and then CDC Director Julie Gerberding tours of the disaster zone. "So," said the Commissioner, "there was already a relationship there. I could get on the phone and talk to him."

In considering their next steps, state and federal officials turned to a matrix featured in both the state and national pandemic plans. This tool detailed actions and interventions appropriate for each level of an outbreak, from a Category 1 low-grade event to a Category 5 full-blown pandemic.[28]

Commissioner Lakey explained, "Your interventions are based on that categorization. And so for things like closing schools, you would definitely do it if it was a Category 4 or Category 5 outbreak. You wouldn't do it if it was a Category 1."

To know what outbreak category they now faced, public health officials first needed to determine the disease's case–fatality ratio and the total number of H1N1-related deaths. But that proved highly challenging early on, given the paucity of good data. As a result, authorities said, they ultimately treated the matrix more as a guide than a fixed plan. "I think it gave us a good framework to consider options, to consider scenarios and say, don't forget about this," Valadez explained. But as for the recommended interventions, "they really had to be honed and tuned to that specific incident at that point in time."

Controlling H1N1 at the Border?

Among the first actions state and federal officials considered was controlling traffic or monitoring incoming travelers for flu-like symptoms along the Texas–Mexico border. On Saturday, April 25, CDC issued an outbreak notice regarding travel to Mexico. But although it advised travelers about precautions they could take, the agency did not warn the general public to avoid the country altogether.[29] All the same, senior officials in Texas, as well as in Atlanta, Georgia, and Washington, DC, were seriously weighing the risks travel to and from Mexico posed. As Roger Sanchez, a senior epidemiologist with San Antonio's Metropolitan Health District pointed out, "It's a concern.... We've got daily flights from Mexico City."[30] And flights were not the only worry, given the high

---

28. David Lakey, *Panel 2: Standardized Protocols for School Districts*, Testimony to the Senate Committee on Health and Human Services (Austin, TX: February 24, 2010).

29. Finley, "Flu Strain Matches Mexico's."

30. Ibid.

volume of traffic that crossed the more than 1,200-mile-long border between Mexico and Texas via foot and ground transportation. In 2008 alone, more than 29 million vehicles and 2 million pedestrians had entered the state from points south.[31]

Calls for closing the border escalated once news broke that H1N1 had appeared in Texas. New York Representative Eric Massa led the campaign in Congress, urging a total shutdown. He was joined by several California anti-immigration groups, and Arizona Senator John McCain announced that he was open to the idea "if it would prevent further transmission of this deadly virus."[32] But even as the case count mounted in Mexico, officials in a position to close the border rejected the idea, deeming it as hasty, counterproductive, and simply too late. Speaking just a week after the first Texas cases of H1N1 had been identified, Governor Rick Perry said closing the border "obviously would be an option, but I think playing the 'what if' game of escalation without indicators is premature."[33]

According to Texas's Director of Emergency Management, Jack Colley, restricting border traffic failed to gain much traction for several reasons. To start with, it would have inflicted a devastating economic toll. In 2008, $367 billion in trade had crossed the Texas–Mexico border, while total exports from Texas to Mexico had surpassed $62 billion.[34] In addition, Colley observed that with dozens of international air and seaports and thousands of miles of interstate borders, travelers and goods could find their way into Texas via multiple ports of entry. Meanwhile, from Washington, President Barack Obama argued that as H1N1 had already appeared in Texas and California, clamping down on travel and other crossborder exchanges was pointless. "It would be akin to closing the barn door after the horses are out," he said.[35] Added US Homeland Security Secretary Janet Napolitano, "The real focus needs to be now on what do we do to reduce the spread of the disease within our border."[36]

A School Year Disrupted

Without a vaccine that could provide immunity against H1N1 and with border closure off the table, health officials in Texas and the United States had only a few options at their disposal as they sought to control the disease's spread. One such tool, social distancing, had at times proven effective in controlling outbreaks of infectious disease in the past, and state and federal authorities decided that it was well worth a try now.

31. Terri Langford, "Swine Flu Arrives Here; World Alert Level Raised, State Reacts," *Houston Chronicle*, April 30, 2009, A1.
32. Editorial, "Border-Closure Talk Is Premature," *San Antonio Express-News*, April 30, 2009, B6; Richard S. Dunham, "Officials Dismiss Calls to Close Border," *Houston Chronicle*, May 1, 2009, B7.
33. Langford, "Swine Flu Arrives Here."
34. Editorial, "Border-Closure Talk Is Premature."
35. Dunham, "Officials Dismiss Calls."
36. Ibid.

In particular, they focused on implementing the measure in school settings, where the first cases of H1N1 in Texas had emerged. According to Commissioner Lakey, the decision did not come easily. But, he continued, "In this situation, where we don't have all the information we would like to have, a decision still has to be made. And the decision was: we're going to err on the side of protecting the students as we figure out what's going on." Added Valadez:

> We didn't know where we were on this scale initially. So in these first few days, we're going to assume we're here, at Category 5, until we get better data.... I think we had to make that assumption because if we were wrong it would have been disastrous.

Following confirmation on April 23 that the two teenagers attending Byron Steele High School in Guadalupe County had contracted H1N1, state health officials pursued an aggressive course of action. First, Dr. Sandra Guerra, the medical director for the DSHS Health Service Region covering the area,[37] immediately advised the superintendent of the Schertz-Cibolo-Universal City Independent School District (ISD), Dr. Belinda Pustka, to notify parents of the identification of H1N1 at Steele. A day later, Guerra recommended that the district close the high school, which administrators agreed to do. And when, on Saturday, April 25, CDC confirmed additional cases of H1N1 in Guadalupe County, the ISD, again in consultation with Dr. Guerra, decided to shut down all 14 of its schools.[38] In announcing their decision, school and public health authorities emphasized the importance of students keeping away from each other throughout the hiatus. The point of shutting down the schools, Guerra explained "is to reduce the risk to students, staff and the community," warning that out-of-school contact at malls, at each other's homes, and the like, would only "defeat the purpose."[39]

Reports of influenza-like illness increased rapidly throughout the state, and by the end of April at least 10 school districts across Texas had closed, affecting more than 130,000 students and their families.[40] Speaking to the public on Wednesday, April 29, TEA Commissioner Robert Scott echoed Guerra's advice, urging ill children to remain home. "It's not the time to worry about the perfect attendance award," he said. Scott also noted that the University Interscholastic League, which manages academic and athletic competitions in Texas, had agreed to postpone all planned events until at least May 11. "One-act play competitions. Track meets. All of those will be affected," Scott declared.[41]

---

37. Texas's public health system consists of 64 autonomous local health departments, which serve approximately three quarters of the state's population, and 11 DSHS-administered health service regions, which provide public health services to counties without a local health department. See: DSHS, *Novel H1N1: Lessons Learned and Preparedness*, Presentation at the Texas Pandemic Influenza Summit (Austin, TX: August 10, 2009).

38. Lakey, *Panel 1: Vaccine Distribution*; Pustka, *Lessons Learned*. In Texas, the decision to close schools rests with the leadership of independent school districts, or ISDs, not with state or local public health officials.

39. DSHS, *School to Close, Other Flu Precautions Recommended* (Austin, TX: DSHS, 2009).

40. Langford, "Swine Flu Arrives Here."

41. Ibid.

Two days later, on May 1, CDC announced that it was recommending schools with probable or confirmed cases of H1N1 to remain closed for as many as 14 days.[42] The announcement prompted even more schools in Texas to shut their doors, and by May 6, more than 830 facilities had done so, collectively disrupting the school year for almost 500,000 children (more than 10% of the state's student population).[43] But cancelling classes meant far more than a bonus vacation for students. Parents would either have to pay for childcare or miss work to watch over their children themselves, a difficult proposition in the midst of a severe economic recession. Jack Colley and Adolfo Valadez added that as school closures piled up, public officials received considerable pushback from business owners, who worried that their employees would have to miss work in order to stay home with their children, thus possibly contributing to losses in productivity and revenue.[44]

Meanwhile, in Guadalupe County, the continued school closures also resulted in the postponement of important tests, such as the SATs, Advanced Placement exams, the International Baccalaureate, and the Texas Assessment of Knowledge and Skills (TAKS), which the state required students to pass in order to graduate. Additional social distancing measures implemented in the county included the cancellation of various after-school social events, as well as the closure of public parks and libraries.[45]

Despite the extensive disruptions caused by these interventions, health officials defended their actions. Speaking to the trustees of the Schertz-Cibolo-University City ISD, Sandra Guerra explained that DSHS had recommended the sweeping social distancing measures in an effort to stem the further spread of this potentially fatal new strain of influenza. "We took very proactive steps," she said, "and with the leadership of Dr. Pustka [the school district superintendent], we were able to come to an agreement very quickly that the health and well-being of the students and staff and this community was paramount. I believe that what we and what you have done by supporting the school closures in this particular district and in this county, has been to actually protect the rest of the community."[46]

But not every locality or ISD that experienced outbreaks of suspected or confirmed cases of H1N1 took the same approach. In San Antonio/Bexar County, for instance, Metro Health Director Dr. Fernando Guerra (who as the head of an independent local

42. HHS, *Statement by HHS Secretary Kathleen Sebelius and by Acting CDC Director Richard Besser Regarding the Change in CDC's School and Child Care Closure Guidance* (Washington, DC: HHS, 2009).

43. Mary Ann Roser, "1st US Citizen Felled by Flu," *Austin American-Statesman*, May 6, 2009, A1.

44. Communicating to businesses the importance of being flexible in the face of social distancing measures proved difficult for state health officials, but some organizations were more cooperative than others. For instance, the grocery chain H.E.B. allowed employees working in its Schertz store to take paid time off if they had children affected by the school closures in the district. See: Elizabeth Allen and Lindsay Kastner, "Schools Getting Ready for Flu Bug," *San Antonio Express-News*, September 18, 2009, B1.

45. David DeKunder, "SCUC Hoping to Return to Class Monday after 'Flu Break,'" *San Antonio Express-News*, May 7, 2009, NH1; Ericka Mellon, Eric Berger, and Jeannie Kever, "Schools, Parents Find Flu Bad Timing," *Houston Chronicle*, May 2, 2009, A1.

46. DeKunder, "SCUC Hoping to Return."

health department did not have to follow state guidance) made it clear that local officials within his jurisdiction had decided against implementing immediate school closures.[47] This contrasted sharply with the policies enforced next door in Guadalupe County, which did not have its own health department and where the region's public health authority functioned as a state employee acting under DSHS's direction.

The juxtaposition of the neighboring jurisdictions' policies presented public health officials with considerable challenges in delivering a clear message. Because the same media market covered the entire region, newspapers and television programs picked up the seemingly contradictory measures taken in Guadalupe and San Antonio. As Lee Lane, Executive Director of the Texas Association of Local Health Officials (TALHO) observed, this, along with similar situations in other regions throughout the state, led many residents to wonder "Why did they close in this county and didn't close in the contiguous county?" Added Stephen Williams, President of TALHO and Director of the Houston Department of Health and Human Services, "When we operated separately using different guidelines in the communities, which are pretty much closely tied to each other, [that] really caused a lot of confusion.... We really need to band together and look at opportunities for cooperating with each other so that we can have the level of influence that I believe we should have in situations like this."

Valadez acknowledged that the school closure process proved challenging, noting that despite having plans for closing down schools, state and local authorities didn't have much experience in implementing the plans on such a large scale. "We had templates for all of that, but once you're there, it's just different. It's one thing to talk about social distancing, but then when you're forced into 'Well, how does that really work?'—What does that mean?"

A Death and a Disaster Declaration

State and local officials continued to grapple with the best approach for containing the spread of H1N1. But on Wednesday, April 29, the stakes were raised significantly, when CDC informed Commissioner Lakey that the nation's first confirmed death from H1N1 had occurred two days earlier in a 22-month-old toddler at Texas Children's Hospital in Houston. Unlike the Guadalupe teenagers, the boy, who had suffered from several underlying health conditions, had a clear connection to Mexico. A Mexican citizen, he had recently traveled from Mexico City to Brownsville, Texas, where he had been treated for influenza before being airlifted to Children's.[48]

47. Elizabeth Allen and Don Finley, "Harberger Tells Public: 'Let's Don't Panic Just Yet,'" *San Antonio Express-News,* May 2, 2009, A1.

48. Cindy George, "Two More Swine Flu Infections Confirmed in Fort Bend County," *Houston Chronicle,* May 3, 2009, A18; Ericka Mellon, "Schools Set to Reopen as Swine Flu Fears Dim," *Houston Chronicle,* May 6, 2009, A1; DSHS, *Texas Reports Swine Flu in Child from Mexico City* (Austin, TX: DSHS, 2009).

State leaders gathered late Wednesday morning to announce the child's death and to reassure an increasingly anxious public. In addition to Lakey, those assembled included Governor Perry, Chief Colley, Education Commissioner Robert Scott, and senior members of the state legislature. Governor Perry spoke first, announcing that CDC had now confirmed 16 cases of H1N1 in Texas, including, tragically, the new fatality.[49] Yet, he emphasized,

> I think it's very important to note that Texans can be confident that we're making every effort to stay ahead of the curve, to keep them and their families as safe as possible.... Fortunately, we have a detailed plan in place to deal with this very situation, an approach based on extensive research, careful planning, and collaboration with our partners all across the state.[50]

Perry added that the state's leadership was uniquely qualified to respond to this new threat. "We have honed our team approach to disaster management during our response to numerous storms, wildfires, and floods," he said. The governor also announced that he was issuing a disaster declaration for the entire state. The move, Perry explained, elevated Texas's alert levels and allowed for the provision of greater federal assistance.

Following Perry, Commissioner Lakey noted that DSHS was closely monitoring the conditions of two more seriously ill patients, including a pregnant woman. Lakey acknowledged that WHO had yet to classify H1N1 as a full-blown pandemic (in fact, that day WHO raised its pandemic alert level to Phase 5, one step below pandemic status), but he told Texans, "In light of the incomplete picture without all the data, we believe it is prudent for us to operate in this heightened state of awareness."[51] Until the public health community could determine the extent and severity of H1N1, Lakey pledged that the state would continue to respond aggressively.

Adapting Response Plans: Texas Department of State Health Services Improvises With Its Antiviral Distribution Model

Despite the considerable uncertainty that remained, the early epidemiological investigations in Texas, California, and Mexico had revealed useful information. Health officials had quickly learned that the existing seasonal flu vaccine provided no immunity against novel H1N1. But they also discovered that certain antiviral medications, such as oseltamivir (marketed commercially as Tamiflu) and zanamivir (Relenza), helped prevent

---

49. Office of the Governor, "Gov. Perry Addresses Efforts to Combat Swine Flu in Texas," April 29, 2009.
50. Ibid.
51. Ibid.

and mitigate its effects.[52] Thus, in addition to social distancing, antiviral distribution emerged as one of the key countermeasures in Texas's battle to minimize the consequences of H1N1.

Most people could obtain antiviral medications through a routine prescription process. That is, a doctor would first determine whether a patient's symptoms and condition qualified him or her for the drug. The provider would then write a prescription, which a pharmacist would fill. But an emergency procedure was in place if state officials determined that it was in the public interest to make antiviral medications as widely available as possible: they could tap into the state's portion of the federal government's Strategic National Stockpile (SNS) as well as other reserves directly controlled by the state.[53] And, in fact, as soon as H1N1 had appeared in Texas, Governor Perry had moved quickly to procure the state's SNS antiviral supplies, requesting a total of 850,000 doses during the weekend of April 25–26.[54] (In addition, Texas had at its immediate disposal another 840,000 doses, for which the legislature had appropriated funding during the previous legislative session).[55]

To contain the spread of H1N1 and minimize its effects, health and public safety officials wanted to ensure that all Texans requiring antiviral medications, regardless of their financial circumstances, had access to the drugs. (This was an important concern, as Texas had the highest portion of uninsured residents of all 50 states, at about 25%.) Those who could afford antiviral medication would still need to fill their prescriptions through routine commercial channels. But for guidance on putting in place a system for distributing stockpiled antivirals to the uninsured and underinsured, DSHS leaders first turned to the state's pandemic plan. The plan detailed a point-of-distribution (POD) model, in which DSHS, along with GDEM and the Texas National Guard, would directly manage every step of the process, from receiving deliveries of the federal stock to dispensing the drugs at mass clinics.

It soon became clear, however, that the POD model was not particularly well suited to the event at hand. Valadez noted, "We had really done a lot with the strategic national stockpile across the state, and done very well [having scored 100 on CDC's most recent technical assistance review], but I think when we got in the thick of it, we realized that this was just an unsustainable model for H1N1." The POD-based system, he elaborated,

---

52. Antiviral medications can inhibit the growth or reproduction of a virus, although they do not offer long-term immunity and are not effective against every strain of the flu. If they are taken within 48 hours of exposure, they may, but are not guaranteed to, prevent disease. They can also help reduce length of illness and prevent severe complications, if taken within 48 hours of onset of symptoms. See: Cindy George, R.G. Ratcliffe, and Liz Austin Peterson, "The Swine Flu Outbreak: More Antiviral Shipments Expected Soon in Houston," *Houston Chronicle*, May 2, 2009, B1; Lakey, *Novel H1N1*.

53. The Strategic National Stockpile is a federally run program that states can access to obtain medications and medical supplies during health emergencies. The stockpile is intended to augment, but not replace, the existing supply chain. DSHS and Texas Division of Emergency Management (DEM), *Antiviral Medication Distribution*, Presentation at Texas Pandemic Influenza Regional Conferences (August and September 2009).

54. Lakey, *Panel 1: Vaccine Distribution*; Office of the Governor, *Gov. Perry Addresses Efforts*.

55. Office of the Governor, *Gov. Perry Addresses Efforts*.

remained appropriate for a bioterror event—when the state would need to rapidly distribute antibiotics within a defined area over a finite period of time—but it did not seem particularly useful for a statewide and prolonged infectious disease outbreak.

Jack Colley recognized the mismatch of the POD distribution plan and the H1N1 outbreak as well and he soon informed his DSHS counterparts that they could not support a 24/7, months-long operation. In response, health officials threw the POD plans out the window and quickly devised a new system, through which the state would distribute stockpiled medication via private pharmacies, federally qualified health centers, and regional and local health departments. Partnering with the private sector made an enormous amount of sense to state officials. As Colley remarked, "Our structures worked, our systems worked, our infrastructure worked, both private sector and public. So there wasn't any need to go out and build PODs to distribute Tamiflu." Private pharmacies, he continued, "do it for a living." Valadez concurred, deeming the refining of the distribution model a critical learning moment in the response to H1N1. "Don't create new systems during disasters—use existing systems [if you can]," he advised.

Since the state already had a standing contract with Texas retail chain H-E-B for the provision of disaster assistance (put in place as a result of the state's repeated experiences responding to large-scale hurricanes), DSHS turned to the company to serve as its private sector partner for the new antiviral distribution strategy. Coordinating with H-E-B proved easy, as the company already had a representative situated in the SOC in Austin, alongside the government officials leading the response. Colley noted that the company's presence in the SOC helped tremendously as the state developed and rolled out the new model. "There's an immediate situational awareness," he said. "If there's a need to distribute these antivirals . . . they're with us when we make those decisions."[56]

Over the course of the next several months, the state made stockpiled antiviral medications available through 63 H-E-B stores in three areas experiencing particularly intense H1N1 activity—Central Texas, Houston, and the Rio Grande Valley.[57] As with the normal process for procuring antiviral medications, a patient would still need to visit a health care provider and receive a prescription for the drug. But now, based on insurance status, DSHS instructed providers to also (1) determine the patient's eligibility for government supplies, (2) guide an eligible patient to a participating pharmacy, and (3) note on the prescription that the pharmacy should fill the prescription with medication from state stock.[58]

Health officials believed that Texas had adequate levels of antiviral drugs through a combination of commercial and government-purchased supplies. But some initial reports indicated that parts of the state faced shortages. In the Houston area, for instance, pharmacies as well as public hospitals and clinics at first experienced dwindling supplies. In response,

56. Office of the Governor, "Gov. Perry, State Officials: Texas Is Prepared for H1N1 Flu Season," August 24, 2009.
57. Lakey, *Panel 1: Vaccine Distribution*.
58. DSHS and DEM, *Antiviral Medication Distribution*.

several health care facilities rationed the medication they had on hand, prioritizing hospital-ized patients and health care workers.[59] But Kathy Barton of the Houston Health Department quickly dismissed talk of shortages. "We're not going to talk about where it is or how much it is because it hypes up the fear, but there is a lot," she insisted. "It really is a ton."[60] Added Colley, "There were cases maybe of somebody who didn't get an antiviral because a doctor didn't prescribe it, but as far as access [and] availability of Tamiflu—we had it."

DSHS officials acknowledged several shortcomings with the new distribution system, however. For one thing, some providers did not feel comfortable serving as a gatekeeper, having to inform patients whether they qualified for the free government stock or had to pay to have their prescription filled. In addition, several pharmacies that only had government stock on hand refused to service people with insurance—no matter the cir-cumstances. Valadez reflected, "We [originally] said that this is only for the uninsured. But really we should have said, 'it's for anyone who cannot afford *or access* it.' And we changed that and made it clear to all pharmacy chains that if someone with insurance shows up and needs that med, they get it."

Additional Deaths, Relaxed Restrictions

On Tuesday, May 5, DSHS reported Texas's second death from H1N1 and the first involving an American citizen. According to state health officials, the woman, who lived in Cameron County, which borders Mexico, had begun suffering flu-like symptoms on April 14. Like the toddler who had died a week earlier, she had an underlying medical condition.[61] Just a day later, on May 6, a 33-year-old Corpus Christi male, also with under-lying medical conditions, died from H1N1 as well.[62]

But by then, health authorities had begun to develop a better understanding of the disease, thanks in large part to the work of local, state, and federal epidemiologists who had fanned out across the state to investigate cases, as well as the many providers who had sent in samples for laboratory testing. The collected data revealed a case–fatality ratio considerably lower than originally feared. Lakey observed that the process proved enormously helpful, although it also posed some major challenges:

> I guess the good thing about that is that we got a lot of samples … and we were able to get that numerator/denominator [for the case–fatality ratio]. The challenge for us, though, is that our laboratory is a surveillance laboratory, a public health laboratory, and all of a sudden it was getting inundated with laboratory specimens. At one time we were receiving in one day the number of samples we would receive in a year.

59. George and others, "The Swine Flu Outbreak."
60. Ibid.
61. Roser, "1st US Citizen Felled."
62. Elizabeth Allen, "Another Swine Flu Fatality," *San Antonio Express-News,* May 16, 2009, B1.

To meet the surge, the state brought in additional equipment and personnel, reassigning department employees and hiring temporary support staff through standing contracts that it had developed with health care staffing agencies. As with the statewide conference calls conducted from the state operations center and the distribution partnership with H-E-B, the contracts had been put in place as a result of Texas's past experiences with hurricanes. State officials had learned through their responses to large-scale events like Hurricanes Katrina, Rita, Gustav, and Ike the importance of having qualified, credentialed personnel available on-call.

The increased staffing helped expedite the testing process, and state and federal authorities soon had a much better grasp on the nature of the outbreak. Realizing that H1N1 was now widespread and no longer containable—but, fortunately, not particularly virulent among most populations—they relaxed some of their initial social distancing guidelines. On May 5, CDC backed away from the strict guidance it had issued the previous week, announcing that schools no longer needed to close upon identification of H1N1. Instead, it advised them to remain open, except in the most extreme cases, when student and staff absences were so widespread that a school could not function.[63]

"We strongly encourage school officials to reopen schools based on the new advice from CDC," Texas Commissioner of Education Robert Scott declared. He added, "In the early phase of this outbreak, it was appropriate for schools and health officials to act cautiously. Within the last 24 hours, the new information made it clear that we can follow standard procedures."[64] Dr. Richard Besser, acting director of CDC, further noted, "Anyone that closed their school based on a previous recommendation, we no longer feel that school closure is warranted."[65]

School districts across the state immediately announced that they would resume instruction.[66] In Guadalupe County, authorities prepared to reopen schools and return to TAKS testing, effective Monday, May 11. In addition, TEA officials confirmed that students there would not have to make up the two weeks of class time they had missed, allowing the district to begin summer recess on June 4, as originally scheduled.[67]

Despite the reversal in policy over school closures, Health Commissioner Lakey believed that the state's recommendations made sense, given the circumstances. "I think we'll get second guessed related to schools that closed. However, I still think when you have the first pandemic in forty years and you have five, ten, fifteen cases that you know

---

63. HHS, *Statement by HHS Secretary Kathleen Sebelius*; Mellon, "Schools Set to Reopen;" Roser, "1st US Citizen Felled."
64. Roser, "1st US Citizen Felled."
65. Ibid.
66. Mellon, "Schools Set to Reopen."
67. DeKunder, "SCUC Hoping to Return."

about, and you don't have the case fatality rate, that's a hard decision that has to be made. Knowing what happened last century, you had 1918, which was devastating; but then you had the pandemics of the '50s and '60s, which were pretty moderate, and we didn't know which one of those scenarios was going to play out."

EPILOGUE

On Thursday, June 11, 2009, with H1N1 now widespread across several continents, WHO declared a full (Phase 6) pandemic for H1N1.[68] Meanwhile, outbreaks of the virus continued across Texas,[69] and by the end of June, health authorities had identified almost 3,000 confirmed and probable cases in the state, with H1N1 activity occurring in 95 counties.[70] A month later, they had confirmed that approximately 5,200 people had contracted H1N1, although Health Commissioner David Lakey believed that this represented just one-tenth of the total cases.[71]

Despite the ongoing spread of H1N1, the situation had become more manageable, as public health officials had gained significant insight into the disease and its behavior. Consequently, the summer provided state and local health officials in Texas with an opportunity to take a look back at the response they had mounted in April and May and to begin planning for an expected second wave of H1N1 in the fall, once students resumed classes.[72] Reflecting on the spring outbreaks, Commissioner Lakey said in mid-June, "We have learned a lot in the last few months." But, he acknowledged, "H1N1 is not going away." Lakey pledged that the state would use the summer months to "fill in many knowledge gaps" and prepare for the fall. Among other things, he elaborated, DSHS would work on bolstering surveillance and laboratory testing systems, revise antiviral distribution partnerships, and prepare for vaccine distribution.[73]

Strategies Revised, Plans Relaunched

In mid-summer, the state recommended that given the relatively mild severity of the disease, school districts should follow seasonal flu protocols, which in general consisted of encouraging parents to keep sick children out of school and of instructing teachers and nurses to send students exhibiting flu-like symptoms home, as opposed to shutting

---

68. IOM, *Domestic and International Impacts.*
69. Lakey, *Panel 1: Vaccine Distribution.*
70. Mary Ann Roser, "Pflugerville Man Is County's First to Die of Swine Flu; State Toll at 14," *Austin American-Statesman,* June 30, 2009, B1.
71. Lakey, *Novel H1N1.*
72. Ibid.
73. Lakey, *Commissioner's Commentary.*

down an entire facility.[74] Commenting on the shift in policy, Debbie Ratcliffe of TEA said, "We tried closing schools to contain the flu [and] that really did not work very well," pointing out that children simply re-congregated at homes, malls, and movie theaters.[75] Moreover, once H1N1 had been identified in a student, it was likely far too late to stop its spread among classmates and the community in general.[76] The state acknowledged that some districts still might need to close but urged school districts to establish trigger points (based on absenteeism rates and student–staff ratios) for determining when to shut a school down.

Also during the summer, the state ceased case counting and laboratory testing to confirm H1N1 (except in select cases, including for hospitalized patients, pregnant women, and deaths).[77] This was due to a variety of reasons. Testing had evolved into an almost unmanageable task, as providers flooded the laboratories with specimens. All the same, it had served its purpose, and health authorities had achieved a much improved understanding of the disease's severity and its reach. DSHS continued to monitor for flu activity, however. It expanded its sentinel surveillance network and monitored for reports from providers of cases of influenza-like illness, while hospitals in Texas continued to report intensive care unit admissions. Providers, local health departments, and hospitals also kept DSHS informed of any new deaths.[78]

In addition, DSHS focused on refining and extending its antiviral distribution system. In response to sporadic outbreaks, the department continued to utilize the model it had developed with H-E-B. But it also formalized a contract for additional partnerships, eventually bringing another seven pharmacy chains (with a total of 1,348 stores) and 71 independent pharmacies into the program, in addition to federally qualified health centers and local health departments. By expanding this public–private partnership, DSHS ultimately ensured the availability of antivirals in 207 of Texas's 254 counties, covering more than 99% of the state's population.[79]

DSHS also organized the Texas Pandemic Influenza Summit, which took place on August 10 in Austin, as well as a series of 13 regional conferences, which occurred across the state in late August and early September, to discuss lessons learned from the spring outbreak and to overview plans for the fall.[80] More than 2,500 people attended the

74. Cindy George, "Schools Revamp Swine Flu Plans," *Houston Chronicle*, August 2, 2009, A1; Mary Ann Roser, "School Year Looms as Swine Flu Marches On," *Austin American-Statesman*, July 24, 2009, A1.

75. Quoted in Roser, "School Year Looms."

76. George, "Schools Revamp."

77. DSHS and DEM, *Laboratory*, Presentation at the Texas Pandemic Influenza Regional Conferences (August and September 2009).

78. DSHS and DEM, *Laboratory*; Lakey, *Novel H1N1*; DSHS and DEM, *Surveillance: Detection and Monitoring for Influenza*, Presentation at the Texas Pandemic Influenza Regional Conferences (August and September 2009).

79. Lakey, *Panel 1: Vaccine Distribution*. In Texas, some countries are so sparsely populated that they may be serviced by just one or two small independent pharmacies, or in some cases (28 counties), by no pharmacy at all.

80. DSHS, *Novel H1N1*.

summit and conferences. Participants included state and local health and education offi-
cials, political leaders, legislative staff, and representatives from the health care sector. The
Austin summit featured several of the key leaders of the spring response: Health
Commissioner David Lakey; Jack Colley, Director of the Governor's Division of Emergency
Management; representatives of the Texas Education Agency; and Dr. Belinda Pustka,
Superintendent of the Schertz-Cibolo-Universal City ISD in Guadalupe County.[81]

The speakers highlighted some essential lessons learned. Dr. Pustka, for instance,
noted that among other things, school administrators and communities at large needed
to understand that CDC guidance evolves and frequently at a rapid rate. She also stressed
the importance of having clearly articulated plans for communicating with the media
and the public, reminding participants that health and school authorities must often
make decisions in the face of considerable political pressure and public alarm.[82] And in
anticipation of a resurgence of H1N1 in the fall, speakers urged participants to coordinate their planning and response activities with neighboring jurisdictions and other levels of government, to encourage uptake of seasonal flu vaccine while H1N1 vaccine
remained in production, and to prepare for a surge along a number of different lines—
from people seeking care to requests for additional information and resources.[83] For his
part, Chief Colley emphasized the enormity of the task public officials faced with the
upcoming start of the school year, noting that more than 4.6 million children attended
public schools in Texas. "That's more people than live in the state of Oklahoma," he said,
warning, "We've got a lot of work to do."[84]

A New School Year Begins

Students in Texas began returning to school on Monday, August 24.[85] That day, just as
they had in late April following the state's first death from H1N1, senior state leaders
gathered together and spoke to the press, seeking to project confidence in their ability to
handle future outbreaks. "I was thinking it just seems like it was four months ago when
we were having this [same] conversation—and it was.... This virus does not seem to
want to go away," Governor Perry observed. But, he continued, "We are more prepared
than ever to handle the challenge."[86] Meanwhile, Health Commissioner Lakey took a
moment to defend the state's aggressive response during the initial outbreaks earlier

81. DSHS, *DSHS Pandemic Influenza Summit and Regional Conferences*, 2009.
82. Pustka, *Lessons Learned*.
83. DSHS, *Novel H1N1*.
84. Corrie MacLaggan, "Schools, Officials Prepare for Next Wave of Swine Flu," *Austin American-Statesman*, August 11, 2009, B1.
85. Mary Ann Roser, "A Present Danger?" *Austin American-Statesman*, August 23, 2009, A1.
86. Office of the Governor, *Gov. Perry, State Officials: Texas Is Prepared*.

that year. "The precautionary illness control actions we took and the messages we conveyed in the spring were prudent, necessary steps to protect Texans from a virus of unknown severity," he said. "At that time, we did not know how this newly discovered virus would behave; we didn't know how severe it would be."[87]

Lakey also cautioned that although health authorities now had a far better understanding of the disease, Texans still faced a number of challenges. "We still have a population that largely has no natural or built-up immunity," he pointed out. "And we won't have, until about mid-October at the earliest, a vaccine that will protect us from the H1N1 virus."[88] Recognizing the state's heavily decentralized system of government and complex public health structure, Lakey emphasized the need for collaboration. "There is," he said, "a shared responsibility between the individuals, local communities, and state government in order to be prepared.... I believe this flu season will be a challenge, but one that we can effectively manage by all of us working together."

Still, a number of public health officials in the state continued to worry publicly about what lay ahead, with several expressing particular concern about the state's ability to effectively respond to a resurgence of H1N1 in the absence of an effective vaccine. As Dr. John Carlo, Dallas County's medical director, put it: "It's kind of like a carpenter going out to the worksite without a hammer. You are without one of your main tools."[89] Yet despite the many challenges Texas had endured when H1N1 first flared up in the spring and the many it would continue to face in the coming months, especially as the state took on the complicated role of distributing the slow-to-arrive H1N1 vaccine, Adolfo Valadez believed that the state's preparedness efforts largely paid off, pointing to DSHS's ability to ramp up an effective response in the face of considerable uncertainty.

"The planning worked," he observed. "I can only imagine where we would have been without it, especially when it was in our backyard."

---

87. Ibid.
88. Ibid.
89. Scott K. Parks, "Dallas-Area Health Officials Double Their Efforts to Keep Flu at Bay," *Dallas Morning News*, August 24, 2009.

Exhibit 7-1. Chronology of Events: Novel H1N1 Influenza A, March–September 2009

March
- Cases of influenza-like illness began appearing in large numbers in Mexico.

Wednesday, April 15
- Laboratory tests conducted by the Centers for Disease Control and Prevention (CDC) confirmed novel influenza A (H1N1) in a 10-year-old from California.

Friday, April 17
- CDC laboratory tests confirmed another case of H1N1 in a specimen taken from a 9-year-old California resident.

Thursday, April 23
- CDC laboratory tests confirmed Texas's first cases of H1N1 in two students attending Byron P. Steele High School, part of the Schertz-Cibolo-Universal Independent School District (ISD), located in Guadalupe County.
- Dr. Sandra Guerra, Regional Medical Director for State Health Service Region 8, which encompasses Guadalupe County, advised the Schertz-Cibolo-Universal ISD to inform parents of students in the district about the appearance of H1N1 at Steele.

Friday, April 24
- Mexico's Health Secretary, Dr. Jose Angel Cordova, warned of the potentially deadly consequences of H1N1, which continued to spread in his country. Mexican officials acknowledged that hundreds of people had become ill with flu-like symptoms and that close to 70 people may have died from the new strain of influenza. Far-reaching social distancing measures were put in place in Mexico City, home to about 20 million people.
- The Texas Department of State Health Services (DSHS) activated its multiagency coordination center (MACC) in Austin.
- Schertz-Cibolo-Universal ISD authorities agreed to close Steele High School.

Saturday, April 25
- Schertz-Cibolo-Universal ISD authorities decided to close all 14 schools in the district. Within days, at least 10 school districts across the state closed, affecting more than 130,000 students.
- Texas Governor Rick Perry made an initial request for the release of antiviral medications from the federal government's Strategic National Stockpile (SNS).
- CDC issued an outbreak notice regarding the spread of H1N1 in Mexico, California, and Texas.

Sunday, April 26
- Texas's State Operations Center, based out of the Governor's Division of Emergency Management, began facilitating daily statewide conference calls.
- Governor Perry increased the state's SNS antiviral request to 850,000 doses.

Monday, April 27
- The first death in the United States from H1N1 occurred in a 22-month-old boy from Mexico who had recently traveled to Brownsville, Texas, before being hospitalized at Texas Children's Hospital in Houston.

Wednesday, April 29
- CDC informed DSHS that the 22-month-old patient in Houston had died from H1N1.
- Texas public officials held a press conference announcing the fatality.
- Texas Governor Rick Perry issued a disaster declaration for the H1N1 outbreak in Texas.
- Texas Education Commissioner Robert Scott announced that the University Interscholastic League had agreed to postpone all inter-district sport and academic competitions until at least May 11.
- The World Health Organization (WHO) issued a Phase 5 pandemic alert for H1N1, one step below full-pandemic status.

Late April–Mid-June
- The state distributed stockpiled antiviral medications to targeted geographic regions. It partnered with H-E-B, a large retailer and pharmacy chain, to carry out the distribution of stockpiled supplies.

Friday, May 1
- CDC issued guidance advising schools with confirmed cases of H1N1 to remain closed for up to 14 days.

(Continued)

Exhibit 7-1. (Continued)

Tuesday, May 5
- CDC revised its guidance regarding school closures. It no longer called on schools with confirmed cases of H1N1 to immediately close; instead it advised localities to make decisions on a case-by-case basis.
- DSHS announced the second death in Texas (and the United States) from H1N1 in a woman living in Cameron County, near the US–Mexico border.

Wednesday, May 6
- A 33-year-old Corpus Christi man died from H1N1.

Monday, May 11
- Schools in the Schertz-Cibolo-Universal City ISD reopened.

Early June
- Texas public school year ended.

Thursday, June 11
- WHO declared a pandemic for H1N1.

Early Summer
- Texas continued to experience outbreaks of H1N1.
- DSHS began refining its response to H1N1, reviewing its experiences during the spring outbreak. Among other things, it expanded its antiviral distribution program to additional pharmacies, extending geographic coverage significantly.

Friday, July 31
- To date, approximately 5,200 cases of H1N1 had been confirmed in Texas.

Monday, August 10
- DSHS held the Texas Pandemic Influenza Summit in Austin.

Mid-August–Early September
- DSHS convened a series of Pandemic Influenza Regional Conferences across the state.

Monday, August 24
- Texas's public schools reopened.
- State officials gathered in Austin to announce plans for responding to H1N1 in the fall.

Source: Based on Institute of Medicine, *The Domestic and International Impacts of the 2009-H1N1 Influenza A Pandemic: Global Challenges, Global Solutions* (Washington, DC: National Academies Press, 2010); David Lakey, *Panel 1: Vaccine Distribution,* Testimony to the Texas Senate Committee on Health and Human Services (Austin, TX: February 24, 2010); Novel Swine-Origin Influenza A (H1N1) Virus Investigation Team, "Emergence of a Novel Swine-Origin Influenza A (H1N1) Virus in Humans," *New England Journal of Medicine* 360 (2009): 2605–2615; and Belinda Pustka, *Lessons Learned from a School Closure in Response to H1N1,* Presentation at the Texas Pandemic Influenza Summit (Austin, TX: August 10, 2009).

Exhibit 7-2. Cast of Characters: 2009 Novel H1N1 Influenza A

State of Texas

Texas Department of State Health Services (DSHS)

- Dr. Sandra Guerra, Regional Medical Director, DSHS Health Service Region 8
- Dr. David Lakey, Commissioner
- Dr. Adolfo Valadez, Assistant Commissioner for Prevention and Preparedness Services

Other State Officials

- Jack Colley, Chief, Governor's Division of Emergency Management
- Rick Perry, Governor, State of Texas
- Robert Scott, Commissioner, Texas Education Agency

Local Health Departments

- Dr. John Carlo, Medical Director, Dallas County Department of Health and Human Services
- Dr. Fernando Guerra, Director of Health, San Antonio Metropolitan Health District
- Lee Lane, Executive Director, Texas Association of Local Health Officials (TALHO)
- Stephen Williams, Director, Houston Department of Health and Human Services, and President, TALHO

Local School Districts

- Dr. Belinda Pustka, Superintendent, Schertz-Cibolo-University City Independent School District

Federal Government

- Dr. Richard Besser, Acting Director, US Centers for Disease Control and Prevention
- Janet Napolitano, Secretary, US Department of Homeland Security
- Barack Obama, President
- Kathleen Sebelius, Secretary, US Department of Health and Human Services

Government of Mexico

- Dr. Jose Angel Cordova, Secretary of Health

Exhibit 7-3. Map of the State of Texas With Counties, Metropolitan Areas, and Central Cities

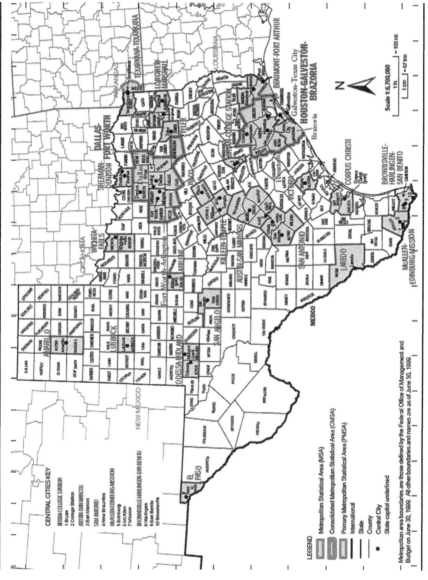

Source: Adapted from US Census Bureau, 1999.

H1N1 at Harvard

Wendy Robison

EDITORS' INTRODUCTION

In early spring 2009, cases of a new strain of influenza—novel H1N1 (or "swine flu")—began to appear in several parts of North America. With no vaccine immediately available to immunize against the disease, many feared that it would take a terrible toll in human lives and cause extensive social and economic disruptions. These worries applied to many different types of communities, including colleges and universities where students, faculty, and staff often study, work, and live together in close quarters, making them particularly vulnerable to outbreaks of infectious disease. In fact, one of the earliest confirmed appearances of H1N1 in the northeastern United States occurred in such a setting, when, in late April, Harvard University administrators learned that a student at the Harvard School of Dental Medicine (located in Harvard's Longwood Medical Area in Boston, Massachusetts) had tested positive for the disease. The situation would only intensify over the next several days, as students from Harvard's other Longwood area schools, the Harvard Medical School and Harvard School of Public Health, also began to report flu-like symptoms.

Although the university was still working on a plan specifically tailored to H1N1, it already had developed and put in place a number of emergency management protocols and tools, including a general pandemic flu response plan. All the same, it was an especially difficult time of year for the university to be confronted by an outbreak

This case was written by Wendy Robison, Research Associate, for Dr. Arnold M. Howitt, Executive Director of the Ash Center for Democratic Governance and Innovation at the John F. Kennedy School of Government, Harvard University. Funds for case development were provided by the Robert Wood Johnson Foundation as part of its State Health Leadership Initiative. HKS cases are developed solely as the basis for class discussion. Cases are not intended to serve as endorsements, sources of primary data, or illustrations of effective or ineffective management.

of a new type of infectious disease: classes were winding down, end-of-semester social events were beginning to ramp up, and commencement and class reunions, which brought families, friends, alumni, and other visitors to campus, were just several weeks away.

This case study describes how, in the face of these and other challenges, senior university and school-level administrators responded to the appearance of the disease on Harvard's campus. It details how awareness of cases of H1N1 first came to the administrators' attention and then explores how they organized themselves and collaborated with key partners, including local and state public health officials, to curtail its spread and treat those suffering from the disease. To this end, they utilized a number of mechanisms, including the activation of university- and school-level crisis management teams and a suite of communication tools. In the face of significant unknowns about H1N1's lethality and contagiousness, they also took the highly unusual step of closing Harvard's Longwood-area schools and developed policies and procedures for isolating and caring for sick students, which involved a number of support services, including housekeeping, the delivery of meals, and identifying and providing appropriate types of accommodations.

The second half of the case begins by exploring how the university spent the relatively quiet summer months reviewing successes and challenges of the spring semester response. It then details how administrators applied lessons learned in preparing for and responding to a second wave of cases during the fall semester. In its final pages, it pays particular attention to the complex challenge of immunizing the university community once a vaccine finally became available.

DISCUSSION QUESTIONS

1. How useful were Harvard's prior emergency preparedness efforts in helping the university deal with the emergence of H1N1 on its campus? What were some of the limitations of these preparations?

2. Are there substantial differences between how a university deals with crises on their campuses and how towns and cities deal with the same type of events within their borders? If so, what are some of the distinctive requirements of ensuring safety within a university community?

3. Harvard administrators settled on three priorities for responding to H1N1. Do you think these priorities made sense? Does it appear that the university adhered to these priorities?

4. If the H1N1 outbreak in spring 2009 had been more extensive and severe, do you think Harvard would still have been able to mount a sufficient response?

Or would certain resources, preparations, and strategies employed by and available to the university prove inadequate?

5. Harvard is an extremely large and resource-rich institution, educating and employing thousands of individuals and owning large amounts of property in Boston and Cambridge, Massachusetts. But it is, in many regards, organized in a decentralized manner. What are the advantages and disadvantages of this decentralization when it comes to crisis response? In reality, how decentralized was Harvard's H1N1 response?

* * *

On the afternoon of April 30, 2009, Dr. David Rosenthal, Director of Harvard University Health Services (HUHS) since 1989, was intently discussing with key university administration members how they would deal with a possible outbreak at Harvard of a new, potentially lethal, infectious disease: "H1N1."[1]

In the past month, media reports of a previously unknown virus in Mexico that seemed to result in alarmingly high death rates had been creating worldwide concern. Because the severity of the viral outbreak was unclear, the general public was growing highly anxious about the disease. Comparisons to the 1918 Spanish flu pandemic that killed 40 million people were circulating on the internet. The Centers for Disease Control and Prevention (CDC) confirmed the first known case of H1N1 in the United States—a 10-year-old boy living in San Diego—on April 17, 2009.[2] Clinical testing soon established that the virus was new to humans. US government officials urged people to avoid nonessential travel to Mexico, and the European Union recommended that people "avoid outbreak areas." The apparently high case–fatality rate and speed at which the virus spread across the globe alarmed the World Health Organization (WHO), which raised its six-phase pandemic alert level from 3 to 4 in late April 2009. (Phase 4 signified that a newly emergent virus was passing from person to person but still in a limited area.)[3] Throughout May and into June, the epidemic accelerated. On June 11, 2009, WHO declared the first global pandemic[4] in 40 years, and by early July 2009 more than 140 countries were reporting cases of influenza A (H1N1).[5]

---

1. The American media used the terms "H1N1 influenza" or "swine flu," WHO called the virus "pandemic H1N1/09," and CDC called it "novel influenza A (H1N1)" or "2009 H1N1 flu."

2. CDC, "The 2009 H1N1 Pandemic: Summary Highlights, April 2009–2010," June 16, 2010, http://www.cdc.gov/h1n1flu/cdcresponse.htm.

3. Tom Randall and Hans Nichols, "Flu Outbreak Doubles in U.S., WHO Raises Alert Level (Update 1)," *Bloomberg*, April 27, 2009; and Martin Downs, "What Is a Pandemic?" *WebMD*, 2005, http://www.webmd.com/cold-and-flu/features/what-is-pandemic?page=2.

4. The two main characteristics of an influenza pandemic are as follows: the virus is a new strain that has never infected people before, and it is global in scale. See: WHO Collaborating Centre for Reference and Research on Influenza, "About Influenza," http://www.influenzacentre.org/aboutinfluenza.htm.

5. CDC, "The 2009 H1N1 Pandemic."

At Harvard, as the April 30 meeting continued, Dr. Rosenthal left the room to answer a phone call and learned that laboratory tests at CDC had shown that a student at the Harvard School of Dental Medicine (HSDM) had tested positive for the H1N1 virus, quite likely the first confirmed H1N1 case in Boston. That raised the strong probability that other students at the university's medical-area schools who had been seeking treatment for flu-like symptoms had also contracted H1N1.

Dr. Rosenthal knew that the university was not being caught unaware. Starting some years before, as part of its overall emergency preparedness efforts, Harvard had developed and subsequently extended and updated plans for an infectious disease outbreak. As a result, there was a structure in place that they could activate in response to this incident. However, as Dr. Rosenthal and other university administrators would find, although they had protocols and guidelines on paper, implementing the plan across the university would be fraught with challenges.

Thoughts racing, Dr. Rosenthal stepped back into the room to share the news and discuss next steps. Over the next five weeks until graduation in early June and then beyond, Dr. Rosenthal and other Harvard leaders had to make their emergency plans operational and effective for addressing the rapidly escalating H1N1 epidemic.

For a chronology of events, see Exhibit 8A-1.

HARVARD'S EMERGENCY MANAGEMENT SYSTEM

Harvard started a process of university-wide emergency planning around 2000 and adopted a formal plan shortly after September 11, 2001. Compared to many other institutions of higher education, Harvard has a highly decentralized administrative structure. Its schools' deans and faculty members have relatively broad discretion over local policies and budgets, while the central administration exercises responsibility for major university-wide matters—although with the authority to step in when it deems that individual school decisions have broader implications for other university units.

That general administrative structure was reflected in the university's tiered emergency management system. Two closely connected teams—the Crisis Management Team (CMT) and the Incident Support Team (IST)—operated at the central level. The CMT was the key policy-making and coordinating body. Led by the Provost, its members included some deans, the University General Counsel, and the Vice President for Government, Community and Public Affairs. The CMT was responsible for setting priorities, making emergency decisions, and communicating information to the President and school deans. The IST, which included other leaders of major administrative units whose work related to emergencies, both provided specialized advice to the CMT and coordinated implementation of important parts of any emergency response. For specialized support, the CMT had created a faculty-based Medical Advisory Committee consisting of medical and policy experts."[6] This and other ad hoc committees allowed the CMT to tap into the deep reservoir of expertise at Harvard.

In addition, Harvard's individual schools and major administrative units had Local Emergency Management Teams (LEMTs) to develop response capabilities at the operating level and to carry out emergency operations during a crisis. If an emergency primarily affected a single school, its LEMT would lead the response; if an emergency affected multiple schools or had university-wide implications, the central administration teams would play the major role. For example, in the Longwood Medical Area, located in downtown Boston separate from the main campus, the Medical School LEMT covered both the Harvard Medical School (HMS) and the HSDM. (See Exhibits 8A-2a and 8A-2b for further information about the structure and functions of the university emergency management system.)

In 2003, due to concerns regarding severe acute respiratory syndrome (SARS), Provost Steven Hyman asked Tom Vautin, the Associate Vice President for Facilities and Environmental Services, to spearhead the development of specific protocols to address an infectious disease crisis. During 2004 to 2005, every school and department developed a local emergency management plan that was coordinated with the university-wide process.[7] In 2005, Vautin's team spent almost a year adapting the infectious disease plan for avian flu scenarios, running two drills with members of the CMT, IST, and LEMTs, and revised the plan based on the results. A broader Pandemic Influenza Response Plan followed.

When H1N1 began appearing in the news in March 2009, Vautin asked Gary Kassabian, Director of Emergency Services, to start adapting these plans for an H1N1 scenario. This was challenging, though, because the H1N1 infection rate and severity of illness were unknown. The H1N1 plan was in draft form when the first case of H1N1 was confirmed at the Dental School on April 30, 2009.

THERE WAS THIS PARTY

Harvard's H1N1 experience began on April 27, when a student at HSDM visited the after-hours health clinic at the main HUHS office in Harvard Square complaining of flu-like symptoms. The intake nurse took his history and tested him for seasonal influenza. But when the student revealed he had recently visited Mexico City, HUHS medical

---

6. Harvard University Incident Support Team, *Harvard University H1N1 Influenza Management, Response, and Recovery Plan* (Cambridge, MA: Harvard University, 2009).
7. Interviews with Gary Kassabian, October 14, 2010, and February 15, 2011. Unless noted, all subsequent quotations from and attributions to Kassabian are from these interviews.

personnel decided to send a sample to a CDC testing center to determine if the student had H1N1.[8] HUHS also informed the Boston Public Health Commission (BPHC), a city government agency responsible for responding to all potential public health threats and emergencies in the city of Boston, including disease outbreaks. BPHC coordinates with the Massachusetts Department of Public Health (MDPH), CDC regional labs, and often the neighboring Cambridge Public Health Commission (CPHC).

While waiting for the first student's test results, other students with similar symptoms started filtering into the health services offices in Harvard Square and in the Longwood Medical Area. Per CDC protocols for potential cases of influenza, HUHS personnel asked students to self-isolate, wear a mask, and take hygienic precautions, such as using antibacterial handwash, when interacting with others.

Many of these students, including the first student, told nurses they had gone to a party—attended by students from Harvard's Medical, Dental, and possibly Public Health Schools—a few days before to celebrate the end of the academic year. HUHS officials wondered if the initial point of infection could be this student party. They also worried that students might not follow requests to self-isolate. Classes were almost over and the summer break was imminent; students, faculty, and staff were all attending parties and celebrating. Intensive social activity increased the chances of additional transmission.

Suspicions of H1N1 were sufficient for Dr. Rosenthal to initiate procedures under Harvard's emergency management system. He notified the university's IST, of which he was a member, and the CMT, and the Harvard Medical School LEMT activated. As described previously, Dr. Rosenthal was attending a meeting of the IST on April 30, three days after the first student came to HUHS, when one of his staff members called to inform him that the Boston Public Health Commission had reported that the regional CDC lab's tests confirmed that the HSDM student's sample was positive for H1N1.[9]

HUHS contacted the student about the results and continued treating him and others with Tamiflu,[10] an antiviral medication. About nine students were sick with flu-like symptoms, and now with at least one confirmed case of H1N1, it was also deemed very important that they continue to self-isolate.[11]

---

8. HUHS, *Emergency Response Report: H1N1 2009/2010 DRAFT* (Cambridge: Harvard University, 2010); HSDM, "HSDM Responds to H1N1 Flu Outbreak," *Harvard Dental Bulletin [Cambridge]* 69 (Summer 2009): 20. In the spring of 2009, many state labs did not yet have the capability to test for and confirm the H1N1 virus. As a result, samples were sent to CDC centers throughout the country. Generally, it took up to three days for confirmation of H1N1 flu infection.

9. HSDM, "HSDM Responds to H1N1 Flu Outbreak," 20.

10. Tamiflu can help alleviate influenza symptoms and treat influenza infection. It is most effective when taken within two days of the symptoms' appearance. See: Institute for Quality and Efficiency in Health Care, "Can Oseltamivir (Tamiflu) Prevent Complications?" *Informed Health Online*, August 1, 2013, http://www.ncbi.nlm. nih.gov/pubmedhealth/PMH0072642.

11. HUHS, *Emergency Response Report*; HSDM, "HSDM Responds to H1N1Flu Outbreak," 24; and Steve Hyman, "H1N1 Flu Update," E-mail Message to Harvard Community, May 1, 2009.

MOBILIZING TO DEAL WITH H1N1

But Dr. Rosenthal and his colleagues' concerns went beyond the treatment of the flu-stricken students. "I immediately started thinking about scaling up treatment for students and others possibly infected with the virus, along with containing the disease. I also was concerned about how this might impact the University in terms of public relations and Commencement," said Dr. Rosenthal.[12] How could the University most effectively—and quickly—coordinate its internal departments and schools to work directly with external public health agencies such as the MDPH, the BPHC, and the CPHC to address this crisis? The school year was wrapping up, final exams were about to begin, and very soon families, alumni, and guests would flock to the university for graduation events. Commencement was scheduled for June 4, 2009, approximately five weeks away. Parties, social gatherings, and formal events would provide ample opportunity for people to mingle in close quarters and spread a highly contagious disease like the flu.

THE BOSTON PUBLIC HEALTH COMMISSION AND HARVARD WORK TOGETHER

Events moved very quickly on April 30. Earlier that afternoon, Dr. Anita Barry, Director of the Infectious Disease Bureau of the BPHC, had been wrapping up a meeting with officials at Logan Airport about contagious disease control. As Dr. Barry left the meeting, her office called and asked her to return immediately: a student at the HSDM had tested positive for influenza H1N1.

Officials at BPHC were uncertain about the severity of the illness and how quickly the virus might spread. The risk of transmission was high. They knew that the Harvard Longwood Medical Area campus in Boston, which housed the Medical, Dental, and Public Health schools, often hosted patient clinics, and its personnel were integrated within area hospitals and the surrounding community.

Once back at her office, Dr. Barry, who had been with the BPHC since 1984, was met by colleagues who had convened a rapid response team. They had created a survey to administer to students that would enable them to conduct a network analysis of relationships and interactions among students, faculty, and staff and help identify who might have been exposed to the virus. Professionals at BPHC were also in contact with CDC regarding the latest treatment and prevention protocols to use in the situation. While the rapid-response team headed to the Dental School, Dr. Barry called Dr. Rosenthal, whom she knew well from their work on public health issues in the Boston area.

---

12. Interview with Dr. David Rosenthal, July 14, 2010. Unless noted, all subsequent quotations from and attributions to Dr. Rosenthal are from this interview.

"When Anita called, she told me that Harvard had achieved another first—the Dental School had the first confirmed case of H1N1 in Boston," recalled Dr. Rosenthal.

Representatives from the MDPH and BPHC joined in the open discussions on the Harvard-supported conference bridge line. At this point, not much was known: a sick student was suffering from a confirmed case of H1N1; a handful of other students had flu-like symptoms; many of the symptomatic students had attended a private, student party; and most Dental School students—including those who were symptomatic and/or at the party—were supposed to conduct clinical rounds with patients, which might expose others to the virus.

The BPHC rapid-response team worked directly with many Dental and Medical School officials, including Mary Cassesso, Dean for Administration and Finance, and Anne Berg, Director of Admissions and Student Affairs. They convened students in an auditorium to inform them of the situation, administer the student survey, and conduct interviews. From late afternoon through late evening on April 30, the same day CDC confirmed a student had H1N1, BPHC officials conducted interviews with and took samples from more than 80 students.[13] More students were becoming symptomatic, and others confirmed the story about a recent graduation party that the infected student had attended.

That evening, at the invitation of university leaders,[14] Dr. Barry participated in a call convened by the leaders of the Medical School LEMT on a conference bridge line—a telephone line that can be left open for an extended time period that allows multiple people to participate in a single call.[15] This bridge line was a virtual room in which people could confer about the latest developments and next steps. The initial call included representatives from the Harvard Office of the Provost, HUHS, HSDM, HMS, Harvard School of Public Health (HSPH), and various departments including the Harvard News Office, Emergency Management Services, and Operations and Facilities Management. Many of the university officials on the call were also members of the university-wide IST.

Participants discussed the strong probability that the Dental School had a "cluster of people infected with H1N1 [and that] the virus presented the potential to spread among various groups in the population … especially among dental and medical caregivers and … patients."[16] Dr. Barry strongly recommended that Harvard close the Dental School, the Medical School and, possibly, the School of Public Health through the

---

13. Interview with Mary Cassesso, Elsbeth Kalenderian, and Catherine Lane, September 28, 2010. Unless noted, all subsequent quotations from and attributions to Cassesso, Kalenderian, and Lane are from this interview.

14. Harvard Medical School, Harvard School of Dental Medicine, and Harvard School of Public Health are located in Boston. As a result, BPHC was primarily responsible for addressing the initial incident at the Dental School.

15. HUHS, *Emergency Response Report.* Emergency Management Services had created conference-call bridges in 2003 at every level of the university, internally as well as externally, to facilitate communication.

16. HSDM, "HSDM Responds to H1N1 Flu Outbreak," 24.

following Wednesday, May 6 (seven days), to reduce transmission of the virus.[17] By limiting contact with potentially infected individuals, BPHC and Harvard hoped to reduce the risk of transmission of the disease throughout the Harvard community and beyond.[18] Harvard officials also reached out to the New England Association of Schools and Colleges and directly to other universities, including MIT, to learn about their institutional protocols for similar infectious disease situations.

After several hours of discussion among university officials and representatives of BPHC, MDPH, and CDC, Harvard leaders decided that evening to close the Dental, Medical, and Public Health Schools as recommended.[19] The *Harvard Dental Bulletin* subsequently reported that it did not appear that the Dental School had ever closed due to a disease outbreak and that "the only other potential closure of [the Medical School] could have been during the Spanish flu outbreak in 1917 and 1918."[20]

The decision to close the schools, made very quickly on the day that H1N1 was confirmed, had many ramifications. BPHC and Harvard strongly encouraged dental and medical students, as well as faculty and staff who worked closely with students in clinical and on-campus settings, to refrain from group activities for the next seven days. Closing the three schools meant canceling classes and all student educational activities in hospitals and other clinical settings, both on and off campus. There are 17 HMS-affiliated hospitals and institutions where medical students typically conduct clinical rounds, including Beth Israel Deaconess Medical Center, Children's Hospital Boston, Brigham and Women's Hospital, and Massachusetts General Hospital, which are major regional and national centers of health care. Dental School students typically see patients on campus and conduct clinical rounds at the Harvard Dental Center, located in the Longwood Medical Area.

PRIORITIES

Harvard leaders had three main priorities during the emerging H1N1 crisis: (1) protecting the health and safety of members of the Harvard community, (2) protecting the larger community of which Harvard was a member, and (3) managing the institution's reputational risk. University leaders pursued these priorities in an environment of high uncertainty with potentially serious public health consequences.

---

17. Ibid.; CDC, "The 2009 H1N1 Pandemic." CDC recommended that infected or exposed health care providers remain out of contact with patients for seven days.

18. There were approximately 753 students enrolled at HMS, 244 students enrolled at HSDM, and 928 students (not including cross-registrations such as PhD students) enrolled at HSPH for the 2008–2009 academic year.

19. HSPH remained closed for only one day. By Monday, May 4, the HMS closure was rescinded and the school reopened. The HSDM remained closed through May 6, 2009. This decision was based on CDC recommendations.

20. HSDM, "HSDM Responds to H1N1 Flu Outbreak," 24.

University leaders wanted to take all necessary precautions and responsibility to inform members of the Harvard community, including students, faculty, staff, and parents, about the situation and start treatment and prevention activities as soon as possible. But no vaccine for H1N1 existed (and would not be developed, manufactured, and made available in sufficient quantity until the fall). This increased the importance of prevention and treatment practices throughout the community. In addition, Harvard leaders felt responsible to communities outside of Harvard, people living and working in Boston and Cambridge near university facilities. As much as possible, Harvard leaders wanted to offer the university's resources in terms of treatment and knowledge about the disease and support prevention activities beyond the university's institutional borders. At the same time, leaders recognized that their resources were limited. By coordinating with external agencies such as BPHC, CPHC, and MDPH, Harvard sought to meet its second priority to protect the health and safety of the greater community in which it was a member.

Finally, university officials were concerned about damage to the public reputation of the institution. The Boston-area press regularly covered Harvard activities, and sometimes the national and international press did as well. Though the care of infected individuals and prevention of the spread of the disease were paramount, Harvard officials were also concerned about potential negative publicity stemming from the fact that the incident at the Dental School was the first confirmed case in the Boston area and therefore very visible. Already, by mid-afternoon, press vehicles started appearing on the streets and in the parking lots around the Longwood Medical Area. Television crews and reporters stopped students and staff for interviews. Officers at the Harvard Public Affairs and Communications (HPAC) Department realized the news of the H1N1 case was spreading and that as an institution Harvard University needed to communicate clearly about the situation directly to the press. In particular, HPAC officials wanted to avoid contributing to the fear and uncertainty about H1N1 and provide clear and consistent information about the situation at the Dental School. "During a tense time of speculation and uncertainty, we were very careful to only say what we knew to be true at the time," said Kevin Galvin, HPAC Director of Media Relations.[21]

At the time the university decided to close the medical area schools, Cassesso felt strongly that she was responsible for communicating to the Dental School community and patients and that they should know about the situation before leaving for the day. Cassesso, who had worked at Harvard for 17 years, wanted to send a community letter via e-mail to inform all involved about the H1N1 case and what the Dental School and Dental Center were doing to ensure the safety of staff, students, and patients. Cassesso wanted to assure everyone—staff, faculty, students, and patients in the community—that they were doing their best to address the issue.

---

21. Interview with Kevin Galvin, February 15, 2011. Unless noted, all subsequent quotations from and attributions to Galvin are from this interview.

The Provost's Office and the Public Affairs and Communications Department under-stood Cassesso's position, but they wanted to ensure that messages remained consistent across campus out of concern for possible legal and reputational risks. Though the inter-nal Harvard community might recognize that an e-mail from a specific school did not speak for the whole institution, university leaders were concerned that most external audiences would interpret communications from any level as an official statement from Harvard University. After further discussion, all involved agreed that there needed to be an approval process for communications.

During the first 24 hours, therefore, the central administration, including the Provost's Office, HPAC, and the General Counsel's Office, vetted communications to ensure that a clear, consistent message was sent to all audiences. Some public relations officials at the individual schools were frustrated at times with what they perceived to be too tight con-trol by HPAC. Although central administrative offices at Harvard did not typically exer-cise such control, if an issue could impact the entire university, they made decisions and communicated in a more top-down manner.

The university also had to communicate with a broader public. Thus, in the evening on April 30, the day that Harvard's first case of H1N1 had been confirmed, the BPHC took the lead at a press conference to announce the decision to close the schools publicly and share H1N1 treatment and prevention information. Members of the CMT and other Harvard leaders decided that Dr. Rosenthal, the Director of HUHS, would represent the university at the press conference as an official spokesperson for the university.[22] Dr. Rosenthal and the Deans of the Medical, Public Health, and Dental schools sent joint communications about the situation via e-mail to students, faculty, and staff throughout the Longwood Medical Area that evening and updated them the next day. The Provost's Office sent a similar communication via e-mail to the entire Harvard community. Members of the CMT asked Dr. Rosenthal to act as the Harvard-wide coordinator of all H1N1 activities, and Harvard Provost Steven E. Hyman called into action the University H1N1 Preparation Plan to guide communications, decision making, and implementa-tion activities moving forward.

COORDINATING H1N1 TREATMENT AND PREVENTION ACTIVITIES

Harvard University has facilities, departments, and schools "on both sides of the [Charles] river" in Cambridge and Boston.[23] The Dental, Medical, Public Health and Business schools are all located in Boston. Many of the other professional and graduate schools—such as

---

22. Interview with Kevin Galvin, September 22, 2010.
23. It is common to hear students, faculty, and staff use the colloquial phrase, "both sides of the river," when referring to the entire Harvard University campus.

the Harvard Graduate School of Education, Harvard Kennedy School, and Harvard Law School, plus the Faculty of Arts and Science and Harvard College—are located in Cambridge. To serve the students, faculty, and staff more conveniently at all locations, HUHS operates small clinical offices in the Longwood Medical Area and at the Business School in Boston, in addition to the larger main HUHS clinical office in Harvard Square in Cambridge.

Despite the existence of the smaller, satellite offices, a majority of students at Harvard use the main HUHS office in Harvard Square. The main office also serves approximately 40% of the faculty and staff. As a result, the HUHS main office located in Harvard Square became the clinical and operational center of treatment of members of the Harvard community with flu-like symptoms. Harvard coordinated with the Cambridge Public Health Commission regarding prevention strategies and treatment provided at the clinic in Harvard Square.

"Throughout the first 24 hours and then into the following weeks," said Dr. Rosenthal, "we were constantly asking: 'How do we get prepared? How do we treat students and prevent an outbreak? What are we going to do about graduation? What are we going to do about the influx of alumni [at class reunions]?' It was almost a day-to-day decision about what to do." But the university's emergency response system and preparations proved important. "Already having some sort of infectious disease response plan in place made a huge difference in the quality of our response," Dr. Rosenthal recalls.

Harvard's draft H1N1 Preparation Plan was part of the university's overall Emergency Management Plan. That plan provided an organizational framework, including the university-level CMT and IST, plus the school- and administrative department-level LEMTs and the Medical Advisory Committee. Taken together, the plan elements sought to guide university officials in effectively communicating and coordinating activities during emergencies within Harvard and with external agencies.[24] (See Exhibits 8A-2a and 8A-2b.)

In the first days, the CMT formed an ad hoc H1N1 Policy Group to help direct Harvard's response. The H1N1 Policy Group was chaired by the Provost, and included the Dean of the School of Public Health, the Dean of Harvard College, and the Director of HUHS (Dr. Rosenthal), in addition to the General Counsel; the Vice President for Government, Community and Public Affairs; and Tom Vautin, the Associate Vice President for Facilities and Environmental Services. Dr. Julio Frenk, the Dean of HSPH, was a former Mexican Minister of Health and had served at the United Nations' WHO as Executive Director of Evidence and Information for Policy.[25]

---

24. Harvard University Incident Support Team, *Harvard University H1N1 Influenza Management, Response, and Recovery Plan.*

25. HSPH, "Julio Frenk Named Next Dean of Harvard School of Public Health," http://www.hsph.harvard.edu/news/press-releases/2008-releases/julio-frenk-named-next-dean-harvard-school-of-public-health.html.

To support its response structure, the university could draw upon recently-acquired database and communications technologies—specifically, WebEOC systems software, an internal emergency preparedness Web site (E-prep), the Harvard University Emergency Notification System, and the emergency messaging system (MessageME). These technologies helped in implementing the decision to close the schools and coordinate activities during the emergency response.

WebEOC is a Web-enabled information management system that is designed to facilitate real-time information sharing during a crisis and to create an archive of data about the decision-making process.[26] The WebEOC system potentially serves as an information source for emergency situations of all kinds—such as severe weather, illness, fires, or utility outages—allowing those linked through the system to share documents, photographs, videos, and other resources. The robust networking capabilities of WebEOC permit cross-organizational information sharing (e.g., from Harvard to the cities of Boston and Cambridge, which had also adopted WebEOC), with individuals' access to specific, limited-circulation information controlled through a system of user permissions. Among other purposes, the system serves as a historical repository of communications and reports pertaining to specific incidents, such as the H1N1 spring incident at the Dental School, through an incident report function. This functions almost like a blog, in that people can access the system and add to a running stream of information. Someone with the proper access could log onto the WebEOC system, search for a specific incident, and find in one place a record of all the postings and guidance materials consulted or available to manage the incident.

E-prep was a restricted-access internal Harvard Web site, which at the time of the H1N1 outbreak served as a repository for official documents and as a source of reference materials. E-prep was managed by the Harvard Emergency Management Office and available to members of the CMT, IST, and LEMTs through a password-protected URL.[27] Emergency planning resources, such as the university and local emergency management plans and procedures, were available through the Web site. University emergency response personnel could post the latest plans, guidelines, and tools on the site. These resources provided a common standard for information, practices, and terminology for protocols and plans developed by the LEMTs and other emergency groups across the university. For example, E-prep hosted a pandemic planning tools section where members of LEMTs could download the latest pandemic plan and other useful documents and fact sheets such as one-page cleaning procedures for contractors to guide how they disinfected rooms while attending to their own health. These protocols could be downloaded directly from the site in various languages, including English, Spanish, and Haitian-Creole.

---

26. Interview with Gary Kassabian, October 14, 2010.
27. Personal communication with Nicholas Hambridge, Associate Director of Emergency Management, Harvard University Environmental Health and Safety, March 25, 2015.

The emergency messaging system MessageME focuses on sending messages about incidents to the general Harvard community: students, faculty, and staff. MessageME is designed for campus-wide emergencies such as a potential active shooter, a security incident at a dormitory, or other major emergencies at the Harvard schools, when near-instantaneous communication to the entire university community is desirable.[28] During the H1N1 emergency, MessageME sent text messages and voicemails through mobile phones to more than 20,000 people on the university campus, as well as via e-mail, Facebook, and Twitter.[29]

IMPLEMENTATION OF THE INITIAL H1N1 RESPONSE PLAN: MAY–JUNE 2009

Once the decision to close Harvard schools was made, the CMT, IST, and LEMT members devoted their attention to planning the university's response to H1N1 over the next five weeks leading to commencement and alumni reunions. How could they address the needs of infected individuals and prevent transmission? How could they best communicate decisions and other information to the Harvard community, as well as external audiences, including parents? Finally, would they need to cancel commencement?

University leaders had many decisions to make. The H1N1 Preparation Plan had frameworks and guidelines but did not address many implementation details or challenges. In general, the plan addressed isolating infected individuals, surge capacity planning, supporting HUHS clinics, communication protocols among responders at the university level as well as with external parties, and educating students, faculty, staff, and guests on prevention and treatment. Members of the CMT, IST, and LEMTs, along with other university leaders, had to work through the plan's general guidelines and create detailed implementation plans to address these major areas. These implementation plans were constantly revised based on feedback and experience.

Though the university offered care and support to all members of the community suffering from H1N1, leaders believed Harvard College undergraduates might be particularly vulnerable to an H1N1 outbreak. Nearly 99% of the 6,650 undergraduates lived in university-operated housing and used campus facilities and services.[30] Meanwhile, all graduate and professional students and staff infected with H1N1 were instructed to return to their homes with guidance from HUHS or a health care provider.[31]

---

28. Interview with Gary Kassabian, January 28, 2011.
29. Interview with Gary Kassabian, February 15, 2011.
30. "H1N1 Influenza Management Response and Recovery Plan," PowerPoint Presentation for LEMT Leaders Meeting, Harvard University, September 21, 2009.
31. HUHS, *Emergency Response Report.*

Isolation Policies

Harvard's patient isolation policies were initially based on CDC, state, and local public health officials' recommendations, which included isolation for the period of the illness plus 24 hours after the fever ended. Later, BPHC recommended isolation for a minimum of four days for the general public and seven days for hospital workers, including medical and dental students.

At first, there was some confusion regarding the meaning of isolation. Did that mean students were free to self-isolate if they lived in a single-occupant dorm room? Was the university in a position to force isolation on infected students and staff? Students seemed to interpret the instruction to self-isolate in a variety of ways, and, possibly, the message was unclear. For example, one student remained in a single room and never left, even to use the bathroom. Another student thought it was a good time to leave the campus and went on a trip alone but traveled by commercial airline on a full plane. When some students were told by HUHS personnel to return to their rooms and self-isolate, they continued to see friends and socialize in their dorm areas.

Harvard provided transportation, dining services, and housekeeping to sick students who were isolated on campus.[32] An HUHS triage and case management decision-tree outlined steps to take when a patient was diagnosed with an influenza-like illness, which included entering basic information into a case registry for tracking purposes and determining the patient's living situation and group activities.

The university central administration worked with Harvard College on a housing strategy to provide space for sick students. If the patient was in a single, s/he was held at Stillman infirmary while HUHS provided information to suitemates and coordinated with Harvard University Dining Services to work with vendors to arrange food delivery services. Once support services were arranged, the student was sent to her or his room and ordered to self-isolate, using masks when in shared, public spaces, and given information about hygiene and disease transmission. If the student lived in a shared room or a dormitory with shared bathroom facilities, s/he was encouraged to go home if s/he lived within 150 miles of Harvard. HUHS and deans at Harvard College would contact the family. If the student could not return home and lived in a shared space, s/he stayed in Stillman infirmary (located at the HUHS offices in Harvard Square) for seven days. If Stillman was at capacity, the plan was to send the student for isolation and treatment to Harvard-owned residential property with available empty rooms.

Surge Capacity Planning

IST, in partnership with other university departments, such as Emergency Management, HUHS, Facilities Management and Operations, and Environmental Health and Safety, created and implemented a plan based on five levels of demand for isolation.

---

32. Ibid.

The five-level framework helped leaders plan for scenarios during which available space was exhausted (Exhibit 8A-3).

At Level 1, all sick students could either go home because they lived within 150 miles of the university or stay in Stillman infirmary (10 beds). Once these spaces were exhausted, Level 2 of the plan provided for sick students to stay in residence halls. Once the residence halls were full, Level 3 required maximizing space at Stillman infirmary by adding five more beds for a total of 15.

In the event that HUHS was in danger of exceeding surge capacity in the dormitories, the infirmary, and residence halls, at Level 4 IST would recommend the use of the Harvard Square Hotel, which has 73 guestrooms and capacity for 130 beds. Collegiate Hospitality, LLC, a hospitality company owned by the university, manages the Harvard Square Hotel. In the case of overflow into the hotel, CMT and IST decided that Harvard would assume responsibility (including financial) for moving regular hotel guests to another location. It would provide medical care, meal service, trash removal, housekeeping, and transportation, and a vendor would assume responsibility for front desk operations and laundry service.[33]

If all available spaces were maximized at Stillman, dormitories, residence halls, and the hotel, Level 5 recommended that students return to their rooms with treatment and prevention instructions and additional guidance. Fortunately, in the five weeks between the initial case and commencement, the available space in dorms, Stillman, and the residence halls proved adequate to house all patients.

Case Tracking System

One of the most useful strategies that emerged from the initial response to H1N1 in May through June 2009 was the establishment of a case tracking system. This was not a strategy outlined in the H1N1 response plan. It developed out of a need for real-time data on infection and recovery rates, as well as accurate, current data on the number of students who needed to be isolated and cared for by the health services, food services, facilities maintenance, transportation departments, and vendors. This type of real-time information helped Harvard leaders keep track of how many students were currently in need of isolation services and treatment. The numbers from the case tracking system fed directly into capacity planning and helped leaders know if they had exhausted space at one level of the framework and needed to move to the next level. The data also informed leaders managing treatment resources so they could order (or stop ordering) more supplies as numbers of sick students, staff, and faculty fluctuated.

As part of the case tracking system, all HUHS clinicians were asked to notify the lead nurse on duty when a patient was diagnosed with an influenza-like illness. The lead nurse entered the information into a detailed spreadsheet that provided identifying

---

33. HUHS, *Emergency Response Report;* "H1N1 Influenza Management Response and Recovery Plan."

information on the patient, including age, patient type (e.g., student, employee, other), residence, date of onset of symptoms, location after diagnosis, follow-up, and discharge date. Nurses were assigned to follow-up on all patients not admitted into the infirmary. The tracking sheet was updated twice daily and distributed to response teams at HUHS and Harvard College, with patient identifiers blocked. The response teams used this information to keep track of the number of cases, including increases and decreases over time. This information informed strategies regarding housing and service provision and helped BPHC and state authorities keep track of incidents at the local level. Students were informed that information would be shared with the college in an effort to contain the public health threat.[34]

Conference Calls

Dr. Rosenthal and his management team at HUHS, including the Chief of Medicine and the Chief of Nursing, held conference calls twice a day (in the morning and evening) with university officials throughout the five-week spring response. The management team also spoke regularly with Dr. Barry at BPHC; Dr. Alfred DeMaria, MDPH's Medical Director of the Bureau of Infectious Disease, Prevention, Response, and Services and State Epidemiologist; and officials at the CPHC to coordinate policies, communicate on the volume and status of illness within the community, coordinate internal and external communication strategies, and discuss any changing recommendations or evolving policy.[35]

Communication Policies

Dr. Rosenthal and University Provost Hyman, a physician and neurobiologist, remained the only official spokespersons for the university. HPAC regularly posted updated information and communications online so members of the Harvard community and the media were informed of current policies and situations.[36]

The Harvard Provost's Office, HPAC, and the General Counsel's Office worked closely with the local press offices at the Medical and Dental schools on communications regarding H1N1—from official statements to e-mails. Once the initial public announcements were made, leaders at the central and school levels worked together to create a communications protocol regarding the H1N1 situation. Officials at the Office of General Counsel and HPAC reviewed official communications coming from the Dental and

---

34. HUHS, *Emergency Response Report.*
35. Ibid.
36. "H1N1 Influenza Management Response and Recovery Plan."

Medical schools before release, but internal e-mails were not as tightly controlled. Though this slowed the communication response, it allowed university leaders to review and coordinate messaging across the institution for internal and external audiences.

Eventually, the CMT created a communications committee consisting of officials from several departments (e.g., HPAC, Medical School deans, student affairs, and individual schools' communications offices) through which the individual schools' news offices would send communications. This group reviewed the statements and then sent them to the General Counsel's Office and the Harvard University News Office.

In addition to managing information for the media, which focused mostly on external audiences, the university also coordinated communications to internal audiences. Internal communications to the Harvard community focused on education about transmission of and treatment for H1N1, similar to public health information campaigns, as well as coordinating response activities. For example, on the Harvard University homepage, as well as the HUHS main Web page and school Web sites, there was a link connected to a new Web site created specifically to provide information about H1N1. This Web site was the central area where the university, HPAC, HUHS, and the schools directed community members to approved H1N1 materials and information. HUHS also established a telephone hotline for similar information. Within a few days, one-page educational handouts on good hygiene to prevent illness were posted throughout the university and within HUHS (Exhibit 8A-4). The HUHS Web site was regularly updated to include information on H1N1, and information for parents and roommates was also included on the Web site. Dr. Rosenthal provided interviews to several Harvard publications, during which he focused on treatment and prevention behaviors.[37]

Harvard leaders used the internal WebEOC and E-prep systems for communication among university departments. Gary Kassabian and his staff regularly updated the incident log within the WebEOC system to share information centrally with emergency team members. LEMT members could also update the log so that a real-time, running history of the situation from the perspective of each location was recorded and could be accessed by members of the emergency management network (i.e., members of the CMT, IST, and LEMTs).

COMMENCEMENT

From May through early June 2009, a relatively small number of flu-like cases appeared across the university. However, the feared widespread outbreak of H1N1 never occurred. Cases were managed according to CDC protocols; the community-at-large was given

---

37. HUHS, *Emergency Response Report.*

instructions on prevention and self-care through Web updates, posters, and handouts; and the university placed antibacterial hand sanitizer dispensers throughout the campus.

Ultimately, leaders at Harvard decided to proceed with commencement, as planned, on June 4, 2009. High traffic areas were cleaned more regularly and extra antibacterial hand sanitizer dispensers were placed at all food service areas. Throughout the week, informational handouts were provided to all people participating in commencement events.[38]

After the confirmation of the first case of H1N1 on April 30 and the rapid emergency response in May through to commencement in early June, members of the CMT, IST, and LEMTs breathed a collective sigh of relief that an initial crisis appeared averted. But was there another on the horizon? Thankful that H1N1 did not appear as deadly as first feared but wary that a new surge of the disease was possible, Harvard leaders planned to use the summer months to review the spring response and plan for a potential pandemic in the fall. What did they do well? What could they do better? How might a greater surge of infections and the added complication of distribution of a new H1N1 vaccine expected to be available in the fall affect operations and staffing at the university? With some trepidation and considerable weariness, the emergency response teams collected themselves for an intense summer of planning and preparation for fall 2009.

---

38. Ibid.

Exhibit 8A-1. Chronology of Events: Harvard H1N1 Outbreak, April 2009–June 2009

April 27
- Harvard dental student has sore throat, body aches, and fever. The student goes to After Hours Urgent Care Clinic at the Harvard University Health Services (HUHS) main office in Harvard Square. A culture is sent to the Massachusetts Department of Public Health (MDPH), which in turn sends it to a Centers for Disease Control and Prevention (CDC) testing facility to be tested for the new H1N1 flu virus.

April 29
- Two additional dental students report mild symptoms and are being tested for the H1N1 virus.

April 30
- Boston Public Health Commission (BPHC) reports to HUHS that the dental student's flu test is positive for influenza A (H1N1) virus. Dr. Rosenthal and other Harvard leaders are informed that there is a confirmed case of H1N1 at the Harvard School of Dental Medicine (HSDM).
- Members of BPHC's infectious disease division arrange a visit to HSDM to administer a survey to students to gather information for a network analysis to help identify who was exposed to the virus. They also isolate symptomatic students for treatment and to prevent transmission.
- The Harvard Medical School (HMS) Local Emergency Management Team (LEMT) convenes a conference call to discuss the situation and response strategies. BPHC and MDPH representatives, Harvard University leaders, including representatives from the Provost's Office, General Counsel, HUHS, Harvard Public Affairs and Communications, HMS, HSDM and Harvard School of Public Health (HSPH), as well as leaders from Facilities Management and University Operations Services, participate in the call.
- Dr. Anita Barry, Director of BPHC's infectious disease division, strongly suggests to Harvard leaders that they close HSDM, HMS, and HSPH through May 6, 2009, to prevent transmission of the virus. Harvard leaders agree with her recommendation and decide to close the schools for the CDC-recommended period of seven days.
- BPHC arranges a press conference to announce the decision to close the schools and inform the public about treatment and prevention of H1N1. Dr. David Rosenthal, the official university spokesperson, represents Harvard at the press conference.

May 1
- HSDM appears in an above-the-fold, front page *Boston Globe* headline article about H1N1.
- HMS, HSDM, and HSPH are closed, which means all classes and educational activities in hospitals and other clinical settings—both on and off campus—are suspended.

May 4
- The HMS closure is rescinded. HSDM remains closed.

May 5
- HMS classes and public activities resume. Clinical rotations and student activities in hospital settings will resume pending coordination with affiliated hospitals.

May 6
- HSDM reopens to students and patients. A total of 11 probable cases of influenza A/H1N1 virus occurred.

Early May–Early June
- The high number of anticipated sick students, staff, and faculty never materializes. Smalls clusters of students from various areas around the campus are seen and safely isolated in private rooms until resolution of fever.
- Cases are managed according to CDC protocols and instructions on prevention, treatment, and self-care are disseminated to the Harvard community through Web updates, posters, fliers, and handouts, and the University places anti-bacterial hand sanitizer dispensers throughout the campus.

June 4
- Harvard Commencement

Exhibit 8A-2a. Emergency Response Team Structure and Responsibilities During the H1N1 Response

The Harvard Emergency Management Plan has three levels of management responsibility:

- **Crisis Management Team (CMT)**—Responsible for developing policy and making high-level decisions. Members include the Provost (who serves as the chair); Deans of the College and other graduate schools; University General Counsel; Vice President for Government, Community and Public Affairs; and the acting Vice President for Administration, who also serves as the leader of the Incident Support Team. In the case of the university's response to H1N1, the Director of Harvard University Health Services (HUHS) was also on the CMT.
- **Incident Support Team (IST)**—Responsible for coordinating the emergency response by developing plans and supporting both the decision making of the CMT and the implementation activities of the LEMTs. Members of the IST include leaders of departments and functional units who provide essential services to schools and other parts of the university.
- **Local Emergency Management Teams (LEMTs)**—Responsible for implementation activities at the school and department level. Members of the LEMTs are essentially the first responders in a crisis and directly interact with students, staff, and faculty at the local level. There are multiple LEMTs across the university, as many schools, departments, and functional units have an LEMT.

CMT responsibilities include:

- Making decisions concerning the university activities and essential staffing during an emergency, including closure of schools or departments during extraordinary events;
- Prioritizing actions and allocating resources among the schools or departments;
- Establishing and maintaining direct communication with the President and the Deans to ensure full information exchange with the schools;
- Establishing financial policies to ensure sufficient resources for rapid response to emergency situations necessary for health and safety.

IST responsibilities include:

- Coordinating health resources to the university community;
- Developing and implementing plans for educating the university community on emergency preparedness, response and recovery strategies, and plans;
- Forecasting and monitoring the scope of the emergency and consequences to the university;
- Coordinating support and communicating with external agencies (including public health, hospitals, public safety, utilities, municipal services, and other non-governmental organizations) during an influenza outbreak;
- Serving as the university's communication and information clearinghouse and to coordinate official interaction with news media regarding information provided to internal and external audiences.

LEMT responsibilities include:

- Establishing effective communication with their Deans and other senior leaders to ensure a coordinated response;
- Identifying effective means of disseminating recommendations on personal preparedness and hygiene practices throughout their school or department;
- Overseeing effective case management of student illness in conjunction with HUHS;
- Managing employee absences in compliance with university policies;
- Coordinating (through local Public Information Officers) with the Harvard Public Affairs and Communications Department any information or internal communication that has the potential to become public;
- Acquiring supplies, materials, and service providers necessary to maintain essential operations.

Source: Reprinted from Harvard University Incident Support Team, *Harvard University H1N1 Influenza Management, Response, and Recovery.*
Note: The responsibilities of the CMT, IST, and LEMTs all come from this document.

Exhibit 8A-2b. Relationship of Crisis Management Team, Incident Support Team, and Local Emergency Management Teams

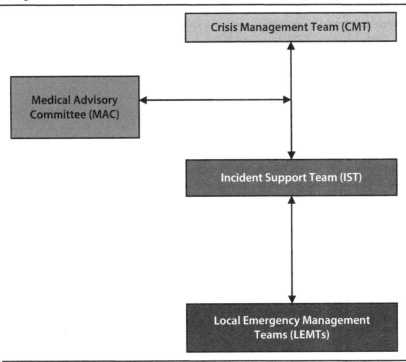

Source: Reprinted from Harvard University Incident Support Team, *Harvard University H1N1 Influenza Management, Response, and Recovery Plan*, 5.

Exhibit 8A-3. Five-Level Isolation Framework

- Level 1: Isolate patients in existing single rooms and recommend those living within 150 miles of the university (or with close family or friends in the area) to go home or stay in a private residence. For patients with roommates, use the existing capacity at Stillman infirmary (10 beds).
- Level 2: Relocate patients to existing empty rooms throughout the university, such as DeWolfe and Leverett dormitories.
- Level 3: Maximize the capacity at Stillman (15 beds total).[a]
- Level 4: Move all sick patients to Harvard Square Hotel and maximize its capacity (~130 beds). Then return to Levels 1 to 3 as new patients are diagnosed. (Existing university space was never exhausted, so no patients were ever housed at the hotel.)
- Level 5: Stillman, Harvard Square Hotel, and other available space at the university maximized. If no isolation space is available, students are told to return to their rooms and given clinical guidance regarding transmission and self-care.

[a]The University received permission to add five additional beds in Stillman, bringing the total number from 10 to 15 beds.

Exhibit 8A-4. Harvard School of Dental Medicine H1N1 Flu Prevention Guidelines

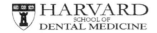

HARVARD
SCHOOL OF
DENTAL MEDICINE

Your health and safety is of the utmost importance to us.

Please help us prevent the spread of the H1N1 Flu.

- **Avoid contact** with ill persons.
- When you cough or sneeze, **cover your nose and mouth** with a tissue or your sleeve (if you do not have a tissue). Throw used tissues in a trash can.
- After you cough or sneeze, wash your hands **with soap and water,** or use an **alcohol-based** hand gel.
- **If you think you are ill with flu,** avoid close contact with others as much as possible. **Stay at home. Seek medical care if you are severely ill (such as having trouble breathing). There are antiviral medications for prevention and treatment of H1N1 that a doctor can prescribe. Do not go to work, school, or travel while ill.**

Symptoms are similar to regular flu and include:

- Sudden fever, cough, muscle aches, headache, chills and general weakness.
- Some people have also had diarrhea and vomiting.
- These symptoms can range from mild to severe.
- If you experience any of these flu-like symptoms, please contact your primary care clinician or HUHS immediately.

Source: Reprinted from Harvard School of Dental Medicine H1N1 Flu Prevention Guidelines.

H1N1 at Harvard

Wendy Robison

As the summer of 2009 began, Harvard University leaders were relieved that the emergency response to an outbreak of H1N1 at the end of the spring semester had gone well. Fortunately, the confirmed H1N1 cases in the Longwood Medical Area did not evolve into a flu epidemic, and infected individuals recovered. Harvard Commencement had occurred as scheduled in early June, without a surge in H1N1 cases among guests attending the celebrations.

Looking to the future, however, Harvard University leaders wanted to identify "lessons learned" and strengthen the university's policies and implementation plans regarding H1N1 for the coming fall semester.[1] Already, University leaders and members of the emergency response teams were anticipating a possible surge of flu cases and complications with distributing the new H1N1 vaccine.

Gary Kassabian, the Director of Emergency Services at Harvard, who had led the drafting of the H1N1 emergency response plan in March 2009, also led the after-action review and revision of the plan in preparation for the fall. The plan had provided guidance and scaffolding for the university's response from late-April through early-June 2009. Kassabian and his team had worked closely with the members of the three main levels of the university's emergency management structure—that is, the Crisis Management Team (CMT), Incident Support Team (IST), and Local Emergency Management Teams (LEMTs)—to implement the response. (See Exhibit 8A-2 for a more complete description of this structure.)

This case was written by Wendy Robison, Research Associate, for Dr. Arnold M. Howitt, Executive Director of the Ash Center for Democratic Governance and Innovation at the John F. Kennedy School of Government, Harvard University. Funds for case development were provided by the Robert Wood Johnson Foundation as part of its State Health Leadership Initiative. HKS cases are developed solely as the basis for class discussion. Cases are not intended to serve as endorsements, sources of primary data, or illustrations of effective or ineffective management.

1. Fall semester started on September 2 and ended on December 18, 2009. Registrar's Office, "2009-2010 Academic Calendar," Harvard School of Public Health.

Many elements of the response went well. All of the patients who were treated at Harvard University Health Services (HUHS) for suspected-H1N1 infection had fully recovered. The isolation plan for sick individuals, along with an aggressive education campaign, seemed to help reduce the transmission of the disease, as the anticipated number of sick students, faculty, and staff never materialized. However, university leaders wanted to review performance in the spring response in preparation for the fall flu season. Some members of the LEMTs involved in the spring, such as the Harvard Medical School LEMT, expressed some confusion about their roles and responsibilities. This confusion resulted in miscommunication and some duplication of efforts. Some team members were also frustrated with the technologies used during the response—including E-prep, WebEOC, and multiparty conference call systems—which they did not feel confident using during the emergency situation.

A timely after-action review was typical for projects administered by Emergency Services and the University Operations Services Department. University leaders had offered several key questions to guide the review effort: What worked well in the spring, and what could we improve? What activities do we continue from the spring response into the fall? What do we discontinue or change? How do we better sort out roles, responsibilities, and decision-making authority? How do we manage the process for administering the new vaccine—especially if there is a shortage? What do we do if there is a massive surge in cases? When do we know that the majority of H1N1 cases are over so that we can downgrade or even stop our response?

For a chronology of events, see Exhibit 8B-1.

SUMMER 2009: HARVARD REVIEWS THE SPRING RESPONSE[2]

Throughout the summer, Kassabian and his team spoke with colleagues and facilitated meetings with representatives from the IST and the LEMTs to review the protocols and strategies used to respond to H1N1 in the spring. The main priorities of the review team (which included representatives from the IST and LEMTs)[3] were to review and identify best practices and lessons learned in the spring response and "plan for a possible pandemic in the fall."[4] University leaders anticipated an increase in H1N1 cases across Harvard due to the timing coinciding with the annual flu season and the influx of students at the beginning of the academic year.

To conduct the after-action review, Kassabian and his team communicated through e-mail, conference calls, and in-person meetings with leaders and members of the

---

2. Unless otherwise indicated, most information regarding implementation processes and systems is from HUHS, *Emergency Response Report: H1N1 2009/2010 DRAFT* (Cambridge: Harvard University, 2010); Harvard University, "H1N1 Influenza Management Response and Recovery Plan," PowerPoint presentation for LEMT Leaders Meeting, September 21, 2009; and "H1N1 After-Action Assessment Outline" created by the Harvard Medical School and Harvard School of Dental Medicine LEMTs.
3. Harvard University, "H1N1 Influenza Management Response and Recovery Plan."
4. HUHS, *Emergency Response Report.*

Harvard Medical School LEMT, as well as with leaders in various university departments responsible during the response for communications, facilities management, and operations. The review team requested memos and other documents outlining best practices and recommendations for improvement from people heavily involved in the spring response, such as Jane Garfield, Director of Operations at the Medical School, and Mary Cassesso, Dean for Administration and Finance at the Dental School.

Based on the feedback, university leaders and directors of departments who played vital roles in the emergency response revised departmental policies and procedures. Kassabian folded these changes into a revised version of the H1N1 emergency response plan, as well as updated protocol documents posted on WebEOC and the internal Harvard E-prep systems. The departments and LEMTs could then easily download the current version of the H1N1 emergency response plan and accompanying documents for use in their departments and schools across the university.

FALL 2009: HARVARD LAUNCHES REFINED H1N1 RESPONSE POLICIES AND PROCEDURES

As the fall semester began, the University hoped to "reduce the health impact [of H1N1] by managing the anticipated surge and maintaining normal activities and the [overall] academic mission" campus-wide.[5] In late September 2009, Kassabian and Tom Vautin, the Acting Vice President of Administration, pulled together university leaders, members of LEMTs from across Harvard, and other emergency response personnel for a meeting in which members of the review team presented their findings and recommendations to other emergency response personnel. The university had already started to implement the revised policies and procedures the review team had worked on over the summer.[6] The meeting agenda covered issues regarding medical care and treatment, communications, residential isolation strategies, public health and hygiene, feeding plans, human resource policies regarding staff and vendors, and special concerns regarding Harvard College such as ensuring academic continuity with regard to class attendance, lectures, assignments, and exams and maintaining positive parent relations.

Relationships

Early in the review process, Kassabian and his team had discovered that many people who implemented the emergency response cited their long-standing professional relationships as a valuable asset. Several key leaders at the university, including Dr. Rosenthal and

---

5. Harvard University, "H1N1 Influenza Management Response and Recovery Plan."
6. HUHS, *Emergency Response Report.*

Provost Hyman, had known both internal and external stakeholders (including Dr. R. Bruce Donoff, Dean of the Dental School; Dr. Anita Barry, Director of the Infectious Disease Bureau for the Boston Public Health Commission (BPHC); and Dr. Alfred DeMaria, Medical Director of the Bureau of Infectious Disease, Prevention, Response and Services and State Epidemiologist at the Massachusetts Department of Public Health) for years from working at Harvard and in the public health sector in the Boston area. These preexisting relationships helped facilitate an effective and rapid response to the incident in the spring and paved the way for a planned response in the fall.

Case Tracking System

The review team found that the case tracking system was one of the most successful processes created and used during the spring response. From the perspective of medical professionals at HUHS, keeping records of infected individuals helped in monitoring and sharing information in a way that facilitated treatment, increased understanding of the progression of the disease, and provided perspective on the extent of infection across the university. The case tracking system helped the emergency management office and LEMTs plan better and implement actions in response to the emerging crisis. Information from the case tracking system informed the patient isolation system and helped with the preparation of food and cleaning services, identification of additional facilities for treatment and isolation, and adequate inventory of supplies.

Areas of improvement for the case tracking system centered on issues of patient confidentiality. Initially, some patients could be easily identified by the information in the tracking system. Particularly at the Dental School, a small community,[7] students found the loss of anonymity stressful. As a result, HUHS and LEMTs needed to figure out a way to preserve the privacy of patients (in accordance with HIPAA regulations[8]), yet still retain essential information useful for treatment and planning.

In the fall, HUHS personnel revised and formalized the case tracking system developed in the spring, specifically improving patient privacy and confidentiality. Per the after-action recommendations, HUHS personnel also implemented a more formal triage system to manage cases. To respect privacy rules, the university informed students at the beginning of the fall semester that HUHS might share information on patients diagnosed with influenza-like illnesses with university and public health officials due to public health concerns. The lead nurse on-duty remained responsible for entering patient

---

7. There were approximately 244 students enrolled in the Dental School in 2008–2009 and 2009–2010.

8. HIPAA "stands for the Health Insurance Portability and Accountability Act, a US law designed to provide privacy standards to protect patients' medical records and other health information provided to health plans, doctors, hospitals, other health care providers" and third parties. See: "Definition of HIPAA," *MedicineNet.com*, June 14, 2010, http://www.medterms.com/script/main/art.asp?articlekey=31785.

information on the spreadsheet. Information recorded included "age, patient type—such as student, employee, faculty, other—residence, date of onset of symptoms, location after diagnosis, follow-up, and discharge date."[9] Throughout the fall semester, the tracking system was updated twice a day and distributed to Dr. Rosenthal's expanded case management team. Names and other identifying information, such as student identification numbers, were now systematically removed from the versions shared with the expanded HUHS management team.

The case tracking system was one of the cornerstones of the university's response in the spring and remained so in the fall of 2009. It provided information over time that allowed leaders to make important, institution-wide decisions based on current data and trend analysis. It also directly informed the isolation system of care for undergraduate students suspected of having H1N1.

Open Conference Bridge

During the after-action review, Kassabian noted that many people talked about how important the initial telephone conference bridge line was for facilitating communication across the university's schools and departments during the first few days of the H1N1 incident. The bridge line allowed representatives from various departments, as well as representatives from outside organizations such as the Boston Public Health Commission (BPHC), the Cambridge Public Health Commission (CPHC), and the Massachusetts Department of Public Health (MDPH), to connect to the same conference call. They could then communicate with one another directly and in real time about a dynamic, uncertain situation. The conference call line acted as a virtual command center, where participants could call in and debate the advantages and disadvantages of various decisions and develop inclusive, representative response protocols and guidelines. A communication system that enabled many people to speak with each other at one time was very useful.

In the same breath, several people also discussed frustrations with the initial conference bridge call that occurred on April 30, 2009. On that call there were simultaneously 20 to 25 people on the line, and it lasted over an hour and a half. Figuring out who was on the line was awkward and time-consuming. During the call, people spoke over each other, making it difficult to hear and communicate effectively. Due to the large number of participants, there was a high level of background noise and distractions on the call— for example, people typing, background conversations, phones ringing. This resulted in gaps in the conversation and confusion. Finally, the conference-call number was distributed widely, which decreased confidentiality.

---

9. HUHS, *Emergency Response Report.*

As part of the after-action review, these issues were considered and included in the Harvard Medical School LEMTs' on-boarding process for new members. Suggestions included designating a notetaker who would not be the LEMT leader, creating an agenda prior to each call that would include summaries from previous calls, establishing a call leader who would manage the flow of the call, agreeing on norms and participating in trainings for conference-call etiquette, arranging alternative conference bridges for different groups, and scheduling specific times for phone conferencing, such as hourly or semi-hourly calls with specific agendas or topics. Thus, those involved could accomplish tasks in between calls and those who needed to discuss a particular topic could join upcoming calls.

Harvard University Health Services Conference Call

At the end of August, Dr. Rosenthal (Director of HUHS) and other members of the IST decided to continue holding the daily conference calls that Dr. Rosenthal's management team at HUHS had held during the spring response. Participation on the calls included the Executive Vice President of Harvard, Assistant Dean of Harvard College, Chief of Medicine, Chief of Nursing, the Director of Stillman infirmary, and representatives from the Provost's Office and the Harvard Public Affairs and Communications Department (HPAC). The calls occurred twice daily at 8 a.m. and 5:30 p.m. and lasted through late December. The purpose of these calls was to coordinate and implement policy decisions regarding the care and treatment of patients, communicate on the status of H1N1 infection among the Harvard community, discuss changes in the situation, and allow for the evolution of policy and recommendations.

"The twice daily calls throughout the fall semester were key in our ability to manage the flow of students and understand the landscape of the situation," said Dr. Rosenthal. Through the calls, leaders were able to more effectively treat patients, plan for potential surges in the infection, uphold the isolation policy, and coordinate activities across the university.[10]

Roles and Responsibilities

Although members of the three main levels of emergency management (i.e., the CMT, IST, and LEMTs) had run several exercises before the H1N1 incident in the spring, the review team had discovered that some people involved in the spring response were still confused about roles and responsibilities during an emergency response. Representatives from the Medical and Dental schools identified several priority issues (listed here) to address in preparation for the fall.

---

10. Ibid.

Improved LEMT member orientation

Harvard leaders needed to improve the orientation of new LEMT members. During the H1N1 incident, there were several new staff members involved who had not served on the Harvard Medical School LEMT before. As a result, they had little knowledge of the university's basic emergency response protocols and had not met other people on the Medical School LEMT. At times during the response, this lack of knowledge, as well as new relationships among team members, contributed to murky communication and some confusion around roles and responsibilities.

Revision of implementation procedures

To reduce confusion in implementation, the review team recommended revising and clarifying procedures (i.e., individuals' responsibilities, decision-making authority, communication protocols, treatment), as well as holding more regular trainings on the most current policies and protocols for all involved.

Clarification of decision-making authority between the Dental and Medical schools

Though those involved felt that the emergency response from the Medical School LEMT and Dental and Medical schools was excellent, they felt that the organizational relationships between the two institutions needed to be addressed in preparation for future incidents. The Dental School did not actually have its own LEMT. Instead, both Dental and Medical school representatives were part of the Medical School LEMT. At times, the H1N1 incident created stress in the relationship between the two schools. The roles, responsibilities, and relationships of members of the Medical School LEMT and within the Dental and Medical School administrations were sometimes unclear. Who had ultimate authority? Who had ultimate responsibility? Which institution covered specific costs?

Communication Strategies

The university's communications strategy was divided into external and internal communication. Audiences for external communications included the general media, agencies such as the BPHC and the Massachusetts Department of Public Health, and the greater Boston and Cambridge communities. The Harvard News Office was responsible for managing information in cooperation with communication officers at the individual Harvard schools, especially regarding external communications. Internal communications targeted the Harvard community, including students, faculty, staff, and contractors across the university.

In the spring, university leaders both in the central administration and at the schools agreed that there needed to be some kind of approval process for communications during emergencies. Harvard leaders decided that Dr. Rosenthal and Provost Hyman would serve as the official university spokespersons regarding H1N1. In drafting local messages about H1N1 from the Dental and Medical schools, the Director of Harvard Medical School's Communications Office worked with leaders at the Dental School to draft communications for the Longwood Medical Area community (which included Harvard Medical School, the Harvard School of Dental Medicine, and the Harvard School of Public Health). These communications would go the Dean of the Medical School and leaders at the Dental and Public Health schools before release to the Longwood Medical Area community. The Medical School's Communications office would also send communications to officials at the Harvard Office of General Counsel and HPAC so everyone was aware of the content of the messages.

This process was put in place specifically for the spring. But response personnel agreed that communications were sometimes delayed and that in the future they needed to find a way to turn around communication drafts and distribute messages more quickly. Additionally, internal communication among the various response teams—CMT, IST, and LEMTs—was a struggle at times. Members of the Harvard Medical School LEMT suggested that in the future, to ensure that the exchange of information occurred as frequently, directly, and accurately as possible, the group should establish a schedule and criteria for messages. Additionally, they recommended that school and department LEMT representatives join the IST for extended incidents.

In the fall, university leaders acted on the recommendations and refined the process through which communication officers at individual schools would send communications to school leaders and contacts at HPAC. During a pandemic, HPAC would coordinate all Harvard-wide communications so that the messaging would be consistent.[11] Officials at HPAC would write messages and send them to officials at schools and departments who would repurpose the messages for their own needs. The schools and departments were responsible for any additional communications at the local level, such as instructions or specific information, but they would keep HPAC updated on local communications. As a general rule, the institution continued to centralize interviews regarding H1N1. Dr. Rosenthal remained "the single university spokesperson to ensure a unified public message"[12] and Provost Hyman continued acting as the university spokesperson for

---

11. Harvard University, "H1N1 Influenza Management Response and Recovery Plan."
12. Ibid.

institutional announcements. Each school self-designated a dean to communicate "School-specific information."[13]

Members of Dr. Rosenthal's management team continued to communicate regularly with public health officials, including Dr. Barry at BPHC and Dr. DeMaria at MDPH. According to Dr. Rosenthal, Dr. Soheyla Gharib, Chief of Medicine, and Maria Francesconi, Chief of Nursing, the relationships built among members of the management team were critical in making quick, appropriate decisions and communicating effectively with external and internal audiences. The members of the team on the university side had worked together for years, and Dr. Rosenthal, Dr. Barry, and Dr. DeMaria had positive relationships from years of public health collaboration.

The membership of the management team remained constant throughout the semester, as did their main systems of communications: twice daily conference calls or meetings and regular summary e-mails sent to all members. The summary e-mails were based on current information about H1N1 from the Centers for Disease Control and Prevention (CDC) and the case tracking system used at HUHS to manage and monitor patients. The e-mails maintained in real time a running catalogue of H1N1 management and implementation issues that developed over the semester. A log of information about cases and decisions was also kept in WebEOC. The team discussed a number of issues throughout the semester, including status of cases, surge capacity, and vaccination availability and distribution.

Regarding internal communications to the Harvard community, the individual Harvard schools remained responsible for communicating with their specific audiences.[14] LEMTs at specific schools and departments met regularly and also kept in touch as necessary with HUHS. Kassabian's Emergency Management Team, located at the University Operations Center, improved the resources for school leaders based on the after-action review. For example, the URL "www.harvard.edu/h1n1" was redirected to the University Health Services Web site, and an FAQ document was posted prominently on the site. Additionally, HUHS established a dedicated H1N1 hotline. "The number was also linked through the main HUHS line as an option and was part of the University's large H1N1 hotline."[15] Calls to the number peaked at 120 a week during November 2009.[16]

The university continued the aggressive H1N1 education and outreach practices from the spring into the fall. Overall, these outreach efforts had received high marks from those involved in the spring response. The team recommended enhancing the outreach measures used in the spring through additional posters and handouts, as well as holding flu clinics and making nurses and health care personnel more accessible.

During the fall, HUHS distributed information to the tutors and proctors in undergraduate housing and asked them to help monitor the health of students isolated in

---

13. Ibid.
14. Ibid.
15. HUHS, *Emergency Response Report*.
16. Ibid.

their rooms. The university posted educational handouts all over the campus and at HUHS. The HUHS and Harvard Web sites were updated regularly with information on H1N1 and vaccinations. New initiatives included posting videos of Dr. Rosenthal providing information on H1N1 treatment and prevention on the HUHS Web site. On Wednesdays in October from 5:30 p.m. to 8 p.m. nurses were stationed in the freshman dining hall to distribute information about the flu and answer students' questions. In general, the message to use antibacterial handwash, wash hands, and practice other forms of good hygiene blanketed the university from the college to the graduate schools.

Technology

Members of the response teams agreed that the technologies used during emergencies—including the WebEOC software system, internal Emergency Preparedness Web site (E-prep), Harvard University Emergency Notification System (HUENS), and the emergency messaging system MessageME—were useful to provide updates and facilitate communications and knowledge-sharing among emergency response personnel, as well as communicate important information to students and other members of the university community. During the after-action review, however, responders recommended updating site materials more regularly. Additionally, they strongly recommended that new LEMT members and others responsible for using the technologies receive more extensive and regular trainings on how to access and maximize the usefulness of the technologies.

As part of its regular operations, the emergency management team had previously conducted a more general training for 500 people on how to use the university's emergency technologies. At the September meeting, Kassabian walked through the WebEOC, E-prep, HUENS, and MessageME technologies to outline how these technologies would be specifically used as part of the H1N1 response in the fall. He showed people how to log in and navigate the systems to find information, such as the newly revised H1N1 Emergency Response Plan. Emergency Management granted access to WebEOC and the E-prep systems to all newly approved emergency response personnel. The latest emergency response plan for H1N1, along with guidelines and protocols, were posted on the E-prep system. In preparation for the fall, members of an individual LEMT could go the E-prep site and download guidelines for distribution to staff and contractors instead of creating their own.

Moving forward, those who joined emergency response teams at any level would receive training on how to use the systems as part of a locally revised on-boarding procedure. The university emergency management department created online tutorials to address the growing need for immediate trainings. The department continued to offer in-person follow-up and refresher trainings, and individual departments and schools could request trainings as well.

Surge Capacity Planning and Operations Support

Fortunately, in the spring the infection rate never outpaced the availability of beds in Stillman infirmary or the residence halls. However, with the expected surge in the fall, university leaders wanted to strengthen the service structure supporting the isolation system. The recommendations from the after-action review called for a more formal HUHS triage and case management system, including protocols and guidelines for inter-acting with food and cleaning vendors, as well as a more concrete plan regarding surge capacity for the fall. Additionally, after issues with students not following prevention and treatment protocols, the team recommended a clearer definition of what self-isolation meant for students with suspected H1N1, including strong recommendations regarding behavior and transmission risks.

The isolation and service support system was a major element in the university's H1N1 treatment strategy for undergraduates.[17] The main concern in the fall was creating and sus-taining a robust enough system to address the expected higher number of cases. Tom Vautin, Acting Vice President of Administration, asked the leaders of each of the major depart-ments involved in the service system—including Harvard Real Estate Services, Harvard Transportation Services, Harvard University Dining Services (HUDS), and Facilities Maintenance and Operations (responsible for cleaning and housekeeping)—to revise their H1N1 practices and prepare a presentation for the September meeting to outline their roles and responsibilities in supporting the student isolation system. (See Exhibit 8B-2.)

During the fall term, Harvard leaders created a five-level isolation framework to guide housing decisions for sick students (Exhibit 8A-3). Level 4 called for housing stu-dents at the Harvard Square Hotel, which was owned by the university and managed by Harvard Real Estate Services. The use of the Harvard Square Hotel for housing sick stu-dents was incredibly expensive, as it required covering the costs of moving guests to another hotel, canceling and refunding reservations, sanitizing rooms and common areas, removing hazardous waste, and coordinating with Harvard University Transportation Service, HUDS, and other vendors for the care of sick students. Some tension developed between leaders in the university's central administrative offices and the Harvard Real Estate Services Department over which department was responsible for covering the costs of the plan. Officials at central administration and Harvard Real Estate Services eventually agreed on a plan to share costs and responsibilities to cover Level 4 of the isolation plan.

Regarding transportation of sick students, Harvard leaders decided that HUHS would identify students who needed to be isolated outside of Stillman and contact Harvard

---

17. All graduate and professional students and staff were instructed to return to their home with guidance from HUHS, including flu kits and information on self-care and transmission; Harvard University, "H1N1 Influenza Management Response and Recovery Plan."

Transportation Services to shuttle patients to a surge facility (i.e., university housing such as DeWolfe or Leverett dormitories). HUDS was the primary provider of meals to patients in the infirmary. (If the university had needed to engage surge facilities such as the hotel, HUDS would have provided food there, as well.) HUDS was responsible for preparing and delivering food, as well as identifying specific dietary needs. HUDS and HUHS jointly created two menus for these Get Well Meals: the acute-phase menu and the later-phase menu. Food service began as soon as a student was diagnosed with an influenza-like illness and isolated.

HUDS also developed contingency plans in case of a surge of patients. For example, if "large-scale distribution" was required, HUDS would prepare the food at a larger facility on JFK Street.[18] HUDS leaders asked vendors to have "shelf-stable menu items and paper goods available at short notice."[19] HUDS even had a multitiered service continuity plan in case 10% to 50% of its workforce fell ill. HUDS also developed a communication plan to guide regular interactions with sick students as well as HUHS and the college.

Facilities Maintenance and Operations is the main cleaning service at the university and is responsible for trash removal and cleaning rooms according to HUHS-established sanitation protocols. Facilities Maintenance and Operations required staff to use Environmental Protection Agency–approved cleaning products and disinfection procedures for frequently touched surfaces and strongly urged all other cleaning service providers working for the university to follow similar procedures. The department also recognized that custodial and cleaning staff might be at greater risk of exposure to H1N1. It provided training on how they could effectively use personal protective equipment, including surgical masks and gloves to control exposure. Harvard Environmental Health and Safety worked with university staff and contractors to establish protocols for workers providing food, cleaning, laundry, and trash removal services to protect their safety as well as that of the patients.[20]

Harvard leaders conducted extended discussions regarding the purchase and distribution of N95 masks to any service personnel who might come into contact with people infected with H1N1. N95 face masks offer a high level of protection against the spread of airborne diseases such as influenza and can be adjusted for a custom fit. They are also considerably more expensive than regular surgical masks. Ultimately, Harvard leaders decided that in this case, since the H1N1 virus seemed to be acting much like a common flu, the typical face masks that dentists and surgeons wear during routine examinations and operations adequately reduced the chance of transmission of H1N1. However, they did create policies through which certain personnel would receive N95 masks, depending on the health emergency.

---

18. Ibid.
19. Ibid.
20. Ibid.

Harvard Emergency Condition Levels

When Kassabian and his team developed the avian flu emergency response plan in 2005, it specifically mirrored the World Health Organization (WHO) and CDC response plan guidelines for certain university actions regarding avian flu. For example, according to the WHO/CDC phase five response guidelines, the university should limit or not allow large public gatherings due to concerns about avian flu disease transmission.

The guidelines put forward by WHO and CDC related to avian flu were different from those needed for H1N1. By late spring 2009, it was apparent that the H1N1 virus was similar to a severe seasonal flu and did not have the same infection and mortality rates as the avian flu. However, WHO and CDC had not yet adapted the guidelines for the avian flu to a less severe infection such as the H1N1 flu. In the spring when WHO declared a phase five pandemic, university leaders realized that their emergency condition levels, based on the previous avian flu guidelines, were overresponsive to the H1N1 situation. As a result, the after-action review team revised the university's system of emergency levels and triggers to more effectively and efficiently address H1N1.

Vaccines

Unlike previous years, *two* vaccines would be necessary for the upcoming flu season: one for seasonal influenza and another for H1N1. However, as the fall semester began, the amount of H1N1 vaccine likely available for distribution was highly uncertain due to production delays. The lack of H1N1 vaccine was a problem across the country. Representatives of vaccine production companies, including Sanofi Pasteur, Novartis, MedImmune, GlaxoSmithKline, and CSL, reported that it took longer to grow the vaccine inside chicken eggs than expected.[21] State and local authorities were struggling with how to manage the limited supplies of the vaccination.

Moreover, when Dr. Rosenthal called state health officials early in the fall semester to ensure that Harvard was included in the production and delivery estimates, he discovered, to his dismay, that the university had been miscategorized and not included in initial projections. As a result, Harvard, like many institutions, did not have enough H1N1 vaccine at the start of the fall semester. Leaders realized by early October that allotments might not arrive until later in the fall or even early winter.

Harvard received enough seasonal influenza vaccine for the fall semester and started offering seasonal flu clinics in early September. Although the seasonal flu vaccine was not specifically tailored to protect against H1N1, there was some speculation that it might help guard against it, as well. The vaccination clinics were held on Mondays and

---

21. Michael Shear and Rob Stein, "Why Such a Shortage of Swine Flu Vaccine?" *Washington Post*, October 27, 2009, http://www.washingtonpost.com/wp-dyn/content/article/2009/10/26/AR2009102603487_2.html.

Tuesdays from 12 p.m. to 3 p.m. and were open to all members of the Harvard community.[22] Clinics were also held at various locations around the campus and graduate schools. By late October, more than 15,000 people had received the seasonal flu vaccine.[23]

Harvard received a limited supply of H1N1 vaccine at the end of October but would not receive enough vaccine in time to properly inoculate all members of the Harvard community against H1N1 during the fall semester. Because of the meager supply, Harvard leaders were put in the awkward position of having to ration the vaccinations. Based on BPHC recommendations (which were based on CDC recommendations), the university prioritized certain populations as initially eligible for the vaccine. For example, pregnant women and children were deemed a high-risk population and were given the vaccine during the first round of clinics. Individuals with compromised immune systems and breathing difficulties such as asthma and emphysema were also considered high risk and prioritized.

Some in the Harvard community took issue with the university's decision to ration the vaccine. Though Harvard leaders shared frustration about its availability, they were not sure how else to address the supply issue. If H1N1 had been a more severe disease, the lack of adequate supplies of the vaccine could have become an extremely difficult situation.

More H1N1 vaccine did slowly become available during November. The university continued to follow Massachusetts Department of Public Health recommendations regarding prioritizing recipients. Only in late December did Harvard start receiving large allotments of the vaccine. By then, however, it was clear that H1N1 was generally not more dangerous than seasonal flu. Ironically, the university started having a tough time convincing students to take the vaccine during exams, as it sometimes made recipients sluggish or tired. Many chose to wait until they returned to campus at the beginning of spring semester. By the end of December, only 3,275 individuals had received the H1N1 vaccination.[24]

Human Resources Planning and Policies

Harvard had several priorities regarding Human Resources (HR) and staffing throughout the fall flu season. First, university leaders recognized the increased need for medical support at HUHS. Patient volumes in internal medicine increased by 10%, after-hours urgent care increased by 15%, and Stillman infirmary saw a 300% increase during the fall semester. In anticipation, the university temporarily hired a registered nurse to work 32 hours a week during the academic year, which helped alleviate some of the capacity issues.[25]

---

22. HUHS, *Emergency Response Report.*
23. Ibid.
24. Ibid.
25. Ibid.

The university was also concerned about illness among its employees and contractors' employees. Accordingly, the central Harvard administration worked with HR officials at all of the schools and departments across the university to revise the HR policies developed in the spring during the initial H1N1 incident. These policies included additional sick leave during flu season, not just for employees to heal, but also to allow staff to take care of sick family members. Harvard leaders encouraged employees not to come to work if ill and explored options for staff to work from home. Harvard also asked vendors to provide information regarding H1N1 sick policies to contracted employees. Policies were extended through the fall after approval by deans and directors responsible for HR functions. Central HR at Harvard worked with HR officials in the various schools to create and distribute an information document to managers about Harvard's H1N1 workplace policies, which was stored on the Harvard E-prep system.

To keep track of the infection among staff, central HR tracked Harvard employees using sick days for the flu, and the information was presented to the IST on a monthly basis. Though there was an increase in employee illness in the fall, most likely due to H1N1, the care of patients was not impacted through medical personnel and other staff absences, and regular university operations continued throughout the fall.

OVERALL LESSONS LEARNED

HUHS reported treating 940 patients with flu-like illness from late-August through December 2010. The total number of patients peaked in November, which mirrored the national trend. The majority of cases tracked by HUHS were undergraduate students (~500/55%), and most were told to self-isolate in their rooms. The next highest number of cases of H1N1 appeared to be graduate students at the Graduate School of Arts and Sciences (<100/~9%) and the Business School (<100/~8%). Not far behind were Harvard employees (<75). Stillman and DeWolfe had sufficient capacity to house students who needed to be isolated, and the university never had to use surge facilities such as the Harvard Square Hotel.[26]

Harvard leaders, including Provost Hyman, Dr. Rosenthal, and Vautin, felt that a number of valuable lessons were learned in the response in the spring and subsequent planning and implementation in the fall. The use of preexisting emergency plans for infectious diseases provided a solid place to start in terms of the university's response to H1N1. The team-centered approach used across the university at multiple levels was also cited as critical to the success of the response. The regular and timely communication among members of the emergency response teams and school leaders, as well as daily conference calls, Web updates, the use of the extensive technologies available, and the

26. Ibid.

hotline helped keep members of the Harvard and external communities informed about processes, guidelines, and recommendations. The educational outreach campaigns focused on prevention, along with access to antibacterial stations, may have helped lower the transmission of the virus.[27]

Areas of strength included a deep pool of professional staff across the university to address treatment and logistical issues, faculty willing to be flexible with academic assignments and requirements, a robust case tracking system, and the financial, infrastructure, and human capacities to develop and manage an intricate patient isolation system.

Delay in the availability of the H1N1 vaccine complicated the response in the fall. Due to the limited initial supply of the vaccine, university leaders struggled with how to distribute it. Another issue was the expense of the response effort—in time and resources—considering that the initial fear about the severity of H1N1 never materialized.

---

27. Ibid.

Exhibit 8B-1. Chronology of Events: Harvard H1N1 Outbreak, July 2009–December 2009

July–August

- Harvard Emergency Management leads an after-action review of the spring response. Members of the Incident Support Team (IST) and the Harvard Medical School Local Emergency Management Team (LEMT) meet to review the response to the virus in the spring and plan for a possible pandemic in fall 2009 when students return to school.

August 5

- The Centers for Disease Control and Prevention recommends isolation for seven days for health care workers and isolation until 24 hours after the resolution of fever for the general population.

August 26

- First clinically presumptive case of influenza-like illness in a newly arriving undergraduate student at Harvard College is seen at Harvard University Health Services (HUHS). The revised policies and procedures established over the summer are initiated.

September 8

- Seasonal flu clinics begin.

September 21

- Meeting of three levels of emergency response groups at the university—Crisis Management Team, IST, and LEMTs—to review revised Emergency Management Plan in preparation for expected surge of H1N1 cases in fall 2009.

October

- Nurses present at the Harvard College freshman dining hall from 5:30 p.m to 8 p.m. every Wednesday to distribute information about the flu (self-care, what to do if ill) and answer general questions from students.

Mid-November

- University experiences highest surge of students with influenza-like illness and influenza cases.

September–mid-December

- H1N1 vaccine allotments are limited through most of the fall and Harvard starts receiving high volumes of vaccine by mid-December. The community-at-large is given instructions on prevention and self-care through Web updates, posters, handouts, e-mails, etc., and the university places antibacterial hand sanitizer dispensers throughout the campuses. There is an ongoing health education, prevention, and outreach campaign throughout the university aimed at students, faculty, and staff. The educational communication campaign focuses on basic hygiene practices to prevent the spread of the flu, vaccination information, and self-care practices.
- HUHS in regular (sometimes weekly) communication with the Massachusetts Department of Public Health, the Cambridge Department of Public Health, and the Boston Public Health Commission.

Exhibit 8B-2. Operations Support Roles and Responsibilities Matrix

Group	Role	Responsibilities
Harvard University Health Services	Health care provider	Establish protocols for isolation, medical care, guests, food service, cleaning, etc.
Harvard University Dining Services	Food service provider	Prepare and deliver meals, identify dietary needs
Environmental Health and Safety	Worker safety, training, and compliance	Establish protocols for workers performing food service, cleaning, laundry, etc.
Facilities Management Operations	Cleaning service provider	Clean rooms according to Environmental Health and Safety/Harvard University Health Services established protocols
Transportation Services	Student transportation provider	Transport ill students to surge facility

9

Tennessee Responds to the 2009 Novel H1N1 Influenza A Pandemic

David W. Giles

EDITORS' INTRODUCTION

Tennessee, like several other states, experienced two waves of the H1N1 influenza A pandemic in 2009—one in the spring and another that started in late summer and lasted for much of the fall (the typical start to flu season in the northern hemisphere). This case study profiles how state health officials approached these two distinct phases of the pandemic, while also highlighting how they reorganized and bolstered their response capacity during a brief mid-summer lull, when cases of H1N1 continued to surface, but at a slower rate.

   The case recounts how following H1N1's emergence, state health commissioner Susan Cooper and her deputies organized the initial response to the outbreak amidst a high degree of fear and uncertainty about the disease and its virulence. As they did so, they had to overcome several significant challenges, not least of which was the fact that one of the most effective tools for combating infectious disease—a vaccine—was not yet available for H1N1. (Manufacturers would spend another several months developing, testing, and producing a vaccine that would be safe and

This case was written by David W. Giles, Assistant Director, Program on Crisis Leadership, for Dr. Arnold M. Howitt, Executive Director of the Ash Center for Democratic Governance and Innovation at the John F. Kennedy School of Government, Harvard University. Funds for case development were provided by the Robert Wood Johnson Foundation as part of its State Health Leadership Initiative. HKS cases are developed solely as the basis for class discussion. Cases are not intended to serve as endorsements, sources of primary data, or illustrations of effective or ineffective management.

effective for use against H1N1.) Moreover, state public health leaders faced the complicated task of coordinating their response with an array of partners. On the one hand, they had to align their actions with a set of local counterparts—Tennessee's hybrid public health system consists of the Tennessee Department of Health, which serves much of the state, as well as several independent metropolitan departments that answer to local governments. On the other hand, they also found themselves working closely with representatives of the media, school officials, and other state agencies to implement various elements of the response, ranging from the organization of an extensive public communications campaign to determining just how long a school should cancel classes once H1N1 had been identified in its student body.

Meanwhile, as flu activity temporarily subsided during the summer of 2009, state health officials had the opportunity to reorganize and reorient their response to H1N1. Among other adjustments, this entailed moving from a response effort driven by the department's emergency preparedness team to one largely led by its immunization program, with much of the department's efforts focused on developing a process for distributing H1N1 vaccine to Tennesseans once it became available. (During the 2009 H1N1 pandemic, the federal government directed manufacturers to distribute vaccine to the states, which then worked out systems of delivery to their own populations.) Over a period of just a few weeks, the Tennessee Department of Health created a system through which health care providers and institutions could pre-order their supplies. This proved highly valuable once doses of the vaccine became available in the fall, enabling state health officials to base their distribution decisions on data about estimated demand, demographics, and geography, which they had collected over the summer.

Tennessee's Department of Health was subsequently recognized for its innovative work in preparing for the arrival of H1N1 vaccine, and federal authorities encouraged other states to consider Tennessee's approach to distribution. All the same, the case illustrates just how complex a task this was.

DISCUSSION QUESTIONS

1. Compared with their counterparts in Texas, at Harvard University, and in other places hit hard in the earliest days of the outbreak, what advantages did Tennessee public health officials have in addressing H1N1? In what ways (if any) did Tennessee improve on the earliest experiences with the disease, including its own?

2. When H1N1 first emerged, the Tennessee Health Commissioner convinced the governor that the state-wide response to H1N1 was best managed through the Department of Health, as opposed to the state's emergency management

agency. And in summer 2009, the Department of Health moved internal command of its H1N1 response from its emergency preparedness team to its immunization program. Do these decisions make sense to you? Would you have a different opinion if H1N1 had been more severe?

3. State health officials determined early on that it was important to regularly engage with the media. Do you think there is value in communicating with the press and public when officials have little or no updated news to share, or when they do not yet have answers to urgent questions?

4. Tennessee was recognized for its innovative strategies in preparing for the distribution of H1N1 vaccine. How would you assess its approach? Could it work in other states, where the manner in which the public health system is organized and governed might be different than in Tennessee? How well do you think this approach would stand up in the face of a more deadly and widespread pandemic?

* * *

In April 2009, news emerged that an unknown strain of influenza had appeared in Mexico and the southwestern United States.[1] The number of cases of the virus, eventually termed 2009 novel H1N1 influenza A (or more simply, H1N1), mounted quickly, and on June 11, 2009, with the disease now widespread, the World Health Organization declared the world's first flu pandemic in more than 40 years.[2]

In the United States, state and federal health authorities moved rapidly to respond to the growing threat. The Centers for Disease Control and Prevention (CDC) played a leading role, developing and issuing guidance on a range of issues, from when to close schools to the appropriate application of infection controls and the prioritization of who would receive limited supplies of vaccine. But how states responded varied dramatically and depended on a number of factors, including the extent of disease spread, the timing of outbreaks, and the design of their public health systems.

As in most states, Tennessee's public health community feared that the new disease would soon appear within its borders. And indeed, by the end of April 2009, cases of H1N1 had surfaced in the state. To confront the emerging pandemic, health officials implemented and adapted a series of response measures. But the peak of H1N1 activity in Tennessee occurred in late summer and early fall, and by then, data from the initial outbreaks in Mexico, Texas, and elsewhere—including Tennessee itself—had provided state health officials critical information and lessons learned. With this information in hand, they set about creating, revising, and implementing strategies to respond to the pandemic's expected second wave. State health officials hoped that their preparations

---

1. Case 7 explores Texas's experience dealing with early outbreaks of H1N1 in spring 2009.
2. Institute of Medicine, The Domestic and International Impacts of the 2009-H1N1 Influenza A Pandemic: Global Challenges, Global Solutions (Washington, DC: The National Academies Press, 2010).

would help them respond effectively to the extensive disease burden they anticipated when schools opened for the fall term.

For a chronology of events and a cast of characters, see Exhibits 9-1 and 9-2.

EARLY MEASURES IN TENNESSEE'S RESPONSE TO H1N1

A Response Structure Takes Shape

In late April 2009, upon learning that cases of a previously unidentified strain of H1N1 influenza had appeared in Texas and California, health officials in Tennessee quickly moved into emergency response mode. As a first step, they activated the State Health Operations Center (SHOC), located in Nashville, the state capital. Senior leaders of the department convened at the SHOC on a daily basis in the first few weeks following H1N1's emergence. Those regularly on-scene included State Health Commissioner Susan Cooper, State Epidemiologist Dr. Tim Jones, Deputy State Epidemiologist Dr. David Kirschke (who oversaw the department's emergency preparedness program), the state's Strategic National Stockpile (SNS) Coordinator Dr. Paul Petersen, and Immunization Program Medical Director Dr. Kelly Moore.

Among other functions, the SHOC served as a conduit for coordinating communications between the state and its local health partners—an important task, given the hybrid nature of Tennessee's public health system. Although the state facilitates the provision of public health services through seven regional offices, six metropolitan (or metro) health departments operate under local governments, independent of the state and each other.[3] With this new and potentially virulent strain of influenza spreading rapidly, Commissioner Cooper and her leadership team determined it essential that the state, its regions, and the independent metros operate in a coordinated manner. According to Cooper, the state tried to impart a very simple message in its discussions with the metros: "We're not going to micromanage you at the local level, but we all need to agree that these are the parameters under which we are going to work."[4]

Health officials also knew that to implement an effective response, they would have to closely coordinate with several other state agencies—especially the Tennessee Emergency Management Agency (TEMA), which plays a leading role in all major emergencies. TEMA had opened its own statewide emergency operations center at the same time that the Department of Health had stood up its SHOC, anticipating that the state might

---

3. Just under 6.3 million people live in Tennessee. Approximately two million Tennesseans live in or around the state's three major cities—Knoxville, Memphis, and Nashville—while roughly half the population is distributed across largely rural counties, some of which are staffed with just one nurse (US Census, *State and County Quick Facts: Tennessee*, 2010).
4. All statements and quotations attributed to state and local officials are from interviews conducted by the author in February and March 2009, unless otherwise noted.

confront a full-blown, devastating crisis. But as the state prepared for H1N1's arrival, Tennessee Governor Phil Bredesen asked Cooper for her thoughts on how the state should manage its response. She had a simple response: "This is a health event."

Cooper believed that TEMA's early reaction made sense, given that emergency management (and public health, for that matter) had been planning and drilling for an extreme, 1918-like pandemic. Moreover, she added, if the pandemic had worsened, TEMA would certainly have assumed greater responsibilities, particularly when it came to logistics and security concerns. But based on the epidemiological evidence emerging from Texas and other areas battling some of the earliest outbreaks, health authorities quickly concluded that the pandemic would likely fall well short of the worst predictions. According to the commissioner, it thus made no sense to automatically ramp up to the most extreme response levels, which inevitably would have strained resources, not to mention intensified public concern. And as it turned out, TEMA's emergency operations center never scaled up to full capacity, and the agency largely deferred to the Tennessee Department of Health as the lead in the state's response.

With Governor Bredesen putting the response in her department's hands, Cooper and other senior state health officials worked hard over the ensuing weeks and months to make clear to state and local partners, the media, and the public that the state would adapt its pandemic response plan to the particularities of H1N1.

H1N1 Appears in Tennessee

It did not take long for the virus to reach Tennessee. On Wednesday, April 29, the Tennessee Department of Health identified the state's first case in a resident of Williamson County who attended school in Nashville.[5] (That same day, Texas health officials announced the country's first confirmed death from H1N1, in a toddler who had been visiting from Mexico). As news of the Williamson County case spread, the state's public health leadership sought to provide the public with guidance and reassurance. Commissioner Cooper immediately advised Tennesseans, "People should be alert to developing news and information about the virus, but should not panic …. The more you know, the more you can do to ensure your family's health."[6] Governor Bredesen joined in as well. "All states, certainly Tennessee, [have] spent a long time thinking about what you would do in the case of a pandemic and making sure there are supplies properly positioned and those kinds of things," he said on Thursday, April 30. "So we actually are, I think, very well prepared for this, and I think we'll get through it just fine."[7]

---

5. "State Identifies Additional Novel H1N1 Virus Case in Williamson County," *US State News,* May 6, 2009.
6. Emily Bregel, "First 'Probable' Case of Swine Flu in Tennessee," *Chattanooga Times and Free Press,* April 30, 2009.
7. Emily Bregel, "Swine Flu Causing Stir, but Not Panic," *Chattanooga Times and Free Press,* May 1, 2009.

Meanwhile, senior state health officials decided to make themselves available to the media as much as possible. On April 30, the department held a conference call with representatives of news organizations from across the state. During the call, Cooper sought to make clear that H1N1's arrival in Tennessee should not come as a surprise, given the virus's quick spread through Mexico and the southwestern United States. "As we've been telling you all along, we've expected to see cases in Tennessee," she told participants. "We expect to see more cases in the state over the coming days and weeks and months."[8] Health officials considered regular communication paramount in maintaining an open relationship with the press—and in ensuring that the public received accurate information—and they soon made the call a daily event. The commissioner elaborated on how the department approached the calls: "We'll tell you what we know. And if we don't have anything to tell you, we're still going to get on the call and [say]: we don't have anything to tell you, but we'll be happy to answer your questions."

Early Countermeasures Taken

Cases of H1N1 continued to pile up in the state. Within a week, health authorities had identified at least 20 probable and two confirmed cases of the virus, all either in or near the state's three major population centers: Memphis in the west, Nashville in the center of the state, and Knoxville in the east.[9] Fortunately, all appeared relatively mild.[10]

On May 7, the state's ability to test for H1N1 significantly improved when its public health laboratory received precision analytical kits allowing it to confirm the virus itself. (Previously, the state had to rely on the CDC labs in Atlanta, Georgia, to confirm H1N1, a time-consuming process.)[11] As a result, the number of confirmed cases of H1N1 in Tennessee spiked, reaching 114 by the second week in June.[12] By the end of July, the state had confirmed more than 300 cases, as well as two H1N1-related deaths.[13]

But with no H1N1 vaccine yet available (and with the seasonal vaccine ineffective against the new strain), public health authorities were limited in the countermeasures they could deploy to lessen the spread and severity of the virus. Consequently, they settled on implementing a mix of interventions, ranging from basic preventive

---

8. Ibid.
9. Associated Press, "Tenn. to Begin In-State Swine Flu Testing," *Associated Press State and Local Wire,* May 6, 2009.
10. Mary Powers, "4 Tennessee Schools Closed by Suspected Swine Flu Can Re-open in 7 Days," *Commercial Appeal,* May 5, 2009. Although the second person identified as having H1N1 in Tennessee—another Nashville student—was initially hospitalized, the patient recovered without incident.
11. Associated Press, "Tenn. to Begin."
12. Associated Press, "Tenn. Health Officials Confirm 114 Swine Flu Cases," *Associated Press State and Local Wire,* June 11, 2009.
13. Bob Benton, Emily Bregel, and Kelli Gauthier, "Child Dies of Swine Flu, School Officials Take Precautions," *Chattanooga Times Free Press,* August 28, 2009, A1.

measures, such as encouraging people to cover their coughs and sneezes, to various forms of social distancing and the distribution of antiviral medications, such as osel-tamivir (Tamiflu).

Antiviral medications

Antiviral drugs do not provide long-term immunity against the flu, but they can alle-viate symptoms and, in some cases, help prevent it from worsening. Although state health officials determined that the medication was available in adequate numbers commercially through local pharmacies in Tennessee, they realized that the uninsured and underinsured could face considerable financial obstacles in obtaining it, leaving them vulnerable to the virus and its effects.[14]

As the state considered the best way to make the medication as widely available as possible, it looked to what had been put in place in Texas, which had been on the front lines of the battle against H1N1 throughout the spring. There, public health authorities had piloted a distribution program built around a partnership with a private pharmacy chain. Instead of the uninsured reporting to government-run clinics to receive their anti-viral medications, they could fill their prescriptions at a participating pharmacy, which then provided them with medication obtained through the federal government's SNS.[15] Tennessee health officials determined that Texas's model made sense, especially in comparison to the existing plan, which called for a heavily centralized, state-run distri-bution process. As Dr. Paul Petersen, the state's SNS coordinator, put it, this centralized approach was simply "not sustainable" over a long period, given the nature of the out-break and the already high demands placed on the public health infrastructure. All the same, Tennessee made some significant changes to the Texas model. Instead of partner-ing with just one chain, as Texas originally had done, health officials in Tennessee opened their program to all pharmacies, including both small independent businesses and large corporations. State health leaders pointed out that this inclusive approach had some important long-term benefits, such as leading to a significant expansion of Tennessee's medical countermeasure distribution infrastructure.

But in rolling out the program, the health department's emergency preparedness group encountered several substantial challenges. To start with, communicating with

---

14. In addition, commercially available pediatric oseltamivir suspension and compounding agents were in short supply, causing concern for parents, pharmacies, and state officials. Luckily this supply disruption was short-lived, and pharmacies were soon able to produce pediatric compounds statewide. But, state health offi-cials said, the shortage highlights the need for the state and federal government to engage in a thorough review of pediatric medical countermeasures and identify barriers to bringing these products to market.

15. The SNS is a federally run program that states can access to obtain medications and medical supplies during health emergencies. The stockpile is intended to augment, but not replace, the existing supply chain. Thus the state decided not to make SNS antivirals available to those whose insurance covered the medication.

pharmacists initially proved difficult, as the state had no system in place for quickly disseminating information to all health care professionals. Additionally, Tennessee (along with other states) experienced a number of complications with delivery logistics, due, state officials said, to the rapid push of medical assets by CDC. But over time and with some adaptation, the state and federal government managed to overcome these initial hiccups. They eliminated after-hours deliveries, and, in an effort to link as many pharmacies into the distribution system as possible, they communicated through mass mailings and professional associations, such as the Tennessee Pharmacy Association and the Tennessee Medical Association. In addition, the department's emergency preparedness team adapted a Web-based inventory management system, the Tennessee Countermeasure Response Network, to perform several critical functions in support of the distribution effort: provider registration, inventory allocation, and inventory reporting. The state also developed a Web-based pharmacy locator that served as a reference to providers. Despite the early challenges, department leaders believed that they had identified a best practice (Texas's pilot) and improved upon it, pointing to the widescale distribution their program ultimately achieved. By January 2010, the state had partnered with 284 different pharmacies, eventually ensuring availability in 93 of its 95 counties.[16]

School closures

School closures constituted another key countermeasure in the earliest days of the pandemic. Within just days of the identification of H1N1 in Tennessee, at least four schools had cancelled classes due to confirmed or suspected cases of the disease.[17] One of these schools was in Knox County. There, health officials had first identified a case of H1N1 in a student attending West Valley Middle School during the first weekend in May.[18] Upon learning the news, school superintendent James McIntyre immediately turned to the county's health director, Mark Jones, and its chief medical officer, Dr. Martha Buchanan, for advice. (The Knox County Health Department is one of the state's six independent metro health agencies.) Jones and Buchanan, in turn, conveyed to McIntyre the guidance issued by CDC, which at the time called for a school to shut down for up to 14 days upon the identification of a suspected case of H1N1. With their support, the superintendent decided on Sunday, May 3, to close West Valley for the

---

16. Paul Petersen, *Tennessee Department of Health H1N1 SNS After Action Review and Comments* (Nashville, TN: Tennessee Department of Health, 2010).

17. Jacqueline Fellows, "Tennessee Schools Remain Closed Because of Swine Flu," *Nashville Public Radio*, May 4, 2009.

18. Kristi L. Nelson, "Second Knox County School Shutters for Flu; Blue Grass to Reopen Thursday; CDC Downgrades Closing Advice," *Knoxville News-Sentinel*, May 6, 2009.

entire week and instructed the school's more than 1,000 students to remain home and avoid public gatherings.[19]

Jones and Buchanan had planned to appear on a radio show that Sunday morning to discuss general H1N1 preparedness. Instead, they spent the day explaining to the public the rationale for shutting the school down. That night, Buchanan and McIntyre appeared with Knox County Mayor Mike Ragsdale at a press conference to address the decision yet again. They tried to project a calming tone. "There is no reason for anyone to change what they're doing now," Buchanan said, adding, "Most people have recovered without treatment, honestly."[20] For his part, McIntyre stressed that the decision to close West Valley was made "out of an abundance of caution."[21]

But just two days later, on Tuesday, May 5, CDC revised its guidelines, adopting a more flexible approach. It no longer called for immediate school closure, instead recommending that local authorities focus on keeping ill students and staff at home and that they only shut down an entire facility in the event of "special circumstances."[22] Buchanan said that the shift reflected the rapidly changing context in which authorities at all levels of government were operating as they tried to respond to H1N1. "The situation was evolving pretty quickly," she pointed out, "It was almost hourly [that] you needed to check and see what was going on." And indeed, just as CDC issued its new guidelines, health officials determined that another child, attending a different school in Knox County—Blue Grass Elementary—had also likely contracted H1N1.[23] Authorities faced a dilemma. Just a few days before, they had followed the more stringent guidelines that had been in place at the time. Would the public understand if they followed CDC's latest, more relaxed recommendations and kept the second school open?

In the end, McIntyre, in consultation with the county and state health departments, settled on implementing a "hybrid" policy: he would close the second school as well, but for just a few days, as opposed to the full week. Following a cleaning of Blue Grass, classes there would resume on Thursday, May 7.[24] Buchanan said county and state health leaders stood behind McIntyre's decision. "It wasn't exactly verbatim what CDC recommended, but it was what he felt like was reasonable to do, to try and decrease some confusion among the parents and the community. And, you know, it seemed to work out OK, but it required a lot of messaging from him and from us." The challenge of managing competing school closure policies soon faded, however, as the pace of changes to CDC's recommendations eased. And within the week, both West Valley and Blue Grass had reopened.

19. Nelson, "Second Knox County School Shutters;" J.J. Stambaugh, "Authorities: Knox School to Be Closed Because of Suspected Swine Flu Case," *Knoxville News-Sentinel,* May 3, 2009.
20. Stambaugh, "Authorities: Knox School to Be Closed."
21. Ibid.
22. HHS, *Statement by HHS Secretary Kathleen Sebelius and by Acting CDC Director Dr. Richard Besser Regarding the Change in CDC's School and Child Care Closure Guidance* (Washington, DC: HHS, 2009).
23. Nelson, "Second Knox County School Shutters."
24. Ibid.

A LULL IN THE STORM: TENNESSEE PREPARES FOR A SECOND WAVE OF H1N1

Tennessee's first death from H1N1 took place on Monday, July 6, in a 48-year-old patient with a preexisting medical condition at Vanderbilt University Medical Center in Nashville.[25] But although cases of H1N1 continued to appear across the state, flu activity subsided somewhat over the summer. As a result, the state health department decided to stand down the SHOC. In its place, department leaders held a meeting every Friday morning with staff involved in the response. Immediately afterward, they conducted a conference call with key stakeholders from across the state, including representatives of the department's seven health regions and the six independent metro health departments.

State health leaders also shifted internal command of the response. Initially, the health department's emergency preparedness program had taken the lead. But as it became increasingly evident that the pandemic would not be as severe as initially feared—and that vaccine distribution would likely represent the most important element of the response—the state's immunization program medical director assumed a more prominent role. Explained State Epidemiologist Dr. Tim Jones:

> At the beginning there was a lot of confusion among states about whether our immunization programs or our preparedness programs ought to be running the show.... It was a National Catastrophe, and so I think the natural inclination was our emergency preparedness people had the communication structure.

But, he continued, in Tennessee at least, the immunization program best understood the issues that would likely dominate response efforts in the fall. All the same, because the program did not have the infrastructure necessary for carrying out the response, it would still rely heavily on the department's preparedness group and its emergency management partners for resources, staffing, and other forms of support. According to Susan Cooper, the department's organizational structure helped ease potential coordination challenges. "Our immunization program manager and that team work in the same division as the hospital preparedness folks, who sit next to other epidemiologists," she noted. "And so these folks were already used to talking to each other."

Preparing to Distribute H1N1 Vaccine

By the beginning of the summer, the immunization program's staff had begun preparing for the distribution of H1N1 vaccine once it became available. This was by no means an easy task. For one thing, states are usually only responsible for distributing vaccine to a

---

25. "Tennessee Has First Swine Flu Death in State," *News Channel 5,* July 15, 2009.

limited number of medical clinics that participate in the federal Vaccines for Children program (which provides free vaccine to eligible children). Otherwise, manufacturers normally supply private distributors, who in turn deliver the vaccine to providers, including hospitals, clinics, and physicians. But facing a pandemic, the federal government had decided that the manufacturers would work through the states to distribute vaccine to all interested providers. In addition, no one could predict when, exactly, H1N1 vaccine would become available and in what quantities.

Learning from the past

Fortunately, the immunization program's medical director, Dr. Kelly Moore, had acquired valuable experience with emergency influenza vaccine distribution during the vaccine shortage crisis of 2004 and 2005, which had followed the British government's suspension of the Chiron Corporation's manufacturing license in early October 2004. [26] The suspension had put a stop to the production of roughly half of the United States' seasonal flu vaccine supply, and forced federal authorities to suddenly try to find other manufacturers who could fill the gap. Eventually, the United States received about 61 million doses of vaccine—a significant amount given the circumstances, but substantially less than originally anticipated.[27]

During the Chiron crisis, CDC had tasked state immunization programs with taking over vaccine distribution for the remainder of the 2004 and 2005 flu season. Moore described the enormity of the task she and her colleagues had faced at the time:

> What happened was, on no notice, in the middle of flu season, when distribution was already underway, suddenly it was plopped in our lap. And we had never done any of this before…. It was a completely new process [for us].

To ensure that available vaccine would reach select high-priority populations (mainly the elderly and those with underlying medical conditions), state health officials had contacted hospitals, nursing homes, and other providers caring for high-risk patients to notify them that they should order vaccine through the state. Given the tight timeframe and the state's limited resources, Moore's team had concluded that there was no way they could distribute vaccine directly to target populations. But by the time these deliveries finally began to arrive in Tennessee in late November 2004, vaccine demand had diminished significantly. Moore observed, "At the end of the day, with all of that effort and very limited supply of vaccine, we had millions of doses left over, unused."

---

26. For an exploration of how CDC managed vaccine distribution during the 2004 flu season, see Case 15.
27. Andrew Pollack and Lawrence K. Altman, "Troubled Flu-Shot Maker Is Allowed to Resume Work," *New York Times*, March 3, 2005, A26.

Planning in advance

Nearly five years later, this time facing a widespread pandemic, the federal government planned once more to make state immunization programs responsible for distributing vaccine. With this in mind, Moore spent the early summer of 2009 reflecting on her experience during the Chiron shortage, asking herself what she would have done differently. To begin with, she realized that the state needed a quick way to get in touch with providers interested in receiving vaccine. Because the department still lacked a comprehensive e-mail list for health care providers, Moore concluded that vaccinators would have to identify themselves to the state, as opposed to the state trying to reach them through multiple letters and countless phone calls. The Chiron experience had also taught her that the state needed to have in place a way to distribute vaccine quickly, so that doses didn't arrive too late and go unused. With the general population not experiencing widespread death or morbidity from H1N1, health authorities couldn't assume that there would be sustained demand for the vaccine, particularly by late fall, when people's attention turned toward Thanksgiving and the winter holidays.

As she continued contemplating her strategy, Moore attended the National Influenza Vaccine Summit, which took place that year in Dallas, from June 29 to July 1. At the summit, Moore talked with Lance Rodewald, director of CDC's Immunization Services Division, to gain a better sense of the federal government's plans for distributing H1N1 vaccine. During their conversation, Moore began thinking that it might be worthwhile for the state to put in place a preregistration system for providers and others to express interest in receiving H1N1 vaccine. Learning that the vaccine would likely not be available until mid-October, Moore thought,

> Great. If I can get the word out now that anybody who's interested in vaccinating people in Tennessee can sign up in advance, and give me their e-mail addresses, their fax numbers, their shipping information so that I can create a shipping profile for them without having to go back and ask for anything else, then what would that look like?

Upon returning to Nashville, she discussed the idea with the manager of the state's Web-based immunization registry, the Tennessee Web Immunization System (TWIS). He told her that he could easily build a preregistration function into TWIS's existing infrastructure. This came as welcome news, as it offered a simple way of ensuring that only authorized vaccinators could preregister for vaccine (department staff verified medical licenses and status of all providers registered in TWIS). And by using the existing system, the state could also capture immunization data and be prepared if the federal government requested documentation of administered vaccinations.

As immunization program staff set about designing the preregistration tool, Moore herself focused on notifying providers and professional associations about the new system.

> We didn't presume that it was [just] going to be general practitioners, pediatricians, family physicians, and hospitals. We sent [word out] to everybody. And in fact, we had a couple of dermatologists who signed up, oncologists, rheumatologists, and others who had high-risk populations that they wanted to protect.... We included pharmacies and pharmacists as full partners as well.[28]

Given that the federal government had identified health care workers and various patient populations as high-priority recipients of vaccine, Moore also held a series of conference calls with hospitals to ensure that they were aware of the program. As per recommendations issued by CDC's Advisory Committee on Immunization Practices (ACIP) in late July, the federal government advised states to target initial doses of H1N1 vaccine to five high-priority populations: (1) pregnant women, (2) people living with or caring for children younger than six months, (3) health care and emergency medical service workers, (4) children and young adults between the ages of six months and 24 years old, and (5) people between the ages of 25 and 64 with medical conditions that "put them at higher risk for influenza-related complications."[29]

State health officials also discussed preregistration with representatives of the regional and metro health departments during their weekly conference call to ensure that they, too, understood the parameters of the process. In these discussions, the state tried to make clear that preregistration constituted just a first step—and that it entailed no commitments on either the part of the state or the provider. Emphasized Commissioner Cooper: "There was no guarantee that once you preregistered you would be the first on the list, last on the list, or anywhere on the list. This was strictly the preregistration piece." And, she continued, providers had no obligation to order vaccine or accept it once it became available.

The concept rapidly gained steam. For one thing, it attracted the attention of federal health officials, who asked Moore to present her idea to fellow immunization program managers from across the country on a July 15 conference call. In the weeks following Moore's presentation, other states developed similar initiatives, with at least 26 other states eventually adapting Tennessee's prototype. Meanwhile, back in Tennessee, the immunization team completed the integration of the new tool with TWIS, and on Wednesday, August 5, the system went live. Providers began preregistering immediately. Among other things, they submitted contact names, e-mail addresses, information on facility type, name of the authorized immunization provider, and shipping addresses.

---

28. In Tennessee, pharmacists can be certified as immunizers, as long as they are working under a standing order from a physician.
29. CDC, "Use of Influenza A (H1N1) 2009 Monovalent Vaccine: Recommendations of the Advisory Committee on Immunization Practices (ACIP), 2009," *Morbidity and Mortality Weekly Report* 58 (2009): 1–8.

Because CDC had told Tennessee that it had allotted the state 1,500 ship-to sites, Moore's team limited the number of providers participating in the preregistration program to just over that number, knowing that some would end up not ordering vaccine, while others might share the same ship-to site.[30] Added Moore: "We weren't bureaucrats about it. If you were a significant provider, we'd make an exception."

The state next turned its attention to designing and implementing the remaining steps in the ordering process. In September, it began e-mailing preregistered providers a six-character PIN, along with a link to an online order form managed through the SurveyMonkey polling tool. In placing their orders, providers selected the quantity of vaccine they wanted and in what form, based upon the age ranges of the intended recipients. During this time, Moore also conferred with other epidemiologists and physicians within the department who had volunteered their time to work on the H1N1 vaccine distribution team to determine which preregistered providers would receive vaccine first. A team led by Dr. Marion Kainer, the director of the department's hospital infections program, provided extensive input and direction in data management, filling a critical gap, as the immunization program staff lacked sufficient expertise in the area. Having learned from the vaccine shortage of 2004 and 2005 that it was best to avoid micromanaging how individual providers administered vaccine, the team decided it would rank providers by facility type, which could serve as a proxy for the target populations they served. Based upon ACIP's recommendations, the state would first focus on getting vaccine to hospitals, pediatricians, and select specialists treating high-risk patients, such as obstetricians. Pharmacies and commercial mass vaccination companies would fall lower on the list.

Said Moore of the state's decision to allow providers and facilities to determine who among their patient populations received vaccine: "Part of the principle for this network was: We trust you, and we need you.... We're not the providers, we don't have the staff to do this. You guys know your patients, you know your business." She added, "If I can get an internist a box of 100 doses of vaccine, he knows who his highest risk patients are.... And he's happy, because he has some control now over the situation instead of the state dictating everything."

Despite the time the vaccine distribution team put into preparing for the ordering process, it still encountered a number of challenges. For one thing, the software it used to generate provider PINs began creating duplicates. By chance, an epidemiologist assigned to support the team happened to notice one set of duplicates—luckily before the system had generated many others—and department staff moved quickly to address the error.

In addition, some providers failed to complete the full preregistration process, while others assumed that by preregistering they had submitted their actual order. Fortunately, for most of these challenges, staff could turn to the contact data they had

---

30. For instance, although Walgreens has about 300 outlets in the state, they were given just two ship-to locations. The company was then responsible for redistribution among individual pharmacies. Said Kelly Moore, "That made a lot of sense, because there was no reason for their individual outlets to be subject to what the state's decision was to where vaccine needed to go. They could look within their own system and see, well we have high demand in this area and low demand in that area, and move it around."

collected during preregistration and quickly follow-up with providers via e-mail and phone. And when some individuals, including a county mayor, tried to preregister even though they were not licensed health care providers, having the preregistration tool integrated into TWIS proved particularly helpful. Since TWIS already verified the medical qualifications of anyone who registered, it flagged those not qualified to receive and distribute vaccine.[31]

Coordinating With Partner Groups

As the vaccine ordering process took off, the Department of Health also worked on building connections with the media, and on Thursday, July 30, it hosted a roundtable discussion with members of the press from across the state. Participants included news executives, individual reporters, and senior state officials.[32] At the roundtable, the state stressed the need for good government–media collaboration. As Susan Cooper explained, "We tried to encourage them to see themselves as a major player in getting information out to the residents of our state," asking them to report "true, credible, helpful stories." The department also took the opportunity to clarify what types of information it could and could not provide news organizations. Because of the Health Insurance Portability and Accountability Act (HIPAA) regulations,[33] for instance, the state would not be able to verify personal details about individuals with confirmed or suspected cases of H1N1.

The Tennessee Department of Health also partnered in late July and early August with the Tennessee Hospital Association in organizing a series of full-day meetings at hospitals across the state. The sessions explored medical disaster plans in general but also served as venues to discuss pandemic preparedness in advance of the anticipated second wave of H1N1 in the fall. Explained Mike McKeever of Chattanooga's Erlanger Hospital, "The purpose is to bring all the players—health care facilities, emergency response agents, and public health—all together in one venue to share the same information."[34]

H1N1 ACTIVITY PEAKS; TENNESSEE RESPONDS

In Tennessee, public schools reopened the week of August 10.[35] And although CDC and state health officials now advised schools to close only in the most extreme cases, the resumption of classes translated into intense influenza activity throughout late

---

31. In the case of the county mayor, state health officials followed up with his office, explaining the guidelines for distribution, noting that he could partner with a licensed health care provider if he wanted to obtain vaccine.
32. Tennessee Department of Health, *H1N1/Swine Flu Information for Tennessee Residents: Information for the Media*.
33. A federal law, HIPAA restricts the amount of information that can be shared about a patient and his or her medical history and conditions.
34. Adam Crisp, "Hospital Leaders Review Prescription for Disaster Readiness," *Chattanooga Times Free Press*, August 5, 2009, B1.
35. Joy Lukachick, "Schools Urged Not to Panic over Flu," *Chattanooga Times Free Press*, August 15, 2009, B2.

summer and into early fall.[36] Most cases of H1N1 remained generally mild, but the state's public health community realized it faced something out of the ordinary. Dr. Janara Huff, a pediatrician at T.C. Thompson Children's Hospital in Chattanooga, observed, "The really odd part about it is that we're having it now—August and September. This is not the typical influenza season. In fact, there has been a trickle of cases all summer, and it's not something we usually see in the summer at all."[37]

Le Bonheur Children's Hospital Handles the Surge

The Memphis area experienced a particularly bad outbreak among children, who began flocking in large numbers to the city's Le Bonheur Children's Medical Center.[38] By mid-September, Le Bonheur's emergency department, which on an average day saw between 160 to 180 children, was seeing more than 350 per day.[39] But hospital administrators determined that the vast majority of those seeking emergency care did not need to do so and that they were undermining the hospital's capacity to deal with the most serious cases. According to Le Bonheur's chief medical officer, Dr. William May, "These are people who are coming to our emergency room without emergency conditions.... It has put a stress on our space."[40]

To handle the surge, in mid-September hospital administrators implemented a triage system that they had designed as part of their ongoing pandemic planning activities. As per the plan, health care workers screened people for flu-like symptoms in a 2,400-square-foot tent placed in the hospital's parking lot. The scene, according to one account was "straight out of MASH"—albeit significantly more modern, with climate control and wireless communications technology.[41] By erecting the tent, health care workers managed to reserve the hospital's emergency services for the most urgent cases. Dr. May noted that the tent improved conditions for everyone—hospital staff and people seeking care. "We think it makes it more efficient and more comfortable for patients," he said.[42] State health authorities applauded Le Bonheur's efforts at creatively responding to the surge, pointing to the effectiveness of prepandemic planning. "That is the kind of thing [where] certainly all the preparedness activities in previous years paid off," said State Epidemiologist Tim Jones.

---

36. Benton et al., "Child Dies of Swine Flu;" Pam Sohn, "Swine Flu Widespread in Southeast; Cases Said to be Mild," *Chattanooga Times Free Press*, September 9, 2009, A1.

37. Sohn, "Swine Flu Widespread."

38. Marilynn Marchione, "McTriage: Hospitals Use Drive-Thrus for Swine Flu," *Associated Press*, September 26, 2009.

39. Tom Charlier, "Hospital Erects Tent to Hold Children with Flu Symptoms," *Chattanooga Times Free Press*, September 13, 2009, 1.

40. Ibid.

41. Ibid.

42. Ibid.

Vaccine Arrives

Toward the end of September, seasonal flu vaccine—distributed through traditional channels—began arriving at county health departments, health care providers' offices, and pharmacies.[43] With it coming at the height of the outbreak, the state managed to vaccinate an impressive number of residents, achieving a seasonal flu vaccination rate of 42.1% among people six months and older. This was higher than the national average of 39.7% and substantially higher than the regional rate of 36.9%.[44]

But although public health officials stressed the importance of getting vaccinated against the seasonal flu, the vaccine provided no immunity against the dominant strain, H1N1, which continued to cause widespread disease and severe health complications among the most vulnerable populations. In early October, however, State Health Commissioner Susan Cooper received a long-awaited call. Federal authorities asked her if Tennessee was willing and prepared to receive the country's very first batches of H1N1 vaccine. Cooper immediately agreed, and a shipment soon arrived at Le Bonheur, which continued to treat some of the most severe cases of H1N1. The very next day, small quantities of vaccine began to become available for ordering and distribution to priority recipients across the state. Yet for much of the population, the H1N1 vaccine would not be available in large supply for at least another month.

Distributing H1N1 vaccine

Due to production delays, H1N1 vaccine slowly trickled into the state throughout October and into November. Therefore, the state at first focused on distributing the small amounts of available vaccine to providers and health care facilities treating ACIP priority groups. The limitations on who could initially receive vaccine proved both frustrating and confusing for the public, however. In an effort to demonstrate the importance of prioritization, when Commissioner Cooper fell ill (believing at first that she might have contracted H1N1 herself), she made a point of indicating that she had not gotten vaccinated, as she did not fall into any of the priority groups. This, she says, was a small but meaningful way to simplify the message about who needed vaccine and who didn't while supplies remained scarce.

At the same time, public health officials also struggled to convince skeptical segments of the population that the vaccine was safe. In mid-October, a poll conducted by Middle Tennessee State University found that approximately 50% of Tennesseans would

43. "Health Commissioner Receives Flu Vaccination, Stresses Importance to Prevent Flu," *State News Service,* September 25, 2009.
44. CDC, "Interim Results: State-Specific Seasonal Influenza Vaccination Coverage—United States, August 2009–January 2010," *Morbidity and Mortality Weekly Report* 59 (2010): 477–484.

decline receiving the H1N1 vaccine once it was available.[45] The poll's findings were not unique to the state, but they revealed the significant challenges health authorities encountered in getting people vaccinated against H1N1. Speaking on an October 14 conference call with health officials from across the United States, Cooper bemoaned: "We've been spending an inordinate amount of time lately saying the vaccine is made just like seasonal flu vaccine…. There's this misperception that keeps getting heightened in the media that this vaccine was rushed to market, that corners were cut, that there's some special way this was made that's different from seasonal flu." She continued, "[When] you get a talking head saying 'well, they're lying to you,' that then complicates the messaging."[46]

Although the state health department never physically received vaccine itself (through the preregistration system, providers had selected a shipping site, to which the department directed the distributor's shipments), its H1N1 vaccine distribution team was quickly consumed by the demands of managing the vaccine allocations. State Epidemiologist Tim Jones noted that initially, despite all the careful planning conducted over the summer, managing the distribution process threatened to overwhelm department staff:

> A Target or a Walmart could do this with their eyes closed—they have trucks, they have logistic experts, and computer systems. But health departments nowhere in the country have any of this. So we had people here until 3 a.m. cobbling together spreadsheets and software. You know, once it was working, it was working, but it was painful getting it started.

Other senior health officials agreed that the first few weeks in October were particularly challenging. Throughout the distribution process, department staff had to take into account a complex mix of factors, given the multiple companies producing multiple types of vaccine, each appropriate for different age groups and populations. But complicating matters even more, the first batches of available vaccine arrived in the form of FluMist, which is not appropriate for several priority group populations, including pregnant women, children under two years old, and children and adults with chronic disease. "So," explained Commissioner Cooper, "there was a mismatch between the type of vaccine and the priority groups that you were trying to give it to."

Filling orders ended up involving a combination of automated software functions and human decision making. At the start of each day, Kelly Moore would review a series of spreadsheets, which indicated each provider's order balances and their priority rankings (based on facility type). Knowing the types and quantity of vaccine that CDC had made available to Tennessee that day, she would work backward, filling the most restrictive orders first, updating balances as she went along. In addition, she tried to ensure a

---

45. Kevin Hardy, "Supplies of H1N1 Vaccine Plentiful," *Chattanooga Times Free Press,* October 15, 2009, A4.
46. Robert Roos, "State Health Leaders Busy Battling Myths about H1N1 Vaccine," *Center for Infectious Disease Research and Policy (CIDRAP),* October 14, 2009.

geographic balance in distributing vaccine, dividing the available formulations proportionally among Tennessee's 13 public health regions and then allocating each region's doses to providers located in that region.

Despite the difficulties in managing distribution, state health officials ultimately succeeded in getting at least 100 doses of H1N1 vaccine out to every provider who ordered it, including to more than 1,300 of the approximately 1,600 private sector locations that had preregistered. But the delays in the vaccine's arrival meant that throughout October and into November, few health departments could organize mass vaccination clinics, as many had originally planned. According to Moore, "When we were only getting small quantities each day, we were more focused on getting frequent shipments that may not be that big out, rather than sending a big shipment to one big provider who was going to do some mass event."

Knox County and FluMist

In Knox County, however, H1N1 vaccine distribution proceeded somewhat differently than in much of the rest of the state. There, the metro health department made H1N1 FluMist vaccine available to the public as soon as it arrived, beginning Monday, October 12.[47] County health officials and other providers in Knox County had made a point of ordering large quantities of FluMist vaccine, which, it turned out, many other parts of the state had less interest in receiving. Explained Moore,

> I had hardly any orders for FluMist from any private providers or the health department [in one metro area in particular]. And so, as a result, I had their regional allocation sitting there, not being able to be placed, and I just had to reallocate it…. Because I wasn't going to let it sit. The bottom line was: everything's going out the door today.

Accordingly, Moore's team began filling FluMist orders from Knox (along with other regions with high FluMist demand) in larger quantities than originally planned. This allowed the county to make vaccine available on a wider scale than elsewhere in the state and contributed to the fact that Knox never ran out of vaccine. "We had vaccine all the way through," remarked the county's health director Mark Jones. "Sometimes it was only the mist, but we had it and we made it available to everybody."

Jones and his chief medical officer, Dr. Buchanan, said that the county's willingness to accept the mist arose from its experience partnering with the school system for the previous five years in holding free school-based flu vaccination clinics. For a variety of reasons, the clinics only distributed FluMist vaccine, and because of this, said Buchanan, the community already had a level of comfort with the product. She added that as the county

---

47. "H1N1 Vaccine Available at Knox County Health Department: Intranasal Mist Being Offered for Free to the Public," *Knoxville News-Sentinel,* October 13, 2009.

geared up to organize H1N1 vaccination clinics, its five years of experience helped the process unfold smoothly.

> We had a previous existing relationship with a temporary medical staffing group that has worked with us in two or three of those years, and so they are familiar with the program and were able to step in and help us get back into the schools with H1N1 after we had already completed our first phase of seasonal FluMist.

Jones also pointed to the importance of having several years of experience with vaccinating in the schools. "Teachers were used to it. Principals in the school were familiar with what we were doing. So we felt like we had a great advantage in administering that vaccine."

Yet even in Knox County, vaccine distribution ran into substantial obstacles. Although the health department had placed health care workers at the top of its list of target groups, it encountered resistance to the FluMist from some hospital employees afraid of taking a live-virus vaccine, despite reassurance from public health authorities at all levels that it was safe and effective. Additionally, as vaccine demand began to diminish, the health department could not even give away much of its remaining stock. Despite organizing mass vaccination clinics at sporting events and other public forums, uptake remained extremely low. Jones and Buchanan acknowledged that they had more research to do to understand what venues, beyond school settings, might be most appropriate for distributing vaccine to the general population.

Vaccine Demand Slows

H1N1 activity in Tennessee began to subside in late October,[48] and doctors' offices and hospitals across the state soon reported a marked drop in the number of people being treated with influenza-like illness. (Almost all cases of flu experienced in 2009 were H1N1.) At Le Bonheur Children's Medical Center in Memphis, for instance, weekly positive tests for H1N1 fell to less than one-fifth the level seen in early September, and daily visits to its emergency department dropped by half, from more than 400 to about 200.[49]

In early November, through communication with providers and its weekly conference call with regional and metro health departments, the Tennessee Department of Health learned that the demand for H1N1 vaccine from high-priority populations was ebbing. And after a series of discussions with local and regional partners, state officials decided to begin opening up access to the general population. Thus, in an e-mail sent out on

---

48. Tom Charlier, "Swine-Flu Cases Slowing Down, But It's Not Over," *Commercial Appeal,* October 30, 2009, A1; Christina E. Sanchez, "Tennessee Keeps H1N1 Crisis Plans Flexible, Health Officials Say," *Tennessean,* November 2, 2009.
49. Charlier, "Swine-Flu Cases Slowing Down."

Friday, November 20, the Tennessee Department of Health informed participating private providers that it no longer recommended that they limit distribution to ACIP's priority groups, if their supplies were sufficient to expand use to others who wanted it. Recalling the Chiron vaccine shortage, Kelly Moore stressed, "The last thing we want is vaccine sitting unused.... Don't let it sit on the shelf." Shortly thereafter, on December 1, all public health departments across the state also dropped their restrictions, making Tennessee one of the very first states in the country to open up H1N1 vaccine access to the population at large.[50]

CONTINUED CHALLENGES

By January 2010, flu activity had significantly diminished in Tennessee, as it had across much of the rest of the country. By and large, state health officials believed they had managed an effective response. To start with, the vaccine distribution preregistration program had served as a model for other states, winning a national award for its innovative design.[51] As for its antiviral distribution system, the state had identified and—health department officials asserted—improved upon a best practice from another state. Communications had been an ongoing struggle, but state and local health departments had made considerable effort to keep the public informed and up to date, regularly participating in press conferences and maintaining an open channel to news reporters, which helped minimize misinformation.

But when it came to vaccine administration the results were mixed. Although the state had exceeded national and regional seasonal flu vaccination rates, its results (as of January 2010) with H1N1 vaccine (22.5%) fell short of the national average (23.9%).[52] State health leaders believed that the variance reflected the different ways H1N1 played out across the country. Data provided by CDC to Tennessee showed that by Thanksgiving (while H1N1 was still active in the state), the percentage of Tennesseans vaccinated was, in fact, 46% higher than the percentage of US residents vaccinated against H1N1

---

50. CDC recommended that the rest of the country follow suit in mid-December. See: Blake Farmer, "More States Follow Tennessee in Offering H1N1 Vaccines to All," *Nashville Public Radio*, December 17, 2009; Jim Matheny, "H1N1 Vaccine Restrictions Lifted; Free Clinics Scheduled," *WBIR*, November 30, 2009; National Association of County and City Health Officials, *Story from the Field*, 2010.
51. In November 2009, the Association of Immunization Managers awarded its Bull's-Eye Award to Moore's group for the preregistration system it had designed in advance of H1N1 vaccine distribution. In announcing the award, Claire Hannan, the association's executive director remarked, "What Tennessee did was really innovative.... The concept definitely caught on." See: Christina E. Sanchez, "Tennessee's H1N1 Immunization System Is Model for Other States," *Tennessean*, November 16, 2009. Tennessee's H1N1 vaccine distribution team also was awarded the Honorable Mention for Overall Influenza Season Activities by the CDC/AMA National Influenza Vaccine Summit in May 2010.
52. CDC, "Interim Results: State-Specific Influenza A (H1N1) 2009 Monovalent Vaccination Coverage—United States, October 2009–January 2010," *Morbidity and Mortality Weekly Report* 59 (2010): 363–368.

overall.[53] State officials acknowledged that demand in the state waned quickly after Thanksgiving. But, they pointed out, Tennessee had endured its peak in flu activity well before H1N1 vaccine became widely available. By the time it did, H1N1 activity had dropped off considerably. In addition, they continued, many Tennesseans had the time to observe that even at its peak, H1N1 did not appear particularly virulent. Given these circumstances, why should they take the time to hunt down vaccine? All the same, health officials recognized that they could have done more to increase vaccination rates, and among other things, they began exploring alternative sites to host clinics.

And indeed, with H1N1 activity throughout the southeastern United States again rising above national levels in spring 2010, Tennessee health authorities knew they had more work to do.[54] In the meantime, they continued to encourage vaccination as best they could. "We have plenty of it. It's free. Come and get it, please," Knox County's Martha Buchanan implored in late March 2010 as the state reported several more H1N1-related deaths.[55]

Perhaps most significantly, state health authorities realized that H1N1 had not constituted the worst-case scenario. As State Epidemiologist Tim Jones put it, "To be blunt, I think we got really lucky this time around, in that the flu did not blow up." The world's next pandemic could be equally, if not more, contagious than H1N1—and take far more lives.[56] This realization prompted some serious concerns on the part of the public health community. For one thing, with hospital capacity already stretched thin, how would health care facilities handle substantial surge? Commissioner Cooper acknowledged, "If the severity had changed, not just the amount of people we had sick, but if we had really sick people that needed to go to hospitals and be on ventilators, there would have been significant challenges there."

With the federal government's emergency funding for the response to H1N1 tapering off as of June 2010, state and local health officials wondered how the public health system could maintain a sufficiently robust infrastructure to meet the challenges of a more severe pandemic event. Tim Jones observed that once federal funds disappear, "Our infrastructure will be exactly like it was two years ago, before the flu ever happened." Thinking ahead to the next public health emergency, Susan Cooper warned, "The time to build the infrastructure is not in the midst of a crisis."

---

53. CDC, *CRA Novel Influenza (H1N1) 09 Event Summary: Tennessee* (Atlanta, GA: CDC, 2010).
54. CDC, "Update: Influenza Activity—United States, August 30, 2009–March 27, 2010, and Composition of the 2010-11 Influenza Vaccine," *Morbidity and Mortality Weekly Report* 59 (2010): 423–430.
55. Kristi L. Nelson, "H1N1 Suspected in Death; Vaccine Is Available, *Knoxville News-Sentinel,* March 28, 2010.
56. Although this virus was seen as mild largely because it spared the elderly, it should be noted that its effects on children were unusually severe. The state recorded the confirmed H1N1 deaths of 13 children under age 18, far exceeding the two to three childhood influenza deaths reported to the state during a typical flu season.

Exhibit 9-1. Chronology of Events: Tennessee Response to H1N1, April 2009–March 2010

Late April 2009
- Following reports of a new strain of influenza appearing in California and Texas, the Tennessee Department of Health activated the State Health Operations Center (SHOC).

Wednesday, April 29, 2009
- Tennessee's first case of 2009 novel H1N1 influenza A was identified in a resident of Williamson County, in a suburb of Nashville.
- Tennessee received initial shipments of federal medical countermeasures (antiviral medications, personal protective equipment) from the Centers for Disease Control and Prevention's (CDC's) Strategic National Stockpile Division.

Thursday, April 30, 2009
- Speaking to the media, Tennessee Governor Phil Bredesen and State Health Commissioner Susan Cooper sought to reassure the public that Tennessee was well prepared to respond to H1N1.

Sunday, May 3, 2009
- The Knox County School System closed the West Valley Middle School for a week, after preliminary tests determined that a student had contracted a probable case of H1N1. The decision to close was based on recommendation from CDC that schools cancel classes for up to 14 days following the identification of suspected or confirmed H1N1 within a school community.

Tuesday, May 5, 2009
- CDC released revised recommendations regarding school closures, advising school districts to avoid automatically shutting down facilities following the identification of H1N1.
- Knox County Schools closed a second school, Blue Grass Elementary, once health authorities determined that a student there likely had H1N1.

Thursday, May 7, 2009
- After two days of sanitization, Blue Grass Elementary reopened.
- Tennessee's public health lab received kits enabling it to confirm whether specimens were positive for H1N1. With improved testing capabilities, the number of confirmed cases rose dramatically.

Monday, May 11, 2009
- Knox County's West Valley Middle School reopened.

Thursday, June 11, 2009
- The World Health Organization determined that the 2009 H1N1 outbreak had reached global pandemic status.

Monday, June 29–Wednesday, July 1, 2009
- Dr. Kelly Moore, Tennessee's Immunization Program Medical Director, attended the National Influenza Vaccine Summit in Dallas, Texas. There, she came up with the idea to develop a preregistration system for providers interested in receiving H1N1 vaccine.

Monday, July 6, 2009
- The first death from H1N1 in Tennessee occurred at Vanderbilt University Medical Center in Nashville.

Wednesday, July 15, 2009
- Moore presented her preregistration prototype on a CDC conference call with other state immunization program managers.

Friday, July 24, 2009
- Tennessee health officials announced that the state had more than 300 confirmed cases of H1N1 and two deaths from the disease.

Thursday, July 30, 2009
- The Tennessee Department of Health hosted a roundtable discussion with representatives of the media in advance of an anticipated second wave of H1N1 activity.

(Continued)

Exhibit 9-1. (Continued)

Late July–Early August 2009
- CDC's Advisory Committee on Immunization Practices issued recommendations for immunization practices using novel H1N1 2009 vaccine.
- The Tennessee Department of Health and Tennessee Hospital Association organized a series of meetings at hospitals across the state on emergency preparedness and, specifically, H1N1 pandemic plans and protocols.

Wednesday, August 5, 2009
- The Tennessee Department of Health's immunization program launched its H1N1 vaccine preregistration system.

Monday, August 10, 2009
- Public schools in Tennessee reopened.

Late August–Early September, 2009
- The number of people complaining of influenza-like illness increased dramatically. Although most cases were mild, the high case count at this time of year was unusual.

September 2009
- Providers began placing orders for H1N1 vaccine through the state.
- Facing a drastic surge in emergency department visits relating to H1N1, hospital administrators at Le Bonheur Children's Medical Center in Memphis opened a triage clinic in an outdoor tent.

Late October 2009
- The number of cases of influenza-like illness subsided substantially. At Le Bonheur, visits to the emergency department fell by half.

Mid-November 2009
- Supplies of H1N1 vaccine in Tennessee became more widespread.

Friday, November 20, 2009
- Tennessee became one of the first states in the country to make vaccine widely available to the general public, as the state health department began recommending that providers lift restrictions on access to H1N1 vaccine, if their supplies permitted. CDC reports of doses administered indicated that, by this stage, the proportion of Tennessee residents vaccinated was 46% higher than the vaccinated proportion of the US population.

Tuesday, December 1, 2009
- Local and regional health departments in Tennessee joined providers in offering vaccine to the general public.

January 2010
- Through January 2010, Tennessee succeeded in vaccinating 22.5% of its population aged six months and older against H1N1.

March 2010
- Although nowhere near peak levels, the southeastern United States continued to experience sustained H1N1 activity somewhat above the national baseline (although the rise remained limited to localized disease clusters).

Exhibit 9-2. Cast of Characters: Tennessee Response to H1N1, 2009–2010

State of Tennessee

- Phil Bredesen, Governor

Tennessee Department of Health

- Susan Cooper, MSN, RN, State Health Commissioner
- Dr. Tim Jones, State Epidemiologist, and Section Chief, Communicable and Environmental Disease Services (CEDS)
- Dr. David Kirschke, Deputy State Epidemiologist and Director, Public Health Emergency Preparedness Program, CEDS
- Dr. Kelly Moore, Medical Director, Immunization Program, CEDS
- Dr. Paul Petersen, State Strategic National Stockpile Coordinator, Public Health Emergency Preparedness Program, CEDS

Knox County

- Dr. Martha Buchanan, Chief Medical Officer, Knox County Health Department
- Mark Jones, JD, Director, Knox County Health Department
- Dr. James McIntyre, Superintendent, Knox County Schools

Centers for Disease Control and Prevention

- Dr. Lance Rodewald, Director, Immunization Services Division

Hospitals

- Dr. William May, Chief Medical Officer, Le Bonheur Children's Medical Center

III. BIOTERRORISM

10

Anthrax Threats in Southern California

John Buntin

EDITORS' INTRODUCTION

The potential for terrorist attacks on US territory had become readily apparent in the 1990s as a result of the initial bombing of the World Trade Center in New York City in 1993 by international terrorists and the destruction of the Murrah Federal Building in Oklahoma City in 1995 by Timothy McVeigh, a domestic terrorist. The Japanese cult Aum Shinrikyo's sarin attack on the Tokyo subway in 1995, moreover, made palpable the possibility of an attack with a chemical or biological weapon in the United States and underscored the vulnerability of ordinary people going about their daily business.

An attack with anthrax seemed one of the more likely scenarios, and one of the most frightening. Anthrax could kill an individual who absorbed it through her/his skin, and airborne anthrax—perhaps sprayed by a small plane—could potentially kill thousands or more if they inhaled the spores.

Stoking growing public concern was the wave of hoaxes that law enforcement, public health, and emergency medical professionals had to deal with. These were usually triggered either by telephoned warnings that anthrax had been placed in a public place or by calls from agitated citizens, business people, or government workers worried that white powders found in their homes or workplaces might be anthrax. These incidents aroused deep fears among both those directly involved

This case was written by John Buntin for the Executive Session on Domestic Preparedness, directed by Dr. Richard Falkenrath, Assistant Professor of Public Policy, and Dr. Arnold Howitt, Executive Director, Taubman Center for State and Local Government, for use at John F. Kennedy School of Government, Harvard University. Funding was provided by the Office of Justice Programs, US Department of Justice. (0500)

and others who learned of the threats through sometimes sensational media coverage; they also created tremendous pressure on senior public safety and health officials who had to devote valuable person-power, time, energy, and equipment to respond.

These circumstances posed a difficult dilemma for public safety and health leaders. On one hand, they had to treat these threats seriously because a deadly biological agent might genuinely have been sent or planted where vulnerable individuals would be affected. On the other hand, as a near epidemic of such anthrax incidents broke out in Southern California in late 1998 and 1999—with every one proving to be a hoax—these officials also had to consider the immense disruption of people's lives and the consumption of law enforcement and public health workers' time and resources. To ensure that people were protected, public safety workers had to decontaminate potential victims, having them totally disrobe and be sprayed off with streams of water; people who might have come in close contact with anthrax needed to undergo a course of antibiotics. Treating a hoax seriously, moreover— with the attendant media coverage—could well encourage hoax perpetrators or copycats to engineer further incidents.

But how could officials judge whether a given anthrax threat or suspicious powder incident was a credible danger deserving full-scale investigation and preventive measures, or whether it was a hoax that should be quickly investigated and dismissed with far less intrusive and resource-intensive actions? Under what circumstances could responsible officials conclude that public safety was not at risk in a given incident and thereby forgo decontamination and antibiotic treatment of potentially exposed people?

This case study describes public safety and health professionals' risk assessment and decision making practices as anthrax incidents proliferated in Southern California. It recounts their efforts to develop protocols that could be used to guide decision making in a particular instance and to cope with the risks entailed in making such judgments.

This case permits readers to assess the reactions and decisions of responsible officials both from the perspective of what they knew at the time and viewed with current knowledge that actual anthrax attacks were launched only a few years later.

DISCUSSION QUESTIONS

1. Did responders overreact to the initial anthrax incidents in Perris and Palm Desert?

2. Why did law enforcement and public health officials, respectively, develop different perspectives on anthrax risk assessment?

3. What dynamic drove the emergency response to the 1998 Christmas Eve anthrax threat in Palm Desert?

4. Were the adaptations of practice subsequently adopted appropriate? From the perspective of what was known at the time, why or why not?

5. Does your judgment about these practices remain the same with the benefit of hindsight, particularly considering the real anthrax attacks of 2001?

*   *   *

By the late 1990s, the possibility of a terrorist attack on the United States involving biological or chemical weapons had become a major national security concern. In March 1995, the Japanese religious cult Aum Shinrikyo staged a nerve gas attack on the Tokyo subway system that killed 12 people and injured more than a thousand others, demonstrating that sophisticated terrorist groups were capable of developing and using weapons of mass destruction. In November 1997, Secretary of Defense William Cohen appeared on a Sunday morning talk show to discuss the dangers of chemical and biological weapons. Flourishing a five-pound bag of Domino's sugar for the cameras, Cohen noted that half that amount of anthrax would be enough to "destroy at least half" the population of Washington, DC, or about 300,000 people.

This concern did not go unnoticed by those bent on causing disruption. The Federal Bureau of Investigation (FBI) reported 37 anthrax threats in 1996, the first year in which these figures were recorded. All of the threats proved to be hoaxes. In 1997, the FBI reported 74 anthrax hoaxes. By the fall of 1998, it was clear that the number of anthrax hoaxes was continuing to rise as family planning clinics that provided abortion services in Indiana, Kentucky, and Tennessee received letters that allegedly contained anthrax.

The anthrax threats received in most parts of the country had been isolated events, but in late 1998 in Southern California that would change. There, a series of anthrax threats that began in the small town of Perris in Riverside County and quickly spread to Los Angeles County before culminating in a Christmas Eve "attack" in the resort town of Palm Desert would force public safety officials to reconsider how they should respond to threats involving biological weapons. Public safety agencies used to working together under a well-established unified command system would find that responding to anthrax threats raised perplexing questions about traditional command-and-control arrangements. In the end, public safety officials would develop a new response to threats involving weapons of mass destruction. It attempted to walk the fine line between overreacting to an improbable threat (and thus encouraging still more threats) and ignoring a threat that just might turn out to be real.

ANTHRAX IN PERRIS

Southern California's string of anthrax "attacks" began in the small rural town of Perris in Riverside County.[1] At approximately 2:30 p.m. on December 14, 1998, the director of special education at the elementary school district building in Perris opened a letter and found a moist paper towelette, a small amount of brown powder, and a piece of paper that read: "You have been exposed to anthrax." Several other school officials were in the room as well. They immediately called 9-1-1. Riverside County now faced the challenge of responding to a potential terrorist attack with a weapon of mass destruction.

Public safety personnel reacted quickly. A fire department dispatcher immediately contacted Captain Larry Katuls, one of the Riverside County hazardous materials (hazmat) team's two co-commanders and directed his unit to respond to the incident in Perris.[2] Katuls, though alarmed, felt prepared for the task before him. Just one week earlier, Katuls had taken part in a special state training session that included an exercise simulating an anthrax attack on a shopping mall. As a result, Katuls was familiar with anthrax. He knew it was a spore-forming bacterium that could, in skilled hands, be "weaponized" and used as a deadly airborne weapon. He knew that people who had inhaled anthrax could be successfully treated, as long as they received antibiotics quickly.[3] He also knew what would happen to people who were exposed to anthrax but did not receive treatment: within one to five days of the exposure, people would develop flu-like symptoms and then approximately 85% of them would die. With the worksheets from the class in hand, Katuls and the hazmat unit immediately set off for Perris, 40 minutes away.

En route, Katuls called the state Office of Emergency Services, as well as the FBI, to inform them of the possible attack. He also called the fire department unit that had first responded to the incident and was already at the school to instruct them to don Level B protective gear—essentially, full-protection suits with self-contained breathing apparatuses—and to isolate everyone who had been exposed. But he was too late. Two firemen wearing oxygen tanks but no protective suits had already gone in to survey the scene.

---

1. Riverside County (1992 population: 1.3 million) is California's fourth largest county; its physical area is slightly smaller than Massachusetts. The densely populated western portion of the county is adjacent to Orange and Los Angeles counties and centers on the city of Riverside. Moving east, the character of the county changes from hilly scrublands to desert. This portion of the county centers on the resort town of Palm Springs and its satellite cities farther to the east and ends at the Colorado River, almost 200 miles away from the county's western border.

2. Riverside County's hazmat unit consists of 11 specially trained officers, drawn from the California Department of Forestry and the environmental health division of the Riverside County health department. Three to five hazmat personnel are on call to respond to hazardous materials incidents at all times. "We have the busiest hazmat unit in the state," says Larry Katuls, one of the unit's two captains. "LA has three teams; all three put together are slightly busier than us."

3. Experts believe that people who receive antibiotics within 24 hours of an exposure to aerosolized anthrax are not at risk of developing the disease. However, it is not clear how successful prophylaxis received more than 24 hours after an exposure would be. See: G. Marshall Lyon, "Internal Memorandum," National Center for Infectious Diseases, Centers for Disease Control and Prevention, January 21, 1999.

Katuls concluded that two other people had now potentially been exposed to anthrax. He directed the remaining firemen to suit up and form two quarantine groups, one for the four people who had been in the room when the letter was opened (and for the two firefighters who later entered that room), the other for the other 15-odd people in other parts of the building. The postman who had delivered the letter purporting to contain anthrax was also isolated.

The Chief Is Informed

Just two blocks away from the elementary school district building in Perris, Riverside County Fire Chief James Wright and a group of other fire department officers were looking at a piece of equipment in the fire department shop when an ambulance pulled in to ask where the staging area was for the incident. Unaware that there was "an incident," Wright rushed back to the command center, where he was informed that there had been a possible anthrax attack at the Perris school district office.

At the command center, Wright's first, involuntary thought was, "Are we upwind or downwind of this thing?" His next thoughts turned to the situation itself: "I was thinking, 'Are there people lying dead over there right now? How quick does this attack and you get the effects of it?'" Given the potential magnitude of the situation, Wright decided to send a division chief, Michael Brown, to the scene to serve as the fire department's senior official.

Making a Decision on How to Proceed

Meanwhile, Katuls and the hazmat unit had arrived at the school building in Perris where the incident had taken place. As instructed, the firemen already at the scene had divided the people in the building who were potentially exposed into two groups, one for the people in the room when the envelope was opened, the second for the people in other parts of the building. Law enforcement officials had also arrived at the scene and had cordoned off the entire area.

At most incidents where coordination across agencies was required, public safety personnel established a unified command using the Incident Command System (ICS).[4] (See Exhibit 10-1 for a diagram of the ICS structure.) Firemen, hazmat personnel, and police officers in Riverside were accustomed to coordinating their activities using ICS.

---

4. Created in the early 1970s to help multiple agencies respond to wildfires and other natural disasters in California, ICS set forth a command template that could be used to respond to incidents both large and small. By providing a command structure and a common terminology, ICS allows different agencies to work together smoothly at the scene of virtually any type of incident.

Usually, it worked quite smoothly. The nature of the incident determined which agency would select the Incident Commander and take the lead on the response. At incidents that were purely hazmat situations, the designated Incident Commander was invariably a hazmat or fire department officer and the primary responsibility of the police department was simply to secure the scene. At a crime scene, law enforcement took a much larger role, often appointing the Incident Commander and providing direction to fire department personnel on ways for them to perform their duties without disturbing evidence at the crime scene.

The anthrax threat at Perris, however, did not fall comfortably into an established category. A crime had certainly been committed, but authorities also seemed to be dealing with a hazardous materials situation. Both the law enforcement officials and the fire department consequently needed to be involved in making command decisions, but it was not entirely clear who should be the Incident Commander, much less what the response should be.

When Captain Katuls of the hazmat unit arrived at the scene, both law enforcement and fire department officials alike deferred to him. Katuls, after all, was the expert on this subject. Katuls recommended that everyone who had potentially been exposed to anthrax spores be decontaminated. "If you already have [been exposed to it], you have," says Katuls. "But if it's on your clothes, you could take it home and infect others." Decontamination—a process that would require people to take off their potentially contaminated clothes (which would be sealed in plastic bags until tests could determine whether or not the powdery substance in the envelope really was anthrax) and be hosed down with a bleach-water solution—would ensure that no stray anthrax spores somehow got into circulation. "Since we actually had some sort of substance in the envelope, we looked at the book. We were trying to err on the side of safety," says Katuls.

At approximately this point in the deliberations, an agent from the FBI's Riverside office arrived at the scene. His arrival further confused the command-and-control structure. Many of the public safety personnel at the scene initially looked to the FBI agent to take charge. But the agent explained that his role was not to "take charge" but rather to observe the investigation and advise local officials on their response. The agent arrived with instructions from the FBI weapons of mass destruction coordinator for Southern California, David Baker, to tell local officials that they were dealing with a hoax ("all of these have been hoaxes"), but the agent also made it clear that the decision rested with local authorities. What if officials did nothing and the agent proved to be wrong? It was a chance local officials were not willing to take. Both Chief Brown of the fire department and law enforcement officials decided to carry out Katuls's recommendation. "It was a joint decision," says Katuls.

Katuls directed his men to start setting up for decontamination in the parking lot outside the school building. Decontamination in the parking lot soon got underway. According to Katuls, "it was not a very good scene." With the temperature hovering below 30°F, people were forced to take off all their clothes (which were then placed in plastic bags and sealed up) and stand in small inflatable plastic containers like child-sized swimming pools while they were hosed down with a bleach solution. Most of the people forced to strip down were women; all of the hazmat personnel conducting the decontamination were men. At the end of the process, people were issued temporary Tyvek clothing. However, their valuables—and their car keys—stayed in the plastic bags, inaccessible. Thus, at the end of the process, many of the people who had gone through the decontamination had no way of getting home on their own.

Meanwhile, Katuls and other public safety officials at the scene were trying to decide what they should do with the six people who were in the room in which the potentially anthrax-bearing letter was opened—the people most at risk. Given the potential seriousness of the situation, Katuls decided he needed to get more medical input before making a decision.[5]

Bringing a Public Health Perspective Into the Integrated Command

At around 4:30 p.m., fire department personnel notified the county health officer, Dr. Gary Feldman, of the possible anthrax attack at the school district building in Perris. Feldman immediately called public safety officials at the scene to get more information. However, details about what exactly had happened to the people who opened the envelope were hard to come by, in part because the people who were most at risk (i.e., the people who were actually in the room when the envelope that purported to contain anthrax was opened) were still isolated.

At first, Feldman recommended immediately sending those exposed to the hospital to get started on antibiotics. However, the personnel on the scene managed to convince him that this action was unnecessary, particularly for people who weren't even in the room when the envelope containing the substance purported to be anthrax was opened. Eventually, Feldman agreed that only the people who had been in the room when the envelope was opened should be rushed to the hospital; he then left to meet them there himself.

At the hospital, Feldman quickly concluded that even if the letter had contained anthrax, the risk of exposure was minimal. "It was pretty clear to me that it was not delivered in a credible fashion," says Feldman. "There was a letter and there was like a little bit of powder on a piece of it. As it happened, the guy who handled the letter saw the powder right away [and] didn't really even shake it out of the envelope." Even if they were dealing

---

5. This was fairly unusual. "There aren't a lot of times when we have to seek medical input on an incident," says Captain Tom Hyatt, the other co-commander of the Riverside County hazmat unit. Hazmat personnel normally thought about health considerations in terms of environmental health and deferred to the members of the hazmat team who were employees of the County Department of Environmental Health. On the rare occasions when more medical information was needed, hazmat personnel turned to their mobile medical database or to the paramedics. Prior to the incident at Perris, hazmat personnel had never called the county health officer directly.

with anthrax, it seemed unlikely that anyone, even the person who had opened the envelope, had inhaled it. Feldman decided not to start this group on antibiotics after all.

Tests later confirmed that the substance was not anthrax. However, because the powder was sent to an FBI laboratory on the East Coast, it took five days to definitively establish that the substance was not anthrax. Given the fact that people exposed to anthrax needed to be treated within 24 hours to maximize the chances that the treatment would be successful, this was a problem. After the incident at Perris, Riverside County health officials arranged to have future lab work done at a facility in Riverside County.

The Aftermath

The incident in Perris received considerable media coverage in the Riverside–Los Angeles media market, some of it quite critical. The school district superintendent described the experience as "the most humiliating thing I've ever been through." However, Riverside County officials defended their actions. "In a situation like this where there are some unknowns, I would rather be criticized for overreacting than criticized for underreacting," says fire department head Chief James Wright. Dr. Feldman echoed this sentiment: "If you over-treat and you're wrong, then you waste resources and upset some people. If you under-treat, then you have a tragedy. You've failed to prevent a preventable death or deaths."[6]

David Baker, the FBI's weapon of mass destruction coordinator for Southern California, felt that Riverside County officials had overreacted. Even if Riverside County officials had been dealing with anthrax, there was no way the anthrax could have circulated throughout the entire school building or even in the room in which the envelope was opened; hence, there was no need to decontaminate everyone in the school building. If Los Angeles had a similar experience, Baker wanted to be sure that it did not overreact as well. In order to forestall such an overreaction, Baker called a meeting of a greater Los Angeles terrorism working group to discuss Riverside's response to the Perris incident. Baker recalls: "We said it probably wasn't anthrax in there. All of these have been hoaxes. We don't need a big reaction like this."

ANTHRAX SPREADS TO LOS ANGELES

Three days later, on December 17, Los Angeles got a chance to test its reaction to an anthrax "attack" when a parking lot attendant at a Westwood Village high-rise opened an envelope that was allegedly laced with anthrax. The building was almost within shouting

---

6. "Anthrax Scare Reaction Draws Doubts, Support: FBI Testing Material From Letter That Caused Toxics Emergency in Perris," *The Riverside Press-Enterprise*, December 16, 1998.

distance of the federal office building where Baker worked, and, as soon as Baker was notified of the incident, he rushed over. By the time he arrived, two hazmat teams had already arrived, along with several fire engines. The police had cordoned off the building and, to make space for the fire trucks, several of the surrounding streets.

When Baker arrived at the scene and found out exactly what the note said, he immediately concluded that they were dealing with a hoax.[7] Baker recalls, "I said, 'Let's just take this letter, send it to the lab.'" But when a high-level Los Angeles county health officer arrived on the scene, he rejected Baker's approach. It might not be anthrax, but what if it were something else? According to Baker, "His idea was, well, suppose it's not anthrax? Suppose they put Q fever in there or they put something else in there to fool us and we're testing for anthrax and it's really something else?"

Baker disagreed with this thought process: "I said, 'Look, it's a threat assessment.' Why was he telling us anyway? The most effective way to contaminate someone with an envelope would be to make it a resume or, 'Hey, you won a million dollars,' and everyone would pass it around. You wouldn't say there's anthrax." Biological weapons are particularly dangerous because they are virtually undetectable until people start to fall sick. As far as Baker was concerned, no real terrorist who intended to use a biological weapon would negate its primary advantage by making a warning in advance. Thus, to Baker, the very fact that there was a threat was the first sign that the threat was not real.

But the county health officer's argument carried the day. At his insistence, law enforcement and fire department officials decided to proceed with a full decontamination. Approximately 20 people who had potentially been exposed to anthrax were sent to the UCLA Medical Center and started on antibiotics. Samples were taken at the crime scene and sent to the Los Angeles County laboratory for analysis. (Two days later, the test results came back negative.) Just three days after Los Angeles–area public safety officials had met and decided that Riverside had overreacted, Los Angeles had responded to an anthrax threat even more aggressively than the public safety officials in Riverside County had.

A WAVE OF THREATS BEGINS

The incident at Westwood Village generated big headlines in the Los Angeles area and triggered a wave of anthrax threats. The very next day, on December 18, a bankruptcy court clerk at a federal office building received an anonymous phone call saying that anthrax *might* have been released into the building's ventilation system. Some 90 people were evacuated from the building, and more than a hundred hazmat, police, and rescue workers were soon at the scene.

---

7. The letter said, "You have been exposed to the deadly anthrax virus." The fact that anthrax is not a virus was one of several indications that they were not dealing with a serious threat.

Baker was also notified of the incident. This time, Baker arrived with one of the nation's foremost anthrax experts—a doctor at the US Army's Medical Research Institute of Infectious Diseases (USAMRIID) in Fort Detrick, Maryland—standing by on his cell phone. The USAMRIID expert explained to the Incident Commander, an assistant fire chief, that it would be very hard to successfully disseminate anthrax through a ventilation system and that, even if there had been an anthrax release (which was extremely unlikely), there was no need to react hastily, since anthrax could be treated with antibiotics. In the meantime, Baker's investigation had convinced him that public safety officials were dealing with another hoax: the caller had said there *might* be anthrax in the building.[8]

Ultimately, local officials agreed to a scaled-down response. They decided not to subject the 90-odd people to full decontamination. (They did, however, take their clothes, which were to be held until test results came back, and issued them temporary, disposable clothing). Instead of being started on antibiotics, people were advised that the threat was almost certainly a hoax and given prescriptions that they could choose to fill if they were particularly concerned. Approximately 48 hours later, the tests results came back. Once again, they were negative.

By now, anthrax had become the threat du jour. On December 21, a telephone operator at a Los Angeles County courthouse in Van Nuys in the San Fernando Valley received a phone call claiming that "anthrax has been released in the Van Nuys courthouse." This time, sheriff's deputies and firemen evacuated more than 1,500 from the two courthouses at Van Nuys before concluding that they were dealing with another hoax.

A NEW APPROACH

Soon after the Van Nuys incident, Los Angeles–area public safety officials held a meeting to discuss how they should respond to anthrax threats. Baker made a strong argument that the public safety response to any particular incident should be guided first by his risk assessment.[9] Since Baker was extremely skeptical that authorities would ever have to deal with a real anthrax threat, relying on Baker's threat assessment would in practice mean that public safety officials would treat almost all anthrax threats as hoaxes.[10]

---

8. In a matter of days, FBI officials arrested a man who had been scheduled to appear in bankruptcy court that day and charged him with threatening to use a weapon of mass destruction. The man was later convicted.

9. The FBI itself had a behavioral science group that was available to help assess any threats received; however, when the threat seemed to Baker to be obviously not credible, Baker himself felt comfortable making that assessment.

10. Baker believed that any anthrax threat was, almost by definition, not credible. The distinctive advantage of biological weapons like anthrax is that they are difficult, if not impossible, to detect until people start becoming sick and dying. Warning authorities that an attack is underway neutralizes biological weapons' primary advantage. In Baker's opinion, the very fact that there was a threat "was your first clue that this was not real."

At first, health department officials resisted the idea that a risk assessment should determine what the response should be. "They didn't like the idea of doing a risk assessment," says Baker. "That was the problem. They didn't like me 'rolling the dice' with these people." However, the Los Angeles Police Department and Los Angeles County Sheriff's Department strongly supported moving in that direction, as did the fire department. These agencies had already spent hundreds of thousands of dollars responding to the three Los Angeles–area hoaxes; they felt they could not keep paying the large sums necessary to deploy hazmat, fire, law enforcement, and ambulance services indefinitely. Moreover, it seemed clear that Los Angeles was in the midst of a series of hoaxes and that big responses only inspired more bogus threats. Eventually, public health officials agreed to support Baker's approach. From then on, law enforcement and the FBI would do the threat assessment. If the threat assessment was that the call was a hoax, then public safety officials would treat it as a hoax.

Two days later, on December 23, Los Angeles got a chance to test the new system when a Time Warner office building in Chatsworth received an anthrax threat. City fire officials evacuated the approximately 70 people in the building, but this time no further steps were taken. Public safety officials handed out pamphlets describing anthrax and its symptoms and collected the names and telephone numbers of everyone in the building. County health officials promised to contact people in the unlikely event that the tests turned up positive for anthrax (which they did not).

WATCHING LOS ANGELES

Public safety officials in Riverside County watched events in neighboring Los Angeles County with some interest. "I remember watching them on the news because I remember [thinking], from the criticism we got, 'What are the big boys doing? … How are they doing their operations,'" recalls Riverside County Fire Chief James Wright. One aspect of Los Angeles' reaction in particular caught Wright's attention: Los Angeles' decision to send people who were supposedly exposed to anthrax home with a brochure explaining what anthrax was and what its symptoms were and a prescription for anthrax-fighting antibiotics that they could fill if they felt sick or didn't want to wait for the test results to come back. Wright directed his emergency staff to start drawing up a similar pamphlet.

For the most part, however, public safety officials in Riverside County did not pay close attention to events in Los Angeles. No systematic effort was made to contact law enforcement or fire department officials in Los Angeles. And FBI agent David Baker didn't give much thought to the way in which Riverside County would respond to an anthrax threat in the future. "I had been so busy here I never really got back to Riverside," says Baker.

A CHRISTMAS EVE ATTACK IN PALM DESERT

The anthrax hoaxes in Los Angeles were big stories in the Los Angeles media market, a market that included the western portion of Riverside County. But in the eastern region of Riverside County known as "the Desert" (an area that included the resort towns of Palm Springs and Palm Desert), the anthrax hoaxes in Los Angeles did not generate big headlines. As Christmas approached and the residents of the affluent town of Palm Desert occupied themselves with last-minute shopping and other holiday tasks, they could never have anticipated that one of Southern California's largest anthrax hoaxes was about to unfold.

On the morning of Christmas Eve, the Mervyn's department store in Palm Desert, like most other stores in the busy commercial strip along Highway 111, was filled with shoppers making their final Christmas selections. More than 200 people were in the store by 10:20 in the morning, when a sales clerk answered the phone and was told, "You have been exposed to anthrax." The sales clerk who fielded the threatening phone call immediately informed the store manager. He in turn called the Palm Desert station of the Riverside County Sheriff. The senior law enforcement official at the station, Lieutenant Craig Kilday, asked the store manager to lock the doors and instruct everyone in the store to congregate at one location. Kilday at once dispatched several officers to Mervyn's to make sure that no one entered or exited the building. He then called the fire department emergency command center to notify it that a threat regarding a weapon of mass destruction had been received.

As with the incident at Perris, the fire department quickly contacted its hazmat unit to respond. Captain Katuls, the hazmat commander who had responded to the anthrax hoax at Perris, was off duty that day, so the responsibility of responding to the incident at Mervyn's fell to the unit's co-commander, Tom Hyatt. Hyatt had not responded to an anthrax threat before, but he had received training on how to respond at a training session earlier in the month and thus felt knowledgeable about the substance he might soon be encountering. The hazmat team was based in the town of Beaumont, roughly 45 miles west of Palm Desert. It expected to arrive at the scene in about one hour.

In the meantime, officers from the Palm Desert Sheriff's station had arrived at Mervyn's at 10:35 a.m. and established a containment perimeter around the building. Regular firemen arrived at Mervyn's at approximately 11 a.m. Captain Dan Miller, the commander of the Palm Desert sheriff's station, arrived soon thereafter. In addition, Chief Wright had instructed Division Chief Mike Brown, who had headed the fire department response to the incident at Perris and who had just happened to be in the Desert that morning, to go to Mervyn's to take command of the fire department response.

During the confusing early stages of the response, law enforcement officials made an important, if essentially unconscious decision to defer to the fire department. This decision was largely a matter of habit. "Here in Riverside County, almost any incident that involves what you would normally consider to be firefighting issues or patient care, [law enforcement] defers to us," says Brown. "If there has been no crime committed, the deference is complete. If there is a crime scene involved, we defer back to them in respect to that crime scene. We tell them what needs to be done; they tell us what they can let us do." The incident at Mervyn's felt more like a hazardous materials situation than a crime scene. It was, of course, a crime to use—or even threaten to use—a weapon of mass destruction like anthrax, but because there was no threatening letter or substance purporting to be anthrax, law enforcement personnel weren't sure what they should do other than continue to maintain a perimeter around the store. They therefore deferred to the more active fire department personnel.

When Chief Brown of the fire department arrived, he became the Incident Commander. High-ranking fire department officials also assumed other important ICS roles: A battalion chief had taken the role of chief safety officer and a fire captain was the head of operations. In keeping with the command structure sanctioned by ICS, Captain Dan Miller of the sheriff's office became the law enforcement liaison to ICS. Once Hyatt and the hazmat unit arrived on the scene, an incident briefing would take place and a decision on how to proceed would be made. Given his expertise with toxic chemicals and the fact that he had been trained to respond to an anthrax attack, it was clear that Hyatt's input would have a major effect on how public safety officials decided to proceed.

Captain Hyatt and the hazmat team arrived at 11:43 a.m. Shortly thereafter, an incident briefing was held. The purpose of the meeting was to sum up what was known about the incident and to decide what the public safety response should be. Captain Dan Miller was there to speak for law enforcement; Chief Mike Brown was the highest ranking fire department officer on the scene and the Incident Commander. But one of the most influential voices was that of Captain Hyatt, who was seen as the expert at hand. Faced with an unknown toxic exposure, Hyatt recommended proceeding with the textbook hazardous materials response—getting everybody out of the store (the exclusion zone) and into a safe refuge area in the parking lot. Law enforcement readily agreed with this idea. Firemen in protective gear began to move the 200-plus people out of the store and into the safe refuge area in the parking lot, where they would be interviewed by law enforcement officers searching for more details about the possible attack.

But Hyatt did not recommend stopping there. He believed that the hazmat unit should proceed with the next step in a by-the-book response to an incident involving exposure to an unknown chemical: it should decontaminate everyone who might have been exposed to the substance. That was both department protocol and, it seemed to Hyatt, the prudent thing to do.[11] "The people could potentially have the stuff on them, in them,

---

11. California's Occupational Safety and Health legislation also required hazmat personnel to decontaminate anyone who had been exposed to an "unknown" substance. While the FBI did not believe this legislation obliged hazmat personnel to decontaminate people involved in anthrax hoaxes, the California legislation did incline hazmat personnel toward a "when in doubt, decontaminate" stance.

or around them, and what are our capabilities to detect that stuff on them? We didn't have any capabilities," says Hyatt.

> What are we going to do? We can tell everyone to go home [and] assume it's a hoax. But this is Christmas Eve; they could take something home to their families. Or we could take a harder approach and go ahead with a field decontamination. Err on the side of caution. I pulled out the reference guide showing that on anthrax exposure, once signs and symptoms occur and patients show up for prophylaxis, 80 to 90 percent [will probably die]. This is a low probability incident but it's a high impact if it's there.

The only way Hyatt saw to make sure that there was no further exposure was to decontaminate all of the people in the store and take possession of all of their clothes until tests could determine whether people had been exposed to anthrax.

A Dissenting Opinion

Although sheriff's department officials had more or less deferred to the fire department in handling the incident up to this point, Captain Miller of the sheriff's department was concerned now that fire department personnel were leaning toward decontaminating everyone in the store. Law enforcement officers had begun to interview the people involved in the incident, including the sales clerk who received the threatening call, and everything they had learned suggested that the threat to Mervyn's was a hoax.

"We interviewed the female that took the phone call; we find out that the female that took the phone call had also been the recipient of two prior bomb threats, which we thought was kind of odd, that the same person would be on the receiving end of now three hoaxes," says Captain Miller. The threat itself seemed vague and generally unconvincing: "The threat was nothing but a phone call to a female in the sporting goods or sportswear [section]. And it was, 'Hey, there's anthrax in the building. You better tell them.' And that was the extent of the threat.... There was nothing that would give any indication of any suspicious device or any residue or evidence of any contamination, I mean, that we knew of." Captain Miller wasn't sure what they should do, but he did not think decontaminating 200 people was the right course of action.

As Chief Brown was weighing these conflicting opinions, he received a phone call from David Baker, the FBI's weapons of mass destruction coordinator for Southern California. Baker had received a call from the Riverside 9-1-1 center informing him of the possible anthrax attack in Palm Desert.[12] To Baker, it sounded like a hoax. Baker wanted authorities in Palm Desert to know that proceeding with decontamination was not the authorities' only option. "I went through, I talked to him about all the things we

---

12. 9-1-1 centers throughout the region had Baker's telephone number and instructions to call him regarding any threats or incidents involving a weapon of mass destruction.

had finally decided here in LA," recalls Baker. "I said that LA is not doing this [i.e., decontaminating people] anymore on these low threats." Instead, Los Angeles authorities were sending people home with informational brochures that explained what anthrax was and instructed people to wash their clothes and shower, and testing any suspicious substances involved. All of the so-called attacks had been hoaxes. Baker also emphasized that there had never been a real anthrax attack in the United States.

The Decision to Decontaminate

Chief Brown agreed that the incident was *probably* a hoax. However, both Brown and Hyatt worried that they could not rule out an incident entirely. "We didn't have any way to really say, 'Yeah, this stuff is here or this stuff isn't here' and be sure about it," says Hyatt. "It's probably a very small probability [that it's really anthrax], but if it were true that they were contaminated, it had very high consequences." Proceeding with decontamination seemed to be the safest course of action.

Chief Brown also felt that his protocol was clear: when confronted with exposure to an unknown toxic substance, hazmat protocol called for proceeding with a full decontamination. "I'll tell you, I struggled for quite a while as to whether or not I should react consistent with our protocols," says Brown. But in the end, says Brown, "the protocol won out." Notes Brown: "The bottom line is although the FBI was telling me I don't need to do this, the FBI is not going to be the one to have to answer for the liability of not doing it." After consulting with Fire Department Chief James Wright, Brown decided to proceed with decontamination. No attempt to contact the county public health officer, Dr. Feldman, was made.

Captain Miller could not believe that the fire department intended to proceed with this step. "We were very adamant and there were some heated discussions," says Miller. "[O]ur concern was that he was making this a successful terrorist event by taking this drastic approach with the decontamination, which would result in huge press coverage, which ultimately we were concerned would result in copycat type hoaxes in the near future." However, fire department personnel did not seem to appreciate this viewpoint. "I was the law enforcement representative to the ICS, but they were not receptive to our recommendations," says Miller. Miller was further angered when Captain Hyatt expressed the sentiment that a full decontamination would, in any event, be good training.

Problems With Decontamination

Decontamination began at approximately one o'clock in the afternoon. The decontamination process itself was fairly simple. Hazmat personnel set up three decontamination corridors, one for men and two for women. (Tarps were set up around the corridors to make the process somewhat private.) Then one by one, people began moving through each corridor. First, they took off their clothes, which were sealed in plastic bags. They then stepped into what resembled a small plastic swimming pool, where they were rinsed off first with a bleach-water solution and then with water. People were issued temporary clothing and moved to a support zone, where they would be examined by paramedics and, if they so desired, sent on to the hospital for further medical attention. Despite the desire of public safety officials to "take no chances," there were no plans to start people in the store on antibiotics.

While people in Mervyn's had at first been genuinely concerned at the potential danger they faced, as the decontamination process got underway, their concern soon changed to annoyance and then anger as people were forced to strip down in a parking lot with temperatures not far above the freezing mark. While hazmat personnel were suited up in protective gear (Level B), law enforcement officers, without any special protection, interacted with people who had potentially been contaminated. This raised doubts about the seriousness of the incident in the minds of many and contributed to a growing restlessness in the crowd. "These people were not happy campers behind the control line in that safe refuge area," says Hyatt.

Hyatt was becoming increasingly worried about public safety officials' ability to maintain the quarantine. If people attempted to leave, Hyatt thought law enforcement officers would need a way to enforce the quarantines, by making arrests if necessary. Consequently, Hyatt decided to contact the county health officer, Dr. Feldman, to ask him to take the unusual step of declaring a public health emergency—a declaration that would empower law enforcement officers to detain anyone who tried to leave without being decontaminated.

The Public Health Perspective

Dr. Feldman had taken Christmas Eve off. He was at a movie when his pager started going off. When he learned that there had been another anthrax threat, Feldman immediately returned to his office. There he was told that more than 200 people had been evacuated from a Mervyn's department store in Palm Desert and that the fire department was now decontaminating all of them in the parking lot. Feldman also learned that fire department officials were requesting an order from the county health official that would allow them to detain people at the scene if the need arose. It was not entirely clear whether the county health officer actually had this power—it had not been invoked since early in the century—but Dr. Feldman offered to go ahead and make the proclamation.

Michael Osur, the head of the county department of public health's special services and the emergency medical services division (one of three major divisions under the purview of Dr. Feldman), had also heard about the incident at Mervyn's—via a phone call one of his subordinates received from her firefighter boyfriend—and had gone down to Dr. Feldman's office. Osur was aghast at what was happening—and at the possibility that Feldman might get saddled with the responsibility for the decision to decontaminate more than 200 people in a parking lot in almost freezing temperatures on Christmas Eve. Feldman saw Osur's point. Ten minutes after declaring a county health emergency, Feldman rescinded his order.

Decontamination

Hazmat and fire department personnel at Mervyn's, however, did not yet know that this order had been rescinded. Hyatt informed Captain Miller that Dr. Feldman had signed a public health emergency that gave sheriff's deputies the authority to arrest anyone who tried to leave. But Miller rejected this authority. "I told him that we would arrest people for any kind of legitimate criminal event that occurred," says Miller, "but he was wanting us to arrest anybody who ... tried to leave. And I said, 'no, we're not doing that.'" Refusing to be stripped and hosed down in the parking lot struck Miller as a sign of common sense, not a criminal act.

Meanwhile, the detainees were becoming increasingly restless. When fire officials approached Miller with a request to go talk to the group and explain why they were being detained, Miller refused, saying that, since hazmat was responsible for detaining people, it should do the explaining. "I'm sure that was probably viewed to a certain extent on their part as a lack of cooperation from law enforcement," says Miller, "but there was a lot of hostility" at that point. Ultimately, despite their disgruntlement, the detainees did not leave.

Decontamination began at approximately one o'clock in the afternoon and was concluded at approximately 7 p.m. Forty-five minutes later, hazmat personnel in full-body protective gear with self-contained breathing apparatuses made a reconnaissance entry into the building to look for signs that they were dealing with a real attack. After making two entries into the building and spending approximately 50 minutes in the building, hazmat personnel could find no signs of anything out of the ordinary—no powder, no suspicious package, no dispersal device, nothing that could even be sent to a laboratory for testing. Hazmat officials concluded that they had been dealing with a hoax. At approximately 11 p.m., public safety officials left the scene.

RETHINKING THE PUBLIC SAFETY RESPONSE TO ANTHRAX THREATS

While press coverage of the public safety response to the incident at Mervyn's was relatively sympathetic, public safety officials nevertheless came in for some harsh criticism from both the public and the county board of supervisors for their decision to decontaminate everyone at the store. In the incident's aftermath, it seemed clear to virtually every public safety official involved in the response that Riverside County needed to change the way it responded to these incidents. The sheriff's department felt that its input had been ignored and that the fire department had responded in a way that would just generate more hoaxes. Fire department officials felt that they had once more been forced to make the tough decision and were now being portrayed as the bad guys. County health officials were frustrated by their lack of input into the decision-making process: "I would say that the fire department and the police department don't consider [public health] part of a unified command," says Michael Osur. "They think that environmental health—the hazmat part—is public health." Clearly, these problems needed to be worked out. Public safety officials agreed to hold a meeting in early January at the Riverside public health center to do just that.

On January 15, 1999, representatives from the sheriff's department, fire department, health department, the FBI, the California Office of Emergency Services, the California Highway Patrol, and other public safety officials met at the Riverside County health complex in Riverside to discuss the best way to respond to anthrax hoaxes. The meeting began with a review of the response to the anthrax hoax at Mervyn's. It soon turned into a discussion about whether or not decontamination was necessary in these situations. Participants eventually agreed that it was not. "We kicked that around and we thought it probably was not, because anthrax, as we know, is inhaled," says Chief Wright. "The only thing decontamination might do is … wash it off the clothing or something of that nature. So the strip-down-and-decontaminate probably wasn't buying us what we needed."

Meeting participants agreed that in the future they should adopt the "LA" approach to anthrax threats. Law enforcement officials, in conjunction with FBI Special Agent David Baker, would assess the threat before making any decisions on what the response should be. In practice, this meant that local law enforcement officers would respond to threats involving weapons of mass destruction in much the same way that they responded to more conventional bomb threats—by sending officers to the scene to look for a dispersal mechanism. If there was no evidence that the threat was real, then it would not be treated as if it were real. No integrated command would be established. If a building had already been evacuated, people would be sent back to work with a brochure explaining what anthrax was and warning them to be on the lookout for symptoms. Participants created a flow chart to capture this new procedure.

Participants at the meeting also agreed to another significant change in operating procedures. If the threat assessment concluded that there was a possibility that first responders were dealing with a weapon of mass destruction, law enforcement and fire first responders agreed to establish a unified command (in keeping with ICS) that included a public health representative.

ASSESSING THE REFORMS

Most of the participants at the January 15, 1999, meeting were satisfied with the new procedures agreed to at the meeting. Some hazmat personnel, however, expressed some concerns—and some uncertainty—about the new policy. They worried that under the new policy of sending deputy sheriffs—who had almost no training in dealing with hazardous materials—to ascertain whether a chemical or biological weapons threat was plausible or not would, sooner or later, lead to a disaster when a threat proved to be real. Some public health officials also worried about whether the county health department, which was not structured to be a first responder agency, would have high-level representation in unified ICS commands at the scene of future threats. However, subsequent events did not provide any insights into whether these concerns were justified: After the January 15 meeting, Riverside County experienced no further threats of an attack with biological weapons.

Exhibit 10-1. Incident Command System Organizational Chart

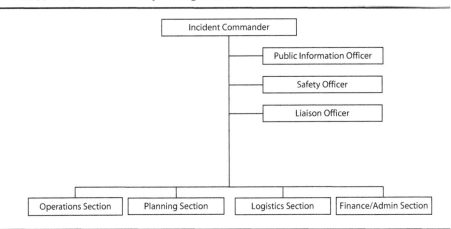

Source: Reprinted from Federal Emergency Management Agency (FEMA), *Basic Guidance for Public Information Officers (PIOs): National Incident Management System* (Washington, DC: FEMA), http://www.fema.gov/media-library-data/20130726-1623-20490-0276/basic_guidance_for_pios_final_draft_12_06_07.pdf.

11

Charting a Course in a Storm: US Postal Service and the Anthrax Crisis

Kirsten Lundberg

EDITORS' INTRODUCTION

Al Qaeda's September 11, 2001, devastating assault on New York City's World Trade Center towers and the parallel attack in the Washington metropolitan area on the nation's military command center at the Pentagon were watershed events in US history. For the American people, the reality of international terrorism struck home with frightful force.

Less than one month later and just as the US retaliatory war against Afghanistan had begun, the public's fears were dramatically accentuated as a series of anthrax letters began arriving at news media and government offices in Florida, Washington, DC, and New York, disrupting NBC News and Congressional office buildings. The crisis intensified as postal workers fell victim, and even ordinary individuals proved at risk from letters laced with lethal, weaponized anthrax.

But federal officials had great difficulty understanding the precise nature of the danger, its extent, who was behind the attacks, and what protective measures might be effective. US Department of Health and Human Services Secretary Tommy Thompson's declaration that "there is no terrorism" in Florida proved absolutely wrong and effectively discredited Thompson as a spokesperson for the health system during the anthrax crisis. That thrust to the forefront the new Centers for Disease Control and Prevention

This case was written by Kirsten Lundberg for Dr. Arnold M. Howitt, Director of the Executive Session on Domestic Preparedness, and Executive Director, Taubman Center for State and Local Government, Kennedy School of Government. Funding was provided by the Volpe National Transportation Systems Center, US Department of Transportation, with additional assistance from the Robert Wood Johnson Foundation. (0503)

Director Julie Gerberding as her agency struggled to grasp the technical and practical issues and develop responses. Scientific understanding of how anthrax behaved was proving inadequate or simply wrong in some respects, and the lack of clear understanding made it very difficult for policymakers to know what they could safely recommend to the public and to workers who might come in contact with anthrax.

The crisis was also a body blow to the US Postal Service (USPS). Not only were the mails the vector for lethal attacks on innocent recipients of seemingly ordinary mail, but USPS's own workers also proved at risk. Several postal workers contracted anthrax—both skin contact and inhalation varieties—and spores were detected in the Capitol building mailroom and in postal facilities in Washington and New Jersey. These developments undercut well-meaning but incorrect reassurances from high-level USPS officials that there was no danger to individuals who handled unopened anthrax letters or simply worked in postal facilities through which the letters had transited. Moreover, the fact that the mostly white workers in Congressional offices had been carefully assessed and liberally offered prophylactic medication contrasted with the much less attentive treatment given to the predominately black postal workers in Washington's Brentwood mail processing center, and this disparity gave rise to charges of racism within and outside the Postal Service.

As the crisis deepened, the very existence of the USPS seemed in question. Could the USPS protect its workers when scientists and public health officials seemed unable to anticipate accurately the behavior of anthrax? If anthrax letters continued to travel through the mail, how could the Postal Service continue operations? Would the public be willing to use the Postal Service if the threat persisted? Indeed, might public fears drive the fiscally challenged USPS out of business?

As days of crisis turned to weeks, senior postal officials organized and got a grip on the realities of the situation, even as many questions remained. This case study tracks their efforts to manage and emerge from crisis, steering a massive public agency with thousands of facilities and millions of employees.

DISCUSSION QUESTIONS

1. What strategic implications did the anthrax attacks have for the Postal Service?
2. What internal and interorganizational relationships and considerations became important as the Postal Service dealt with anthrax-related tasks such as informing and assisting employees, keeping the public apprised of both danger and remediation efforts, identifying and decontaminating affected sites, and maintaining the delivery of mail?
3. How effective were the ad hoc structures that the Postal Service put in place to handle the crisis?

4. Could the employee relations issues that arose during the crisis have been better handled, particularly the charge that black postal workers were treated differently than white Capitol Hill staffers? If so, how?
5. What should the Postal Service do to prepare for possible future bioterror attacks?

* * *

On Sunday, October 21, 2001, a postal worker from a mail sorting facility in Washington, DC, died of inhalation anthrax—a disease virtually unseen for a century. The next day, a second employee from the same facility died. Fear of anthrax had already infected the public: media workers in Florida and New York City had contracted the disease. In addition, Senate Majority Leader Tom Daschle (D-South Dakota) had received an anthrax-laden letter, his staff were all on antibiotics, and Senate and House of Representatives buildings had closed for anthrax tests. Until the deaths of the postal workers, however, the anthrax attack seemed plausibly targeted at the media and politicians. With the deaths of the mail workers, the public perception of risk mushroomed. The recent terrorist hijackings of September 11 had already devastated Americans' sense of safety. This new threat reignited public panic.

Virtually overnight, the US Postal Service (USPS) found itself at the eye of a national security and public health storm. USPS was the nation's second-largest employer after Walmart. Its services reached into millions of American homes. Now it had become a vehicle for terrorism; anyone with a mail slot felt threatened. No one knew who was behind the attacks, how extensive they might be, or much about anthrax. In the midst of this turmoil, learning as it went, USPS shifted into overdrive to accomplish three overriding tasks: reassure and keep the public safe, reassure and keep its employees safe, and deliver the mail.

For a chronology of events and a cast of characters, see Exhibits 11-1 and 11-2.

EARLY DAYS

What would become a defining crisis in USPS history did not, at first, look particularly threatening. The first indication that an anthrax attack was underway came in Florida, where presumably a letter containing anthrax (it was never found) was delivered to the Boca Raton headquarters of American Media, Inc. (AMI), publisher of the *Sun* tabloid. On Sunday, September 30, 2001, *Sun* photo editor Robert Stevens felt ill; the next day AMI mailroom employee Ernesto Blanco was admitted to the hospital with heart problems, coughing, fever, and fatigue. By Friday, October 5, Stevens was dead of inhalation anthrax—the first case of inhaled anthrax in the United States since 1976 and only one of 18 documented cases in a century.

Inhalation anthrax was an ugly disease and, without treatment, fatal. It developed when anthrax spores—which live in soil and travel on hooved animals—settled in the lymph nodes, where they grew into toxin-producing bacteria.[1] The toxins degraded lung tissue and promoted fluid build-up, eventually reducing oxygen supply. Early symptoms resembled the flu: chills, fever, nausea, and vomiting. Once symptoms were present, antibiotics had limited effect. But inhalation anthrax was difficult to contract; the spores ordinarily were heavy, sticky, and difficult to breathe in. The medical consensus was it took 8,000 to 10,000 spores to become infected. Through touch, however, spores could cause a milder form of the disease: cutaneous, or skin, anthrax. Either the antibiotic ciprofloxacin (Cipro) or doxycycline cured cutaneous anthrax and was effective against inhalation anthrax if administered early.

CDC Arrives

The Stevens case swiftly attracted the attention of the Atlanta-based Centers for Disease Control and Prevention (CDC), part of the US Department of Health and Human Services (HHS). Together with state health authorities and other partners, CDC monitored disease outbreaks, implemented disease prevention strategies, and maintained national health statistics. At the request of Florida public health authorities, CDC on October 4 (the day Stevens was diagnosed) dispatched a team of epidemiologists and laboratory scientists. Stevens's employer, AMI, asked CDC whether it should close its building. CDC said no. But the next day the team swabbed the AMI mailroom, as well as Stevens's computer keyboard, and found anthrax contamination. AMI closed its headquarters on October 7. The Federal Bureau of Investigation (FBI) took over the case as a criminal matter on October 8.

Meanwhile, CDC, HHS, and the White House rushed to assure the public that Stevens's was a unique case (Blanco was diagnosed with anthrax only on October 15) and not the work of evildoers. "It is an isolated case, and it is not contagious," HHS Secretary Tommy G. Thompson said October 4. "There is no terrorism."[2] On October 9, President George W. Bush told citizens the Florida case seemed to be "a very isolated incident."[3]

---

1. Diana Jean Schemo, "Postal Employee in Washington Has Anthrax in Lungs," *New York Times*, October 22, 2001, A1.
2. Gina Kolata, "Florida Man Is Hospitalized With Pulmonary Anthrax," *New York Times*, October 5, 2001, A16.
3. Stephanie Kirchgaessner and Richard Wolffe, "Bush Acts to Calm Fears on Anthrax Outbreak," *Financial Times*, October 10, 2001, 6.

USPS PRECAUTIONS

Isolated or not, the USPS vice president of public affairs and communications wanted to take no chances. On Columbus Day, October 8, USPS Vice President (VP) of Public Affairs and Communication Azeezaly Jaffer watched a 9 p.m. television news report associating Stevens's death with a letter. He recalls:

> Three things crossed my mind. Number one, that 800,000 [USPS] employees would all of a sudden become worried about handling the mail. Number two, that it would rapidly turn into a public issue. Number three, it could conceivably … bring this organization that moves 500 million pieces of mail a day to a screeching halt, thereby bringing the economy of the United States to a complete halt.[4]

If the Postal Service even *appeared* to be involved, Jaffer needed to preempt employee and public concerns. So that night, with two staff from his crisis team, he headed straight to the office to write a newsbreak, an internal communication to employees, which let them know there was no confirmation that anthrax had come from a letter but provided guidelines in the event they suspected anthrax. Jaffer worked until 2 a.m. During the following week, his office sent messages to employees three to four times a day, activated a Web site, and launched obligatory informational talks ("stand-up talks") for employees. "I made a conscious decision to have the Postal Service voice louder than everybody else's voice starting on October 8," says Jaffer. "We wanted to make sure that our employees and our workforce were getting information first-hand from us and not hearing it only on the news."

Jaffer's caution paid off quickly. Starting October 12, investigators discovered that the Florida incident was not isolated. That day, NBC News anchor Tom Brokaw's assistant Erin O'Connor, 38, was diagnosed with skin anthrax. Over the following week, other cutaneous cases were confirmed: ABC reported that the 7-month-old son of a producer was ill; on October 18, CBS News aide Claire Fletcher tested positive; on October 19, the *New York Post* confirmed that editorial page assistant Johanna Huden had skin anthrax.[5]

Confirming Jaffer's fears, the common culprit in all these cases seemed to be contaminated letters. On September 18, the FBI learned, anthrax-laced letters had been posted from Trenton, New Jersey, to NBC News as well as to the *New York Post*. (There were probably letters sent to CBS and ABC as well, but they were never found.) An unopened letter containing anthrax was found on October 19 near Huden's work station at the *Post*, and it gave authorities their first opportunity to study firsthand what strain and quality

4. Author's phone interview with Azeezaly Jaffer, September 18, 2002. All further quotations from Jaffer, unless otherwise attributed, are from this interview.
5. Eric Lipton, "Media Outlets, Governor's Office and Postal Center Feel the Brunt," *New York Times*, October 31, 2001, B6.

of anthrax was causing the infections among media employees.[6] The material proved rather coarse, with the consistency of baby powder. Although it could float in the air, the particles quickly settled back on surfaces. Encouragingly, its virulence seemed limited to those who physically touched it. "We see no public health concern," said New York City Health Commissioner Dr. Neal L. Cohen.[7]

THE DASCHLE LETTER

Such calming statements did little to soothe the public, which was already reporting hundreds of cases of suspicious white powder, stockpiling protective masks, and asking for prophylactic doses of the antibiotic Cipro. This anxiety had good cause: four days earlier, on Monday, October 15, an anthrax-laden letter had arrived at Senate Majority Leader Tom Daschle's office in the Hart Senate Office Building. That morning, an intern opened the heavily taped letter postmarked October 9. Like the Brokaw and *Post* letters, it had been sent from Trenton. White powder fell out with the letter, whose return address was an elementary school. A Daschle aide interrupted a staff meeting next door to let those individuals know white powder was in the vicinity. Daschle was not in the office at the time. The Capitol police secured the area, quarantined the staff, and conducted on-the-spot tests, which were positive for anthrax.

By that afternoon, Daschle staff members were all taking Cipro. Later that day and the next, hundreds of Hart Building staffers—many of whom had been nowhere near the Daschle office—were administered nasal swabs to see if they had been exposed to the released anthrax; 28 tested positive, some from a floor below the Daschle suite. All who wanted it were prescribed Cipro. On Tuesday, the Hart Building—which housed the offices of half the Senate members—closed. On Wednesday, the House of Representatives shut down for testing, although the Senate remained open. On Thursday night, all House and Senate office buildings closed.

Capitol police sent samples taken from Daschle's office, as well as the letter itself, not to CDC, as in the Florida and New York cases, but to the US Army Medical Research Institute for Infectious Disease at Fort Detrick, Maryland. By Monday night, Fort Detrick reported in a conference call that its scientists, according to one participant, had been "somewhat surprised by the nature of it ..., that it was a fine powder, that it easily went into the air."[8] Daschle Tuesday confirmed that "[w]e were told it was a very strong form of anthrax, a very potent form of anthrax, which clearly was produced by someone who knew what he or she was doing."[9]

---

6. The NBC letter had been found October 13, but so little material was left that it yielded minimal information for scientists.
7. Eric Lipton, "Anthrax Is Found in 2 More People," *New York Times*, October 19, 2001, A1.
8. Steve Twomey and Justin Blum, "How the Experts Missed Anthrax," *Washington Post*, November 19, 2001, A1.
9. Sheryl Gay Stolberg and Judith Miller, "Officials Admit Underestimating Danger Posed to Postal Workers," *New York Times*, October 24, 2001, A1.

But as the week progressed, Tom Ridge, President Bush's director for Homeland Security, and other spokesmen adopted milder language. CDC called the Daschle letter's anthrax "naturally occurring" and Fort Detrick's commander, Major General John S. Parker, termed it "garden variety." Meanwhile, the hoaxes started. Attorney General John Ashcroft said October 18 that authorities had already received some 2,300 reports of suspected anthrax, many of them hoaxes, and he threatened prosecution of perpetrators.

Despite these reassurances, many federal agencies were on heightened alert. No one could determine the level of threat. Was this a bioterrorist attack by a sophisticated adversary, or the work of a backyard chemist angry at the media and government? The USPS leadership could not answer these questions. For the time being, says then-USPS Senior Vice President for Government Relations and Public Policy Deborah Willhite, "it seemed to be more a targeted media crisis. But it seemed like it could become ours. So we were being very cautious."[10]

POSTAL BUSINESS

USPS had good reason to worry: the anthrax letters were arriving through the mail. Although USPS did not seem to be the target of a bioterrorist attack, it was emerging as the means of delivery for bioterror. If the public did not yet fully realize that, it soon would. In fact, after the Daschle letter, Congress quarantined all mail received at the Capitol from October 12 to October 17. If Congress no longer trusted its mail, how long before the general public would also come to distrust the post?

USPS was no stranger to crisis: it had famously weathered mail bomber Ted Kaczynski (known as the Unabomber), as well as shootings by enraged postal employees. It had a professional communications department well rehearsed in crisis management. Ironically, the Postal Service had for years practiced how to deal with anthrax hoaxes but never how to handle the real thing. The rule of thumb had been that anthrax could never be sufficiently powderized (or weaponized) to send it through the mail. In fact, since September 11, USPS had studied how its vehicles or facilities might be used for a terrorist attack but, according to Deputy Chief Inspector for Security in Technology James Rowan, no one had thought of an anthrax-laced letter.[11] There were no USPS guidelines for managing an outbreak of anthrax.

At this point, USPS could afford no fall-off in public confidence. It was a business in trouble, and it needed every customer it could get. September 11 had already caused a 7% drop in mail volume, the largest decline since the Great Depression of the 1930s.[12] But the Postal Service troubles went back well before September 11. Since the 1970 Postal

10. Author's interview with Deborah Willhite, Washington, DC, September 9, 2002. All further quotations from Willhite, unless otherwise attributed, are from this interview.
11. Author's interview with James Rowan, Washington, DC, September 11, 2002. All further quotes from Rowan, unless otherwise attributed, are from this interview. USPS had worried terrorists might use postal trucks, or postal uniforms, to gain access to homes or mail facilities.
12. Ellen Nakashima and Andrew DeMillo, "What's in the Mail: Many Doubts," *Washington Post*, November 27, 2001, A1.

Reorganization Act, USPS had been quasi-governmental—a self-supporting corporation owned by the federal government.[13] Unfortunately, that had resulted in USPS suffering most of the disadvantages of public regulation while enjoying few of the advantages of a private corporation. USPS received no taxpayer money, but at the same time was not allowed to set postal rates or wages freely. Efforts to close small, inefficient post offices were stymied by a general public outcry. Strikes were illegal.

Given these strictures, USPS had run a deficit of $1.68 billion in fiscal 2001 and projected a 2002 deficit (before anthrax) of $1.35 billion. At the same time, it was a mammoth enterprise, which some argued was too integral to the US economy ever to be allowed to fail. A $70 billion organization, it had 800,000 employees. Its 38,000 retail mail outlets were organized into 85 districts in nine regions and moved 670 million pieces of mail a day. The wider mail industry (catalogues, direct mail, paper mills, printers, etc.) was a critical part of the economy, estimated at $900 billion.

But the congressional decision to quarantine its mail carried a second implication for USPS beyond the threat to business. If the congressional mail were actually dangerous, what did that mean for the safety of USPS employees, who had handled that mail before it ever reached Congress?

SHOULD WE TEST POSTAL WORKERS?

Postmaster General John "Jack" Potter, Willhite, and other USPS leaders had been asking since Monday whether postal workers were safe, particularly at the Brentwood sorting center in Washington, DC. "From the descriptions of the powder that came out, and from the reaction of the Capitol physicians in inoculating and quarantining so much of the Hart Building," says VP Willhite, "we became very concerned that the Brentwood facility and our employees had been contaminated." The same question had arisen in Florida, where on Monday anthrax spores were found at a Boca Raton USPS facility that handled AMI mail.[14] For answers, USPS turned to the public health authorities.

Public Health

Each state had its own public health department, headed by a state health commissioner. Some cities, such as New York and Washington, DC, also had autonomous health departments whose chief health officers were appointed by and responsible to the

---

13. The law (39 USC) defines USPS as "an independent establishment of the executive branch of the federal government."

14. Local health authorities, however, had already put postal workers on Cipro three days earlier as a precaution, and there were no reported illnesses.

mayor. State and local health departments did not answer to any federal authority. State public health authorities were responsible for monitoring the provision of public and private health care services. They also investigated and responded to outbreaks of disease. Doctors or hospitals suspicious about a particular case reported it to the local health department. In the event of a threat to public health, the state or local health department notified doctors and hospitals and mobilized care. The state authority also determined whether or not to involve CDC. CDC could operate in a community only at the invitation of the state health department.

By mid-October, USPS was already working with public health authorities in Florida. It was establishing ties in New Jersey. In New York, the Health Department and USPS had been closely allied since September 11 (when 13 postal facilities were temporarily closed). In Washington, DC, the question of jurisdiction was complicated because it was the nation's capital. The DC Department of Health (DOH) had authority over most of the city, but federal establishments were independent. Thus, the Capitol had its own medical director; likewise, the White House, various military installations, and some other federal agencies. USPS, however, was an independent federal agency, and DOH was its public health partner.

When it learned on October 15 about the Daschle letter, says then-DC Chief Health Officer Dr. Ivan C. A. Walks, DOH activated its standing biohazard response plan, which called for early CDC involvement. DOH requested that, if anthrax were confirmed, CDC dispatch a team of public affairs officers, epidemiologists, and pharmaceutical logistics officials. CDC called with confirmation at 4 a.m. on October 16; the CDC team arrived at 7 a.m. DOH provided the team with workspace to establish a DC operation. But CDC remained in an advisory capacity. "The ultimate responsibility for running things in terms of how you set things up and what you do," says Walks, "those remained local."[15] DOH could have been sidelined, he concedes.

> This actually could have been kept a federal issue, from Daschle's office to the US Postal Service ... and there could have been a very minor involvement from the local Department of Health.... [But] we were involved all the way through with a lot of different things because we had done some thoughtful planning ahead of time and we had very committed people at the Department of Health, particularly in our environmental health area.

There was no written policy or procedure governing DOH interaction with USPS because, explains Walks, "there was just never any thought that you would need to contact the Postal Service." But during the week of October 15, USPS contacted DOH and the newly arrived CDC officials to ask whether Brentwood should be tested for anthrax. USPS officials had ascertained exactly where the Daschle letter had traveled before it arrived at the Hart Building, and Brentwood was on the route.

---

15. Author's phone interview with Ivan C.A. Walks, December 3, 2002. All further quotes from Walks, unless otherwise attributed, are from this interview.

The Route

Timothy Haney was senior plant manager at Brentwood, the sorting center for all mail to the US government in the DC area. On Tuesday, using the letter's barcode, he reconstructed the path of the Daschle letter.[16] He deduced that the letter, mailed from Hamilton Township near Trenton had passed through Brentwood to the P Street mail sorting facility for Congress, then through the mailroom in the Dirksen Senate Office Building, before delivery to Hart. Recalls USPS Manager of Safety Sam Pulcrano: "We were talking to [CDC] and trying to ascertain if [the letter] went through our facilities, what would have been the potential hazard to our employees. Should we be doing something?"[17]

"NO THREAT" REASSURANCES

But the CDC and state officials downplayed any risk to postal workers—at Brentwood or elsewhere. In Trenton, state health officials on October 14 told postal workers that anthrax testing was not "medically necessary."[18] In Washington, DC, Walks confirms, "we were all still operating under the assumption that the only place where there was danger was for the folks in the Hart Office Building." CDC officials assured USPS that anthrax posed no threat to the 1,800 Brentwood workers (some 1,500 of whom "touched the mail," as USPS puts it). CDC refused, says VP Willhite, to swab the nostrils of USPS employees, or to issue them prophylactic antibiotics. CDC had several persuasive arguments:

- Only individuals who had opened or been near when a letter was opened had become ill.
- At least 8,000 to 10,000 spores were needed to infect a human with inhalation anthrax, so traces of anthrax were not a risk. Moreover, the material was heavy and sticky, so it would adhere to surfaces.
- The Daschle letter had been heavily taped and spores could not escape through an envelope.
- No postal worker was sick.

"They said there was virtually no risk of any anthrax contamination in the facility, that without the letter being opened at Brentwood, there was no risk of any anthrax escaping,

---

16. The Postal Numeric Encoding Technique (Postnet) barcodes contain zip code information intended to promote reliable, fast mail sorting. The barcode on the front of a letter tells USPS where the letter is going; the one on the back says where it was mailed. See: Andrew C. Revkin with Paul Zielbauer, "Tracking of Anthrax Letter Yields Clues," *New York Times*, December 7, 2001, B1.

17. Author's interview with Sam Pulcrano, Washington, DC, September 9, 2002. All further quotations from Pulcrano, unless otherwise attributed, are from this interview.

18. Sheryl Gay Stolberg, "A Quick Response for Politicians; A Slower One for Mail Workers," *New York Times*, October 23, 2001, A1.

so neither the facility nor the employees needed to be tested," recalled Willhite.[19] "They didn't think [testing] was necessary because in this situation they followed the science," confirms USPS Senior Vice President for Human Resources Suzanne Medvidovich:

> And the science was that no one had gotten sick [at Brentwood] and that in the past it would take large quantities or a massive exposure to anthrax to kill somebody. So they were going off the historical data.[20]

Press Conference

USPS accepted the CDC assurances. In fact, to send a public message about just how safe the mail—and in particular Brentwood—was, the FBI and USPS (plus its Postal Inspection Service) on Thursday, October 18, held a joint press conference at Brentwood announcing a reward of $1 million for information leading to the arrest and conviction of those behind the anthrax mailings. "I did that," says USPS Communications VP Jaffer, "because I told the Postmaster General that the only way we can demonstrate that this facility is safe to everybody—because that's what the science was telling us—is to actually have the leadership walk in." Some 100 journalists attended, as well as Potter, FBI Deputy Director Thomas Pickard, Chief Postal Inspector Kenneth Weaver, and John Walsh, host of Fox's *America's Most Wanted* show.[21] Potter delivered a reassuring message: "[T]here is only a minute chance that anthrax spores escaped from [the Daschle letter] into this facility."[22]

Despite this public display of confidence, Postmaster General Potter had taken some proactive measures. On Monday, October 15, he announced the formation of a Mail Security Task Force.[23] The task force comprised top USPS leadership plus union representatives, and its charge was to study biological hazards in the postal system. On the public front, USPS announced that it would send postcards to 135 million US homes warning about biohazards and describing how to handle suspect mail.[24] Moreover, it would provide gloves and masks as soon as possible to all employees, with those in New Jersey, Florida, New York, and Washington, DC, getting the first deliveries. Potter on Wednesday also decided to hire a private company, at USPS expense, to test Brentwood on Thursday.

---

19. Kathy Chen, Greg Hitt, Laurie McGinley, and Andrea Petersen, "Trial and Error: Seven Days in October Spotlight Weakness of Bioterror Response," *Wall Street Journal*, November 2, 2001, A1.
20. Author's interview with Suzanne Medvidovich, Washington, DC, September 10, 2002. All further quotes from Medvidovich, unless otherwise attributed, are from this interview.
21. John Lancaster and Justin Blum, "District Postal Worker Seriously Ill," *Washington Post*, October 22, 2001, A1.
22. Chen et al., "Trial and Error."
23. Potter was in Denver addressing a major mail industry meeting, but he flew home immediately after his talk.
24. Spencer S. Hsu and Ellen Nakashima, "USPS to Warn Public on Biohazards in Mail," *Washington Post*, October 16, 2001, A7.

DISTURBING DEVELOPMENTS

For all that USPS wanted to believe CDC and tried in turn to reassure the public, Thursday, October 18, and Friday, October 19, brought a series of disturbing developments. The USPS leadership did not know what to think. At 7:30 a.m. Thursday, Willhite had an alarming conversation. She and other USPS officials were meeting with Senate Sergeant-at-Arms Al Lenhardt to discuss how to handle Senate mail. Casually, someone mentioned that investigators had found four "hot spots" in the mailroom of the Dirksen Senate Office Building—well away from the Hart Building. This was urgent information for Willhite, who knew the Daschle letter had passed through Dirksen on its way to Hart. She reasoned that if spores had leaked at Dirksen, they might also have leaked at Brentwood. After the Senate meeting, Willhite commented to her colleagues: "Did you think that had some implications?"[25]

After the Thursday morning meeting at the Senate, Willhite determined to involve CDC and the DOH—despite their assurances of no risk. She called Potter, who called HHS Secretary Thompson, and by Thursday evening CDC Director Dr. Jeffrey P. Koplan had promised Potter a team would come to test Brentwood on Friday.

Hamilton Township

But even as the Postal Service grew worried about Brentwood, bad news arrived from New Jersey. On Thursday, October 18, Acting Governor Donald T. DiFrancesco announced that Teresa Heller, a West Trenton letter carrier, had developed skin anthrax.[26] Heller's was the first diagnosed case of a postal worker contracting anthrax. Homeland Security Director Ridge identified West Trenton as the location of the postbox into which the Brokaw and Daschle letters had been dropped.[27]

The New Jersey illness did not bode well for USPS. Mail from West Trenton went to the Hamilton Township Processing Center, which handled mail for 46 branches in the Trenton area. Postal authorities had assured workers at Hamilton Township as recently as Monday, October 15, that the facility was not contaminated, but tests on Wednesday found 13 of 23 samples tested positive for anthrax.[28] On Thursday, the day Heller was diagnosed, USPS closed the Hamilton Township Processing Center for further tests.

---

25. Chen et al., "Trial and Error."
26. Ibid.
27. Fred Kaplan, "FBI Eyes NJ Neighborhood," *Boston Globe*, October 20, 2001, A10. It is possible this was not the culprit mailbox, because in mid-August 2002 investigators found another mailbox in Princeton that tested positive for anthrax. See: Karen DeMasters, "Briefing: Security; Anthrax in Princeton Mailbox," *New York Times*, August 18, 2002, Section 14NJ, 5.
28. Michael Powell and Dale Russakoff, "Anthrax Fear Billows at Postal Plants," *Washington Post*, October 23, 2001, A8.

On Friday, it closed the West Trenton post office. Also Friday, Hamilton maintenance worker Patrick O'Donnell was diagnosed with skin anthrax.

As the situation worsened, New Jersey State Acting Commissioner for Health Dr. George T. DiFerdinando on Friday decided to ignore CDC recommendations and advised Cipro for all workers at Hamilton Township.[29] The state health authority was not prepared, however, to provide the medication and suggested that Hamilton workers see their private physicians for Cipro prescriptions. Hamilton Mayor Glen Gilmore was outraged by this lackluster response. With the help of a local hospital, he personally obtained a supply of the antibiotic, which the hospital distributed free to postal workers.[30] The hospital's costs were absorbed by the Postal Service.

Brentwood Tested

Meanwhile, Brentwood was tested as planned. On Thursday night, URS Corp., an industrial hygiene-testing firm with whom the Postal Service had a preexisting contract, took samples. As testing contractors in white protective suits roamed the plant, one worker asked: "Why are you testing the machines instead of us?"[31] Plant Manager Haney assured them that if anything were found, antibiotics would be provided. But results would take three days. So USPS also asked the Fairfax County Fire Department to do a quick, on-the-spot test.[32] That proved negative—but the test's reliability was a poor 50%. On Friday, October 19, CDC also came in to Brentwood to test. As with URS Corp., results would take a few days.

WAITING FOR THE UNKNOWN

As USPS waited for the Brentwood results, it still seemed that the anthrax attack, while serious, could be handled along traditional crisis management lines. The fact that two New Jersey postal workers had skin anthrax was disquieting, but the patients were responding to treatment. Matters were nonetheless sufficiently grave that the new USPS Mail Security Task Force, whose formation Potter had called for on Monday, held its first meeting on Friday, October 19, to discuss biohazards and mail. Task force members were drawn from senior management and unions alike. The group's chief concern during that meeting was to calm the public. That weekend, Communications Vice President Jaffer

---

29. Justin Blum, "Workers Question Response; CDC Says Policy Evolving," *Washington Post*, October 23, 2001, A1.
30. Michael Winerip, "Hail the Mayor (Whose Name Isn't Giuliani)," *New York Times*, November 14, 2001, D1.
31. Chen et al., "Trial and Error."
32. Twomey and Blum, "How the Experts Missed Anthrax."

made sure Postmaster General Potter and Chief Postal Inspector Weaver were on a number of news programs and talk shows assuring citizens that there was no conclusive evidence anthrax posed any general threat.

USPS did not yet know that Thursday night Dr. Cecele Murphy of Inova Fairfax Hospital in Virginia had telephoned the DOH with a report of a suspected anthrax case: Brentwood worker Leroy Richmond, 56.[33] It did not know Mrs. Richmond had tried to reach the mail plant Friday night to say her husband was being tested for inhalation anthrax.[34] But on Saturday, October 20, as he was working out in a gym, Jaffer got a phone call that realized his worst fears: DC health officials were going to announce that a Brentwood employee had anthrax. Willhite was also notified that the mayor wanted to hold a press conference.

It was logical, says Jaffer, that the city should know of a postal worker's illness before USPS did. "We're not medical experts and we're not health experts, so we depended and continue to depend on CDC, HHS as well as local DC help. So a diagnosis of inhalation anthrax would not have come from me or anyone in the Postal Service."

Saturday

Now Jaffer mobilized for a major public relations effort. No one yet understood how Richmond had become ill, or whether others were likewise stricken. Jaffer would have to do his best to ascertain the extent of infection. He summoned his deputy, Irene Lericos, as well as Internal Communications Manager Jon Leonard. They spent Saturday night in the office working.

At the same time, VPs Willhite and Medvidovich headed over to meet with DC Mayor Anthony A. Williams and DC Chief Health Officer Walks. "I was pretty furious," says Willhite, that city officials would hold a press conference with such alarming news at a time when postal employees were not being offered either anthrax testing or prophylactic antibiotics. Willhite even called DC Congresswoman Eleanor Holmes Norton at home to enlist her support. But Mayor Williams informed the USPS officials that he planned to test Brentwood employees at a central DC location and give them antibiotics. Walks, says Willhite, stressed that "we needed to give real time information about what was happening."

The press conference was scheduled for Sunday to allow the public health commissioners from Maryland, Virginia, and Washington, DC, to participate. By Sunday, it was also likely that Richmond's condition would be confirmed. Willhite assured the city officials that USPS would pay for antibiotics for its employees. "The United States Postal

---

33. Richmond turned 57 in the hospital on October 22. See: Kirk Johnson, "By Demanding a Diagnosis, He Lives to Tell of Anthrax," *New York Times*, December 3, 2001, A1.
34. Willhite interview.

Service will pay for it," Willhite recalls saying. "We are not doctors. We cannot write the prescriptions. But we are self-insured and we will pay for it."

Meanwhile, on Saturday evening, Medvidovich, Safety Manager Pulcrano, Manager for Environmental Management Policy Dennis Baca, Chief Operating Officer (COO) Patrick Donahoe, Willhite, and communications officials went to Brentwood to draw up a plan to close the facility if anthrax were confirmed. "We had to go in there, had to assess the situation," recalls Medvidovich. The group, meeting upstairs, drew on a board exactly where the mail would go if Brentwood were out of commission. Pulcrano also contacted the Environmental Protection Agency (EPA) to ask for on-scene coordinators at Brentwood and—because the Daschle letter had been postmarked there—at Hamilton Township. "We needed the expertise," says Pulcrano. "[*B. anthracis*] is not something we would deal with, obviously, on a normal basis. But it turned out it wasn't something that most others had ever dealt with [either]."

BAD NEWS AND WORSE

On Sunday morning, October 21, at 7 a.m., CDC Washington official Rima Khabbaz called Dr. Walks at home on his cell phone and confirmed that Richmond had inhalation anthrax. CDC had not expected this result; its scientists, said Walks's deputy Larry Siegel, were "astounded, really."[35] As investigators would soon learn, Richmond daily brought Express Mail from a facility near Baltimore–Washington International Airport to Brentwood. The Daschle letter had not been sent via Express Mail, but on October 11, Richmond had volunteered to clean a Brentwood mail-sorting machine.[36]

USPS also got the news. Now there was no question: Brentwood would have to close. At 10:30 a.m. Sunday, Safety Manager Pulcrano called Environmental Manager Baca to tell him Brentwood was closing. Baca immediately called John Bridges, the Brentwood environmental coordinator (and the only trained incident commander in the USPS system) who had retired from the military. Bridges and an on-scene EPA coordinator, Marcos Aquino, conducted a 6-hour assessment of Brentwood. By evening, Bridges and Baca had agreed that Bridges would manage day-to-day clean-up operations, while Baca promised to ensure that Bridges got what he needed without undue interference.

On Sunday afternoon, DC Mayor Williams held his planned press conference. "We're going to do everything we can and everything we have to do ... to see that people are getting the treatment they need when they need that treatment," he said.[37] He instructed Brentwood's 1,800 employees to report to a downtown office building on Sunday or, in following days, to DC General Hospital (which had been closed) for nasal swabs and a

35. Twomey and Blum, "How the Experts Missed Anthrax."
36. Johnson, "By Demanding a Diagnosis."
37. John Lancaster and Justin Blum, "District Postal Worker Seriously Ill," *Washington Post*, October 22, 2001, A1.

10-day supply of Cipro. At the press conference, Willhite was by his side because, she says, "I knew there had to be a postal presence from Day One or there wouldn't be a postal presence on Day Two."

But Sunday evening things grew much worse. At 8:45 p.m., another Brentwood worker—Thomas L. Morris, Jr.—died of inhalation anthrax at a Maryland hospital. Morris had tried repeatedly to get medical attention during the days preceding his death, but no one diagnosed anthrax. USPS had not even known that Morris was sick. On Monday afternoon, a second Brentwood employee, Joseph P. Curseen, died in a Maryland hospital after arriving by ambulance that morning. The same hospital had sent him home the night before. The anthrax attacks had just become a USPS crisis of unprecedented magnitude.

STAYING IN BUSINESS

The deaths of the postal workers changed the scientific equation. Until then, all anthrax patients had presumably come into physical contact with an anthrax-tainted letter. While some seemed to have contracted skin anthrax from unopened letters, only opened envelopes had caused inhalation anthrax. But the Brentwood employees had been nowhere near one of the letters, certainly not an opened one. The machines they worked near were automated; mail moved through them at up to 30 miles per hour. How could they have become infected? Until those deaths, anthrax had been considered a killer that could at least be seen (in quantity), touched, and hopefully avoided. As understanding of the threat matured, scientists and the public alike learned that anthrax in fact could be an invisible stalker, spores hanging suspended in air to be unwittingly inhaled. But it was days before that understanding clarified. Meanwhile, USPS was faced with contaminated buildings, dying employees or healthy ones who felt betrayed, and a scared public.

The first question to answer was: Should USPS continue normal operations? As VP Medvidovich puts it: "Are our customers safe? Are our employees safe? What could possibly have happened here?" At CDC headquarters in Atlanta, doctors gathered Monday, October 22, in a conference call with the FBI, USPS, the Postal Inspection Service, the Office of Homeland Security, and local law enforcement officials.[38] Each organization was on the line for a reason. Under Presidential Decision Directive 39, the FBI was the lead agency on any criminal investigation of terrorism.[39] USPS was the affected agency and the Postal Inspection Service was its law enforcement arm. The Office of Homeland Security, created in the wake of the September 11 terrorist

---

38. Eric Lipton and Kirk Johnson, "Tracking Bioterror's Tangled Course," *New York Times*, December 26, 2001, A1.
39. The FBI took precedence over the Postal Inspection Service because, says USPS Deputy Chief Inspector Rowan, the Department of Justice had declared the anthrax attack an act of domestic violence with a weapon of mass destruction—an area where the FBI had jurisdiction. The Postal Inspection Service served, however, as a member of the investigative task force.

attacks, coordinated the federal response to terrorism. Local law enforcement officials were responsible for public safety in their communities. CDC Deputy Director for Infectious Diseases Dr. Julie L. Gerberding led the discussion. Was the postal system itself contaminated? Should it be shut down?

The final decision on USPS operations rested with the Postmaster General, but the verdict from the CDC conference call was to keep the mail moving because there was no evidence of widespread contamination. "This was not just the Postal Service," says Medvidovich. "This was the country and the economy." As Willhite confirms, "only the Postmaster General can stop the mail [and] there was no justification to shut down the Postal Service....[40] It is such a huge system and it has such an incredible impact that to shut it down, you just wouldn't do it." On Tuesday, a White House spokesman confirmed that there were no plans to close USPS.[41]

WHOSE CRISIS IS THIS?

With that issue settled, another critical question loomed: Who should manage the anthrax clean-up? Who would identify potentially contaminated sites, sample them for anthrax, process the samples and then decontaminate where needed? The Federal Emergency Management Agency (FEMA)? EPA? USPS? One potential approach was to initiate the Federal Response Plan (FRP), an interagency strategy for dealing with natural disasters. Under the FRP, FEMA was designated the interagency coordinator, with wide-ranging authority to save lives, protect property, and restore damaged areas. FEMA could provide personnel, equipment, supplies, facilities, and a variety of services, plus the funding for these. But the FRP, authorized by the Robert T. Stafford Disaster Relief and Emergency Assistance Act, could be activated only (1) if the President declared a major disaster or emergency or (2) under Presidential Decision Directive 39, in response to terrorism.

Environmental Manager Baca remembers that USPS senior managers held a meeting on Wednesday, October 24, with Senior Vice President for Operations John Rapp, COO Donahoe, and Vice President for Engineering Thomas Day (Baca's boss).[42] At the meeting, Baca says he suggested that the government initiate the FRP. The request was conveyed by an unidentified postal liaison to a high-level team meeting under the aegis of Homeland Security to consider the broader national security implications of the anthrax deaths. "Within hours," says Baca, the postal liaison to the Homeland Security team delivered the decision: the FRP would not be invoked "because this was not a

---

40. If a national emergency is declared, the President can of course shut down anything, including the Postal Service.

41. Ellen Nakashima and Eric Pianin, "USPS Cleans Truck Fleet, Isolates Mail at Brentwood," *Washington Post*, October 24, 2001, A1.

42. Day was about to leave for San Diego to look at irradiation technology; irradiation killed anthrax spores.

natural disaster."[43] In the end, says Medvidovich, it hardly mattered: "We did exactly what FEMA would have done."

Another candidate to lead the clean-up effort was EPA, which was already in charge of the AMI building in Florida and had taken responsibility for decontaminating the Hart Senate Office Building. There were voices in USPS—notably Deputy Postmaster General John Nolan—who felt EPA should take over the USPS clean-up, especially at Brentwood. EPA anyway was required by law to approve any clean-up plan other agencies proposed. But the majority of the USPS leadership felt that EPA would take too long. Environmental Manager Baca speaks specifically to the question of the Brentwood decontamination:

> It was my recommendation to senior management that we not turn it over, because [USPS] were interested in getting this facility back for our purpose, which is to move the mail. People in EPA wanted it as a living laboratory. They'd never get this opportunity again. They would have kept us out of there for 3 to 5 years performing studies.

On balance, Willhite recalls, most felt that "it was a Postal Service crisis and that we'd better keep control of it."

> We are an independent establishment of the Executive Branch. The only way you maintain your independence is to take care of the situation, get them [EPA] to sign off, and leave.... We're not a science project. Unlike most branches of the federal government, we do something visible every day. We deliver 500 million pieces of mail. If we don't, there are very unhappy citizens.

By Wednesday evening, USPS was confident it would be the lead agency managing the consequences of the anthrax attacks. But that was not much comfort. As the USPS leadership saw it, at least four daunting tasks needed urgent attention:

- Inform and assist employees.
- Inform the public.
- Identify and decontaminate infected sites.
- Deliver the mail.

Pursuing all four simultaneously would require some sensitive decision-making. Throughout the crisis, muses VP Willhite, "there was constantly a balance between health and safety considerations, and movement of the mail. This whole crisis has brought that to everyone's consciousness: the incredible economic and social impact of the mail not moving." Of the four tasks, orchestrating mail delivery was the most straightforward. That responsibility fell to the National Operations Center (NOC). Located on the seventh floor of USPS headquarters, NOC had been set up after September 11 to

---

43. Author's interview with Dennis Baca, Washington, DC, September 10, 2002. All further quotations from Baca, unless otherwise attributed, are from this interview.

make sure the mail kept moving when aircraft were grounded. Now it continued its logistical task, redeploying mail and personnel to ensure timely processing and delivery despite the closing of various facilities for anthrax treatment.

The other jobs were assigned to different groups, with considerable overlap. The Mail Security Task Force formed the nucleus of the crisis management effort. While it coordinated all efforts, it took particular responsibility—with full-time support from the in-house Communications Department—for informing and assisting employees. At the same time Communications, which together with NOC maintained a public hotline, also took on the job of informing the public. Finally, responsibility for identifying, sampling, and decontaminating sites went to a new subgroup created for the purpose—the Unified Incident Command Center (UICC).[44]

MAIL SECURITY TASK FORCE

At the top of the anthrax response pyramid stood the Mail Security Task Force. The Postmaster General and his senior deputies had decided that, to be most effective in this emergency situation, its membership should be comprehensive—including not only top postal management but also union representatives and members of management associations. A liaison from CDC also sat on the Task Force. Potter designated Chief Postal Inspector Weaver to lead the task force. Other senior management members were Deputy Postmaster General Nolan, COO Donahoe, Senior VP Willhite, Senior VP Medvidovich, Manager of Safety Pulcrano, and Environmental Manager Baca.

The Task Force settled surprisingly quickly into a grueling but effective routine. Its members met daily at 10 a.m.—at first for four hours a day. They heard reports from all parties working on the anthrax aftermath. "Everything was discussed every day," recalls Medvidovich. Over the weeks, to stay on top of all its responsibilities, the Task Force created seven subcommittees: mail screening, mail preparation, workplace safety, contingency planning, surface transportation, mail center security operations, and communications.

The group saw its principal job as ensuring a constant and reliable flow of information. Confirms Pulcrano: "We [had to] communicate, communicate, communicate to our employees, as well as to the public, as to what we were finding and what we were doing about it." If sampling showed a site was contaminated, word had to go to field managers and employees and arrangements made to reassign workers during the clean-up. If a site tested clean, that too was reported. Sometimes as many as three official announcements

---

44. In addition, the Postal Inspection Service—the USPS criminal investigation arm—had started after September 11 an Inspection Service Command Center, also staffed 24 hours a day, seven days a week, which continued to operate through December 2001. The Inspection Service was in daily contact with the FBI, and the two agencies exchanged personnel.

a day would go out to the unions and the public. As Medvidovich learned, "[y]ou cannot communicate too much. Because you can't underestimate the fear."

Interagency Coordination

The Task Force also coordinated communications and logistics with other federal agencies involved in various aspects of managing the anthrax attacks. Willhite twice a day participated in conference calls with Homeland Security (liaison Lisa Gordon-Haggerty, succeeded by Joseph Rogan), CDC (liaison Dr. Gerberding), and EPA (the liaison kept changing). Potter was in close contact with HHS Secretary Thompson. For his part, Jaffer briefed White House spokesman Ari Fleischer or his deputy, Scott McClellan, daily. Jaffer also took part in daily Homeland Security teleconferences during which "we would all talk about what was going to be said, how we were going to say it, who was going to cover what, and then we basically deployed."[45] Homeland Security, recalls Medvidovich, "really did help. I can't tell you how many times they cleared pathways, they called people, they got us help."

Such cooperation did not necessarily come easily and required different institutional cultures to mesh. "We had to join together," muses Medvidovich.

> We had to figure out how our organizations worked together, very quickly. The CDC has a culture that says you investigate, you examine, you make a determination based on the health risk and on evaluating things over a longer period of time. Our culture is do something and do it now.

INFORM AND ASSIST EMPLOYEES

The Task Force also closely monitored employee welfare. Unusually, the Task Force provided a forum where union members learned critical information at the same time as management. The Postal Service leadership considered this a remarkable shift from the often hostile union-management dealings at USPS. Recalls Jaffer:

> It wasn't management telling the labor organizations this is what the deal is. They were sitting at the table with us and if they had questions, they went ahead and fired away.

From the start, as USPS officials remember it, Postmaster General Potter emphasized the health and safety of the employees. As Jaffer recalls:

> The Postmaster General made it very clear at the first meeting that we would do what the medical experts asked us to do. If it meant shutting a plant down, we would shut it down. If it meant isolating an area, we would isolate it. If it meant providing medication, we would do so.

---

45. Jaffer's contacts at Homeland Security were Communications Director Susan K. Neely and her staff.

In one of his first measures to improve worker safety, Potter on Monday night, October 22, announced that the standard procedure for cleaning postal machines, known as "blowdown," was being revised on the spot. While there was as yet no proof, there was suspicion that anthrax might have been blown into the air by the powerful jets of pressurized air that cleaned the machinery. Ten days later, on November 2, USPS announced that nationwide it would now clean machinery with vacuums instead of forced air. Postal managers also eliminated the practice of riffling (by running a thumb across the tops) envelopes to separate them. VP Willhite said she would like to make it mandatory that postal employees wear gloves and masks; at a minimum, she strongly recommended their use. In another move directed at public as well as employee confidence, USPS on October 23 announced it would buy ion beam sterilization devices to irradiate the mail.[46]

VP Medvidovich was keenly aware that the Postal Service's four unions and three management associations "could have had a nationwide walkout" if USPS was seen to be taking anything other than the proper safety and health actions on behalf of its employees.[47] In general, she insists, USPS worried about "people first"—the workers and the customers:

> You worry about the employees. You keep them safe. If the Department of Health says close the building, you close the building. Ask for the experts, get them involved, but protect the employees. If you think there's any danger to customers, don't give them the mail.

In the first few weeks, the Task Force paid special attention to identifying and treating any postal employee infected with anthrax. It sent out instructions daily that all employees potentially exposed to anthrax should be tested. Jaffer reinforced that message through his mandatory employee stand-up talks, during which "you gather over 3,000 employees on a workroom floor in a plant and you deliver a specific set of messages." In addition, says Medvidovich, "we literally kept a log of all people who received treatment and we called people who did not receive medication. A few people got called two, three times, and they were mad at us. But we wanted to make sure that everybody got the opportunity to get the medicine."

Logs were maintained for every contaminated facility, and even postal inspectors were pulled into the tracking program. Deputy Chief Inspector Rowan remembers sending inspectors out one weekend "contacting people who had either not reported to work, or we didn't know if they'd gotten Cipro." As for those who were sick, staff from the Employee Assistance Program (EAP) visited them and their families.

---

46. Barnaby J. Feder and Andrew C. Revkin, "Post Office to Install Devices to Destroy Deadly Organisms at Mail-Processing Centers," *Washington Post*, October 25, 2001, B5. The decision as to just which mail would be irradiated was left until later. USPS could not afford to treat all mail.

47. Under the terms of the union contracts with USPS, strikes and walkouts were not permitted—but that might not have prevented such an event.

EAP staff also visited postal sites, talked with employees, met with them in groups and one-on-one, offered counseling, and worked with families. In early November, USPS offered free flu shots to its 800,000 employees so that flu symptoms would not be mistaken for anthrax.[48]

The Task Force focus on employee well-being had at least two powerful motives. One was to allay health concerns, and the second to reestablish trust. The fact was that a chasm of distrust and anger had opened up between USPS and many of its employees in the wake of the Brentwood deaths.

SECOND-CLASS CITIZENS

Many Postal Service workers did not feel they were getting adequate protection. Interviews with the (mostly black) postal workers at Brentwood and elsewhere revealed suspicion that they had received second-class treatment compared to the (mostly white) staff at the Capitol. "They've been playing this down for us, telling us work was safe," said a Brentwood worker after the plant closed. "And we were asking, 'How do we know that?' The Senate's mail comes through here."[49]

William Smith, president of the New York Metro Area Postal Union, insisted that postal workers were subject to a double standard. "When Congress got letters with anthrax, they got checked and got out of town," said Smith. "Our people were left to be the guinea pigs and they feel let down by Congress, the President, and the American people."[50] USPS workers in Florida, too, were complaining that emphasis was on getting the mail out, rather than on protecting workers. "The supervisors and managers aren't doing enough to protect us," said one Florida union official. "They're just worried about the volume of mail."[51] A Brentwood worker agreed. He bitterly rephrased the Postal Service motto about delivering the mail regardless of weather conditions: "Mud, flood, or blood, the mail's got to go," he said. "Anthrax doesn't fit into the rhyme."[52]

Given the significant scientific uncertainty as events unfolded, it was not easy to explain the chain of events, but members of the Task Force tried. On October 22, VP Willhite clarified at a press conference that USPS had followed CDC advice that testing at Brentwood was unnecessary "until there was an evidence chain that indicated there

---

48. Michael Janofsky, "Mail Delays Are Minimal, Despite Anthrax Problems," *New York Times*, November 2, 2001, B8.

49. Sheryl Gay Stolberg, "A Nation Challenged: The Government Response: A Quick Response for Politicians; A Slower One for Mail Workers," *New York Times*, October 23, 2001.

50. Dale Rusakoff and Michael Powell, "N.J. Postal Worker May Have Anthrax," *Washington Post*, October 24, 2001, A15.

51. Powell and Russakoff, "Anthrax Fear Billows at Postal Plants."

52. Francis X. Clines, "A Nation Challenged: Washington Post Office; Being Left in Gloom of Night Over Threat," *New York Times*, October 23, 2001.

was anthrax present in the facility."[53] No one had known until Sunday, she emphasized, that a Brentwood worker had inhalation anthrax. CDC's Dr. Mitchell Cohen, who was supervising the DC anthrax operation, added that "this is really a new phenomenon. At first, we had no evidence that any of the mail handlers were at risk.... How it's actually occurring isn't clear."

If this message was not exactly reassuring to postal workers, it was also not much to offer the public by way of comfort. Yet comforting the public, by clearly and fully informing the media and citizens, was the second task USPS had set itself. Communications VP Jaffer and his team had their work cut out for them.

INFORM THE PUBLIC

Reassuring mail users was a pressing matter. Not only did public hysteria need dampening, but every passing day was costing the Postal Service millions of dollars. It could afford no more loss of business. USPS could restore much confidence by providing the public with concise and reliable information. It could also put the crisis in context: of millions of pieces of mail delivered since September 18, only a handful of letters contained anthrax. Getting that and other USPS messages across was Jaffer's challenge.

Media Relations

To handle the deluge of requests from the media and others, Jaffer created a Communications Command Center with 30 phones and 15 computers open 24 hours a day, seven days a week. Jaffer held daily teleconferences with the DC press corps— anywhere from 30 to 75 reporters. He made available USPS spokespeople to go on camera immediately after the conference calls. But Jaffer decided that he personally would not appear as a spokesman for USPS because, as he told Postmaster General Potter, "in light of the fact that I've got a name [Azeezaly] that comes from the Middle East, I don't think that I should be out there." Instead he recruited others to do the job: Potter, Chief Inspector Weaver, COO Donahoe, and VP Willhite.

Potter, comments Jaffer, "was truly the calming face to the nation." At the same time, the postmaster general had to be careful to preserve his credibility. Thus, during the week of October 22, when postal officials were asked repeatedly if they could guarantee the safety of the mail, Potter on Jaffer's advice told a television interviewer that "I can't

---

53. Sheryl Gay Stolberg, "A Quick Response for Politicians; A Slower One for Mail Workers," *New York Times*, October 23, 2001, A1.

offer a guarantee."[54] COO Donahoe likewise commented that "[s]ince we don't have 100 percent control of the mail that comes into this system, we can't say it's 100 percent safe." At the same time, he demurred, "the mail is safe, has always been safe, and we're going to make it safer." Jaffer urged USPS officials to paint a full picture, pointing out, for example, that during the 10 days following the Daschle letter, the Postal Service had delivered millions of pieces of mail—without incident. "One of the mottos we lived by," says Jaffer, "was keep it simple. Break it down to the most common denominator."

Publications

Jaffer's office also put out USPS publications. Immediately after the Brentwood deaths, he hurried into production the postcards USPS had promised on October 15 with guidelines on how to handle suspicious letters. By Monday, October 22, the cards were being printed and by Thursday and Friday they were delivered across the country to the 800,000 USPS employees as well as to 120 million homes. Jaffer also made sure that any and all anthrax information went onto the USPS Web site. Typically, the Web site got some 1 million hits a day. During the days and weeks of the anthrax crisis, it averaged 12 to 15 million a day.

In addition, Jaffer contributed staff to the anthrax information hotline housed at NOC. Hotline callers could speak to representatives from the Postal Inspection Service, Communications, EAP, Safety, or to a medical professional. The Postal Inspection Service also produced and distributed thousands of mail-security videos and posters to business mailrooms nationwide.

Facing this mountain of tasks, Jaffer on Tuesday, October 23, called an old friend for assistance: Harold Burson of the renowned New York–based public relations firm Burson, Marsteller. Jaffer was afraid his small staff of eight, working 12-hour shifts, could not long manage the 700 to 900 phone calls plus 600 e-mails a day pouring into the Communications Center. During those first weeks, says Jaffer, Burson staff helped out with some of the logistical burden. Burson himself, says Jaffer, was invaluable as a barometer of how the media covered the anthrax events: "He was an independent third party who had no vested interest." The two men spoke regularly for the first month of the crisis.

SAMPLE AND DECONTAMINATE

Meanwhile, the most logistically challenging of the four chief tasks USPS faced was to identify, sample, and decontaminate infected postal sites. The Postal Service had no existing structure prepared to handle this task. Its Environmental Management Policy

---

54. Ben White, "Postmaster General Lauded Despite Mixed Performance," *Washington Post*, October 25, 2001, A29.

department was accustomed to dealing with such problems as asbestos, air quality, or solid waste—not bioterrorism. USPS knew it would have to form a new unit. Safety Manager Pulcrano and Environmental Manager Baca set out to recruit staff for the new unit before they even knew what form it would take.

First to arrive was James Gaffney, who flew in Monday, the day of the Brentwood deaths, from New Jersey, where he worked as an Environmental Compliance Specialist. On Tuesday, Manager for Environmental Compliance for the Northeast Charles Vidich was pulled in from his office in Connecticut. His job typically involved such issues as solid waste, asbestos, or hazardous waste. The third member of what became a leadership triumvirate arrived a week later when, realizing they needed an administrator as well as technical expertise, Baca and Pulcrano asked Environmental Programs Analyst Paul Fennewald (who worked under Baca) to come in and run the new unit. The scene on arrival, they remember, was chaotic.

The newly recruited officials immediately sought advice on what kind of structure would get the job done. EPA was the first to recommend that USPS put together a UICC. The advantage of this model was that it allowed all those with jurisdictional or functional responsibility for an incident to participate day-to-day in jointly managing the situation. Baca briefly looked into whether EPA could run such a center for USPS under an interagency agreement, but such an arrangement proved impossible in the absence of a national emergency. USPS would have to create its own unified command center. Several agencies helped USPS set up the center, including EPA; the USDA's Forest Service, which sent an advisor for two weeks; and Homeland Security (which had its own incident command structure).

Within weeks, there were 15 to 20 people (plus contractor representatives) working at UICC. They came from a variety of agencies and included liaisons from EPA, CDC, the Occupational Safety and Health Administration (OSHA) and, occasionally, the Postal Inspection Service.[55] "Now," says Pulcrano. "you had a pool of people with expertise who also had a lot of contacts." Vidich, Gaffney, and Fennewald reported to both Pulcrano and Baca, who reported in turn to Senior VP for Human Resources Medvidovich. UICC did not report directly to Postmaster General Potter. As for the Task Force, technically UICC reported to it through Pulcrano and Baca. But in practice, most Task Force members wanted constantly to know what UICC was doing—creating a communications challenge UICC would have to resolve.

First it had other problems to address. To do its job, UICC needed outside contractors. But it had no authority to negotiate new contracts. Although USPS had existing contracts with four national environmental companies, UICC would need many more. By exploring the wider resources of the Postal Service, UICC by the end of the first week found a solution. The USPS Office of Inspector General, it emerged, had a standing contract with

---

55. Some stayed longer than others. High turnover in liaisons, especially from OSHA, was a frustration at UICC.

the US Army Corps of Engineers Rapid Response Group. The Corps in turn had authority to contract out both the sampling and decontamination work USPS needed done. Corps officer Timothy Gouger became the fourth (unofficial but critical) member of UICC's leadership team. At first, Pulcrano's safety staff took responsibility for environmental sampling, while Baca's environmental group handled the decontamination. With time, however, Gaffney emerged as the individual in charge of sampling, while Gouger oversaw the decontamination contractors.[56]

Trading Partners

But before it could send teams to sample and decontaminate, UICC had to decide where to do so. VP Medvidovich, Pulcrano, COO Donahoe, and others realized the first week that USPS needed to devise a system for anthrax testing that would clarify the extent of contamination. There were two theories as to how contamination could occur: from a direct hit (a contaminated letter arrives) or from cross-contamination. So far, USPS had tested only at sites where there were proven infections, or where contaminated letters had been known to transit. By mid-week, the idea of "trading partners" came up—postal facilities with which the contaminated sites traded mail. Remembers Medvidovich: "We decided we would test the big plants, and if a big plant was positive, we would go downstream until we all of a sudden started getting negatives."

There were at first only 30 facilities on the list, but as the number of contaminated sites grew, so too did the list of trading partners. "We made a decision," recalls Pulcrano, "that we needed to test throughout the mail stream because no one had any idea what was the potential extent of contamination." Trenton, for example, traded with 151 postal facilities. They would all be tested. Brentwood did not strictly speaking have trading relationships, but it sent mail onward to some 50 retail facilities. Many of the Trenton/Brentwood trading partners in turn had their own downstream relationships. On Thursday, October 25, USPS announced that it would expand anthrax testing to more than 200 facilities across the country.

As UICC geared up to do that, events threatened to overtake any plans it could lay. The week of October 22 would be a difficult one by any measure.

WEEK OF OCTOBER 22

The week started with an encouraging move: Congress signaled its resolve that government would operate as usual by reopening the House on Monday—despite the discovery Saturday of traces of anthrax on mail-bundling machines in the Ford House Office

---

56. These officials were in charge in theory. In fact, UICC did not manage the sampling or clean-up of Brentwood, Hamilton Township, or Morgan Station.

Building, a few blocks from the Capitol. But six congressional office buildings remained closed pending test results (the Russell Senate Office Building reopened Tuesday). Meanwhile, more contamination was uncovered through the week. On Tuesday, anthrax was discovered on machinery at a military base that sorted mail for the White House (though the White House itself tested negative). President Bush felt obliged to tell the nation, "I don't have anthrax." On Friday, the Supreme Court building was ordered closed for anthrax testing (it closed the following Monday) and a small amount of anthrax was found at Central Intelligence Agency headquarters. On Tuesday, the FBI released copies of the Daschle, *New York Post*, and NBC letters in hopes the public might be able to help trace their origins.

Scientific and governmental confusion was palpable. "We're going to act quickly and, if need be, let the science catch up to our actions," HHS Secretary Thompson told Congress Tuesday. "Remember, we have never had cases of anthrax attacks in this manner before. It's a new challenge that we are all facing as a country."[57] Already accusations were flying. Angry words were exchanged in a meeting Tuesday morning at the office of Secretary Thompson because Dr. Anthony S. Fauci, director of the National Institute for Allergy and Infectious Diseases, felt the government had understated the threat in its statements the preceding week.[58] Questions arose also at a Wednesday night meeting Homeland Security Director Ridge chaired in the White House Roosevelt Room as to whether the FBI had properly shared with CDC and Fort Detrick the results of each other's testing, with charges made that the potency of the Daschle letter's anthrax had been concealed.

TERRORISM CONFIRMED

By Thursday, October 25, the tenor of the government's message to the public had changed. Now the alarms were ringing. Ridge confirmed that anthrax from the Daschle letter was highly concentrated, potent, and could hang suspended in the air (i.e., be aerosolized). It was much more finely milled than the NBC and *New York Post* anthrax. Scientists were investigating whether after all such weaponized anthrax could escape through a sealed envelope. Ridge said:

> It is clear that the terrorists responsible for these attacks intended to use this anthrax as a weapon. Clearly, we are up against a shadow enemy, shadow soldiers, people who have no regard for human life.[59]

---

57. Sheryl Gay Stolberg and Judith Miller, "Officials Admit Underestimating Danger Posed to Postal Workers," *New York Times*, October 24, 2001, A1.
58. Judith Miller and Sheryl Gay Stolberg, "Stung by Criticism, Aides Gather to Coordinate Efforts on Anthrax," *New York Times*, October 25, 2001, A1.
59. Sheryl Gay Stolberg and Judith Miller, "After a Week of Reassurances, Ridge's Anthrax Message Is Grim," *New York Times*, October 26, 2001, A1.

On the medical front, events moved swiftly. On Monday, October 22, an employee at a State Department mail sorting facility fell ill and on Thursday he was hospitalized; inhalation anthrax was quickly confirmed. The State Department on Wednesday, October 24, started to hold all mail, and instructed embassies to seal and return to Washington all mail sent in diplomatic pouches since October 11. On Tuesday, Hamilton postal worker Norma Wallace, 56, was hospitalized with a suspected case of inhalation anthrax. On Wednesday, six postal workers from DC were hospitalized on suspicion of anthrax. A *New York Post* mailroom worker was listed as a suspected cutaneous anthrax case. A second NBC News employee, desk assistant Casey Chamberlain, was confirmed to have skin anthrax. On Thursday, a State Department postal worker with no connection to Brentwood was confirmed with inhalation anthrax.[60]

By Thursday, there were 32 cases of anthrax exposure, of which 13 had developed infections—seven cutaneous and six inhaled. In New Jersey, Acting Health Commissioner DiFerdinando recommended all postal workers follow 60- instead of 10-day Cipro treatment regimens.[61] The number of Americans taking antibiotics at government urging for possible anthrax exposure was well over 10,000.[62]

POSTAL ANTHRAX

More anthrax was also found in post offices during the week of October 22. The case that would cause USPS management the greatest union-related trouble emerged on Thursday, October 25, when anthrax was discovered on four high-speed machines known as Delivery Bar Code Sorting machines on the third floor of the Morgan Station postal facility in Manhattan.[63] Morgan processed 2 million pieces of mail a day at a site that took up two city blocks, or nearly 2 million square feet. The presumption was that the letters for NBC and the *New York Post*, which would have been sorted at Morgan, had caused the contamination.

USPS had already late Wednesday night started Morgan employees, as well as workers at five other midtown Manhattan post offices, on 10-day regimes of Cipro.[64] Now USPS decided not to close the facility, but to cordon off and clean the 150,000-square-foot contaminated section—which was all in one area on the third floor. The union reaction at Morgan was swift.

---

60. David E. Rosenbaum and Todd S. Purdum, "Another Postal Worker Contracts Inhaled Anthrax," *New York Times*, October 26, 2001, B6.
61. Steven Greenhouse, "Sorting Machines at Mail Center Are Contaminated," *New York Times*, October 26, 2001, B7.
62. David E. Rosenbaum and Todd S. Purdum, "Another Postal Worker Contracts Inhaled Anthrax," *New York Times*, October 26, 2001, B6.
63. Morgan was located at the corner of 29th St. and 9th Ave.
64. The five post offices were the James A. Farley Building, Ansonia Station, Radio City Station, Rockefeller Center Station, and Times Square Station. By Thursday evening, more than 2,500 employees had picked up the antibiotic.

Morgan Station

The executive board of the New York Metro Area Postal Union voted Friday, October 26, to file a lawsuit to close Morgan completely while it was cleaned. Union President William Smith, who represented 5,500 workers, challenged USPS, saying that "no one piece of mail is worth a human life."[65]

But David L. Solomon, USPS vice president for operations in the New York area, assured workers that health officials had said there was "no danger for employees to continue working in the building." CDC and local health officials, says Pulcrano, "went on the workroom floor with operations management on the shifts to talk with employees and explain what was going to happen, what we were going to do, and answer their questions." No Morgan workers had reported anthrax-like symptoms. Morgan used vacuums on the third floor, not blowers, to clean equipment. Contamination was restricted to the third floor. USPS also gave Morgan workers the option of working across the street in a different postal building. Solomon and Mayor Rudolph Giuliani in a press conference jointly reiterated that "if in the future a determination is made that the building should be closed, we'll do whatever the health professionals tell us to do."

On Friday, November 9, Federal Judge John F. Keenan of US District Court in Manhattan dismissed the postal union suit, saying Morgan employees had not been shown to have suffered "irreparable harm" and that the peak risk period had been mid- to late-September. According to USPS management, the Postal Service had communicated effectively. "We had one union person in New York who tried to stir up the union folks," recalls Medvidovich, "[but] because we had communicated so well with them, they weren't interested."

> I think the key to the whole thing is [to] bring everybody in and they hear everything and they're part of this discussion process.... Our position ended up being, and this was a consensus with all except one union, we would go with the Department of Health's advice.

New Jersey

Anthrax was newly discovered on Saturday, October 27, on a mail bin at the main Princeton, New Jersey, post office in the town of West Windsor. The contamination was judged to have come from the Daschle letter, now identified as highly potent. There was no union antagonism because USPS did close the facility. West Windsor's closing brought the number of shuttered central New Jersey postal facilities to three, along with Hamilton and West Trenton. Samples taken at West Trenton had so far yielded no positive results. But at Hamilton, 19 of 59 samples were positive. Five New Jersey postal workers had

---

65. Robin Finn, "Union Chief's Battle Is With the Postal Service," *New York Times*, November 1, 2001, D2.

developed anthrax-like symptoms: four worked at Hamilton and one in West Trenton.[66] The local health department opened a clinic to dispense antibiotics to all those—as many as 2,500—who had visited Hamilton's public areas since September 18, the day the NBC and *New York Post* letters were postmarked.

Given these developments, there was intense public and internal pressure on UICC to get on the job—and quickly. Sampling teams had been going out to identified sites even that first week on a crisis basis. But before UICC could come up to full speed, it had to put its own house in order. UICC Director Fennewald realized that that would take some doing.

ORGANIZING THE TROOPS

Fennewald recognized that his first job was to create a sense of unity and purpose for the ad hoc interagency group that he was overseeing. He had no model to follow, as this was the first UICC to deal with anthrax. He would have to create an organizational chart from scratch. At least the group now had a dedicated space. By Tuesday, October 30, UICC was able to move into offices at North L'Enfant Plaza across from USPS headquarters. The fourth floor suite had one room for contractors, one for federal agencies, one for USPS staff, and a large conference room.

To create a common culture, Fennewald asked all UICC staff "to take off their [institutional] hat and say 'I am here for the organization.'" That was not always easy, even for those from within USPS. He recalls that Environmental Management Policy [Baca's department] "had a very hard time buying into Command Center support." Environmental Management, which was in charge of the decontamination program, in the early days often failed to send a staff member to UICC. In November, however, an environmental representative was present when anthrax was confirmed at a facility, thereby transforming it from a sampling site to a decontamination site. "Light bulbs went off," recalls Fennewald, "and he said, 'We need to be here all the time in case this stuff happens.' So then it started to change." But most UICC members, says Fennewald, entered quickly into "the atmosphere of cooperation that was there. It was just happening."

Fennewald also tackled process. He asked himself: "How do I organize this thing to accomplish what it is that we want to accomplish?"

> The very first thing that I did is ask: "What is the problem we're trying to solve here?" And I [realized] it's an information flow problem; it's a communications problem. It's not an anthrax problem.[67]

To facilitate the flow of information within UICC, Fennewald began every day with a planning meeting that identified UICC's top five issues of the day. He then posted a daily

---

66. Two had skin anthrax and a third was suspected, while two others might have had inhalation anthrax.
67. Author's interview with Paul Fennewald, Washington, DC, September 10, 2002. All further quotes from Fennewald, unless otherwise attributed, are from this interview.

operations plan, a schedule of the day's meetings and targets. "I literally every day was planning for crisis," he chuckles. He also instituted a situation board where staff could post problems as they arose. A log was kept of the problems, how they were resolved, and how quickly. "What I was trying to do," comments Fennewald, "was document as well as identify where processes were breaking down within the organization."

But he also had to pay attention to how information was flowing from UICC to the outside world, specifically to senior USPS management. Fennewald quickly discerned that senior management was hesitant to let the Command Center operate as it was designed to do. Some of that stemmed from turf issues; some from lack of information. He notes:

> I think there was a reluctance to let go. What we constantly came up against was management's fear of letting the Command Center make the decisions that needed to be made. And so in a time of crisis, the bureaucracy fell back on a very autocratic way of doing business: "I'm going to control this."… What I constantly tried to do was to let my management chain know that there were all kinds of capability here.

Interference sometimes hampered operations. For example the leadership, anxious to move things along, would call contractors directly instead of going through UICC, or ask for instantaneous test results. So Fennewald tried to educate them. He says:

> All that management knew was that as soon as we had taken a sample, they wanted results. No one was telling management it takes a while to do this. So I developed little process flow charts to show how long it's going to take to get a sample back.

To further help senior management understand what UICC was doing and how it was doing it, Fennewald sent them the daily operations plan. He also "put myself on their calendar every day. One o'clock, I would go see Sam Pulcrano. At 1:30, I'd go see Dennis Baca. As opposed to waiting for them to ask for me." Every day at 6 p.m., he also sent senior managers a summary report of testing and decontamination results. But the report caused its own problems. Too often, in the last 15 minutes before it was printed, managers would flood UICC with requests that changed the content and delayed the report. Fennewald tried instead to create a Web site where the status of sampling and decontamination sites could be checked continuously, but it took months to set up due to concerns over cyber-security. Eventually, Fennewald organized a daily teleconference with all senior managers to update them simultaneously.

TESTING AND CLEANING

Fennewald had logistical problems to resolve as well. If a suspicious powder was found in a letter or package in any postal facility, it was the Postal Service's responsibility to have it tested. Some powders were hoaxes; many were simply false alarms. It hardly mattered. As VP Medvidovich recalls, "For every hoax, you had to act as if it wasn't a hoax. You had to call the CDC, the health department, get the thing tested, set up the protocol on how to isolate the mail."[68] At the height of the crisis, postal inspectors were responding to 600 to 700 suspicious mail reports each day.

UICC realized quickly that its existing laboratory partner was overwhelmed by all the samples submitted for testing. Postal samples initially went to PathCon (effectively a branch of CDC), a laboratory with which USPS had a preexisting contract. But by the end of October, PathCon had been deluged with well over 1,000 samples and it was clear the laboratory could not keep up. UICC, with a potential need to test suspicious substances across all 50 states, did not know where to turn. As with the sampling and decontamination contractors, the Postal Service had no authority to contract with scientific laboratories. UICC officials did not see how they could create contractual relationships with individual laboratories across the country.

During UICC discussions, there was a suggestion that USPS ask CDC to contract with labs, but the CDC liaison dismissed that option. There was also a quality issue: using less experienced laboratories to process anthrax samples meant a possible compromise in the quality of analysis. There were no protocols telling labs how to process samples. Many of them had never dealt with *Bacillus anthracis*. Still desperate to find a solution, late on Friday, November 2, UICC organized a conference call with CDC.[69] CDC told the Postal Service officials about the existence of the Association of Public Health Laboratories (APHL)—a not-for-profit corporation. All 50 state laboratories belonged to the association. One contract and one set of protocols could govern all 50 labs. USPS jumped at the opportunity. By Sunday, USPS had a working agreement with APHL to process anthrax samples.

Sampling Plan

UICC simultaneously developed a strategic plan for sampling. There was no protocol for sampling, and creating one was complicated by the continual scientific changes. The technology evolved on a daily basis. As a result, every three to five days, UICC orders to contractors would change. For example, early testers took 32 samples per facility. By mid-November, that number had gone up to 55. Likewise, there were at first no air samples—there was no awareness anthrax spores could be dispersed in the air. UICC also had to decide where to sample. The center developed its own checklist but was open to suggestions. When the unions, for example, asked UICC to sample the small tubs

---

68. The Postal Service was not the only agency overwhelmed by anthrax scares. Across the country, police and fire departments were inundated with requests to examine every variety of suspicious white powder. Nonpostal samples went to local laboratories that, as a rule, had never seen anthrax and were just learning how to identify it. From October to December, according to one estimate, the nation's laboratories processed some 121,000 samples. See Case 12 for an account of how the state of Georgia coped with the rising tide of suspicious powders.
69. Vidich was at the airport, Fennewald in VP Medvidovich's office.

carrying the mail, it added those to the list. Many of the emerging protocols for air sampling and decontamination came from tests conducted at Brentwood.

Cleaning Protocols

Then there was the question, once anthrax was found, of how best to clean it up. As soon as it was realized that two types of anthrax were in play, coarse and fine, different clean-up methods were devised for each. Environmental Manager Baca had charge of cleaning the two largest sites believed contaminated by finely milled anthrax: Brentwood and Hamilton. There the challenge was how to reach and clean lofty bays where aerosolized anthrax had eventually settled. UICC contract teams tackled the remaining, less contaminated, sites—those that were either directly contaminated by the coarser anthrax or by cross-contamination from letters containing the finer grade of anthrax.

UICC, together with EPA, developed protocols for bleaching contaminated surface areas with sodium hypochlorite (a mix of chlorine, sodium hydroxide, and water). But even these procedures kept evolving. At first, bleach solution was left on for a recommended 5 minutes, then 10 minutes, and later 15 minutes. Eventually, based on World Health Organization information, the recommendation increased to 60 minutes of contact time. The 60-minute directive was labor intensive: someone had to keep respraying the area to keep it moist.

Typically, once contamination was found, USPS immediately cordoned off the affected area (if it could be isolated) or closed the building. Then the teleconferencing started. Pulcrano remembers the questions that were posed:

> Who's going to go on the floor? Who's going to be the representative? CDC, who are you going to have there? Who's the Department of Health going to have there? How many days do you have? Give us the names of the people. When are they going to be there? When can we start?

Often a decontamination team came in that same night. Then the area was retested but kept closed until the test results came back negative. Often two or three locations were treated at the same time. Remembers Pulcrano of that time: "There were a dozen linear streams all occurring simultaneously. We were testing and decontaminating multiple facilities, communicating those results."

Interim Guidelines

To codify what UICC teams were doing in case similar efforts should be needed in the future, Pulcrano and Vidich over a six-week period assembled a set of interim guidelines. "We knew that if there were more letters discovered in the Midwest or further out, we were going to have to establish additional area-level incident command operations," remembers Pulcrano. "We developed [the guidelines] with all of the agencies' input, as well as the unions. In fact, for weeks, every day we were meeting to pull this document together." Vidich held meetings nearly around the clock to get comments from other federal agencies and postal unions. As a result, the guidelines were formally adopted in early December. For USPS policy documents, that set a speed record.

PAYING FOR CRISIS

None of these activities came cheaply. As early as October 22, the USPS Board of Governors had approved $200 million for new technology to detect anthrax. The next day, USPS spent some of that, signing a $40 million contract with Titan Scan Technologies to supply eight mail sterilizers (with an option for 12 more) to national mail centers.[70] On October 30, Postmaster General Potter told the Senate Governmental Affairs Committee that USPS would require "several billion" dollars to recover from the anthrax crisis. On November 8, he told a Senate Appropriations subcommittee that USPS needed $5 billion—$2 billion to cover lost revenues (mail volume had dropped 10% since the crisis began) plus another $3 billion for the anthrax clean-up. Potter did not want to raise postal rates to meet the expenses. "Users of the mail should not be burdened with these extra costs through the price of postage," Potter told the committee. "This could quickly threaten the foundation of a universal postal system serving all Americans."[71]

Congress had already granted $175 million (out of $40 billion previously appropriated for recovery from September 11) for USPS to buy respirators, gloves, and other protective equipment. In late December, USPS won another $500 million in emergency funds for anthrax clean-up and security measures. Homeland Security Director Ridge, says Jaffer, "worked with the Administration to get the monies for us ... just to cover the initial costs associated with all of the retrofits and changes that we had to go through." But that was all.

Congress sympathized with USPS. But the Postal Service had been struggling financially for years. Congress did not propose to bail out, under the guise of anti-anthrax funding, an organization with systemic problems. The difficulties besetting the Postal Service were fundamental and required thoroughgoing reform. Temporary cash infusions, Congress believed, would only stave off a day of reckoning.

Nonetheless, the anthrax outbreak forced real costs on USPS. No place proved more expensive than Brentwood.

---

70. Lipton and Johnson, "Tracking Bioterror's Tangled Course."
71. Ellen Nakashima, "Postmaster Asks Senate for Bailout of $5 Billion; Congress Reluctant to Cover Losses," *Washington Post*, November 9, 2001, A30.

UNIQUE CASE OF BRENTWOOD

From the earliest stages, Brentwood was a special case. While Hamilton was also seriously contaminated (the Daschle letter and a suspected second letter went through both facilities), it was at Brentwood that postal workers died. After the sorting facility closed on Sunday, October 21, the first challenge was to figure out what had happened. The test results from the previous Thursday and Friday showed heavy contamination at Brentwood. Where had the Daschle letter gone? Which machines had it touched?

First in the line of suspicion were the Advanced Facer Canceller System (AFCS) machines. When a letter arrived, the AFCS looked for a stamp. If it saw the stamp, it cancelled the letter, then sent it through some rollers toward the next station. If the letter were turned facedown, the AFCS would flip, then cancel, it. As the letter flipped and went through the rollers, it was twisted and pinched. Letters also went through Delivery Barcode Sorters, whose optical scanners read the name and address and put letters in the appropriate bins. To reach the bins, the letters traveled down chutes powered by belts moving as quickly as 30 miles per hour, pinching to keep the letters in place. It seemed likely that at some point during this process, the Daschle letter had released anthrax into the air. The pressured-air blowdown process used to clean the machinery would then have served to aerosolize the anthrax.

For advice, Baca during that first week contacted the US Army Center for Health Promotion and Preventive Medicine at Aberdeen Proving Grounds in Maryland. Baca knew the Department of Defense had experience with anthrax as a potential battlefield weapon, and he wanted to draw on that expertise. The Center, he says, provided six people to help out for three weeks as USPS learned what it was up against at Brentwood. Environmental Coordinator Bridges, who for eight weeks after October 21 never went home, set up a command post. First, the team classified all equipment and mail as suspect or nonsuspect, with the suspect material treated as a biohazard. All the trucks and trailers that had been inside the Brentwood fence line were included in the suspect category. That meant 529 delivery vehicles and nearly 300 trailers would have to be decontaminated. Over the next days and weeks, they were vacuumed using high-efficiency filtration systems and then washed down with a chlorine solution within constructed containment areas.

Cleaning the Mail

Then there was the mail. Three million pieces, or 68 tons, of mail remained on the premises. Engineering VP Day and others had decided that irradiation would be the best way to clean the Brentwood mail before delivering it to customers. But first it had to be packaged for transport to an irradiation facility. The mail that was still in trucks or outside the main sorting area was treated first. Working with the Armed Forces Radiobiology Research Institute, Baca's team came up with a packaging protocol that would allow efficient mail irradiation. USPS contracted with Titan Scan Technologies for its plant in Lima, Ohio, to irradiate the Brentwood mail. Baca was in constant touch with the irradiation experts at Titan "because there were no procedures written for how to handle mail being irradiated. I had to learn about irradiation and they had to learn about mail." After treatment, the letters would reenter the mail stream.

At Brentwood, the team set up tents labeled hot zone, warm zone, and cold zone. As mail was removed from the periphery of the building and from trailers, it progressed through the zones. First, the trays on which mail rested were wiped down with a chlorine bleach solution. Then the trays of mail were put inside a plastic garbage bag, which was wiped down with chlorine solution. Another bag was placed on the outside. The resulting package could not be more than 4 inches high, or it would not fit into the irradiation machine. After problems developed with the bags, they were further placed inside boxes so they would not shift around. Each box was secured, marked with a designation code, and loaded into a trailer. Once the system was up and running, workers could load three to five trailers a day.

USPS contracted with Federal Express Custom Critical for trucks licensed to transport hazardous materials. Each truck had two drivers for the 10-hour drive from Washington, DC, to Titan's Ohio plant. For security, each truck was equipped with an emergency satellite call button on the dashboard. The drivers were certified, the trucks placarded. The first trucks arrived in Lima with packages of Brentwood mail on Friday, October 26—just four days after the second postal worker died.[72] Unfortunately, when the Allen County hazardous materials team examined the first three trucks (containing bags only), it found torn bags inside. Alarmed, they shut the trucks back up and sent them straight back to Washington, DC, for repackaging. The members of the hazmat team went on Cipro. But in the days and weeks that followed, trucks—escorted by state troopers the 200 miles to Lima from the Pennsylvania–Ohio border—arrived without incident.

The preparations for clean-up at Brentwood, however, were just beginning.

Protecting the Clean-Up Workers

As of early November, Brentwood still had a million pieces of mail left on its machines and nothing inside the building had been touched. That was due to the difficulty of deciding under what circumstances to permit clean-up workers to enter the building. Contract personnel (no postal employees were certified for this type of work) at Brentwood bagging the suspect mail at first wore Level A personal protective equipment,

---

72. Jennifer Lenhart, "City Wants Mail Returned to Sender," *Washington Post*, November 24, 2001, A16.

requiring the use of double suits with a supplied air system. By early November, the category was downgraded to Level B (one suit). Not until November 7, however, did CDC and OSHA sanction the entry of USPS contract workers into the building to remove the remaining mail and begin to decontaminate the machines.[73]

Delivery Barcode Sorter (DBCS) 17 was, they determined, the most contaminated. Located in the open area of the workroom floor, it had processed the Daschle letter.[74] The deceased Brentwood workers, Morris and Curseen, had both worked near DBCS 17. Tests in October showed it had spore colonies in the hundreds of thousands. There were spores embedded in the belts and in the wheels. Contract workers wiped it down three times with a hypochloride solution of chlorine and water, reducing the colonies to less than 400 spores. But it was not only heavily contaminated machines that required attention. Workers would have to wipe down every piece of equipment and office furniture in the building. They would need to clean walls, remove ceiling tiles and incinerate them, and remove carpeting and incinerate it.

Just the experience of removing mail revealed what a time-consuming project the clean-up would be. The 15-year-old building had been completely sealed with thermal foam board to prevent contamination leaking out. Its 235 skylights were covered with black plastic, sealed inside and out, and taped. All 17 HVAC systems were sealed, as were gas pipes, water pipes, and electrical conduits. The temperature inside soared. Workers going in wore suits taped all around—sealing gloves and masks. It took up to 30 minutes to suit up, and another 30 to undress and then shower. But these precautions coupled with the heat in the building meant the temperature inside the suits was well over 100°F. Workers at times could remain inside no more than two hours before they had to come out, take a shower, rehydrate, and start all over. Says Baca:

> So we've got 150, 200 people generating two suits an entry. By the end of the fourth day, we had eight dumpsters of personal protective equipment and now we have to figure out where do we dispose of it. So we have to go to the EPA.

EPA's Office of Solid Waste and Emergency Response had to issue a ruling permitting USPS to dispose of the suits. The ruling came in by the first part of December. Next, USPS had to seek State of Virginia Department of Environmental Quality approval to dispose of the suits and other material as medical waste—the most costly disposal method—by incinerating it. But the citizens of Virginia protested, so USPS had to obtain permission to transport the hazardous materials (eventually 98 dumpsters' worth) through Virginia and other states enroute to Georgia and those states that would accept it. Remarks Baca: "We were trying to figure out the rules and write them at the same time."

---

73. Justin Blum and Neil Irwin, "Some DC Mail Still Has Not Gone Through," *Washington Post*, November 8, 2001, B1.
74. It would later emerge that the Leahy letter went through DBCS 17 as well, not far behind the Daschle letter.

Keeping the Records

But while Baca was recording those hard-learned rules, he also made sure they remained in-house. From the start, he kept careful records. He and Environmental Coordinator Bridges had decided from the first day to treat Brentwood as a potential litigation case according to the guidelines set by the National Contingency Plan (NCP). Usually NCP governed hazardous spills, but "[t]here were no specific instructions on how to deal with anthrax," points out Baca, so he modified NCP for anthrax. Utilizing the NCP framework, all information pertaining to clean-up was restricted as if it were evidence for a court case. Baca wanted to protect any data that could have national security implications. He says:

> If we start putting out some of the information that we've generated, and it's made public, then a terrorist will say "Oh, here's where the holes are in their system." So everything that we've done, we've pretty much had to keep under wraps.

Baca instituted a document control numbering system, so he would know who had which documents. Most of them never left Brentwood. This secrecy met with some resentment from, among others, UICC. Its members, who were trying to assemble the national protocols for anthrax removal, could learn little about Brentwood. Fennewald remembers that "at Trenton, they did a good job of keeping us informed … [with information] that would help us in terms of the national protocols. [By contrast] the only information that we got on Brentwood was out of the paper.… They were really sitting on it." This did not bother Baca. The experts he needed were at Brentwood field-testing and implementing, as he puts it, "real-time protocols, not hypothetical conditions."

Not surprisingly, as the dimensions of cleaning Brentwood and Hamilton expanded, Baca's role in other decontamination efforts fell off. He rarely attended UICC meetings and, by default, Tim Gouger of the Army Corps took over responsibility for all the decontamination except the big two (and Morgan, which had its own command center). At the same time, recalls Baca, he was under pressure from management to reopen Brentwood (Hamilton also remained closed; it was slated for clean-up after Brentwood). He comments:

> Here I was, a support function manager, taking away a primary processing facility for the Postal Service, and I couldn't give them dates on which they might get it back or when they might get their mail.

The mail-cleaning operation, however, was proving successful. By November 24, 29 of an expected 45 trailer-loads from Brentwood had gone through Titan at the rate of two truckloads a week and operations seemed on track to work through the remainder. But there still remained the question of how to clean Brentwood itself—particularly its large open spaces where aerosolized anthrax presumably hung suspended in air. As Baca and others studied that question, the anthrax outbreak took a turn as dramatic as it was difficult to explain.

LATE OCTOBER–NOVEMBER

It started in late October. On Monday, October 29, New York Mayor Giuliani announced that a stockroom worker at the Manhattan Eye, Ear, and Throat Hospital was in critical condition with inhalation anthrax. Kathy T. Nguyen, 61, of the Bronx, had felt ill since October 25. The hospital closed and its hundreds of employees and patients were tested for anthrax starting October 30. On October 31, Nguyen died. The same day Nguyen's illness became public, Linda Burch in New Jersey was diagnosed with skin anthrax (2 days after her release from the hospital). The 51-year-old worked as a bookkeeper in an office whose mail bin was found to be contaminated. Mail to both her office and home was processed at Hamilton.[75] The Nguyen and Burch cases alarmed public health authorities because neither woman worked with the mail. The Nguyen case was especially frustrating because there were no clues indicating how she became infected, yet somehow she had contracted the more virulent inhalation anthrax.

Three weeks later, the mystery deepened. On November 21, Ottilie Lundgren, a 94-year-old woman from Oxford, Connecticut, died from inhalation anthrax. Mrs. Lundgren had no connection to the media, to the government, or to the Postal Service. She rarely left her house. Connecticut health officials, CDC, and USPS were baffled. Tests at the nearby Wallingford postal facility found anthrax residue on several sorting machines.[76] But no one else was ill. Traces of anthrax were found on a letter sent to a home 1.5 miles from Lundgren. Cross-contamination seemed likely. But how little anthrax had it taken to kill the elderly Connecticut resident?

The case of Nguyen remained similarly unsolved. There was only circumstantial evidence of cross-contamination: a letter mailed to an address near Nguyen had passed through the same Hamilton sorting machine that handled the Daschle letter.[77] "We have no evidence yet that they actually got [anthrax] from the mail," says VP Medvidovich. "But guess what? We had to act like they got it from the mail and re-start our procedures."

There was pressure to close the Wallingford post office, but contamination was light and localized, and USPS kept it open. Again, the Task Force took pains to communicate fully with the unions and the employees. "We worked with the employees," says Medvidovich. "You can't just dismiss stress. You can't dismiss fear…. We had doctors go out on the workroom floor and talk to them about anthrax…. The key was, you kept the unions involved."

Postal union leaders were not, on the face of it, reassured. On Thanksgiving Day, November 22, President Bill Burrus of the 360,000-member American Postal Workers

---

75. Nicholas Kulish and Jared Sandberg, "Questions of Security: Postal Officials to Face Grilling on Capitol Hill About Anthrax," *Wall Street Journal*, October 30, 2001, A6.

76. Revkin with Zielbauer, "Tracking of Anthrax Letter Yields Clues." Anthrax was found on December 2, after numerous tests by both USPS contract teams and the CDC.

77. Eric Lipton and Judith Miller, "US Says Thousands of Letters May Have Had Anthrax Traces," *New York Times*, December 4, 2001, A1.

Union recommended that members refuse to work in buildings where any traces of anthrax remained. "It's a continuing concern that so much uncertainty continues to exist regarding the source of these infections," he said.[78] The unions did not, however, stop mail delivery. Perhaps they, like the USPS leadership, were waiting to see what could be learned from a second anthrax letter bound for Congress—found only on November 16.

THE LEAHY LETTER

Investigators from the FBI and EPA had believed for weeks that the extent of aerosolized anthrax contamination they were seeing could not have been caused by the Daschle letter alone. They suspected a second letter, perhaps among the mountains of quarantined congressional mail. On Monday, November 5, the FBI had moved all the mail received at the Capitol from October 12 to 17 from a congressional building to a General Services Administration warehouse in a northern Virginia suburb.[79] The 600 bags took up 286 sealed, 55-gallon barrels.

FBI, EPA, and Fort Detrick investigators had started on Monday, November 12, to go through the barrels of congressional mail. At 5 p.m. on Friday, they struck gold: a heavily taped letter, postmarked in Trenton on October 9, with handwriting similar to that on the Daschle letter, addressed to Senator Patrick Leahy (D-Vermont), chair of the Senate Judiciary Committee. Like the Daschle letter, the return address was the nonexistent "4th Grade, Greendale School, Franklin Park, NJ."[80] Like the Daschle letter, it was loaded with anthrax.

The investigators had been extraordinarily careful handling the quarantined mail. Now that it was found, scientists, with help from experts around the world, devised an entirely new procedure to handle the Leahy letter. Their efforts were rewarded. Analyzing this plentiful supply of weaponized anthrax, scientists made significant investigative strides over the next couple of weeks. Just one sample from the Leahy letter, the FBI reported shortly after the letter's discovery, contained 23,000 spores.[81] Just two weeks later, weapons experts restated that estimate, clarifying that the anthrax sent to Congress contained 1 trillion spores per gram, a degree of fineness inconceivable before the recent events.[82] If a deadly dose was close to 10,000 spores, one trillion could potentially kill 100 million people.

---

78. Associated Press, "Postal Union Urges Members Not to Work if Anthrax Is Found," *New York Times*, November 23, 2001, B6.

79. Guy Gugliotta, "Senate Delays Plan to Fumigate Its Hart Office Building," *Washington Post*, November 6, 2001, A10.

80. Judith Miller and David Johnson, "Investigators Liken Anthrax in Leahy Letter to That Sent to Daschle," *New York Times*, November 20, 2001, B1.

81. Ibid.

82. William J. Broad, "The Spores: Terror Anthrax Resembles Type Made by US," *New York Times*, December 3, 2001, A1.

The high quality and specific strain (known as Ames) of the refined anthrax led HHS Secretary Thompson on November 20 to say that the anthrax-tainted letters most likely came from a domestic source. Others speculated more explicitly that it must come from a US defense laboratory. Leahy told NBC's *Meet the Press* that the letter addressed to him contained enough anthrax potentially to kill 100,000 people. Armed with this new information, EPA returned to the AMI building in Florida, the site of the first inhalation anthrax cases. New tests showed far wider contamination than initially thought; EPA announced on December 5 that 88 of 460 swabs on three floors tested positive.[83] As with Hart and Brentwood, anthrax must have spread through the air vents.

For its part, the Postal Inspection Service discovered why the Leahy letter had lain for so long undiscovered. An optical reader had misread the zip code as 20520 instead of 20510. As a result, the letter went to the State Department before being rerouted back to Capitol Hill. That explained why some diplomatic mail may have been contaminated. USPS also discovered that the Leahy and Daschle letters were closely spaced during processing. It was the letters in between (plus some in front and behind) that most likely had caused most of the cross-contamination.

Fewer Patients

Finding the Leahy letter was not the only good news in November. Apart from the anomalous cases of Nguyen and Lundgren, there were signs that the anthrax outbreak was tapering off. On November 1, DC health officials revised their recommendation that all employees of private firms whose mail came from Brentwood—at least 2,000—should take antibiotics. Now they narrowed the category to include only firms whose zip codes started with 200, or firms likely to be targets of terrorism. With no new case in more than a week, DC health chief Dr. Walks cautiously suggested the city was "on the downside" of the crisis.[84]

Meanwhile, some of the afflicted were returning home. As early as October 23, Ernesto Blanco, the Florida AMI employee with inhalation anthrax, left the hospital after 23 days. On November 5, Hamilton postal worker Norma Wallace was released after 2 weeks of hospital treatment for inhalation anthrax.[85] On November 9, a State Department mail handler with inhalation anthrax, as well as a 56-year-old Brentwood postal worker, both went home.[86] On November 19 Leroy Richmond, the first Brentwood worker known to have inhalation anthrax, left the hospital.

83. Ceci Connolly and Ellen Nakashima, "CDC Sets 'Tips' on Handling Mail," *Washington Post*, December 6, 2001, A26.
84. Steve Twomey and Avram Goldstein, "Officials Call Off Antibiotics for Many Who Handle Mail," *Washington Post*, November 2, 2001, A13.
85. Gugliotta, "Senate Delays Plan to Fumigate."
86. Lipton and Johnson, "Tracking Bioterror's Tangled Course."

POSTAL CONTAMINATION LESSENS

Fewer patients did not mean an end to discoveries of contamination. On October 30, traces of anthrax were found at several more DC area post offices—including Friendship and an outlet at Dulles airport. On November 2, testers found contamination on two more machines at Morgan Station in Manhattan. On November 3, the South Jersey Processing and Distribution Center in Bellmawr, New Jersey, which had been closed and reopened the preceding week, closed again after spores were found on a mail-sorting machine.[87] Spores were found November 5 inside two mailboxes inside the Pentagon. On November 9, authorities announced they had found trace amounts of anthrax in four small post offices that fed into Hamilton. None of the four was closed, but they were cleaned overnight.

But encouragingly, the new contamination cases exhibited merely light concentrations of anthrax. With the lessened risk, facilities were able to remain open while contaminated areas were cordoned off and cleaned. On a similarly positive note, UICC sampling teams were finding contamination not because of sick workers, but because the command center was testing facilities according to its trading-partners chart. Of the 230 locations on the list by early November, 200 were included as a precaution, and only 30 because they were known to have handled contaminated letters or had sick employees. As of November 2, VP Jaffer said, 64 had been tested. Of those, 39 were anthrax-free, eight had been contaminated and were closed pending cleaning, while 17 results were not yet available.[88] Slowly post offices reopened. Bellmawr in New Jersey reopened on November 8. The Princeton main post office was also back in business.

Brentwood Revisited

Brentwood, however, remained definitively closed. With the discovery of the Leahy letter and the analysis of the anthrax it contained, the dimensions of contamination at Brentwood were far better understood. The aerosolized anthrax had by now spread through the ventilation system. It was in the high bays. It was in the ventilation ducts. There were close to 100 truck bays to clean. Baca and his team would have to decide how best to kill those spores. For initial guidance, they observed closely what EPA was doing at the Hart Senate Office Building, where aerosolized anthrax had also spread widely. The clean-up of surface contamination at Hart started on November 5.

To clean Hart's contaminated open spaces, EPA had made a choice. Historically, paraformaldehyde had been used to clean up anthrax—for example, at CDC laboratories.

---

87. "Anthrax Discovery Closes Mail Center," *New York Times*, November 4, 2001, B6.
88. Michael Janofsky, "Mail Delays Are Minimal, Despite Anthrax Problems," *New York Times*, November 2, 2001, B8.

But there were fears—although no proof, despite its use for a century—that paraformaldehyde might be a carcinogen. The agent chlorine dioxide had been used at the Ames government laboratory for anthrax decontamination. Although it had no commercial use, EPA selected chlorine dioxide gas as the best agent. Plans to fumigate, however, were put on hold pending tests of the effect of the gas on various materials.

Unbeknownst to the outside world, those tests were conducted at Brentwood. Starting October 29, USPS set up a trailer and ran 10 tests on the effects of chlorine dioxide on such materials as old paintings, leather chairs, plastic, Plexiglas, copper piping, aluminum pipes, steel pipes, PVC, computer monitors, and fluorescent lights. The results: blue and green silks discolored. Otherwise, chlorine dioxide seemed safe. It had been used in decontaminating over 900 water treatment facilities. It was used on food. It had been around for 70 years. The USPS tests also developed protocols on where best to place surrogate spore strips (which test for the presence of anthrax), how to retrieve them, how to package and send them to a lab, plus how to maintain temperature and humidity levels during the administration of the gas. On December 1, EPA (using contractor Saber Technologies and Ashland Chemical) started fumigating the Hart Building with chlorine dioxide gas.

Baca decided that he would select for Brentwood the same cleaning agent that EPA chose for Hart. It was not an easy decision. Since October 22, businesspeople (supported by their congressional representatives) had presented Baca with plenty of options, each salesperson promising his product could solve the problem. For six weeks, the three lines on Baca's office phone plus his cell phone rang constantly. For Baca, it was a nightmare. "Probably the hardest thing was everybody that brought silver bullets ... vendors, congresspersons," he recalls. "Believe me, there were hundreds of companies saying this stuff works and this—but nobody could prove it. [I worried]: Did I miss an opportunity?" But Baca felt chlorine dioxide was the right choice—scientifically and politically. He says:

> My recommendation to the Postal Service was that we had been characterized as second class citizens compared to the Hart employees. Well, we were going to use the exact same processes and science that was used at the Hart. Our employees deserved nothing less.

But cleaning Brentwood would be more challenging than cleaning Hart. At 17.5 million cubic feet, the building covered 14 acres and was 175 times larger than the area that had to be cleaned at Hart. Clean-up would not happen quickly. Baca also continued to fend off attempts from EPA to take over the Brentwood decontamination. "John [Bridges] and I would not let them have it," recalls Baca. "EPA could at any time, if we weren't doing what was right, take it away from us," he adds. "But we are the lead agency and we were doing it correctly."

As Baca geared up for the Brentwood operation, the rest of the USPS anthrax response team was downshifting from full-bore crisis mode to a more manageable state of emergency.

A CALMER DECEMBER

Although false alarms continued to cause occasional scares in offices and homes around the country, by December there had been no new deaths since Lundgren and no new tainted letters since the discovery of the Leahy letter. The crisis seemed to be in retreat. The discovery of anthrax on December 2 at the Wallingford postal facility (after Ms. Lundgren's death) did trigger two weeks of fevered activity for UICC. The problem was that contamination was found only after repeated tests by a variety of methods—dry swabs (Q-tips), wet swabs, and wet wipes. Only the wet wipes revealed the presence of anthrax. This disturbed UICC officials because their contract teams, up to now, had used mostly swabs to test for anthrax. The results at Wallingford called into question the validity of all previous tests that had relied on swabbing. With no new illness, however, UICC worry diminished. As of mid-December, CDC had confirmed 18 cases of anthrax infection since the start of the outbreak—11 cases of inhalation anthrax and seven of skin anthrax. Five people had died, all from inhalation anthrax.[89]

USPS senior management began to dare to think they could start to breathe normally again, although the Postal Service did come under pressure in early December from public health authorities. Because of barcode tracing, USPS could determine precisely which letters had possibly been cross-contaminated by the Daschle and Leahy letters. The numbers would be in the tens of thousands, however, and USPS had no desire to newly alarm the public by sending out notifications. "It's not our decision," Communications VP Jaffer said on December 4. "We have asked the CDC over and over and over.... They have told us repeatedly: 'There is no risk here. No need to do any notification.'"[90]

By Christmas, UICC had lessened its frenetic pace of October and November.[91] Except for Brentwood and Trenton, UICC teams had bleached and reopened all contaminated postal facilities—21 in total (some work remained to be done at Wallingford, but it was open).[92] UICC had sampled 284 sites. Postal inspectors had fielded more than 17,000 reports of anthrax. The 500 to 600 calls a day from the press and the public to the USPS Communications Center had dwindled by December to a dozen a day. On Friday, December 21, UICC closed its doors—at least temporarily. When it reopened in January, it was as a smaller operation.

---

89. The deceased were Stevens, Curseen, Morris, Nguyen, and Lundgren.
90. Ellen Nakashima and Rick Weiss, "Postal Service Seeks to Soothe Fears about Anthrax Letters," *Washington Post*, December 5, 2001, A10.
91. In late November Fennewald urgently needed back surgery, and Deputy Incident Commander Vidich took over.
92. In addition, affected organizations (the State Department, NBC, etc.) had independently cleaned up 27 contaminated nonpostal facilities. Of the 27 nonpostal facilities, 20 were in Washington, DC.

Cleaning the large, open buildings proved a long-term and costly task. EPA did not finish with the Hart Building until February 2002. The agency reported that the final cost of cleaning up Capitol Hill (30 buildings) topped $23 million, twice the original estimate.[93] VP for Engineering Day said USPS learned a lot from the Hart treatment: how much chlorine dioxide gas to use, under what conditions, at what temperature and humidity, and for how long.[94] Still, progress at Brentwood—due to its large size and complex configuration—remained slow and the building was still closed more than a year later. Despite that, confidence in the mail had rebounded. During the crisis, polls showed it had dropped over 15%—only 82% of Americans trusted the mail. By March 2002, 96% of Americans once again had confidence in their nation's postal service.

---

93. Spencer S. Hsu, "Cost of Anthrax Cleanup on Hill to Top $23 Million, EPA Says," *Washington Post*, March 7, 2002, A7.

94. Steve Twomey, "Mail Official Predicts Brentwood's Return," *Washington Post*, January 9, 2002, A11.

Exhibit 11-1. Chronology of Events: Anthrax Crisis, September–December 2001

Tuesday, September 18
- Envelopes containing letters and granular substances are sent to *New York Post* and NBC News Anchor Tom Brokaw. Both mailed from Trenton, NJ, and later tested positive for anthrax.

Thursday, September 20
- Postal worker at Hamilton, NJ, mail processing center Richard Morgano, 39, scratches himself on mail-sorting machine. Sees doctor September 30; given antibiotics. Cutaneous anthrax confirmed October 18.

Friday, September 21
- Editorial page assistant at *New York Post* Johanna Huden has blister on finger. Diagnosed with cutaneous anthrax in mid-October.

Monday, September 24
- Ernesto Blanco, 73, mailroom worker at American Media, Inc. (AMI), in Boca Raton, FL, is sick. Hospitalized October 1. Inhalation anthrax diagnosed October 15.
- Robert Stevens, 63, photo editor at AMI's *Sun*, feels ill. Hospitalized October 2; dies October 5 from inhalation anthrax.

Thursday, September 27
- Teresa Heller, letter carrier at West Trenton, NJ, post office, develops a lesion on her arm. Hospitalized October 3; diagnosed with skin anthrax October 18.

Friday, September 28
- Erin O'Connor, 38, assistant to NBC News Anchor Tom Brokaw, has lesion on collarbone. Diagnosed with skin anthrax on October 12.
- Casey Chamberlain, 23, NBC desk assistant, has rash on leg. Diagnosed October 24 as probable cutaneous anthrax.
- 7-month-old son of ABC producer spends time at the network office in New York City. Hospitalized October 1. Diagnosed with cutaneous anthrax October 15.
- CBS news aide Claire Fletcher, 27, develops two spots on face, then swelling and nausea. Diagnosed as cutaneous anthrax on October 18.

Thursday, October 4
- Authorities confirm AMI's Stevens has inhalation anthrax. CDC sends team to Boca Raton.
- Of Stevens, HHS Secretary Tommy G. Thompson states, "It is an isolated case, and it is not contagious."

Friday, October 5
- Stevens dies. First US death from inhaled anthrax since 1976, and one of only 18 cases documented in the previous 100 years.

Monday, October 8 (Columbus Day)
- FBI takes over the Stevens case.
- USPS Vice President Azeezaly Jaffer prepares memo for employees about anthrax and the mail.

Tuesday, October 9
- Letters postmarked Trenton are mailed to Senate Majority Leader Tom Daschle (D-SD) and Senator Patrick Leahy (D-VT), chair of the Senate Judiciary Committee.
- Bush informs the nation that Florida case appears to be an isolated incident.

Thursday, October 11
- Daschle and Leahy letters arrive at Brentwood mail processing center, which handles all federal government mail. The letters go through Delivery Barcode Sorter Machine 17. Daschle letter sent on to P Street mail facility; Leahy letter misdirected to State Department.

Friday, October 12
- NYC officials announce NBC's O'Connor has skin anthrax; first known case outside Florida.
- Investigators discover the anthrax-laden letter addressed to NBC, which was processed at Hamilton postal facility on September 18. After O'Connor's case is announced, so too are cases at ABC, CBS, and *New York Post*.

(Continued)

Exhibit 11-1. (Continued)

Sunday, October 14
- Norma Wallace, 56, postal worker in Hamilton develops nausea. Hospitalized October 19; diagnosed as suspected anthrax October 23; first NJ inhalation case. Patrick Daniel O'Donnell, 35, Hamilton, NJ, postal worker has rash and trouble breathing. Hospitalized October 16; diagnosed with anthrax October 19.

Monday, October 15
- Letter containing anthrax opened in Senate Majority Leader Tom Daschle's office in the Hart Senate Office Building.
- Postmaster General John "Jack" Potter announces formation of a Mail Security Task Force.

Tuesday, October 16
- Twelve Senate offices closed; hundreds of staffers get tested for anthrax.
- Leroy Richmond, 56, mail sorter at Brentwood, develops fever, chills. Hospitalized October 19, inhalation anthrax diagnosed October 20. Released November 19.
- Brentwood worker Thomas L. Morris, Jr., 55, ill. Hospitalized October 21. Dies same day of inhalation anthrax.
- Brentwood worker Joseph Curseen, 47, ill. October 21 seeks medical treatment, dies October 22 of inhalation anthrax.

Wednesday, October 17
- Anthrax spores found in Dirksen Senate Office Building. House of Representatives closes.
- Linda Burch, 51, bookkeeper at Hamilton-area firm, has pimple on forehead. Hospitalized October 22; discharged October 27; cutaneous anthrax confirmed on October 29.

Thursday, October 18
- House and Senate office complexes close.
- FBI and USPS hold press conference at Brentwood; offer $1 million reward for information leading to the arrest and conviction of those involved with the anthrax mailings.
- USPS hires private firm to test Brentwood on Thursday night.
- USPS closes Hamilton Township mail processing center for tests.

Friday, October 19
- Anthrax-laced letter postmarked September 18 is found, unopened, near where *New York Post's* Huden worked.
- USPS Mail Security Task Force starts meeting
- *New York Post* mailroom worker, 34, notices pimple on left arm. Is listed as suspected cutaneous anthrax on October 27.
- CDC tests Brentwood for anthrax.

Saturday, October 20
- DC Department of Health, Mayor Williams, and USPS learn Brentwood employee Richmond most likely has inhalation anthrax.
- USPS team plans how to shut down Brentwood facility.

Sunday, October 21
- Richmond confirmed with inhalation anthrax.
- Brentwood closes.
- DC Mayor Anthony Williams holds press conference; offers Brentwood workers antibiotics.
- Brentwood worker Morris, Jr., dies.

Monday, October 22
- Brentwood worker Curseen dies.
- Contract postal employee, 59, at State Department mail sorting facility ill. Hospitalized October 25; confirmed with inhalation anthrax.
- House reopens; Senate and House office buildings remain closed.
- CDC headquarters in Atlanta organizes conference call with FBI, USPS, Postal Inspection Service, Office of Homeland Security, and local law enforcement officials; decide to keep USPS running.
- USPS VP Deborah Willhite tells press conference Postal Service followed CDC advice.
- James Gaffney arrives in DC from the USPS New Jersey district to work at Unified Incident Command Center (UICC).

(Continued)

Exhibit 11-1. (Continued)

- Sampling found spores at 14 of 29 Brentwood locations.
- DC offers antibiotics to USPS workers at 36 area post offices.

Tuesday, October 23
- President Bush says: "I don't have anthrax."
- CDC Deputy Director Dr. David Fleming says now investigating whether anthrax could escape from an envelope.
- Charles Vidich arrives in DC to work at UICC.

Wednesday, October 24
- Mark Cunningham, 38, *New York Post* editorial page editor, has pimple on forehead. Diagnosed with cutaneous anthrax November 2. Also, a *Post* mailroom worker, 34, listed as suspected cutaneous anthrax case.
- USPS decides its Environmental Management Policy department will do decontamination of sites, while the Safety Department will conduct sampling.
- USPS announces purchase of ion beam sterilization devices; is buying masks and gloves.

Thursday, October 25
- USPS announces will expand testing to more than 200 facilities that "trade" with infected sites.
- Homeland Security's Ridge confirms Daschle letter was intended as a weapon.
- As of today there are 32 cases of anthrax exposure and 13 confirmed anthrax infections—seven cutaneous and six inhaled. Three have died of inhalation anthrax.
- Anthrax is found on one floor at the Morgan Station mail processing facility in Manhattan.
- Nineteen of 59 samples taken at Hamilton mail center are positive for anthrax.
- Kathy Nguyen, stockroom worker at the Manhattan Eye, Ear, and Throat Hospital, falls ill; hospitalized October 28; dies October 31.

Friday, October 26
- Executive board of the New York Metro Area Postal Union votes to file a suit to close Morgan for cleaning. Judge dismisses suit November 9.
- First trucks carrying mail from Brentwood arrive in Lima, OH, for irradiation.

Saturday, October 27
- Post office in West Windsor, NJ (Princeton), joins Hamilton and West Trenton—all closed for decontamination.

Monday, October 29
- Supreme Court closes for anthrax testing.
- Manhattan Eye, Ear, and Throat Hospital closes.

Tuesday, October 30
- UICC team moves into dedicated space.

Wednesday, October 31
- Nguyen dies.
- Paul Fennewald joins UICC as director.

Thursday, November 1
- DC health officials reduce list of those who should take preventive antibiotics for anthrax.

Friday, November 2
- Supreme Court building reopens.

Sunday, November 4
- USPS concludes working agreement with Association of Public Health Laboratories to process anthrax samples.

Monday, November 5
- EPA begins surface decontamination of Hart Senate Office Building.
- FBI moves Capitol Hill's quarantined mail—received between October 12 and October 17—in 280 sealed, 55-gallon barrels from DC to a Virginia warehouse.

(Continued)

Exhibit 11-1. (Continued)

Wednesday, November 7
- USPS concedes 1 million pieces of mail are still in Brentwood; contract workers begin removing it from sorting machines.

Thursday, November 8
- Postmaster General Potter tells Senate USPS needs $5 billion—$2 billion to cover lost revenues plus at least $3 billion for anthrax clean-up.
- Bellmawr, NJ, postal facility reopens. West Windsor has also reopened.

Tuesday, November 13
- Ottilie W. Lundgren, 94, falls ill in Oxford, CT; hospitalized November 16; died November 21.

Thursday, November 15
- Investigators find anthrax spores throughout the 68,000-square-foot AMI building in Boca Raton on all three floors.

Friday, November 16
- Investigators uncover (but announce only November 19) another anthrax-laden letter addressed to Sen. Leahy. Like the NBC, *New York Post*, and Daschle letters, Leahy letter is postmarked October 9 from Trenton.

Wednesday, November 21
- Lundgren dies.

Thursday, November 22 (Thanksgiving)
- Bill Burrus, president of 360,000-member American Postal Workers Union, recommends members refuse to work in buildings with any trace of anthrax.

Saturday, December 1
- EPA starts fumigating Hart Senate Office Building with chlorine dioxide gas.

Sunday, December 2
- Traces of anthrax found in Wallingford, CT, post office near Ms. Lundgren's home.

Tuesday, December 4
- UICC finishes Interim Guidelines.
- USPS VP Jaffer says CDC has said there is "no need to do any notification" of households that possibly received cross-contaminated letters.

Monday, December 10
- Tests confirm the letter sent to Sen. Leahy's office contained the same grade of anthrax as that sent to Sen. Daschle.

Friday, December 21
- UICC closes down temporarily, reopens in January as far smaller operation.

Exhibit 11-2. Cast of Characters: Anthrax Crisis, September–December 2001

US Federal Government Officials
- Tommy G. Thompson, Secretary of the Department of Health and Human Services
- Thomas Ridge, Director for Homeland Security
- Senator Tom Daschle, Senate Majority Leader (D-SD)
- Senator Patrick Leahy, Chair Senate Judiciary Committee (D-VT)

US Postal Service
- John "Jack" Potter, Postmaster General
- John Nolan, Deputy Postmaster General
- Deborah Willhite, Senior Vice President for Government Relations and Public Policy
- Suzanne Medvidovich, Senior Vice President for Human Resources
- Patrick Donahoe, Chief Operating Officer
- Azeezaly Jaffer, Vice President of Public Affairs and Communication
- Jon Leonard, Internal Communications Manager
- Kenneth Weaver, Chief of the US Postal Inspection Service, Chair of the Mail Security Task Force
- James Rowan, Deputy Chief Inspector for Security in Technology, US Postal Inspection Service
- Thomas Day, Vice President for Engineering
- Dennis Baca, Manager for Environmental Management Policy
- John Bridges, Brentwood Environmental Coordinator
- Sam Pulcrano, Manager of Safety
- Charles Vidich, Manager for Environmental Compliance for the Northeast
- Paul Fennewald, Environmental Programs Analyst
- James Gaffney, Environmental Compliance Specialist
- Timothy Gouger, US Corps of Engineers
- Timothy Haney, Brentwood Senior Plant Manager

Centers for Disease Control and Prevention (CDC) Medical Officials
- Dr. Jeffrey P. Koplan, Director of CDC
- Dr. Julie Gerberding, CDC Deputy Director for Infectious Diseases

New Jersey and Washington, DC, Officials
- Dr. George T. DiFerdinando, New Jersey Acting Commissioner for Health
- Anthony A. Williams, Mayor of Washington, DC
- Dr. Ivan C. A. Walks, Chief Health Officer of Washington, DC

Anthrax Victims (not a complete list; covers those named in text)
Deceased
- Robert Stevens, Photo Editor of American Media, Inc. (AMI) Tabloid the *Sun*; died October 5.
- Joseph P. Curseen, Brentwood Employee; died October 22.
- Thomas L. Morris, Jr., Brentwood Employee; died October 21.
- Kathy T. Nguyen, Stockroom Worker at Manhattan Eye, Ear, and Throat Hospital; died October 31.
- Ottilie Lundgren, 94, Oxford, CT, homemaker; died November 21.

(Continued)

Exhibit 11-2. (Continued)

Recovered Cutaneous Anthrax Cases
- Erin O'Connor, Assistant to NBC News Anchor Tom Brokaw; diagnosed October 12.
- Claire Fletcher, CBS News Aide; diagnosed October 18.
- Johanna Huden, New York Post Editorial Page Assistant; illness announced October 19.
- Teresa Heller, West Trenton, NJ, Letter Carrier; Illness announced October 18.
- Patrick O'Donnell, Hamilton, NJ, Maintenance Worker; diagnosed October 19.
- Casey Chamberlain, NBC News Desk Assistant; diagnosed October 24.
- Linda Burch, New Jersey Bookkeeper; diagnosed October 29.

Recovered Inhalation Anthrax Cases
- Ernesto Blanco, AMI Mailroom Employee; admitted September 30; diagnosed with anthrax October 15.
- Leroy Richmond, Brentwood Employee; diagnosed October 21.
- Norma Wallace, Hamilton Postal Worker; diagnosed October 23.

12

White Powders in Georgia: Responding to Cases of Suspected Anthrax After 9/11

Daniel J. Collings

EDITORS' INTRODUCTION

Beginning in October 2001, weaponized-anthrax letters menaced congressmen, Capitol Hill staffers, media figures, rank-and-file postal workers, and seemingly random individuals in their own homes. Intensely nervous Americans, only weeks before traumatized by the terrorist attacks on the World Trade Center and the Pentagon, absorbed a stream of news reports about deaths and critical illness in Florida, Washington, DC, New York, and New Jersey. The public's anxiety was only accentuated by a spate of anthrax hoaxes generated maliciously or in twisted attempts at humor. As a result, the United States experienced an explosion of fearful calls to local public health, first response, and law enforcement agencies all over the country about suspicious white powders that callers feared might be deadly. For months, these suspected hazardous materials, or hazmat alarms, and the possibility that real anthrax might again be found placed enormous strains on the public health and emergency management systems and required major adaptations in operating routines by the response organizations. Virtually all proved harmless—whether confectioners' sugar, talcum powder, or other innocent

This case was written by Daniel J. Collings for Dr. Arnold Howitt, Executive Director, Taubman Center for State and Local Government, John F. Kennedy School of Government, Harvard University. Funding was provided by the Robert Wood Johnson Foundation and the Volpe National Transportation Systems Center of the US Department of Transportation. (1003)

substances—but each had to be handled with care, investigated, and determined not to be dangerous.

This case study tracks this experience in a single state, examining the interactions among federal, state, and local agencies, and highlighting the interdependencies among law enforcement, emergency response, and public health professionals.

How would authorities handle the rapidly increasing volume of hazmat incidents? Existing practice called for highly trained hazmat technicians, primarily from fire departments, to safely clean up or collect dangerous substances and, where terrorism was suspected, to turn these over to the Federal Bureau of Investigation. The mushrooming number of calls, however, quickly exceeded the capacity of hazmat units, and the volume of materials to be stored while investigations proceeded—not to mention the potential safety hazards if kept in ordinary locations—made rapid adaptations of procedure essential.

The interplay of public health, law enforcement, and first response meant that enhanced interorganizational and intergovernmental collaboration was needed, but frictions inevitably arose. New locations for storage of samples had to be found, questions of bureaucratic precedence and control had to be resolved, augmented numbers of personnel to answer calls from fearful citizens had to be found, and new protocols had to be developed to train responders for handling suspected anthrax. The latter was particularly important. The number of calls to be handled necessitated sending out not just well-trained and experienced hazmat crews but also young firefighters, emergency medical technicians (EMTs), and police officers who had little or no hazmat training and therefore critically needed guidance on how to protect themselves while protecting the public. Their lives might well depend on it.

Effective interorganizational communications were thus critical but also highly problematic. Scientific understanding of how the weaponized anthrax in the deadly letters behaved was evolving rapidly—sometimes from day to day—but not always rapidly enough for the people contending with and potentially endangered by the burgeoning number of suspicious powders. The Centers for Disease Control and Prevention (CDC) struggled to turn out and then update written advisories that reflected the latest guidance from scientific and medical experts. But multiple constituencies had to be informed: physicians, nurses and technicians, first responders, and the general public. Each needed different kinds of information expressed in accessible language appropriate for their tasks and sophistication. CDC was not accustomed to communicating with all of these stakeholders, particularly the first responders. Therefore, senior first response leaders had to find ways of distilling the guidance CDC and other sources sent to high level public health and medical professionals in order to develop safe, practical, operational guidelines for their rank-and-file officers, firefighters, and EMTs.

DISCUSSION QUESTIONS

1. As emergency calls about suspicious white powders began to proliferate in Georgia, what caused the initial confusion and difficulties in handling them?
2. In what ways did various response agencies initially try to cope with the rapidly escalating workload created by anthrax fears? Why did these prove inadequate?
3. What communications issues arose as public health and public safety agencies struggled with the proliferation of suspected anthrax incidents?
4. How did new ways of handling the work flow emerge?
5. What made these innovations effective?

* * *

On Thursday, October 11, 2001, the Fire and Emergency Services of Cobb County, Georgia, were notified that a white powder, feared to contain anthrax spores, had been discovered at a mail processing firm in the north of the county. Just six days earlier, Robert Stevens, a tabloid photo editor in Florida, had died of inhalation anthrax, and coverage of the threat from the disease had quickly gained momentum in the media. In dealing with this suspicious white powder, Cobb appeared better equipped than many of its neighbors. The county had already invested in a fully equipped hazardous materials (hazmat) team, which was immediately dispatched to the scene. Yet, within hours, the situation began to deteriorate rapidly. For as public anxiety over anthrax grew, so did the number of suspicious powders reported. The Cobb hazmat team was used to responding to around eight calls a month, but now, as fear mounted, call volumes reached eight calls an hour at peak times. Try as they might, there was simply no chance that the hazmat team would be able to respond to this level of calls in the timely manner that was so essential.

With hazmat tied up indefinitely, regular fire crews and police officers were dispatched to suspicious powder incidents. However, not having the relevant training, many contaminated themselves with the powder they were supposed to be securing. Others, increasingly alarmed, came close to refusing to respond to the calls altogether. Outside of Cobb County, the situation looked equally desperate. The Georgia state public health authority faced a deluge of calls asking for information and growing demands that it test hundreds of white powder samples. Federal Bureau of Investigation (FBI) agents, detailed by Presidential Directive to investigate alleged domestic terrorism, were often expected to take charge of suspected anthrax samples before they were tested. Yet they too were unprepared for the sheer volume they now faced. Soon, biohazard bags containing suspected anthrax came to litter the personal offices of FBI agents, as they had nowhere else to put them.

As the situation continued to unfold, there was a real risk that both law enforcement and public health officials could be overwhelmed by the wave of emergency calls concerning potentially lethal white powders. The vast majority of these calls were likely to be inconsequential, but any one of them could be extremely dangerous. The challenge for first responders at the federal, state, and local level was to develop and implement new protocols to bring this situation under control, while simultaneously managing an increasingly fearful public and rapidly dropping morale within their own ranks.

EARLY DAYS IN GEORGIA: THE STATE AND THE FBI RESPOND

The Anthrax Attacks Begin

Before September of 2001, there had not been a case of inhalation anthrax in the United States since 1976. Therefore, when Robert Stevens, a photo editor for the *Sun* tabloid in Florida, died of the disease on October 5, 2001, a major investigation was initiated. Unsurprisingly, media interest was intense. On October 10, it was announced that the Stevens case had not originated from natural causes but rather from anthrax spores that had been intentionally planted. Within days, possible new cases were reported in Florida and at NBC News in New York, and an anthrax-tainted letter was soon discovered in Senator Daschle's office on Capitol Hill. The common factor linking many of the victims was contact with mail contaminated with white powder. As reports of anthrax spread throughout the nation, so did heightened anxiety. For many citizens, white powders that previously would have gone unnoticed took on a new and sinister dimension. Very soon, across the country, members of the public began reporting these powders to the authorities.

Existing Protocol in Georgia

In Georgia, as elsewhere, protocol required law enforcement officials to be informed if emergency calls had a potential criminal or terrorist connection. The dispersal or threatened dispersal of anthrax was a crime under both Georgia state law and US federal law. According to Presidential Decision Directive 39, federal responsibility for investigating suspected acts of domestic terrorism rested with the FBI. Consequently, it was the duty of local law enforcement to notify the agency should such an event occur. Prior to 9/11, the bureau had responded to every single such incident and taken charge of the investigation. Furthermore, in Georgia, unlike some states, the FBI had established a working relationship with the Georgia Division of Public Health (GDPH) in relation to the threat from bioterrorism. This originated in Georgia's experience as host of the 1996 Olympic Games but had been maintained through more recent, albeit relatively loose, discussions between the two bodies. The agreed procedure provided that, in the event of the discovery of a suspected biohazard, an FBI agent would go to the scene to investigate.

If the discovery was judged sufficiently credible, a local hazmat responder would package the item and the FBI would then transport it to the Georgia Public Health Laboratory (GPHL), where an authoritative test would be conducted.

Chaos Throughout Georgia

As the first reports of suspicious white powders in Georgia were received immediately after Stevens's death became public, existing protocol came to the fore. In the beginning, the FBI responded as planned. Agents from the bureau arrived on the scene and took a sample back to their offices, before transferring it to the GPHL for testing. However, late in the weekend of October 6 and 7, this approach became unworkable. As public anxiety spread, the volume of suspicious powders being reported exploded, and very soon all available FBI agents were tied up at different locations across the state. Reports of new white powders continued to flood in, and it was clear that the FBI would not be able to respond in person to these reports for days. Given the dangers of anthrax,[1] this sort of delay was simply not an option.

The FBI hazmat coordinator for Georgia was responsible for framing the FBI's response to this unprecedented situation. The FBI knew that eventually most white powder specimens would have to go to the GPHL for testing. However, despite the drain on FBI resources, the FBI decided to continue to act as a filter, investigating the credibility of the suspected anthrax bacteria before transferring it to the laboratory. As the hazmat coordinator recalls: "What we were worried about, more than anything else, was overpowering the laboratory with so many samples that they couldn't actively work on something that might have been really important." It was also important for the law enforcement officials to retain a secure chain of custody in case the powder later ended up in court as part of a criminal prosecution. Nevertheless, says the FBI hazmat team leader: "Public safety was the overriding concern ... the criminal intent side of it became secondary to our real mission at that time."

With these arguments in mind, the FBI changed the response protocols to recognize the practical impossibility of responding to every call, yet retain FBI involvement in processing the samples. In essence, the FBI would continue to respond to as many of the reports as possible, but when there was no agent available to go to the scene in person, first responders would be asked to bring the specimens directly to the FBI office. Yet, even while the FBI formulated this initial response, the protocols were already beginning to evolve in a rather different direction.

---

1. According to CDC, "Anthrax is a serious infectious disease caused by gram-positive, rod-shaped bacteria known as *Bacillus anthracis*.... Although it is rare, people can get sick with anthrax if they come in contact with infected animals or contaminated animal products.... Contact with anthrax can cause severe illness in both humans and animals." See: CDC, "What Is Anthrax?" http://www.cdc.gov/anthrax/basics/index.html.

Bedlam at the Georgia Public Health Laboratory

As possible anthrax spores were reported across the state, the pressure on state agencies to respond increased considerably and, over the weekend of October 6 and 7, differences emerged. The Georgia Emergency Management Agency (GEMA), charged with coordinating responses to emergencies within Georgia, faced a barrage of queries from first responders who wanted to know what to do with the white powder specimens they were collecting. In reply, the agency prepared a fax, which was then sent to the GPHL for approval. Yet, instead of asking for the specimens to be first processed by the FBI, the fax instructed first responders to proceed directly to the state laboratory. Realizing that this contradicted the existing protocols, Dr. Susan Lance-Parker, the epidemiologist on call at the GDPH, contacted GEMA immediately. She remembers:

> We called GEMA and said you can't send this out ..., let us put some language in here that reflects what really should happen, and they said "I don't want to wordsmith with you," and they sent it out anyway.

It later emerged that GEMA believed that it had been given approval by an official lower down in the GDPH hierarchy. In fact, this official had no authority to give such approval and had the impression that he was being asked for a personal opinion. The immediate result was that, as the week of Monday, October 8, began, first responders from all over the state descended upon the GPHL. Of course, the laboratory staff was completely unprepared for such a deluge. It was "absolute bedlam" recalls the director of the laboratory:

> I mean, literally, fire engines pulled up in the parking lot. Emergency vehicles. Guys just kept wandering in and saying, "Here, I've got this stuff for you to test." There was absolutely no sense to it whatsoever. I mean it was everything from sugar to doughnuts, to Cremora, to anything.... It was bizarre.

Within hours, GEMA was made aware of the situation and issued revised guidelines, in line with the FBI protocols, informing first responders that they should take samples directly to the FBI. Considerable use was made of a basic telephone and fax system to communicate this message, allowing the modified guidance to reach first responders across the state very rapidly. Yet, as first responders began to follow these instructions, the pressure that was taken off the public health laboratory was merely transferred to the FBI.

The FBI Overwhelmed

By Tuesday, October 9, the new procedures for transporting anthrax samples to the FBI were being implemented across the state. Consequently, the specimens that FBI agents had been bringing in from the field since the scares began were now joined by scores of new samples, arriving at the office in the custody of first responders. The FBI's task was to process the specimens and try to establish which required higher priority treatment, before transferring them to the state laboratory for testing. Critically, this allowed the FBI to regulate the supply to the laboratory, keeping the test load manageable. Yet it soon emerged that achieving this objective had generated a whole new series of problems.

First, the volume of samples being delivered to FBI headquarters was far greater than the FBI had expected. More importantly, however, FBI headquarters were situated in a regular office building with no facilities for handling suspected biohazards. As the specimens continued to roll in, FBI agents had no choice but to stockpile the sealed biohazard bags containing potential anthrax bacteria on the floor of their offices. Desperate to relieve the backlog, they began to improvise a triage system based on the case history associated with each sample. For some samples, the investigating agents felt confident that there was no anthrax present. In these cases, they would don gloves and open up the specimen for inspection before disposing of it as routine trash. In other cases, the case history suggested that the risk was more serious. These samples were taken directly to the GPHL.

However, before too long the FBI was again forced to rethink its strategy. For one thing, there was increasing discontent at FBI headquarters and among the other businesses in the same office building about the presence of potential anthrax bacteria and the dangers of contamination. The FBI agents involved understood these concerns, which were echoed by the state laboratory director. She recalls:

> I was very concerned when I found out that they were storing and opening triple-bagged packages that had potential anthrax.... I said, "We've got these things called biological safety cabinets where you can safely handle the specimens."... It's for the safety of the persons handling the specimens as well as for the security and the validity of the specimen so you can say, if anything ever goes to court, that there was no opportunity for contamination. I mean, you have to test a valid specimen.

And then, driven by the growing complaints of others in the office, the managers at the Georgia FBI field office intervened. The hazmat coordinator received a call on his cell phone and was advised that it was no longer acceptable to bring samples into the office. Instead FBI management had ordered a large steel CONEX container to be placed outside the FBI offices. From then on, the anthrax operations were to be confined to the parking lot.

Toward a Solution: the FBI and the Georgia Public Health Laboratory Join Forces

While this might have reassured those working in the FBI building, it did little to mitigate the risk to the FBI team. This concern and the prospect of being exiled from his office during a chilly Georgia fall led the hazmat coordinator to reconsider the position once again. Initially, he contemplated the idea of using a nearby FBI warehouse to triage the samples, but realized that this did not resolve the FBI's complete lack of suitable equipment. The only place where such equipment could be found was the state laboratory. Having ruled out all other options, the FBI appealed for help to the lab's director. The hazmat coordinator recalls the conversation:

> I said, "Is there some place here in your laboratory where we can set up, and receive and evaluate and determine what's going to be tested and what's not going to be tested?" And she said, "Yes, we have a training laboratory that's not being used right now and we will be glad to open that up for you and activate phone lines." And, I was ecstatic because the Bureau wasn't at that point geared up to help us in that regard. They were involved in investigations and interviews and a lot of other type of things.... So basically, we became autonomous from the office and set up our own operation.

Consequently, the CONEX container in the FBI parking lot was never used. Instead, beginning on Wednesday, October 10, there began an unparalleled cooperative effort between the GDPH and the FBI.

A Secure Triage Operation

Over the latter part of that week, an FBI hazmat team physically moved into the building housing the GPHL. The training laboratory became the base for a secure triage operation, which allowed the FBI to assess the threat posed by each suspicious powder before deciding whether to pass it to the main laboratory for testing. The first stage of this threat assessment took place over the telephone. Four telephone lines were activated to deal with anthrax-related calls from local first responders and the public. To determine the level of risk associated with each call, an interview process was developed. Callers would first be asked whether there was actually a substance present, as sometimes people reported envelopes and packages they considered suspicious, even if there was no white powder evident. If there was a white powder, thought was given as to whether there was a plausible innocent explanation for its presence. If not, the caller would be asked if there was a written threat accompanying the powder and whether anyone who had come into contact with it was displaying medical symptoms. Consideration was also given as to whether the supposed victim was a likely target for terrorists.

Threats were deemed to be most credible if all these questions were answered in the affirmative. However, on many occasions there was no threat, no symptoms, and maybe even no powder. In this case, the FBI would reassure callers, explain that the item did not need to be tested and advise them of how to dispose of it to put their mind at rest. This helped calm the public and saved the FBI team from evaluating in person every single suspicious powder. Toward the end, once they had mastered the phone triage process, the FBI team was rejecting upward of 75% to 80% of powders. The specimens that were considered more credible threats were brought to the training laboratory and handed over to the FBI.

Newly arriving samples had to be accompanied by a chain of custody form and an official police incident report, detailing the circumstances under which the sample was discovered, which was important background information for a more detailed threat assessment. To assess the sample, an agent would gown up and enter the laboratory's secure area. A biological safety cabinet would be activated and the agent would start opening the package to evaluate whether or not the sample was a powder and whether or not it could be explained. Only if no explanation could be found and the substance was not obviously something other than anthrax spores, would the specimen be deemed sufficiently credible to be tested by the GPHL staff.

In implementing the secure triage operation, the FBI initially received substantial support from the GPHL. The laboratory director recalls: "We provided them with lab coats, masks, gloves, all the laboratory equipment they needed, a technologist who was familiar with using biological safety cabinets, and training." Once implemented, the FBI completed the required training in just a day. However, the laboratory staff continued to work with the FBI agents on a regular basis. "We wanted to keep an eye on them" says the laboratory director, who arranged for technologists to monitor agents when working under biological hoods. The agents, new to these techniques, were grateful for the oversight. All in all, it took around five days for the basic procedures to be established and two weeks to ensure things were running smoothly.

Testing only those powders judged credible helped ensure that the workload for the laboratory remained manageable. While anthrax became a priority, the GPHL also had to continue in its usual role, providing screening, diagnostic, and reference laboratory services for a range of health care professionals in Georgia. The laboratory's regular workload included testing clinical human samples for sexually transmitted diseases, tuberculosis, and HIV, as well as providing laboratory support for epidemiological investigations into a range of diseases more common than anthrax, such as influenza and rabies. Overall, the GPHL performed around 2.4 million tests each year. Numerically speaking, therefore, the tests they were asked to conduct on suspected anthrax bacteria, which eventually numbered around 600, were insignificant. Nevertheless, testing for anthrax bacteria was not something the laboratory was used to doing every day. Setting up and implementing new testing procedures required staff members to put in grueling hours. Ultimately, however, this did not prove an insurmountable task. Recalls the lab director: "There were two or three nights when several of us didn't get much sleep ... but we absorbed [the anthrax testing] into our regular workload. Everything went out on time. There was no delay in our routine work."

THE CRISIS COMES TO COBB COUNTY

Cobb County: Background

Cobb County is one of 159 counties in the state of Georgia. Cobb is located directly north-east of Atlanta, Georgia's capital city, with much of the county considered metro-Atlanta. Encompassing some 345 square miles, it was Georgia's 81st largest county geographically; yet with around 615,000 people in the early 2000s, it was the state's third most populous. Marietta, Cobb's main city, was situated in the center of the county and had a population of some 58,000. Cobb's other major cities included the second most populous city, Smyrna, Acworth and Kennesaw in the north, and Powder Springs and Austell in the south.

The county had one of the largest fire and emergency departments in Georgia. In 2001, Cobb County fire headquarters, the nerve center for 27 fire stations up and down the county, was located on a newly constructed government parkway in Marietta. The department employed around 600 men and women and was headed by the Fire Chief, who answered to the Public Safety Director. Through the County Manager, the Public Safety Director was ultimately accountable to the Board of Commissioners. Law enforcement in Cobb was split between a police department whose Chief was also accountable to the Public Safety Director and a Sheriff's department. The Sheriff was directly elected by the people of Cobb but accountable to the Board of Commissioners for budgetary purposes.

Dealing With Biohazards Prior to 9/11

Prior to September 11, 2001, there had never been a report of suspected anthrax in Cobb County. During the late 1990s, there had been a handful of anthrax hoaxes at abortion clinics in the counties that bordered Cobb and 1999 had seen a well-publicized scare at the offices of NBC News in Atlanta. Ultimately, however, no anthrax spores had been found. Although Cobb had been largely unaffected by these events, the county's emergency management officials had still given considerable attention to the dangers posed by hazardous materials.

Cobb's fire department was one of the very few in Georgia with a hazmat division, made up of 36 highly trained technicians. These technicians were prepared to deal with a variety of hazardous materials, from gasoline spills right through to radioactive material, chemical agents, and biohazards. Established procedures required that whenever a suspected hazardous material was reported, the 12-member hazmat unit on duty would be dispatched to the scene. Past experience suggested that incidents involving hazardous materials would be rare, allowing them to be handled by one hazmat team. Indeed, before 9/11, the team was called out to about eight calls concerning potential hazardous materials of any nature each month. Although Fire Chief Rebecca Denlinger had considered investing in more teams, analyzing the costs and benefits of allocating more of the fire department's limited budget to this purpose led her to conclude that a second team could not be justified. In 1998, however, Denlinger decided to upgrade the basic hazmat training all firefighters received, admitting that the possibility of a terrorist attack was one of the driving forces behind her decision.[2] This operations level training was not designed to be comprehensive but instructed firefighters on the need to isolate any suspected hazardous materials and wait for the full hazmat team to arrive.

The Lason Company: Cobb's First Incident

The emergency services of Cobb County received their very first white powder call on Thursday, October 11, about a week after the nation's first anthrax fatality. An employee at the Lason mail processing plant, in the city of Kennesaw, became alarmed by an apparently inexplicable white powder on a piece of mail. 9-1-1 was notified and, following the existing procedure for the discovery of potentially hazardous material, the Cobb hazmat team was immediately dispatched. Given the potential terrorist connection, Cobb police were also informed. Those who may have come into contact with the powder were ordered to remain in the building. Once the 12 hazmat technicians were on the scene, some donned fully protective moon suits, respirators, and oxygen tanks and entered the building to take samples of the white powder. Others set up decontamination shower units and verified that proper safety procedures were being followed. Meanwhile, detectives from Cobb Police notified the FBI and started to interview those at the scene. Initial onsite tests carried out by the hazmat team proved negative for anthrax. However, given the potential for error in onsite testing, the powder was still handed over to the FBI, to be assessed and tested at the GPHL if required.

From the point of view of the Cobb County fire department, this response, which took about four hours in all, was highly successful. Existing procedures had been followed to the letter. The suspicious powder had been effectively isolated, tested, and had proved negative. But this was only the beginning. In a matter of days, the Cobb hazmat team would be stretched to the breaking point and the emergency response system confronted with an entirely new and frightening dilemma.

Rapid Escalation

Within days of the successful response at the Lason Company, the deluge of white powder calls reached Cobb. Chief Denlinger recalls the sheer magnitude of the situation: "We went from zero to 100 almost overnight.... We experienced the highest sustained

---

2. Doug Payne, "Hazardous Materials Training Gets Upgrade," *The Atlanta Journal and Constitution*, May 28, 1998, 3JG.

level of calls for service in our history." Existing protocols required the full hazmat team to respond to each call, but faced with such volume, there was no way that the team would be able to respond in a timely manner: "People would have been waiting for months." With the hazmat team tied up indefinitely, managers on the ground began to improvise their own responses, leading to regular fire crews and police officers being dispatched to white powder calls. Very soon, these improvised responses began to cause serious problems.

With little training and only their regular firefighting equipment, many firefighters became increasingly alarmed. Deputy Chief Sam Heaton headed operations for Cobb fire department at the time and remembers the anxiety that began to develop: "Earlier on, I think all of our people were concerned, because they were really no different from the citizens that were being potentially harmed by whatever." Lieutenant Chris Sobieski, who was further down the command hierarchy, yet would eventually play a key role in finding a solution to the crisis, puts it more bluntly:

> We had [fire] engine crews that were ready to rebel because they were going to these white powder calls.... These guys aren't trained hazardous materials technicians, and they said, "It's not our job." And, I agreed with them. It's not their job.

By Sunday, October 14, Heaton faced persistent questioning from an anxious staff, desperate for information on how to deal with white powder calls. Firefighters were unsure as to what protective equipment they should use, whether they could keep their uniforms after coming into contact with a white powder, and what they should tell concerned citizens. At this early stage, Heaton was frustrated that he had little firm guidance to give them. He feared that the situation was getting out of hand: "I felt that if we didn't do something that night, right away, that our people were going to, well, I didn't know what they were going to do."

However, if the situation was alarming for regular firefighters, there was even greater concern at the Cobb police department. While firefighters had basic training and equipment, the police department had none. Yet they too were being asked to respond to cases of suspected anthrax and, in the minds of some, risk their lives in the process. Recalls Major John Howser:

> The problem with the white powder calls, first of all, was lack of training on behalf of the Police Department. We really didn't have any protocol on how to handle white powder, really what the risks were, how to gather that evidence, once it was gathered, whether or not it would be tested and where to test it.

One consequence of this was that in responding to calls, police officers regularly contaminated themselves with the white powders that they were supposed to be investigating. During a response to an early white powder incident, Deputy Chief Allred of Cobb Police's detective division recalls a disturbing phone call: "One of the detectives called me and said, 'we can't leave. They won't let us leave.' They didn't know what to do.... At that time our detectives were kind of semi-quarantined up there. So it was quite alarming." While some officers continued to respond to the calls, others began to have serious second thoughts.

Immediate Steps

As Chief of Cobb Fire Service, the agency charged with addressing hazardous materials within the county, Denlinger felt a responsibility to find a way to respond. She had been out of town from October 11 through October 13 and so was not made aware of the situation until Sunday, October 14, when Battalion Chief George Lehner, the hazmat team leader, reported the immense backlog facing his team. Her immediate reaction was one of frustration: "I was made aware of the problem without the team suggesting a solution." Denlinger then consulted with other fire command staff, including Sam Heaton, and soon understood the growing severity of discontent amongst her firefighters. She tried calling fire chiefs in neighboring counties, but she discovered that they were having the same problems and also had no solutions. Cobb fire department was on its own and the situation was deteriorating rapidly. Already, Denlinger was running into new problems, many of them with an increasingly anxious police department. She recalls:

> It was immediately apparent that one of our biggest operational problems was that the police department trusted no one.... In fact that first evening I spent some time on the phone with a sergeant who was running the evening shift in East Cobb trying to convince him that they should take a sample for us to the public health laboratory. And they didn't want anything like that anywhere near any of their police cars.

Denlinger soon realized that such ad hoc interventions would be far from sufficient to resolve the crisis. It was clear that a more creative and fundamental solution was required. Among the top staff, Denlinger had the most hazardous materials experience and so she resolved personally to lead the search for this solution. Aware of the urgency of the situation, she told Lehner and Heaton to bring whatever guidance they could find and meet at her house later Sunday evening.

Dual Main Priorities

At the time of this meeting, Cobb's protocol for responding to white powders remained based on the need for the hazmat team to respond in full to each and every incident. Although no real anthrax bacteria had been discovered in Cobb so far, the volume of calls reporting suspicious substances had increased so that, at peak times, several reports were being received each hour. Attempts to use regular firefighters or police officers to respond to such unprecedented volume appeared unworkable and risked mutiny among first responders. Meanwhile, the white powder calls continued to roll in.

Given this situation, the task facing the group was twofold. First, it had to decide how to address the immediate situation. Heaton argued that it was imperative to get as much information out to his firefighters as soon as possible. In particular, his staff needed to know what measures they could take to mitigate the risks to their personal safety. The group sorted through the guidance in front of them and distilled the more useful elements. This included basic information concerning the nature of anthrax infection, the ability of firefighters' equipment to provide protection against the disease, and the importance of washing with copious amounts of soap and water after dealing with suspect items. Details such as this helped counter the wilder speculation in the media concerning the threat from anthrax and were communicated immediately. Says Heaton:

> It seemed like it was 9:00 at night that I was sending things out to the field that we had so far.... I felt a lot of pressure from the field to put something out there.

Yet, the group realized that while the provision of information was a vital start, at best it would calm anxious firefighters, giving them some confidence in responding to minor incidents.

The second task, therefore, was to develop new protocols for an efficient, yet safe response to more credible reports of anthrax, allowing samples to be collected and fed into the FBI triage system at the state laboratory. Here, Denlinger took the lead. Her premise was that the vast majority of suspicious white powders were probably the result of over-anxious citizens rather than a genuine terrorist attack. Nevertheless, there remained a risk that there could be anthrax out there and so no report could be simply ignored. The heart of the problem was that the existing procedures only provided for two extremes in responding to a suspicious powder: either a regular first responder could attend or the full 12-member hazmat team would be sent. Denlinger believed that the key was to introduce a new way to respond, which would fit in between these two extremes.

In seeking a solution, the group drew on a number of sources. These included the protocols from the FBI, the existing guidelines followed by George Lehner's hazmat team, and a wealth of ideas that Denlinger had picked up during her participation in the Executive Session on Domestic Preparedness at Harvard University. Taken together, these sources led the group to the idea of carrying out an initial threat assessment of supposedly suspicious white powders before deciding how to respond to them. This process of threat assessment could be based on similar principles to those being used by the FBI. Thus, an envelope considered suspicious by a member of the public but with no white powder present would be considered the least dangerous threat, whereas a white powder accompanied by an overt threat would be taken far more seriously. Instead of simply dispatching the full hazmat team to every incident, assessing the threat first would allow only the more credible reports to receive such a resource-intensive level of response.

At this stage, Denlinger envisaged some form of fire department response for every suspected anthrax call. For the least credible threats, essentially those with no powder present, regular firefighters could respond, while the most credible reports with a substance and a clear, overt threat would still require a full hazmat response. However, many calls fell between these two extremes, featuring some sort of powder, but no overt threat. For these calls, Denlinger suggested a new approach, based on a response protocol already operating in New York City. Months earlier, this had been explained to her during a meeting of the Executive Session on Domestic Preparedness by Jack Fanning, who had been head of New York's hazmat team before losing his life in the 9/11 attacks. Following Fanning's approach, Denlinger proposed the creation of a team comprised of one trained hazmat technician and a representative from the law enforcement community. Once on the scene, this biological response team (BRT) could carry out a more detailed assessment of the potential threat and law enforcement could determine whether a criminal investigation was warranted. If the team judged the threat to be particularly high, they would be able to call in the full hazmat team for support. If they considered the threat to be of a lower order, the hazmat technician could take a sample of the powder and the law enforcement officer would liaise with the FBI to feed this specimen into their testing operation.

The next day, Denlinger mentioned the basic element of her proposal at a meeting at the County Manager's Office, which had been called to discuss a broad spectrum of potential terrorist threats to Cobb County. Present were David Hankerson, the County Manager; James Arrowood, the Director of Public Safety; and high-ranking officials from a wide range of Cobb's governmental agencies, including the police department, the 9-1-1 service, and the water authority. Denlinger's contribution was only one of many, but little objection was raised by those present, and she resolved to flesh out the concept in more detail. In doing this, there was a number of contacts that Denlinger wished to consult.

INTERACTING WITH OTHERS: COBB LOOKS FOR GUIDANCE

Liaising With the Georgia Division of Public Health

During her meeting at the County Manager's Office, Denlinger had stressed the importance of involving the GDPH. Her next step was to do just that. In seeking guidance from the GDPH during the week of October 15, Denlinger's timing was fortunate. By this stage, the GDPH staff had been dealing with requests for information from other first responders, already inundated with white powder calls, for around a week. As a consequence, Denlinger found the situation at the GDPH to be busy, but under control. Yet, during the previous week, things had been very different. Dr. Susan Lance-Parker, charged with responding to the first calls for information over the weekend of October 6 and 7, remembers a chaotic time:

> I mean, it was really incredible, they were coming in through our answering service.... And you know, I would hang up the phone and I'd have [more calls waiting], and while I was on the phone call, my pager would go off three or four times. There would be lines of people.

First responder after first responder wanted to know how to collect specimens, what sort of personal protection was needed, and what they should do with the specimen. Yet, initially, Dr. Lance-Parker and the other experts at the GDPH had little clear information to provide. Normally, the GDPH would look to the Centers for Disease Control and Prevention (CDC), a federal agency based in Atlanta, for guidance, but on this occasion CDC remained silent.

A Quiet CDC

Dr. Kathleen Toomey, who had worked at CDC before her appointment as Public Health Director for Georgia, describes the problem as she saw it:

> There was not quick easy information flow from CDC to us as to what to do. And part of that just had to do with the way CDC works. CDC is a bureaucracy. You have to pass information up and get it approved.

Structural issues aside, CDC officials explained that at the beginning of the crisis, the FBI had refused to release important information, fearing that it might prejudice the criminal investigation. This, it was suggested, had made it difficult to issue reliable guidelines in the early stages.[3] However, in reality, the roots of CDC's slow initial response went far deeper. Dr. Rich Meyer, the head of CDC's rapid response laboratory, suggests that, on one hand, CDC was more prepared to deal with anthrax than practically any other agent. Anthrax was considered a likely agent for bioterror and prior to 9/11 there had been hoaxes, largely at abortion clinics, with false claims of anthrax propagation. CDC had investigated these hoaxes and learned from them. Yet, now CDC faced an entirely new situation, which few had foreseen. Says Dr. Meyer:

> Nobody ever had an idea that someone would simply take *Bacillus anthracis* spores, place them into a postal envelope, and then put it into a mailbox. And that's what they did. I mean, how simple can you get?

Existing preparedness programs had been largely based on military modeling, which envisaged large-scale releases. Addressing the very different complications associated

---

3. Charles Seabrook, "Backgrounder: CDC: Germ Hunters' Home Base Is Leader in Anthrax Fight," *Atlanta Journal-Constitution*, October 23, 2001, 6A.

with anthrax in the mail would take time. Eventually, considerable progress was made. Later in October, CDC mounted a substantial information campaign with top officials making numerous public appearances. They also produced a special broadcast dealing with the anthrax threat, which was viewed by 100,000 health professionals.

As the scare began, however, CDC had little to offer the first responders, the medical workers, and the members of the public who were desperate for information. In Georgia, citizens were looking to the GDPH for help, and Dr. Toomey felt her department had to respond: "We were the State. And if we weren't going to get clear guidance from CDC, *we* were going to have to do it and set the parameters." Prior to the white powder crisis, she had worked tirelessly to impress upon traditional first responders the importance of involving the GDPH in addressing the terrorist threat. Her appointment to the Georgia Homeland Security Taskforce, a body that brought together different agencies from across Georgia to consider the terrorist threat, suggested that her efforts had paid off. But now she faced a real challenge. She says: "I felt like this was our chance to step up to the plate. And we either would do a good job and have credibility or we would not be trusted again."

The Georgia Division of Public Health Steps Up to the Plate

Dr. Toomey's first step was to ask Dr. Cherie Drenzek, an epidemiologist at the GDPH, to conduct her own study of the medical literature on the issue, which would then be fed into the guidelines that were being given out over the phone. However, the GDPH staff felt they could do more. Specifically, they were eager to find a way to diminish the torrent of anxious phone calls, rather than dealing with each one as it came in. They had noticed early on that the phone inquiries they were receiving were largely the same questions, but coming from different people across the state. Building on this, Dr. Drenzek suggested that they could issue written guidelines, with answers to all the common questions, which could then be widely disseminated. While reluctant to implement this idea early on because they feared contradicting any similar offering from CDC, when CDC seemed unwilling to act, they decided to go ahead.

Therefore, around a week after the GDPH had first been inundated with requests for information, Dr. Drenzek drafted three separate documents for the GDPH's three main audiences. The first was for hospital clinical laboratories, which were increasingly concerned as to how to conduct primary clinical work-ups on suspected anthrax patients. The second was for physicians and contained advice on how to treat patients who claimed exposure to white powders, and the third was for use by first responders. The first responder document was based on the threat assessment approach being used by the FBI to determine the level of risk involved. It thus contained two main sections, which distinguished between how to respond to suspicious letters and packages, accompanied or unaccompanied by white powders and written threats, and how to respond to suspicious substances not associated with letters or packages. To this framing, Dr. Drenzek added information "from the literature primarily about hazardous materials response or personal protective equipment … and from laboratory diagnosis." The result was a document that made specific recommendations, ranging from disposing of substances as routine garbage, should the risk be very low, through to the details of personal protective equipment needed for taking a sample, should the risk be high. These protocols were then distributed using e-mail and personal contacts and were also posted on the GDPH Web site.

DEVELOPING COBB'S APPROACH

Conveniently for Cobb, the early versions of these protocols became available in the week beginning October 15, around the same time that Denlinger was seeking the GDPH's guidance. As she reflected on the protocols, Denlinger became increasingly encouraged. The GDPH's decision to adopt an approach based on threat assessment fitted well with her proposals for a BRT. During the week, she continued to refine the idea through liaising with her own staff, especially George Lehner and his hazmat technicians, as well as studying the latest guidance coming from the GDPH and other outside sources such as the FBI. Later that week, Denlinger decided to seek the input of her second Deputy Chief, Mike Ellington. One of Ellington's responsibilities was to chair a working group, bringing together Cobb's first responders, to address the threat from terrorism. Denlinger wanted to ask the group for their opinion of the BRT idea. Little did she know that they were already working on a solution almost identical to her own.

The Planning and Intelligence Working Group

Shortly after 9/11, the Cobb County Manager had brought together department heads and other key individuals involved in preparing for the threat of terrorism in Cobb County to establish the Cobb County Domestic Preparedness Task Force. Early on, the Task Force decided to create a smaller Planning and Intelligence Working Group in order to deal with the details of responding to the terrorist threat. This working group was to be convened and headed by Deputy Fire Chief Ellington and responsible to Cobb's Director of Public Safety, James Arrowood. From the start, Ellington was clear on the sort of people he needed on the group. He suggests that he was looking for "individuals that I knew had particular expertise [and] that I thought were very intelligent within the disciplines that they represented." Critically, the working group was to be broad enough to ensure all views were represented, but small enough to enable it to remain manageable. The eventual size of the group was six people, with representation from Cobb Fire, Cobb Police, Cobb Sheriff, Public Health, and the fire department from the nearby city of Austell.

The Parallel Development of the Biological Response Team

As the problems of the white powder scare became all too clear, Ellington's first thought had been to involve the working group. Its mandate was broad and he believed they were exactly the right people to come up with a solution that would address the concerns and needs of all of Cobb's first responders. During the first week of the crisis, while Denlinger had been searching for a solution with Heaton and Lehner, Ellington and the working group had begun to move toward their own solution.

Although the group made some effort to pull together new information that might help them, its main asset was the experience of its members. According to Major John Houser, who represented Cobb Police on the group: "We did go out and research it over the internet and call other departments, but this was so new, we really didn't have anything else to go by." Other members of the group brought ideas that they had come across more by chance than careful research. Recalls Lieutenant Sobieski, the group's expert from Cobb fire department:

> I was watching TV one night, and I saw New York City [was] getting hit with white powder calls as well. They paired a firefighter hazmat technician with a police officer, and they were going out and investigating all these themselves ... [so] I brought that back to the working group.

Coincidentally, this procedure was the very same one that had been described to Chief Denlinger months earlier by Jack Fanning. Therefore, although they did not know it at the time, both Denlinger and the working group were looking to the same model for guidance. As chair of the group, Ellington took the lead. He began by identifying the problem with the pre-9/11 protocols for dealing with biohazards. Given the evident reality of the situation, his diagnosis was very similar to the one being simultaneously offered elsewhere by Denlinger. In essence, the assumption that reports of suspected biological agents would be few and far between had been exposed as naive. He pointed out that, given the volume of white powder calls, it had become impossible for the hazmat team to respond in full to each incident. However, despite the fact that the vast majority of white powders appeared to be false alarms, the calls could not be ignored as any one of them could still unearth real anthrax bacteria. A new response protocol was needed, which would enable the emergency services to respond to these calls in a swift, yet safe, manner.

In asking the group for ideas, Ellington tried to focus the discussion by asking exactly what the hazmat team did when they responded to a white powder:

> And I finally said, "So what do they do when they go out there? What do they *do*? What is the basic element? What is occurring as a result? What's the end result when they leave?"

Having generated a list of the functions currently carried out by the 12-member hazmat team, the group began to consider the circumstances under which it was necessary to have the team perform these functions and when it might be possible to have a less resource-intensive response.

Toward a New Protocol

Like Denlinger, the working group embraced the need to incorporate the principle of threat assessment into Cobb's response to suspicious white powders. According to John Houser, it was simple common sense to require an initial evaluation of the threat and the risks involved. This evaluation would be based on the FBI's distinctions between the high threat situations, where a powder was accompanied by an overt threat and medical symptoms, and the low threat scenarios where a powder might not even be present. The results of the threat assessment would form the basis of a new tiered response system, with a different level of response depending on the perceived risks involved. As more was found out about the threat, the response level could be swiftly escalated or reduced. A tiered response would also allow every citizen, if sufficiently worried about a white powder, to have his or her concerns addressed in person by the emergency services. Addressing public anxiety was a key goal for the new system. Says Ellington: "The citizens were really afraid. And without some sort of official response, it would have a damaging effect on the community." Having agreed to this principle, the group moved further than Denlinger had done in determining the most appropriate contribution from each of Cobb's first responder agencies to the various levels of response.

To Sobieski, it was clear that regular firefighters should have no role in responding to potential anthrax. He recalls:

> We needed to take those responsibilities completely away from the engine companies.... You would have as many as seven, eight engines tied up on these white powder calls. Somebody's having a heart attack down the street, and they're handling talcum powder.... That was probably one of my biggest concerns, as well as the feeling that we're asking people to do something that they're not trained to do.

In contrast with Denlinger's initial assumption that all suspicious white powder calls would need a fire department response, the working group agreed that calls assessed as posing a very low or noncredible threat would receive a Level 1 response, which required only the dispatch of a regular police officer. If the police officer felt uncomfortable when arriving on the scene, or if the threat was judged to be more credible, the response would be escalated to Level 2.

To handle reports designated as Level 2, Sobieski argued for the creation of a new BRT, along the lines of the response adopted by New York that he had seen on television. This was essentially the same concept that was being developed independently by Chief Denlinger. The working group agreed that the fire department's contribution to this team would be one trained hazmat technician, the police department would contribute one police officer, who would take charge of any investigation and liaise with the FBI, and the Sheriff's Office would provide one crime scene technician. The involvement of a crime scene technician was crucial, as the dispersal or threatened dispersal of anthrax bacteria is a crime under both federal and Georgia state law. Taking photographs of the scene and preserving the necessary evidence is thus essential. While the Cobb Police department did have some crime scene technicians, there were far more available in the Sheriff's department. Making use of them helped reduce the strain on police resources. All members of the proposed team would be given appropriate training and upgraded personal protective equipment.

Sobieski's original idea called for a permanent BRT, with the required personnel together in a car all day long, waiting for and responding to the white powder calls. However, this idea met strong resistance on the grounds that it would be too demanding on resources. Instead, the group agreed that the BRT would come together only when calls demanded it. Although each department would always have a specific staff member on call for the BRT, this staff member would only assume his or her BRT duties once a call came in. The pool of staff who served on the BRT would be kept small to concentrate the risk on a few carefully trained personnel and ease the fears of the vast majority of first responders. Once notified of the call, each BRT member would convene on the location of the white powder. If the BRT agreed that the threat was credible, they could either collect samples for the FBI and Georgia state laboratory to process, or in a particularly high-risk scenario, they could escalate the response further and call in the full hazmat team.

IMPLEMENTING COBB'S NEW APPROACH

Early Difficulties

While the details of this proposal were not finalized for several days, the working group's main ideas were already clear when Denlinger checked in with Ellington, later in the week of October 15. Although surprised to learn that Ellington had launched his own efforts to solve the crisis without eliciting her views first, Denlinger was pleased to discover that she and the working group were essentially of one mind. She also welcomed their attempts to draw on the resources of all of Cobb's first responder agencies. In her opinion, the obvious next step was to put these ideas into practice. Yet, she soon discovered that it was not quite as simple as that. Implementing the BRT proposals would require considerable cooperation between Cobb's first responders, and not everyone was ready to make the new commitment. At this early stage, Denlinger recalls significant resistance to the idea from Cobb police, who were still attempting to come to terms with the threat posed by anthrax. On the ground, few officers were ready to cooperate. "It was a new area for us," says Detective Steve Brawner. Cobb police had no protective equipment, but more importantly, no training or experience in dealing with an invisible killer. Armed suspects were usually the most deadly threat officers could expect to face. In this situation, recalls Brawner, the procedure was clear: "I confront [and] I neutralize if I can.... But something you can't see, you can't confront." Addressing the threat from anthrax required an entirely different mindset and this would take time to develop.

Furthermore, new operating procedures that involved first responders from different jurisdictions working together would require the approval of Denlinger's boss, James Arrowood, Cobb County's Director of Public Safety. In the beginning, the urgency of implementing the BRT concept seemed a hard sell. Denlinger recalls:

> The difficulty was, of course, I don't have authority over the police officer and the crime scene technicians, so I needed the Director to tell them to do this. That was very difficult. He did immediately agree that we needed to talk about it, but it didn't seem to be a pressing concern.

The reluctance of the Director of Public Safety to agree to immediate implementation became a source of intense frustration to Denlinger. "I started chasing him around," she recalls. "I began to despair that he was ever going to see the light." Yet, while attempts to implement the BRT from the top stalled, lower down the first responder hierarchy change was already underway.

The Evolution of a New Response Protocol

Although the BRT proposals were not officially sanctioned for several weeks, the idea soon took on a life of its own. As reports of white powders continued to flow in, the excessive burden on the hazmat team began to show. Says George Lehner, hazmat team leader: "We were getting slammed. The guys were getting fatigued and it was affecting morale." For the fire department, doing nothing was no longer an option. "Everybody on the ground knew something had to change," recalls Denlinger. She resolved to push ahead with the BRT idea with or without her director:

> We used the concept before it had been fully approved. We went ahead and used it ... and so, bit by bit, it began to take hold. But, because it hadn't become part of doctrine or anything, there were people who resisted it, people who weren't aware of it, and we couldn't put it out, this is what we're going to do, because I didn't have the authorization to do that....
> So it was remarkable to watch it happen.

As the BRT response slowly evolved, Mike Ellington's working group became critical to bringing other first responders besides the fire department on board. Not only were the members of the group the authors of the BRT but they also became its key proponents within Cobb's different first responder agencies.

The first element of a tiered response system was implemented on October 18, when the Cobb 9-1-1 service began to conduct some elementary triage on calls concerning suspicious substances. If a caller reported a suspicious letter or package, the call would be designated 54T, which required only the dispatch of a regular police officer. However, if the letter or package was accompanied by an unknown substance, the call would be designated PDFD, signifying the need for a response from both the police department and the fire department. In the case of a very credible risk, 9-1-1 was able to dispatch the full hazmat team. This system incorporated the element of threat assessment directly into the emergency response system, exactly in line with the tiered response idea put forward by the Planning and Intelligence Working Group. Although the 9-1-1 tiered system made no mention of a BRT, through informal channels, the PDFD level of response gradually evolved into something very similar to the BRT concept. According to Mike Ellington:

> There were numerous white powder calls that were managed with the BRT before BRT was formally established.... In many instances, [9-1-1 operators] were contacting me when they had white powder calls. And I would say "Go ahead and send the BRT," or "Contact the following individuals. And they will manage this situation." It took a while to formalize it.

Critical to persuading other first responders to participate in the BRT response was the provision of information concerning the dangers posed by anthrax. As more information became available, first responders would be more aware of how to handle potential anthrax bacteria safely and be more confident in managing the associated risks. In ensuring this occurred as swiftly and efficiently as possible, the Planning and Intelligence Working Group soon took center stage.

Improving Information Flow

By Friday, October 19, two weeks after the first death from anthrax had sparked heightened anxiety nationwide, Cobb County was beginning to bear up to the crisis. Although the BRT concept had not been approved by the county's senior hierarchy, the 9-1-1 service had officially implemented a tiered response system for reports of white powders, which were being received at the rate of around 10 each day. On the ground, attempts to provide first responders with the latest information on how to handle the threat from anthrax continued, but this effort was becoming increasingly difficult. The essential problem concerned both the quantity and the nature of the information that was now being received.

While early on information may have been scarce, by this stage the volume of guidance being received by Cobb's first responders had increased massively. Many senior staff, who faced pressure to provide information to those on the ground, simply did not have the time to sort through everything they were sent. For example, Denlinger remembers receiving a deluge of information from the FBI, GDPH, CDC, GEMA, the US Postal Service, US Fire Administration, and the International Association of Fire Chiefs among others. While she was grateful for the information, she was often critical of the form in which it appeared:

> It would be blah, blah, blah, blah, negative information. Blah, blah, blah, blah, blah, negative, and a lot of it was written in government language, and it was just very difficult to make sure that you picked all the plums out of it.

Furthermore, as more became known about the threat from anthrax, the guidance that bodies such as the GDPH were providing needed to change to reflect this. Often, the GDPH had to reissue its guidelines on a daily basis. While they used color and other formatting tricks to draw attention to the most recent changes, it was still often difficult for those receiving the information to keep up.

It was here that the Planning and Intelligence Working Group stepped in and assumed the burden of processing information concerning the threat from the disease. By the start of the week beginning October 22, this effort was in full flow. "Initially we met every morning to review some of the intelligence that was coming in," says Ellington, "and for Cobb County's purposes, we would issue an opinion." This opinion was included in a situation report (SITREP) that the group would put out as often as necessary. From October 22 right through to early November, the SITREP appeared every day and was circulated widely amongst all the first responder agencies in Cobb County. In the police department, for example, the SITREP was sent directly to each precinct commander who then disseminated the latest information to the officers in the field during their daily briefing.

The working group also had a role in providing information to an increasingly anxious public. One of its first steps in this regard was to compile a short pamphlet addressing the threat from anthrax and describing what constituted a suspicious package and how it should be handled. However, in general, Cobb's information policy sought to deal with requests for information rather than actively distributing the latest news. "Typically, we would primarily just respond to inquiries from the media," says Ellington, with the key aim being to reassure people that the anthrax threat was being taken seriously and there was a plan in place to deal with it. In the police department, contact with the media was also carried out judiciously. On occasion, involving the media was crucial. "If there is something to it," says Steve Brawner, "we'll take steps, and the media will be the first one we call." Yet Brawner was conscious that media reports of the latest white powder calls would be "food for thought for tomorrow's calls." Unless the public needed to know specific information about the anthrax threat, Brawner did not encourage media coverage of the situation.

Formalizing the Biological Response Team Response

By early November, call volume had reached a new level of intensity, with some 30 or more white powders being reported in Cobb each day. Although under strain, the system continued to function. The reality was that through Ellington's informal network, a BRT-style response had begun to operate within the 9-1-1 center's tiered system for dealing with white powder calls. Officially, the BRT had still not been implemented, but calls designated PDFD by 9-1-1 now usually received a response that was the BRT in all but name.

Meanwhile, attempts to inform, educate, and persuade those higher up in the county hierarchy continued. Throughout the end of October and beginning of November, the Planning and Intelligence Working Group held a series of meetings with heads of departments and agencies to push their plan and continued to build support. On October 26, Director Arrowood took some time away from Cobb to attend a conference, leaving Chief Denlinger in the role of Acting Director of Public Safety until his return on November 2. Given the growing support for the BRT proposal, Denlinger was eager to use her new temporary position to formalize the protocols. However, she soon discovered that as Acting Director she had "responsibility but no authority." Those managing Cobb's first responder agencies seemed unwilling to make the change officially until they had heard it from Arrowood himself. Therefore, deeply frustrated, Denlinger resolved to make herself Arrowood's first appointment on his return to Cobb to explain the need for the BRT once again. After this meeting, she began to press her case with a new intensity, talking to him on a daily basis. Soon these efforts paid off. On November 6, Denlinger was attending a Citizen's Academy Graduation Ceremony, along with Arrowood, and once again presented her argument. She recalls:

> I was standing out in the hall with him. And, all of a sudden, it just turned. I can't even remember what I said … I could see the light come on in his head. "Well, sure, of course we should be doing that." You know, "get right on it!"

With blessing from the top, the BRT-style response was swiftly made explicit and formalized. Finally, it became possible to recruit members to the BRT on an official basis. Participation in these duties was strictly voluntary and members were eligible for overtime pay as required. In the case of the fire department, off-duty hazmat technicians were hired back during the day to run BRT calls. During the night, the lower call volume made it possible to use the regular technicians who were already on duty. There was only ever one BRT in operation at any point and the pool of people who could be drawn on to serve on the team was deliberately kept small. This made it easy to communicate updated information on the anthrax threat to those dealing with the powders as well as concentrating the risk and taking the anthrax burden away from the vast majority of first responders. The fire department provided hazmat training for the law enforcement officers, and specific procedures for handling suspected biohazards were codified. A range of personal protective equipment was provided for BRT members, starting from a basic HEPA mask and nylon gloves right up to full body suit. Those serving on the BRT could decide which pieces of equipment were most appropriate for each incident.

Once formally implemented, the BRT was considered a major success across first responder agencies. "What they did was wonderful," recalls George Lehner, who was grateful that the BRT response left the full hazmat team with only the most credible anthrax threats to deal with. The new BRT fitted neatly into 9-1-1's tiered response system. Says John Houser: 'There was very little tweaking. It worked well." Ann Flynn, the 9-1-1 manager, worked with Houser to explicitly incorporate the working group's proposals within the procedures followed by 9-1-1 operators. In essence, a 54T designation matched a Level 1 response. A Level 2 response, or PDFD, would now require the formal dispatch of the BRT, a Level 3 response required the hazmat team, and a Level 4, signaling the confirmed presence of a biological agent, would require federal involvement. Once the personnel dispatched by 9-1-1 arrived on the scene, they retained the option of either raising or lowering the response level as they saw fit. On the ground, the BRT members soon added experience to their training and were ready and able to change the way they operated accordingly. The fruits of experience were also passed back to the 9-1-1 service, allowing them to fine-tune their triage abilities and gather information that would be useful to those responding to the incident. Ann Flynn recalls that, as a result of feedback from ground: "We added a series of questions … to help identify what was really going on on the scene."

New Relations and New Linkages

Toward the end of November, following her active role in developing Cobb's new protocols, Chief Denlinger was asked to join the Georgia Homeland Security Taskforce. This allowed her to communicate directly with officials at the state level and ensure that the fire department perspective, as she understood it, was expressed. Furthermore, once on the taskforce, Denlinger struck up a close friendship with Dr. Toomey, the only other woman present. "We were natural allies," recalls Toomey. As early as December 4, Dr. Toomey used this new association to try to understand why first responders in the field were not always responding in line with the GDPH protocols. She recalls: "And I thought, well, something's wrong here. Either they're not reading it, they're not getting it, or whatever we're writing isn't making sense." Her solution was to call Chief Denlinger. "And I said, 'Can I come out and see you?' And Dr. Lance-Parker and I went out there. And I said, 'Look, you've got to help us. How can we reframe this in a way that makes sense?'"

Through building on her relationship with Denlinger, Dr. Toomey was able to establish a dialogue between the first responders at the local level and the state department of public health and make changes to the GDPH guidelines as a result. In particular, recalls Dr. Toomey: "We actually changed the language [so that] the document for first responders actually read like something a first responder would understand, rather than something the medical epidemiologist wrote." As the white powder scares began to fade, the relationship between Toomey and Denlinger endured.

Calming Down

By early December 2001, reports of suspicious white powders had dropped dramatically. On average, Cobb County 9-1-1 now received just two such calls each day, a far cry from the 30 or so that were coming in only a month earlier. And during January of 2002, the calls gradually all but petered out. A similar picture was evident at the state level. By December 14, the volume of white powders had diminished sufficiently to allow the FBI to shut down its operation in the public health laboratory. Although the bureau would still be asked to investigate suspicious white powders from time to time, the number of requests was low enough to permit the response to be determined on a case-by-case basis. First responders were still asked to take the specimen directly to the state laboratory but also to notify the FBI, which would then determine whether a criminal investigation was warranted.

As the situation normalized, a startling fact emerged. Despite the hundreds of calls in Cobb County and thousands of calls across Georgia, not one spore of anthrax bacterium had been discovered. Every single reported white powder had either been judged a non-credible threat, or had made it through the FBI triage only to test negative at the state laboratory. Some of those involved in the process wondered how things might have been different had real anthrax bacteria been discovered. In conducting triage, the FBI agents continually had to make judgment calls as to which white powders should be considered credible and which could be dismissed without a laboratory test. The gravity of this decision was not lost on the agents involved, who were well aware of the potentially devastating consequences should they make the wrong choice.

Ultimately, Chief Denlinger believed that the specifics of the situation had played a key role in the successful outcome. In particular, she says: "It helped that there really was no threat to life and limb." Despite the enormous challenges in dealing with anthrax, the bacterium poses fewer problems than many other weapons of mass destruction. Unlike some chemical agents, exposure to anthrax spores does not result in instant death or irreversible harm. Instead, following the infection, the disease develops over a period of days and, in the early stages, remains treatable with antibiotics. "Even if it had been anthrax," says Denlinger, "you still have an opportunity, a window of opportunity, to make up for an error. That won't always be the case."

When Prevention Can Kill: Minnesota and the Smallpox Vaccination Program

Kirsten Lundberg

EDITORS' INTRODUCTION

In the aftermath of the 9/11 jetliner attacks and the anthrax letters in 2001, the United States was on high alert against potential threats. For many, the most glaring bioterrorism vulnerability was the possibility of a devastating epidemic of smallpox—the historic "scourge of mankind" that had been declared eradicated in 1980 after a comprehensive, worldwide public health campaign. No smallpox virus was supposed to exist except for samples kept under tight security at the Centers for Disease Control and Prevention (CDC) in Atlanta, Georgia, and in a similar facility in Russia. However, senior US officials feared that a US enemy—whether a hostile country or nonstate terrorists—might somehow have acquired and weaponized the virus and would use it to launch a deadly attack on the United States. Since Americans had not received routine childhood vaccinations for smallpox since 1972, this meant that a large portion of the population had no immunity to a highly contagious disease that killed about one-third of those who contracted it. No available intelligence indicated that an enemy actually had weaponized smallpox, let alone that an attack was imminent. But it is highly likely that the Bush Administration, pondering the invasion of Iraq that did occur in mid-2003, feared that Saddam Hussein's regime might have that capability, which it could use itself or share with nonstate terrorists.

This case was written by Kirsten Lundberg for Dr. Arnold M. Howitt, Director of the Executive Session on Domestic Preparedness and Executive Director, Taubman Center for State and Local Government, Kennedy School of Government. Funding was provided by the Volpe National Transportation Systems Center, US Department of Transportation, with additional assistance from the Robert Wood Johnson Foundation. (0803)

Vigorous public discussion therefore began in 2002 inside President George W. Bush's administration and among outside advisers about whether the United States should establish a precautionary vaccination program. This case study recounts the national policy-making story and how the president's program played out in a single state.

During much of 2002, as the administration and public health officials considered the smallpox threat, a number of strategic questions arose. How great was the risk of a smallpox attack? How many people should be vaccinated? Fifty thousand public health workers? Five hundred thousand public health and public safety personnel? All Americans? Was such a program wise given the fact that a relatively small percentage of Americans—but a large aggregate number of people—could well experience deadly side effects from the vaccine itself because of adverse reactions or immune system weakness?

By the end of 2002, however, the administration seemed to be resolving those broad questions in favor of a vaccination program. In late November, CDC asked states to submit full plans for pre-event vaccination programs for medical and public health vaccination teams. Then in mid-December, the president formally proposed that 500,000 health workers be vaccinated through a program administered by the states.

The states, however, had the independent authority to decide whether or not they would participate. The program raised many doubts within the country's public health community. As a former director of CDC lamented, noting that the national security justification did not seem strong enough, "if you are going to ask people to use a vaccine with known and significant side effects, then you've got to make a very good case that the risk of exposure to the disease is real, tangible, quantitative and worth the risk you are going to take with your patients."[1]

Moreover, even states that agreed to participate had to confront unresolved program design problems: What would the extent of liability for negative outcomes be—and under what circumstances—for vaccine manufacturers, the hospitals that administered the administration's program, those people who gave vaccinations, and vaccinated individuals who inadvertently shed virus? Who would cover the costs of running vaccination clinics or of time that workers would not be able to report because they might be shedding virus or had become ill?

Beyond these issues, a host of operational problems had to be dealt with. Who would train the health care workers who would administer the vaccinations? Who would develop and supply training materials? Who would care for patients who contracted vaccinia or experienced other side effects of the vaccine? Would adequate supplies of vaccine be available in enough time to meet the federal schedule for completing immunizations? How would liability issues be resolved? Notwithstanding

---

1. Ceci Connolly and Dana Milbank, "US Revives Smallpox Shot," *Washington Post*, December 14, 2002, A1.

language in the new Homeland Security Act about liability, a wide range of detailed questions arose about legal responsibility and compensation that gave states, hospitals, and practitioners pause in agreeing to participate.

More and more doubts accumulated as the program was supposed to be accelerating in early 2003. Labor unions representing health care workers advised their members not to be vaccinated. Prominent medical groups called for a pause in implementation while looming questions were answered and operational issues were resolved. Would the Bush Administration and state-level officials work through and resolve these problems? Would the vaccination program achieve its goals? Or were mounting doubts likely to stifle the program?

DISCUSSION QUESTIONS

1. From the federal perspective, what considerations shaped the way the smallpox vaccination program was designed?
2. How did the smallpox vaccination program look from the perspective of state and local officials and private health institutions?
3. Describe the implementation system—stretching from the federal government to the states and to health care institutions and workers—that Bush Administration officials envisioned would result in achieving the smallpox vaccination program's goals.
4. At each step of this implementation process, what positive and negative incentives faced organizations and individuals responsible for carrying out the program?
5. Could the Bush Administration have improved the program design to increase the likelihood that implementation would prove successful? If so, how? If not, why not?

* * *

In early 2003, the Minnesota Department of Health (MDH) had implemented, on short notice, an ambitious program that deployed public health officials in the fight against terrorism. Despite the misgivings of some key MDH officials, Minnesota had gone ahead with Phase 1 of a federal smallpox vaccination program and inoculated a core group of some 1,400 health care workers, who could vaccinate the general public in the event of a terrorist attack that used smallpox as a weapon.

By mid-March, despite substantial obstacles, Phase 1 was essentially over, and the chief emotion at MDH was relief. The all-out push had exhausted MDH and its local health care partners. Phase 1 had also proven expensive in terms of time, effort, and money. MDH was looking forward to a hiatus during which it could evaluate the effectiveness of Phase 1. MDH did not yet know, for example, whether Phase 1 had even achieved the goal of medical preparedness for a smallpox attack.

But as Phase 1 drew to a close, pressure mounted to move directly into Phase 2: vaccination of first responders (police, fire, and other emergency personnel). In Minnesota, that could mean upward of 200,000 vaccinations. The federal government had announced that states were free to move to Phase 2 at will. The issue came to a head for MDH when the sheriff of Ramsey County, seat of the state capital, St. Paul, demanded that his public safety officials be vaccinated without delay. Failure to do so, he charged, would demonstrate that MDH would protect its own but not those who protected the public.

Minnesota Assistant Health Commissioner Aggie Leitheiser was worried about how those in her department who had handled Phase 1 would respond to the sheriff's request. Virtually no one at MDH wanted to embark yet on Phase 2. While Leitheiser respected the professional judgment of the doctors and public health experts at MDH, she could also see the sheriff's point of view. Leitheiser called a meeting for March 13, 2003, of top MDH officials to discuss the Ramsey County situation. Implicit in the question of how to respond to the sheriff were larger issues. MDH needed to ask itself what constituted preparedness? How many vaccinated people was enough? What job categories were essential? How would MDH define success for the smallpox vaccination program?

SMALLPOX VACCINE POLICY: BACKGROUND

The smallpox vaccination program that Minnesota had implemented had its roots in the events of September 11, 2001. After the suicide hijackings that day and the anthrax attacks of October 2001, the federal government stepped up efforts to prevent terrorist use of biological weapons. The Bush Administration suspected that terrorists, or hostile states like Iraq, might already control stocks of smallpox—a highly contagious disease that the World Health Organization declared eradicated in 1980 but samples of which were preserved in laboratories in the United States and Russia. The US general population was vulnerable to smallpox. Routine vaccinations had stopped in the United States in 1972.[2] Without vaccination, the disease killed one-third of those infected.

In November 2001, the Centers for Disease Control and Prevention (CDC)—which is a branch of the US Department of Health and Human Services (HHS)—published *Smallpox Response Plan and Guidelines*, which it updated in January and again in September 2002. That document laid out what various agencies should do in the event of a smallpox attack. Essentially, it called for mass vaccination against the disease. Even before September 11, HHS had begun to build up its stockpile of vaccine; this process

---

2. The last known case occurred in 1977 in Africa.

accelerated in October 2001. By the end of 2002 or early 2003, HHS expected to have available over 285 million doses.[3]

ACIP Report

Meanwhile, a debate began within government about whether the United States should inoculate—in anticipation of a smallpox attack—some number of health care workers who could vaccinate everybody else if the need arose. This was known as a pre-event vaccination program because individuals would be vaccinated even though there had been no outbreak of disease. Under existing US policy, only scientists and laboratory workers testing smallpox-related viruses received vaccines. Since 1983, only 11,000 Americans had been vaccinated against smallpox.[4]

Some in the health care community advocated immunizing *everyone* in advance of an outbreak because they felt the traditional ring vaccination control and containment model would not work. Under that model, doctors isolated the patient and vaccinated those who had had direct contact with him/her. William J. Bicknell, a Boston University School of Public Health physician and former Massachusetts health commissioner, objected that "ring containment in a terrorist situation has been thoroughly discredited ... and that has not been recognized by CDC."[5] He pointed to Yale University research, which predicted that 1,000 infections would lead to nearly 100,000 deaths in three months if handled by ring containment but to fewer than 1,000 deaths if mass vaccination took place. Yale public health specialist Edward H. Kaplan agreed, commenting that "[u]nless the initial attack is very small and the infectiousness of the agent is quite mild, ring vaccination is not going to do much good."[6]

In search of expert opinion, the government in the spring of 2002 asked a prestigious advisory group to consider whether a pre-event vaccination program made sense and, if so, on what scale. On June 20, 2002, the Advisory Committee on Immunization Practices (ACIP)—which routinely advises CDC and HHS—recommended that a small number of volunteer health care and law enforcement workers in each state be vaccinated against smallpox.[7] This core cadre of smallpox response teams would provide initial care and

---

3. The government still had 15 million doses frozen. It was buying 209 million doses from the Cambridge, England, firm of Acambis. The drug company Aventis Pasteur additionally donated 80 million doses it had kept frozen since 1958, which the government said it would keep as an emergency supply. See: Lawrence K. Altman, "Smallpox Vaccinations Urged for Health Care Workers," *New York Times*, June 7, 2002, A24; and William J. Broad, "US Guide for Mass Smallpox Vaccinations," *New York Times*, September 24, 2002, A19.
4. William J. Broad, "US to Vaccinate 500,000 Workers Against Smallpox," *New York Times*, July 7, 2002, A1.
5. David Brown, "Limited Smallpox Vaccine Use Eyed," *Washington Post*, June 21, 2002, A1.
6. Broad, "US to Vaccinate 500,000 Workers Against Smallpox."
7. The National Vaccine Advisory Committee also deliberated over vaccine policy, but the ACIP recommendations are the ones that drew the greatest public attention.

vaccinations in the event of a smallpox outbreak.[8] At least one hospital per state would be designated as a referral center for smallpox. The ACIP report gave no official target number, but individual committee members estimated that 15,000 to 20,000 people nationwide would suffice. The option was the most limited of several the panel considered; it outright rejected the proposal to inoculate every American.[9]

In developing its recommendations, ACIP had to weigh the advantages of having an immune group, combined with the likelihood of an attack using smallpox, against the risks posed by the vaccine itself. The difficulty was that, because smallpox had been eradicated, the risk of getting smallpox was actually zero until the moment that an attack occurred. So the risk of an attack was part of ACIP's equation. But so far, the government—to protect intelligence sources or because it did not know—had provided no firm evidence of a planned attack. The vaccine, on the other hand—while safe for most people—carried the highest risks of any vaccine in use.

Vaccine Drawbacks

Made from the smallpox-related vaccinia virus, or cowpox, the smallpox vaccine worked because the body considered it identical to smallpox and manufactured antibodies to both.[10] But the vaccine could cause serious complications. Fully 30% of Americans were advised not to take the vaccine because they suffered from conditions—such as eczema or compromised immune systems—that increased their risk of complications.[11] Of the remaining 70%, studies from the 1960s indicated that 14 to 52 people per million would suffer serious reactions such as encephalitis (brain inflammation) and blindness, while another 50 to 900 would suffer complications like fever, sore arms, swollen lymph nodes, and other aches. One or two per million would die. Interestingly, in the fall of 2001, CDC vaccinated some 200 staff members against smallpox but canceled plans to vaccinate more once they saw the severity of the reactions.[12]

The smallpox vaccine was classified as investigational or experimental because, while it had been widely used in the past, the standards under which it was made were no longer current. Anyone receiving the vaccine had to sign in advance a consent form of the

---

8. A typical team would include a doctor, nurse, public health adviser, epidemiologist, disease investigator, diagnostic laboratory scientist, vaccinator, and security and law enforcement workers. See: Lawrence K. Altman, "Traces of Terror: the Bioterror Threat," *New York Times*, June 21, 2002, A16.

9. Brown, "Limited Smallpox Vaccine Use Eyed."

10. The vaccine was made from pustules that formed on the bellies of calves infected with vaccinia. Scientists extracted fluid containing the vaccinia from the pustules, cleaned it up, treated it with antibiotics, and froze it. See: Josephine Marcotty, "Smallpox Vaccinations; Ready or Not," *Minneapolis Star Tribune*, January 27, 2003, 1A.

11. Studies showed that among eczema sufferers, the rate of complications could be one per 100,000 vaccinations, higher than the risk of paralysis from oral polio vaccine—administration of which the government halted due to the high risk. See: Lawrence K. Altman, "Action Delayed on Vaccination Advice," *New York Times*, August 25, 2002, A22. On the other hand, in the event of an outbreak of smallpox, these individuals would have been vaccinated without hesitation.

12. Altman, "Action Delayed on Vaccination Advice."

sort typically used in drug trials.[13] Not only did the vaccine itself cause reactions, but for 19 days after the vaccination, the vaccinia virus could spread (in a process known as shedding) from those who had just been vaccinated. Proper bandaging and a careful change of dressings could prevent this.

In response to the ACIP recommendation, HHS Secretary Thompson said he would "now review the recommendation with experts … as the Administration works toward a policy on the smallpox vaccine."[14] He added: "We plan to move as expeditiously as possible so that we have a policy in place as more vaccine becomes available later this year."[15] HHS had never rejected or significantly modified an ACIP recommendation.[16] The ACIP chair and Dr. Julie L. Gerberding, acting deputy director of CDC, said it would take several months to carry out the ACIP recommendations if they were adopted.[17]

WHY SMALLPOX? WHY NOW?

As it was, it took nearly half a year for HHS and CDC to decide on the structural design of a pre-event smallpox vaccination program. During that time, state public health departments—frustrated by the lack of definite instructions but fearful of being unprepared—struggled to stay on top of the situation. As early as July 7, 2002, reports began to surface that the government intended to vaccinate not 15,000 to 20,000 but 500,000 public health and emergency workers. HHS Acting Assistant Secretary for Emergency Preparedness Jerome Hauer predicted that vaccinations could start within eight weeks.[18] But then nothing happened. "It's much more complicated than one might imagine," said Dr. Donald A. Henderson, chairman of the HHS Secretary's Council on Public Health Preparedness.[19] Those who would inoculate others needed training. The newly inoculated could be out of work for up to 10 days. There was also debate over whether to require an HIV or pregnancy test for all who wanted the vaccine, due to the known danger it posed to expectant mothers and people with compromised immune systems. Other questions included:

- Who would have legal liability if the vaccine produced an adverse reaction? The hospital or clinic? The doctors/nurses who administered it? The manufacturer?
- Who would pay those vaccinated for time lost from work?
- Who would pay to screen those who wanted to be vaccinated?

---

13. The government did have an antidote to the more dangerous side effects, called vaccinia immune globulin.
14. Brown, "Limited Smallpox Vaccine Use Eyed."
15. Lawrence K. Altman, "Panel Rejects Immunizing All Against a Smallpox Outbreak," *New York Times*, June 21, 2002, A16.
16. Altman, "Action Delayed on Vaccination Advice."
17. Altman, "Panel Rejects Immunizing."
18. Ceci Connolly, "Smallpox Vaccine Program Readied," *Washington Post*, July 8, 2002, A1.
19. Connolly, "Smallpox Vaccine Program Readied." Henderson had led the worldwide smallpox eradication effort in the 1970s.

Pros and Cons

Inside and outside the Administration, supporters and opponents of a pre-event vaccination program took to the op-ed pages and the airwaves with their views. The chief argument of those who opposed it was that the government had failed to identify any specific threat. They speculated that the Bush Administration was using the smallpox vaccine for political purposes. The Administration had embarked on a campaign against Iraq—accusing it of harboring terrorists and building weapons of mass destruction—that seemed likely to end in a war. US public support of a war was, however, far from ensured. The critics wondered out loud whether the smallpox vaccine program was meant to stir up public anxiety and thus support for the war.

Vaccine supporters accepted the Administration's claim that terrorists and hostile states, such as Iraq, were capable of manufacturing and using smallpox in a biological attack. They felt it was only a matter of time before the United States would have to confront the consequences of such an attack. Prudence alone, they argued, dictated a pre-event vaccination program.

On the medical front, opponents pointed out that, because the vaccine was effective up to four days after exposure, the government could wait to vaccinate until after a smallpox outbreak. Supporters argued that because incubation lasted an average of 12 days, individuals might not realize they had been exposed. Moreover, weaponized smallpox, such as terrorists might develop, could spread much faster than the standard virus. Multiple, simultaneous infections could dwarf the ability of public health authorities to conduct a post-facto vaccination program.

MINNESOTA'S DRAFT PLAN

Public health officials in Minnesota followed—and participated in—this debate closely. By August 2002, they concluded that some version of the ACIP recommendations would be adopted and that they had better prepare. Responsibility for vaccinations at MDH rested with the Infectious Disease Epidemiology, Prevention, and Control Division, headed by State Epidemiologist Dr. Harry Hull. Within the division were two sections that could logically manage a smallpox vaccination program. The Acute Disease Investigation and Control Section had already been working on smallpox as part of a broader bioterrorism prevention program. The Immunization, Tuberculosis, and International Health Section handled vaccinations.[20] Richard Danila was the head of Acute Disease (and deputy state epidemiologist), while Kristen Ehresmann directed the Immunization Section.

---

20. Two other sections had little role to play: the Epidemiology Field Services Section and the AIDS/STD Prevention Services Section.

In an effort to stay ahead of the curve, Ehresmann, Danila, and a few colleagues drew up a preliminary pre-event smallpox vaccination plan for Minnesota. Dated August 30, the draft plan presented four scenarios:

1. Obtain vaccine supplies but vaccinate no one.
2. Vaccinate some 1,000 medical personnel as per ACIP (e.g., smallpox response teams, a laboratory response team, regional patient care teams, plus a few security staff).
3. Vaccinate some 100,000 health care personnel (e.g., public health staff, emergency management staff, medical teams, and others such as law enforcement and public utility operators).
4. Vaccinate 1 million people (e.g., all possible contributors to a smallpox response).[21]

The draft plan noted that, at the moment, no smallpox vaccine was commercially available. It also raised a number of MDH concerns. Is Minnesota *required* to vaccinate? Does MDH have a policy regarding workmen's compensation after vaccination? Who would meet with staff to explain vaccination options? Who would indemnify the state for associated costs? How would MDH monitor whether each vaccination "took" (was working) or not? Would members of response teams receive extra compensation?

The plan circulated within MDH on a limited basis but, because there was no movement at the federal level, MDH took no further steps for the time being.

GATHERING SPEED

In September, debate continued to simmer on the advisability of a pre-event vaccination program. According to press reports, Vice President Dick Cheney was said to want rapid, universal vaccination while HHS Secretary Thompson preferred a voluntary program that would wait at least two years for an improved vaccine.[22] Thompson's advisor Dr. Henderson argued for more limited vaccinations.[23] "If you look at the vice president's office, they're thinking strategic [policy], not public health," one insider told a reporter. Thompson's concern, he continued, was that "if something bad happens [as a result of smallpox vaccine], the public is not going to be blaming Dick Cheney, they're going to be blaming Tommy Thompson."[24]

But by October, there were signs that discussion had moved on to the more practical matters of liability, compensation, and logistics. On October 4, HHS gave the states a heads-up that some kind of pre-event vaccination program was in the offing. In a conference call, HHS urged state public health officials to begin planning—while they waited

21. Minnesota has a population of some five million.
22. Barton Gellman, "4 Nations Thought to Possess Smallpox," *Washington Post*, November 5, 2002, A1.
23. Connolly and Milbank, "US Revives Smallpox Shot."
24. Ibid.

for a policy recommendation from Secretary Thompson—how to do pre-event vaccinations. Under current consideration, HHS told the states, was a three-stage program: first up to 500,000 frontline health care workers, then some 10 million first responders, and finally the general public. When and if a public announcement were made, HHS said, states would have 60 days to prepare for Phase 1 and 90 days to implement it. The conference call, says MDH Immunization Section Leader Ehresmann, "was a wakeup call." She realized that the job of coordinating MDH's response was likely to be hers, so "I took the approach of I better get going with this, because I knew it was going to fall on me."[25]

Ehresmann and her colleagues had an additional source of information on federal intentions. Dr. Michael Osterholm had been Minnesota state epidemiologist and now served both as director of the Center for Infectious Disease Research and Policy at the University of Minnesota and on the HHS Secretary's Council on Public Health Preparedness. Osterholm, without violating any confidences, was telling Minnesota state officials that the threat of a smallpox attack was real. Recalls Robert Einweck, director of the Office of Emergency Preparedness (OEP) within MDH: "He said this is a moving train, and we'd better start catching up with it. We took it very, very seriously [thinking] it could happen as soon as next month."[26]

Advisory Committee on Immunization Practices

Further confirmation that a decision was approaching came on October 16, 2002, when ACIP revised its earlier recommendation and endorsed the idea of immunizing 500,000 public health and hospital workers across the country. A committee member said the number of first-stage vaccinations was revised upward because it became apparent that individual hospitals were reluctant to be designated as smallpox centers.[27] The solution was to ask any hospital with a negative air pressure isolation room—a room for respiratory patients constructed to prevent air inside from circulating outside—to form a smallpox care team.

The ACIP meeting also affirmed that the Administration was moving forward with plans for a second phase of vaccinations for up to 10 million first responders. ACIP voted down, however, a suggestion that the 10 million should be vaccinated immediately.[28] Dr. Paul A. Offit, head of the vaccine center at Children's Hospital of Philadelphia and the only member of ACIP to vote against the 500,000 proposal, said later that the Bush

---

25. Author's interview with Kristen Ehresmann in Minneapolis, MN, March 27, 2003. All further quotes from Ehresmann, unless otherwise attributed, are from this interview.

26. Author's interview with Robert Einweck, St. Paul, MN, March 26, 2003. All further quotes from Einweck, unless otherwise attributed, are from this interview.

27. David Brown, "Panel Alters Advice on Smallpox Shots," *Washington Post*, October 17, 2002, A3.

28. It also voted not to make AIDS or pregnancy tests mandatory for those to be vaccinated.

Administration did not pressure the panel but that "the sense was that the course was already set and we wouldn't make any difference."[29]

By late October, more signs accumulated of a looming decision to launch a smallpox vaccination program. CDC guidelines to states on smallpox preparedness (Announcement 99051), issued on October 28, did not announce a pre-event vaccination program but did specifically mention the need to vaccinate response teams in anticipation of an outbreak of smallpox. At the same time, the Food and Drug Administration relicensed the first 117 million doses of vaccine, removing another hurdle to a pre-event vaccination campaign.[30] With these developments, state public health officials from HHS Region V decided it was time they conferred about the pending federal program.[31] Five states scheduled a meeting for October 30 in Chicago.

Region V Meeting

From Minnesota, Commissioner of Health Jan Malcolm went to the Chicago meeting, along with Ehresmann, a department lawyer, and an MDH mass clinic planner.[32] Each state, remembers Ehresmann, "was questioning whether or not they could or should do vaccinations.... There were liability issues. There were ethical issues." At the end of the meeting, the state officials presented HHS and CDC with a list of questions, what Ehresmann terms "showstoppers—all the things that make us say we don't know if we can do this." They included: Who should be vaccinated pre-event and in what order of priority? Who would train the first-round vaccine givers? Who assumes liability—for the vaccine manufacturer, the vaccine givers, vaccinated persons who inadvertently infect others by shedding vaccinia, and hospitals where the vaccine is administered? Who compensates hospitals for the time personnel spend running vaccination clinics? Who pays compensation for vaccinated individuals who miss work or who become seriously ill?

Most of the Region V officials' questions had not been answered when, just three weeks later, the request for action plans arrived. On Friday, November 22, CDC instructed states to submit—by December 9—full-fledged plans for pre-event vaccinations of medical and public health smallpox response teams. CDC could not compel states to submit such plans; the agency's authority over state health departments was quite limited. CDC can send personnel to a state experiencing a disease outbreak, for example, only by invitation. But it did have the power of persuasion, and it owned the vaccine stocks. Any state that ordered vaccine from CDC thereby agreed to administer it.

---

29. Marie McCullough, "So Far, Only 687 Vaccinated for Smallpox," *Pittsburgh Post-Gazette*, February 7, 2003, A1.
30. Ceci Connolly, "President Reviving Program to Provide Smallpox Vaccine," *Washington Post*, December 12, 2002, A1.
31. Region V comprises Minnesota, Michigan, Indiana, Wisconsin, Illinois, and Ohio.
32. The other two were MDH legal counsel Steven Shakman and MDH planner Luanne McNichols.

Once the state plans were in hand and approved, the federal government would announce the program to the public. Not only would states have barely two weeks to prepare their plans, but the speed of implementation had been significantly increased since October. Instead of 90 days from the time of announcement, CDC recommended states should complete all vaccinations within 30 days.

Homeland Security Act

The CDC request came just before President George W. Bush signed into law, on Monday, November 25, the Homeland Security Act of 2002. The much-debated Act created a new Department of Homeland Security, combining 22 government agencies into one mammoth department. Bush nominated Homeland Security Adviser Tom Ridge as head of the new agency. One section of the Act laid to rest some of the concerns raised by the Region V states. Section 304 provided legal protection for smallpox vaccine manufacturers and anyone who administered the vaccine, including hospitals. To recover damages, anyone harmed by the vaccine would have to sue the federal government and prove negligence on the part of the accused. The Act made no mention, however, of compensation for those *taking* the vaccine who might as a result miss work or incur medical bills, nor of liability for secondary infections.

MINNESOTA OVERDRIVE

The news that HHS wanted detailed pre-event smallpox vaccination plans from each state hit MDH hard. One issue was logistical—how would the state put together a comprehensive plan in little more than two weeks? Once the plan was set, how would it be implemented? What about the outstanding questions of liability and compensation? The other was ethical—how would those within the department who questioned the nation's need for and the Administration's motivation for a vaccination program be able to work on it?

The CDC requests for information were considerable. It wanted to know who would manage the vaccination program; what the timeline and the organization chart would look like; how many public health and medical response teams were needed and what kind of experts would be included on each team; what the number of participating hospitals, state policy on hospital responsibilities, and clinic sites and times would be; how states would train vaccinators; and what the number of days and hours per clinic, plus the number of personnel required to run them, would add up to. It wanted to know how clinic staff would screen potential vaccinees, as well as how they would monitor the after-effects of the vaccine.

States also had to guarantee the security of the vaccine itself because there was considerable fear that terrorists might capture the vaccine and infect people with vaccinia. CDC asked Minnesota and other states to provide contact numbers and places for delivery of the vaccine, to stipulate the number of required doses, and to devise a strategy for safeguarding the vaccine. It also asked them to establish data management and communications programs, plus a plan to report their progress on a semiweekly basis (Mondays and Thursdays) to CDC.

Yes or No?

Minnesota, before taking any further steps, asked CDC whether the state's Scenario 1 of August was viable: to stockpile vaccine but not vaccinate anyone until after an outbreak. That, says State Epidemiologist Hull, "would have been my preferred plan."[33] But the answer was no. CDC would provide vaccine only to states prepared to vaccinate.

So the question became: how to respond? At a meeting the same day the CDC request arrived (November 22), MDH staff raised multiple questions and concerns. The conversation continued on Monday, November 25, during a two-hour meeting called by Dr. Hull. As Ehresmann remembers: "There was a lot of dissension within our division as to whether or not we should do this." She adds:

> People felt that in public health we're used to doing things that are pretty purely for the good. You've already established that the benefits outweigh the risks before you do it in a public health setting. We're just not used to contemplating a public health activity in which people may die, there may be negative consequences.

In a memo, Hull attempted to answer some of the more pressing staff questions. When asked how many people MDH would vaccinate, Hull indicated that the number would be up to 10,000. That number was arrived at rather imprecisely, just as the federal 500,000 number had been. CDC had multiplied 5,000 qualifying hospitals nationwide by 100 personnel per hospital to get a target number of 500,000 vaccinees across the country. Ehresmann and her colleagues similarly multiplied what they thought was the number of qualifying hospitals in Minnesota, 62, by 100 to arrive at 6,200 hospital personnel to vaccinate.[34] To that, they added nine public health teams, one for each MDH region in the state, as well as a few security personnel to guard the vaccine and the clinics. That gave them a rough estimate of 10,000 potential vaccinations.

---

33. Author's interview with Dr. Harry Hull, Minneapolis, MN, March 25, 2003. All further quotes from Hull, unless otherwise attributed, are from this interview.
34. As Danila points out, the number 62 was a "guesstimate in the dark" of how many Minnesota hospitals had functioning negative pressure rooms. The actual number was 66, but not all of those were able to contribute to the smallpox effort.

MDH staff also worried about liability issues, but Hull assured them that the Homeland Security Act would take care of that. Some staff feared that health workers might feel coerced to accept the vaccine. Hull tried to reassure them that the program was entirely voluntary. They asked about training materials (CDC would provide some; MDH would develop others) and about the timeline (it depended on when the president announced a program, but Hull anticipated that MDH could be vaccinating health care workers by mid-December 2002).

Finally, Hull and the department grappled with the question of the purpose behind the vaccination program. Was it motivated exclusively by public health concerns, or were there political considerations? An Administration intelligence assessment made public in November, which concluded that four nations—Russia, Iraq, France, and North Korea—had covert stocks of smallpox, did little to persuade the skeptical.[35]

"Several of us here," says MDH Acute Disease Section Leader Danila, "felt really strongly that this was merely a political ruse to support a war effort, rather than a public health preparedness effort."[36] Others at MDH, however, suspected that "there were people who were using objections to the smallpox vaccination program as a way of expressing their dissent from the decision to go to war." In his memo to staff, Hull said that "if the federal government announces that vaccination is necessary because of a threat to the country, MDH will not be in a position to say that the threat is not real.... We have to accept that, for security reasons, we may never know all of the facts." At the same time, Hull expressed the hope of many that "the risk of a smallpox attack may be clarified with the announcement of the program." As Ehresmann puts it: "We wanted to have evidence of a credible threat."

The debate continued to percolate internally, but top MDH officials decided that, for practical purposes, the process of planning had to be considered separately from that of implementation. It was essential the state at least have a plan in place. So for the next two weeks, some 30 MDH staff worked overtime to complete a 48-page proposal plus appendixes, which provided all the information CDC required.

WHO DOES WHAT?

MDH officials first had to map out what needed to be done and then to decide who should do it. The "what" was fairly clear-cut: MDH would ask for volunteers to join teams that would deploy in the event of a smallpox outbreak and vaccinate these volunteers. There would be two kinds of smallpox response teams: public health and medical.[37] Public health teams would draw volunteers from state and local public

---

35. Gellman, "4 Nations Thought to Possess Smallpox."
36. Author's interview with Dr. Richard Danila, Minneapolis, MN, March 25, 2003. All further quotes from Danila, unless otherwise attributed, are from this interview.
37. This characterization is only for purposes of general description. Of course there were medical doctors and nurses on the public health teams, as well as hospital doctors well trained in public health.

health departments. In the event of an attack, these teams would have two jobs: vaccinate the public and trace the contacts of smallpox patients (and vaccinate those contacts). Volunteers for the medical teams would come from hospitals. If there were a smallpox outbreak, these teams would provide 24-hour care for the patients.[38] To vaccinate team members, MDH would run two categories of clinics: (1) public health clinics to vaccinate public health volunteers and a few public safety officials and (2) hospital clinics (located there for the convenience of hospital staff) to vaccinate medical workers. Public health doctors and nurses would administer the vaccinations at both kinds of clinics.

To make this happen, MDH needed managers. But deciding who was in charge of the smallpox vaccination program was not straightforward. On the one hand, MDH Section Chiefs Ehresmann (Immunization) and Danila (Acute Disease) had already taken responsibility for preliminary plans, participated in conference calls, and attended meetings. On the other hand, in June 2002, the state had created an OEP as part of an antibioterror effort mandated and funded by the federal government. It was only logical that OEP take a lead role in the smallpox vaccination program. At least OEP, headed by Robert Einweck, was part of MDH. But, housed in an MDH building in St. Paul, OEP was not physically close to Ehresmann and Danila, who were in Minneapolis.[39] In terms of hierarchy, Einweck reported directly to Assistant Commissioner for Health Protection Aggie Leitheiser, while Ehresmann and Danila reported to Hull, who reported to Leitheiser.

In the end, the MDH plan proposed that both OEP and Infectious Diseases together run the smallpox vaccination program. Ehresmann was made Smallpox Vaccination Officer with Danila as her back-up, but OEP stood at the top of the organization chart. "We created this unbelievable work chart," says Danila. "What we learned is that when you put everybody in charge, nobody's in charge…. It just gets quite complicated."

Decentralize

The work chart became more complex when the plan drafters decided to decentralize the vaccination program. This was atypical for Minnesota. An outbreak of hepatitis, for example, would be managed at the state level. The decision to decentralize was driven in part by the allocation of funding and in part by the structure of public health in the state. On the funding front, the federal bioterror prevention program (which had created OEP) had brought Minnesota public health $18 million.[40] Of that, $2 million were Health

---

38. Hospital teams could include emergency department staff, intensive care unit staff, medical subspecialists (dermatologists, anesthesiologists, etc.), radiology technicians, respiratory therapists, and security personnel.
39. Minnesota is unusual in that its two main cities are neighbors separated by a river. St. Paul is the state capitol, while Minneapolis is its commercial center. Together they are known as the Twin Cities.
40. This constituted Minnesota's share of a $918 million national appropriation for bioterror defense.

Resources and Services Administration funds earmarked for hospitals for preparedness. The remaining $16 million went to MDH, which disbursed a little over $5 million to local public health authorities.[41] Typically, local health departments provided basic services: environmental health, sanitation, public health nursing, simple vaccinations. Now MDH decided that pre-event smallpox vaccinations would be the local health authorities' first antibioterrorism activity. Explains Danila:

> Vaccines would come to us [at MDH], and we'd deliver it out. We'd be responsible for developing policy, developing materials, developing training. But locally they would be setting up the specifics: size of clinics, where the clinics were, how many clinics and so forth.

Decentralization also made sense given the structure of Minnesota public health. Public health policy was formulated at the state level, but services were delivered at the local level. There were nine public health regions across the state, subdivided further into 51 Community Health Boards charged with local public health service delivery. The smallpox program designers decided to organize smallpox clinics by region. This allowed them to tap existing resources. For example, OEP had already hired a bioterrorism coordinator for each region. Those coordinators, some of them hired only a week before the Bush smallpox vaccination announcement, were quickly co-opted for the new project.

At the same time they were designing the program and its management structure, Ehresmann and Danila had to organize the participants. As early as the week of December 2, MDH sent out general advisories to district and local public health staff, to hospital CEOs, and to regional hospital coordinators. During that week, agency officials held three conference calls with local public health officials and four calls with hospitals to discuss the program and ask for feedback. "We got very specific very quickly," recalls Hull. Typically during those conversations, an OEP official would give an overview, then Danila would provide details about smallpox, the vaccine, and infection control issues.

Dealing With Hospitals

There was a special challenge in dealing with hospitals. MDH had to engage their cooperation at the same time it built relationships with them. Hospitals, most of them privately owned, were under no legal obligation to take part in the vaccination program. In the past, MDH dealt with hospitals only infrequently—usually over infectious disease outbreaks. It licensed hospitals but had no fiscal authority over them. "We had to build a relationship with hospitals out of nothing," says Einweck. OEP had recently created—for

---

41. The allocation depended on population, so the most sparsely populated county received $15,000, while the most densely populated one got $900,000.

the mass smallpox vaccination program—a position of liaison with hospitals. This coordinator now became involved in the pre-event vaccination program.

In the conference calls with hospitals, MDH discussed how to develop criteria for hospital involvement, how to identify the number of staff necessary to care for patients in each hospital, and how to decide who would be vaccinated and who would monitor wound care afterward. Hospitals were asked to submit the proposed composition of their health care teams by December 6. For their part, the hospitals had numerous questions about liability, compensation, funding, and furloughs for employees. "All these were unanswered at that time," remembers Danila.

Dressings

MDH during the first week of December also tackled the question of what kind of bandages to provide for the vaccination site wound to prevent shedding. Unsurprising to some, the CDC guidelines failed to mention details like this. MDH decided to research available bandages to find the safest product available. In meetings with bandage manufacturers, MDH eventually spoke with representatives from Smith & Nephew, Inc., a British firm. Their product combined in one piece a semipermeable membrane and gauze. That meant a person could change the dressing by himself, rather than requiring two people. Moreover, the bandage could be left on for two to three days, reducing the maceration to the scab that daily changing—recommended by CDC—would have caused. Minnesota was the first state to contact Smith & Nephew and, in placing its order for 50,000 bandages, depleted the firm's worldwide inventory.

Despite such additional distractions, as December 9 approached, MDH was on target to complete its plan. Just to complicate matters, the department was also preparing, as part of federal bioterrorism defense efforts, a required plan for steps it would take in the event of an actual smallpox attack. The 175-page smallpox response plan was filed with CDC on Monday, December 2. One week later, on Monday, December 9, MDH submitted its plan for Phase 1 of the smallpox pre-event vaccination program.

PROGRAM ANNOUNCEMENT

Events continued to move quickly. Within the week, on Friday, December 13, 2002, President Bush announced that the nation would start vaccinating against smallpox. "To protect our citizens in the aftermath of September the 11th, we are evaluating old threats in a new light," said Bush. "Our government has no information that a smallpox attack is imminent. Yet it is prudent to prepare for the possibility that terrorists who kill indiscriminately would use diseases as a weapon."[42] Some 500,000 members of the military would be vaccinated immediately. In addition, Bush clarified, states would start as soon as possible to implement individual plans to inoculate an estimated 500,000 health care workers nationwide. Those emergency workers would be responsible, in the event of a smallpox outbreak, for tracing and treating smallpox patients, as well as for conducting the first of the mass vaccinations to follow. The program, which was voluntary, would later expand to include 10 million first responders, and the general public could be vaccinated within a year.[43] Bush declared that as commander-in-chief he, but not his family, would be vaccinated.[44]

Deadline Relaxed

At the same time that Bush announced the smallpox vaccination program, federal health officials extended the deadline for completing it. Just before Bush's announcement, CDC realized that states could not complete their vaccination programs within 30 days of the announcement because, inadvertently, the Homeland Security Act–Section 304 did not include an effective date for the liability protection it conferred. That meant the protection would not come into legal effect until January 24 (60 days after the bill's signing) and, even then, only if Secretary Thompson made an emergency declaration. For state planning purposes, that meant no vaccinations could begin until January 24, nor could states be certain they were covered for liability until Secretary Thompson made his declaration. Time was still short but not as desperately short as initially thought.

The deadline extension, while it undeniably brought relief, also produced something of a letdown at MDH, which had been working flat out to be ready for the 30-day implementation. Recalls Hull: "We took them at their word. And we were prepared to do it. And so we felt a little bit foolish for believing that." OEP Director Einweck remembers the abrupt interruption to momentum. He says:

> We thought we were going to be implementing a smallpox vaccination program in December.... We literally stopped everything. People canceled vacations, we were working really hard at the local and the state level. Then all of a sudden, it was like—well, sorry.... I felt like I was a little steel ball on a pinball machine.

On the plus side, more time allowed MDH to deliberate once again over whether or not to join the vaccination program.

---

42. Connolly and Milbank, "US Revives Smallpox Shot."
43. Bush mistakenly said that members of the public who wanted it could demand a vaccination immediately. In succeeding days, public health officials clarified that vaccination was not recommended for the general public and that, while members of the public might be able to get the vaccine in mid-2003, it would be only as participants in clinical trials of new types of vaccine.
44. Bush was vaccinated in private on December 21, 2002.

DEBATES IN THE MINNESOTA DEPARTMENT OF HEALTH

President Bush's announcement meant that MDH either had to move ahead with its December 9 plan or declare publicly that it would not take part. Many at MDH had hoped that Bush would provide a stronger rationale for moving forward. "We did expect a stronger statement: that there is an imminent risk, there is an imminent health threat, something like that," recalls Danila. "What we got was less than that.... There were still lingering doubts among us whether or not we should participate." Health Commissioner Malcolm, remembers Ehresmann, "was really pulling back, asking 'Do we really want to be doing this?'"

The doubts of public health officials in Minnesota were mirrored on the national level. But others, such as Senator Bill Frist (R-Tennessee), a surgeon who had recently written a book on bioterrorism, supported the plan. "A vaccinated population, even a partially vaccinated population, is a protected population," he told a bioterrorism conference on December 11.[45] CDC Director Julie Gerberding also endorsed the plan: "Although the possibility of an intentional release of smallpox is not quantifiable, the consequences of an outbreak would be great and we must be prepared."[46]

In Minnesota, MDH held staff meetings on Monday, December 16, and again on December 17 to discuss participation. A few staff, notes Danila, expressed their view that "this is against all public health principles that I have" and refused to take part in the vaccination program. "This was a very emotional time," he comments. But eventually, says Danila, most of the resisters realized "that the program was going to occur anyway.... We decided that, if we were going to have the program and if anyone was going to get vaccinated, then we were going to make it the safest program possible." Remembers Ehresmann: "It got to the point where it just felt like there was a national push and we were riding the wave.... It was a patriotic thing, too.... Public health was unable to 'just say no' in this situation even though the debate raged." There was also an issue of responsibility, she adds.

> You are responsible for the health of the citizens in Minnesota, and if you had the opportunity to plan and you did not take it, or by having people vaccinated that's going to make you more prepared and you didn't do it—then you're screwed. It was truly a lose-lose situation.

It was also important, though perhaps more so to the political appointees running the department than to the doctors in the Infectious Diseases division, that Governor Jesse Ventura very much supported the smallpox vaccination program. By Christmas, MDH was fully committed to implementing its plan to inoculate some 10,000 health care workers.

---

45. Connolly, "President Reviving Program to Provide Smallpox Vaccine."
46. CDC Press Release, "CDC Initial Review of State Smallpox Vaccination Plans Complete," December 12, 2002, https://www.cdc.gov/media/pressrel/r021212.htm.

Amending the Centers for Disease Control and Prevention Template

Mid-to-late December continued to be busy for Ehresmann and her team. They recruited MDH staff for the wide variety of tasks at hand: to liaise with local public health coordinators; to manage administrative functions such as finance, technology, legal issues, and tribal health; and to take charge of adverse event (negative reaction to the vaccine) surveillance. Ehresmann also filled positions for data management, vaccine handling, communications, clinic operations, and a Web site, as well as positions that linked with the health alert network. Finally, she appointed individuals to liaise with field epidemiologists, with hospitals, and with federal agencies. A core team led by the Commissioner of Health met regularly to review progress, although there was a change of personnel on January 5, 2003, when Commissioner Malcolm stepped down with an outgoing administration and Assistant Commissioner Leitheiser became Acting Commissioner.

Meanwhile, MDH took advantage as much as possible of materials and training CDC provided. On December 5 and 6, health workers had watched a CDC smallpox vaccination education program. The week of December 16, a doctor and four nurses prepared to fly to Atlanta to learn how to give smallpox shots.[47] CDC scheduled another nationwide satellite broadcast on smallpox vaccine risks for Friday, December 20, which MDH staff attended.

But there was much MDH felt it had to invent for itself. For example, in late December it occurred to MDH officials that someone would have to handle negative reactions to the vaccine. The department hastily created a network of physicians who would be on call around the clock. CDC suggested a similar system to all states only later and offered training for clinicians in early February. Minnesota by then had organized a group of some 75 doctors who would take calls from vaccinated persons worried about a rash or other symptom. In addition to general practitioners, the network included ophthalmologists, dermatologists, and infectious disease specialists.

Minnesota became the first state to point out that CDC could not require vaccination of those who checked smallpox vaccination dressings. ACIP, in its October recommendations, had insisted that dressing checkers be vaccinated. But hospitals, MDH informed ACIP members, could not afford this measure. Were it insisted on, the hospitals would drop out of the program. As a result, ACIP in its January recommendations amended its earlier stance and suggested that checkers be vaccinated only if feasible.[48] Minnesota also was one of the first states to raise the question of how to care for vaccinia patients—those infected by the vaccine or secondary infections. The Minnesota officials were particularly

---

47. Maura Lerner, "State's Plan for Smallpox Takes Shape," *Minneapolis Star Tribune*, December 13, 2002, 1A.
48. Oddly, ACIP never required vaccinations of those caring for vaccinia patients.

concerned about infection control. Lacking guidance from CDC, MDH developed its own protocols for the care of vaccinia patients.

While it was satisfying in some ways to be out ahead of CDC, State Epidemiologist Hull would have preferred clear, well-conceived directives. "On a number of occasions," he muses, "my feeling was that the advice we were given was from a couple of people who didn't have a clue about how state health departments work, sitting in a bar and writing out the solutions on a napkin."

> They've not been thought through. They don't reflect an understanding of our relationship with the local health departments, and how local health departments work.

The CDC hadn't considered practical details, says Hull, such as "who's going to cover the patients [while hospital workers are vaccinated]? Who's going to pay for the transportation? Who's going to pay the salary time?" In a state the size of Minnesota, it could take a day to drive to a designated regional clinic site and back.

Target Date

Despite these difficulties, by late December, Minnesota felt sufficiently prepared to tentatively schedule its vaccination clinics to begin on January 27. In early January, however, MDH learned it need not have rushed. By then, the department was already nervous about the January 27 date. In a memo dated January 10, 2003, Acting Health Commissioner Leitheiser asked the Association of State and Territorial Health Officials (ASTHO), which monitors federal public health policy, whether it could confirm that Secretary Thompson would issue his declaration on January 24, thereby activating the Section 304 liability protection. Also, there were rumors that vaccine would not ship until February 3. With clinics scheduled for January 27, Minnesota needed to know what the schedule was. "Canceling clinics at the last minute will waste time and money, discourage participation, and make it very difficult to go through another round of planning," wrote Leitheiser.[49]

Before that letter could arrive at ASTHO, however, a neglected fact came to light. Many states had continued to believe that, although the earliest smallpox clinic start date had been pushed back to January 24, they were still expected to complete the vaccination program within 30 days. In Minnesota, says Einweck, "we were under the impression that we had 30 days to do all of our vaccinations because the liability protections would only be in place for 30 days." However, on January 10, Minnesota and other states learned in a conference call that the vaccination program did not have to wrap up within 30 days of starting after all; in fact, the states had a year's liability coverage.[50]

---

49. Memo from Leitheiser to George E. Hardy, Jr., January 10, 2003, 9:34 a.m., "Smallpox Pre-event Issues."
50. Secretary Thompson clarified the liability schedule two weeks after the conference call.

CDC Director Gerberding explained in an interview the following week that the 30-day deadline was "another complete misunderstanding. The bottom line ... is that there is no end date for this program."[51] She also pointed out that the smallpox vaccination program had no set goal for numbers vaccinated: "We need to get away from this notion of a number." Federal officials, she added, had deliberately overestimated to make sure sufficient vaccine would be available: "We knew full well that we did not need to vaccinate that many people." She noted that safety, not speed, was CDC's priority. "Because the smallpox threat is not imminent, we can put safety as our highest priority," Gerberding said.

Meanwhile, the January 10 CDC conference call also confirmed Leitheiser's worry about getting vaccine on time. MDH learned that CDC had concerns over liability if it started shipping before January 24. It told the states that it *could* start shipping as early as the week of January 13 but would not confirm that it *would* ship then. The reaction at MDH, recalls Einweck, was resignation: "In Minnesota, we were really trying to be good soldiers, get all our plans in place, only to find out later, oh, well—we really didn't mean that.... So we said let's just get this over with." MDH rescheduled the first clinic for February 12.

But before it would vaccinate even one volunteer, MDH—like other public health departments nationwide—wanted to settle to its own satisfaction the liability and compensation questions that had beset the pre-event vaccination program from its conception.

LIABILITY AND COMPENSATION

By January, there was a groundswell of anxiety from states about the unresolved liability and compensation issues. On January 9, Secretary Thompson sent a letter to states assuring them that liability issues had been taken care of and they should not worry. But this did not reassure MDH. Acting Commissioner Leitheiser's January 10 letter to ASTHO also posed specific questions about liability and compensation. Minnesota wanted to know about (1) liability coverage under the Homeland Security Act for clinicians who were not vaccinators but who screened, managed adverse events, or cared for secondary transmission cases; (2) coverage for hospitals that did not host clinics but permitted vaccinated employees to work; (3) compensation for vaccinated persons who did not have workers' compensation or were otherwise incompletely covered for missed work or medical treatment; and (4) arrangements for compensating and providing medical care for those with secondary infections.

---

51. Vicki Kemper, "States Lag at Start of Smallpox Program," *Los Angeles Times*, January 17, 2003, 1. The other quotes in this paragraph are also from this article.

MDH also contributed to a document compiled by a number of states under the auspices of ASTHO, along with the National Association of County and City Health Officials (NACCHO). The ASTHO/NACCHO document listed state concerns over liability and compensation. It noted, for example, that because the smallpox response teams benefited society, "any attendant costs should be borne by society-at-large and not by the local community or individual."[52] It called for a "uniform national solution" to state concerns over institutional and personal liability for ill effects of the smallpox vaccine and a "comprehensive national approach" to injury compensation.

The document identified a number of shortcomings in the Homeland Security Act–Section 304, such as the fact that individuals must prove negligence—a heavy burden—in order to sue the federal government for injury from the vaccine. It pointed out that workers' compensation schemes differed from state to state and were therefore not equal, that workers' compensation in most cases did not cover a waiting period nor provide full salary, that compensation for minor side effects was not provided, that workers' compensation payouts would result in higher premiums, and that no reimbursement was provided for furloughs. The document wanted no-fault compensation for any person injured by the vaccine. It also asked that the definition of "covered entities" be broadened to include public health departments, hospitals, and other organizations that participated in any way in the vaccination program.

The Bush Administration did respond on January 14 with a ruling that those who administered vaccine or those who received a vaccination would not be held liable if someone else became ill.[53] The Administration refused, however, to create a compensation fund for those who suffered complications from the vaccine. "We are looking at ways to work with all of the involved parties to address issues related to compensation," said CDC Director Gerberding. But, she added, "we are certainly not going to delay this program because of concerns about compensation."[54]

In the midst of this debate, two of the nation's largest unions on January 16 asked President Bush to postpone smallpox vaccinations until the Administration could pay for medical screening of volunteers and compensation for anyone injured. The Service Employees International Union, with 750,000 members in the health care sector, and the American Federation of State, County and Municipal Employees, with 350,000 health care and emergency workers, advised their members not to take the vaccine.[55] The American Nurses Association also sought delay. On January 17, the Institute of

52. ASTHO/NACCHO Smallpox Liability and Compensation Working Group, "Smallpox Pre-event Vaccination: Liability and Compensation Concerns [draft]."
53. Ceci Connolly, "Caregivers Protected Against Smallpox Lawsuits," *Washington Post*, January 15, 2003, A14.
54. CDC Telebriefing Transcript, "CDC Smallpox Vaccination Update," January 17, 2003, https://www.cdc.gov/media/transcripts/t030117.htm.
55. Ceci Connolly, "Unions Call for Changes in Smallpox Vaccine Program," *Washington Post*, January 17, 2003, A13.

Medicine (IOM), a division of the National Academies of Science and an advisory body to the federal government, urged CDC to proceed cautiously. It said the government should answer questions about liability and compensation and should clarify the risks. The IOM also suggested a pause between Phases 1 and 2 to allow time to evaluate lessons learned.

These accumulating doubts and unresolved issues began to have an effect. By mid-January, some half-dozen prestigious hospitals around the country, including Grady Memorial in Atlanta and Virginia Commonwealth University Health System in Richmond, Virginia, had decided not to participate in the vaccination program. Minnesota hospitals were starting to make the same choice.

PARTICIPATION RATES

MDH had long since realized it would not attract the 10,000 volunteers envisioned in the December 9 plan. In late December, when it set January 27 as a target starting date for clinics, MDH planned to ask CDC for 4,500 doses of vaccine. But as Minnesota drew closer to the revised clinic start date of February 12, even that number began to look optimistic.

MDH in mid-December had identified 66 of the state's 142 hospitals as qualified to treat smallpox patients. That number soon emerged as too high. It included some hospitals that did have the required negative pressure isolation room but that were otherwise small and/or rural and unequipped to deal with an influx of smallpox patients. Seven of these hospitals informed the state by early January that they would not participate; a couple of others dropped out for other reasons. As of early January, however, 52 had agreed to participate.[56]

But as January progressed, a number of qualifying hospitals declared their intention not to vaccinate any staff. The number of nonparticipating hospitals was small, but their publicity impact was high. On January 9, North Memorial Medical made headlines with its decision to delay any action. North Memorial was the first hospital in the St. Paul/Minneapolis metropolitan area to pull out. The hospital's vice president expressed concern over the risk of the vaccine to staff members and to patients. On January 26, another three hospitals from one network opted out: St. Joseph's in St. Paul, St. John's in Maplewood, and Woodwinds in Woodbury. They cited health threat concerns. On January 30, United Hospital in St. Paul said it had not decided whether to participate. If United dropped out, only two hospitals—albeit large ones—in St. Paul would be

---

56. Maura Lerner and Jill Burcum, "Metro Hospital Is Opting Out of Smallpox Plan," *Minneapolis Star Tribune*, January 9, 2003, 1A.

prepared for smallpox patients. By early February, 42 Minnesota hospitals still agreed to participate; 24 had said no.[57]

At the same time, the sign-up for the vaccine even at participating hospitals was considerably lower than expected. At St. Cloud Hospital, only 22 of an expected 210 health workers had volunteered by January 18.[58] Fairview Health Services, operator of seven hospitals, also had fewer volunteers than projected. Some hospitals, however, reported volunteers in line with expectations. Abbott Northwestern in Minneapolis and Hennepin County Medical Center in Minneapolis were close to meeting their goals. Of those medical workers who chose not to participate, many cited children at home—who might become infected—as the reason for declining. Some doctors dropped out because, as self-employed persons, they didn't carry workers' compensation insurance.

MDH had few tools at hand to increase participation rates. Persuasion was its strongest suit. After that, it could only try to make the best of the situation at hand. State health officials repeatedly reassured the public that lower numbers of vaccinees would not leave the state unprepared. "What we're trying to do is make sure that the entire state is prepared," Hull said, by putting "a team in every appropriate hospital. But one of the key points that has to be made here is that a vaccination can occur after exposure for up to four days. In most scenarios, we would be able to protect the people even after exposure."[59] Buddy Ferguson, communications staff member at MDH, said that "I don't think we are concerned at this point that we won't be able to vaccinate enough people."[60]

> The idea is to have minimal numbers of people vaccinated in advance of an actual event so they could respond to it. But again, you can vaccinate people even after they've been exposed to smallpox. That's the backup.

Hull also felt that participation rates were driven lower by overreaction to the perceived risk. People did not properly understand risk ratios. A risk ratio of 1 in 50,000, for example, "is the risk of dying on the way to work if you drive to work five days a week, 50 weeks a year for 200 years," says Hull. "So a 1 in 50,000 risk is something that we take virtually every day without thinking about it." The smallpox vaccine, given after careful screening, carried something closer to a miniscule 1 in 500,000 risk.

---

57. Maura Lerner, "Homeland Security: Osterholm Defends National Smallpox Program," *Minneapolis Star Tribune*, February 10, 2003, 1A. By way of comparison, Johns Hopkins Hospital in Maryland announced January 30 that it would go slow, vaccinating five or six workers a week on a voluntary basis for six to nine months and keeping them away from patients as they reacted to the vaccine. The hospital would provide its employees medical treatment and compensation for time off work, if needed. See: Erika Niedowski, "Hospitals Outline Smallpox Vaccination Plan," *Baltimore Sun*, January 31, 2003, 2B.
58. Josephine Marcotty and Maura Lerner, "Smallpox Signup Is Less Than Expected," *Minneapolis Star Tribune*, January 18, 2003, 1A.
59. Lerner and Burcum, "Metro Hospital Is Opting Out of Smallpox Plan."
60. Marcotty and Lerner, "Smallpox Signup Is Less Than Expected."

The federal government, for one, was convinced the risk was justified. On Friday, January 17, CDC finally announced it would begin shipping vaccine on Tuesday, January 21. Eleven states, said CDC Director Gerberding, had requested shipment. "We intend to make this program happen on time," she told a press conference. "We live in a dangerous world these days where a terrorist attack with smallpox is possible…. We have to be prepared so that we can protect the American people."[61] Gerberding also spoke to some of the doubts expressed about the purpose of the smallpox vaccine. "Sometimes," she said, "it is difficult for people who are thinking of this from a totally public health perspective to recognize that this decision is not just a public health decision. This is an issue of homeland security and an issue of national defense."

National Program Launches

On Friday, January 24, Secretary Thompson made his long-promised emergency declaration, which allowed Section 304 of the Homeland Security Act to take effect. To mark the official launch of the smallpox program, four doctors in Connecticut that day became the first in the nation to be vaccinated. Four was far fewer, however, than the 20 participants Connecticut had advertised. Most of the no-shows, according to press accounts, were worried about compensation.

GET IT OVER WITH

With the green light given, MDH finalized its preparations for clinics to start February 12. The same day the national program launched, MDH secured a pledge from the Minnesota Department of Labor and Industry that any state worker made ill by the vaccine would be covered by workers' compensation. That ruling would not cover nonstate employees. But the state ruling established a precedent and would, MDH officials hoped, set an example for the roughly 400 private sector workers' compensation programs across the state.

MDH also finalized the packet of materials sent to each prospective vaccinee. CDC was still revising the documents it wanted included. But MDH decided it could wait no longer. The department wanted vaccinees to receive their packets at least a week in advance and thousands of copies had to be made. "At a certain drop-dead date," remembers Danila, "we said it doesn't matter if the CDC is revising it at this point. We're going to make our copies now." MDH also added its own original documents to the packet, such as a warning on latex allergies, one on dressings, and some state-specific privacy forms.

---

61. CDC Telebriefing Transcript.

During the last weeks of January, MDH held vaccination training by satellite for over 800 individuals, mostly nurses. On January 29, MDH ordered 4,500 doses of vaccine, less than half the amount proposed in the December 9 plan. It arrived on February 4. At this point, the department expected to vaccinate 2,700 volunteers—1,700 hospital personnel and 1,000 public health workers—over a period of several weeks.[62]

The Minnesota pre-event smallpox vaccination program opened on February 12 with a clinic at the state emergency operations center in the Department of Public Safety building in St. Paul. Because of security concerns, MDH had kept the location secret until the last moment. Television cameras were invited to witness the first vaccination, that of State Epidemiologist Hull. Hull, who had been vaccinated three times already, said afterward, "I couldn't even feel it."[63] Only five volunteers were vaccinated in front of the cameras; others were inoculated in another, confidential location. Dr. Gregory Poland, a smallpox expert at the Mayo Clinic in Rochester, Minnesota, who had long been immunized himself, administered the televised vaccinations.

For the next five weeks, clinics were held regularly in unpublicized sites around the state. Eventually, local public health departments hosted nine regional clinics, while another 30 or so satellite clinics were held at hospitals. The vaccination procedure was time-consuming, taking up to an hour per patient, because the protocols for administering the smallpox vaccine were closer to those required in drug trials than to standard immunization clinics. Much time went to screening each volunteer to discover if s/he had any reason not to take the vaccine. Counter-indications included pregnancy or a desire to become pregnant soon, eczema, a recent case of skin disease of any kind, allergies to medications, or an immune-compromised system due to treatment for cancer or other illnesses. Any borderline case was referred to a second screener. The potential vaccinee was then shown a CDC-produced film warning of the risks of the vaccine. Finally, each vaccinee had to sign a consent form acknowledging agreement to be vaccinated.

Eventually the vaccine was administered. The vaccinator unwrapped the two-pronged needle, dipped it in the vaccine vial to trap drops between the prongs, then pricked the skin on the upper arm 15 times. The spot was covered with the two-layer bandage MDH had special-ordered. The site had to be kept covered for roughly two weeks to prevent shedding. Next, a nurse showed the vaccinee how to care for the wound site properly, including bandage changes. Finally, a public health worker conducted an exit interview. Over the next 19 days, each vaccinee also reported for regular checks to a health care worker who ascertained that the vaccine had "taken."

---

62. Marisa Helms, "Smallpox Vaccinations Begin This Week," February 10, 2003, http://news.minnesota.
publicradio.org/features/2003/02/10_helmsm_smallpox.
63. Maura Lerner, "US Prepares on Multiple Fronts: State Smallpox Effort Starts With Both Secrecy, Publicity," *Minneapolis Star Tribune*, February 13, 2003, 1A.

As the program unfolded, problems inevitably surfaced. Some had been foreseen; others took officials by surprise.

KINKS AND COSTS

The organizational structure arrived at so hastily in early December proved one obstacle to smooth operations, at least in the eyes of some. A few state officials felt they gave up too much policy authority, while locals complained of contradictory instructions from too many masters. Many clinics, for example, decided to inoculate laboratory technicians because the number of volunteer health care workers was small. The original MDH guidelines had allowed for this local discretion, and many MDH officials, says Ehresmann, continued to believe that was a good strategy. But Deputy State Epidemiologist Danila, for one, came to feel that such autonomy was an error. "I'd say that's wrong," comments Danila, noting that ACIP specifically prohibited vaccinating lab technicians.

> Locally they'd say, "Well, you gave us flexibility to make local decisions." I would say that was a mistake on our part. We should not have had flexible policy decisions. There should have been a clear line of authority.

Danila would have preferred to see a master list of all potential vaccinees and their roles, with a central authority deciding yes or no in each case. "That," he notes wryly, "was not done." From the other end of the spectrum, Jane Norbin, director of the Health Policy and Planning section of the Saint Paul-Ramsey County Department of Health, feels that local health officials' autonomy was constrained: "You have a lot of autonomy to do it your way as long as you follow the way you are told to do it."[64] She complains that state responses to local inquiries were not consistent: "You'd get an answer from one person, and another one would contradict it. That was very difficult." Danila agrees that the chain-of-command was poorly conceived. A single hospital with a single question had to send its query through multiple layers of authority. "By the time it gets to us, it's like telephone tag. What gets said and what gets done is not clear," he says.

Diverting Resources

Another problem, anticipated but nonetheless real, was the diversion of resources—both people and money—from other health needs. Public health nurses who normally did clinic immunizations or visited at-risk mothers had been diverted to smallpox. Nurses who worked for the federal Women, Infants and Children (WIC) program, which

---

64. Author's interview with Jane Norbin, St. Paul, MN, March 27, 2003. All further quotes from Norbin, unless otherwise attributed, are from this interview.

provides nutrition and health care advice to low-income families, were now doing smallpox training. Elderly people experienced delays in screenings for admission to nursing homes. Minnesota was not alone; states across the country reported trimming services such as prenatal care, AIDS prevention, water testing, and tuberculosis tracking. Public health nurses had been diverted to smallpox from childhood immunization, new mother visits, and diabetes screening.[65]

OEP Director Einweck told the House Health and Human Services Policy Committee on January 29 that "we're very concerned about being able to meet all our other grant requirements at the state and county level."[66] MDH, for example, had hired experts to help plan for radiological or chemical terrorism but these people had been diverted to smallpox. Another program to train all health workers in bioterrorism emergency procedures had been put on hold.

As for expenses, it was hard to estimate how much the smallpox vaccination program cost the state because most of the expense came in the form of diverted personnel. State employees such as Danila had devoted weeks to smallpox. It was impossible to put a value on the other tasks they had not accomplished. But there were hard costs as well. The 50,000 specialty bandages MDH ordered, for example, cost 74 cents apiece.

The federal government had suggested that states simply redirect to the smallpox program the bioterrorism monies they had received in the spring. But after MDH officials did just that, says Einweck, the accountants at CDC asked for exhaustive accounts of where the money had gone and why. Not that the $18 million Minnesota had received was sufficient. Mary Wellick, director of the Olmsted County Public Health Department, complained to the House Health and Human Services Policy Committee that "no local health department has adequate funding for [smallpox] clinics at this point."[67]

Our services are right against the wire. We had planning money, but no implementation money. And even the planning money is running out.

Einweck testified that while not all 87 Minnesota counties were experiencing budget problems, those running the vaccination clinics were hard hit. Unanticipated expenses included the price of security details. These were arranged, Einweck explains, because CDC had required them. To MDH dismay, CDC in March said that that was incorrect; security coverage had always been a local decision "based on your own internal risk assessment." But by then the money was spent.

Hospitals, meanwhile, incurred their own costs, with no prospect of reimbursement from the state. They had to pay for time to educate vaccinators and vaccinees, for time

65. Ceci Connolly, "Smallpox Campaign Taxing Health Resources," *Washington Post*, March 10, 2003, A4.
66. Jean Hopfensperger, "Anti-smallpox Effort Is Strapping Counties," *Minneapolis Star Tribune*, January 30, 2003, 1B.
67. Ibid.

both groups spent away from their customary work, and for time staff spent checking the bandages of those vaccinated. There was also the cost of setting up the clinics and taking them down. A few hospitals reported bills in excess of $100,000.

Other states also complained about costs and diverted resources. In a NACCHO survey of 539 health departments released in February, some 79% said the smallpox vaccination campaign was using up staff time and money meant for other antibioterrorism programs, such as upgrading laboratories, building secure communications, training staff, and planning for chemical or radiological attack. Even at CDC, almost all of the 350 immunization division staff had been reassigned to smallpox.[68] As for money, in December ASTHO Executive Director Hardy had called the smallpox vaccination campaign "the ultimate unfunded federal mandate.... We can't afford to do this at the expense of all other preparedness."[69] Patrick Libbey, executive director of NACCHO, added that "states and localities already are diverting significant resources to smallpox vaccination and there is no end in sight."

> We urge that the program be kept at minimal levels and grow only as rapidly as threat assessments demand, so as not to disrupt other basic community health protections or cause unnecessary harm.

So it was with considerable relief that, by mid-March, MDH officials concluded that all health care workers who would volunteer for the smallpox vaccine had done so. Minnesota had vaccinated some 1,400 people, ranking the state fourth in the nation for absolute numbers vaccinated. Turnout among public health employees, as at the hospitals, had been lower than anticipated. "A lot of interest," Ramsey County Health official Norbin characterizes the situation, "but very few at the end actually got vaccinated." Out of the 330 people in her department, for example, fewer than 10 were vaccinated. Phase 1, MDH officials hoped, was officially drawing to a close. But the federal government had other ideas.

PHASE 2 ALREADY?

It had been clear for some time that the federal government was not happy with the slow pace of inoculation. By early March, with the compensation issue holding so many states and hospitals back, only 12,404 health care workers had been immunized out of the 500,000 Thompson had hoped for by March 1. Hundreds of hospitals across the country had refused to participate.

So the Bush Administration on March 5 finally agreed to a limited compensation plan for those injured by the vaccine. Drafted by HHS and the White House, the

---

68. Connolly, "Smallpox Campaign Taxing Health Resources."
69. Ceci Connolly, "Smallpox Plan May Force Other Health Cuts," *Washington Post*, December 24, 2002, A1.

proposal offered $262,100 in benefits to those who died or suffered a permanent disability from the smallpox vaccine. Moreover, HHS would pay two-thirds of lost wages, up to $50,000 a year, for those temporarily or partially disabled up to a cap of $262,100. Those payments would begin only after missing five days of work. The same benefits would go to those with secondary infections. The plan would now have to go to Congress for approval. In a caveat, however, the plan covered only those vaccinated in the first 120 days after the bill's passage, not those who participated later.[70]

One day later, Secretary Thompson took a second step to jumpstart the smallpox program. There had never been a firm timetable for starting Phase 2, just as CDC had never provided any definition of what constituted success in Phase 1—number of teams successfully vaccinated, caregivers per hospital, or other measures. But on March 6, HHS gave states permission to move into Phase 2 of the vaccination program. The decision seemed to be driven by the low numbers of health care workers vaccinated so far. The government needs, said Thompson, "to make sure we have enough people prepared" for a smallpox attack.[71] "There is no question," he said, "we wish there were more people willing to be vaccinated."[72] On March 7, Thompson arranged a conference call with the public health commissioners of all the states to discuss moving into Phase 2.

Minnesota was one of several states dismayed at the prospect of moving into Phase 2 with little guidance or advance planning. There was no question of hospitals doing any more vaccinations; public health staff would have to assume the full burden of running clinics. MDH wanted to assess what had been accomplished in Phase 1 before moving on to Phase 2.

RAMSEY COUNTY WANTS IN

Yet starting in early March, pressure began to build to do just that. It began with the sheriff of Ramsey County, home to the state capital, St. Paul. Back in February, Sheriff Bob Fletcher had called the Ramsey County health department to ask for smallpox vaccinations for two top officials from his office. Those two were vaccinated on February 21 under the provisions of Phase 1 to inoculate a few public safety officials. The Ramsey County public health clinic also vaccinated a third official from the sheriff's office and a police officer from St. Paul on March 3 as part of Phase 1. But then the sheriff spoke with the mayor of St. Paul, who upped the ante; he asked for vaccinations for all city police and firefighters.

---

70. Rick Weiss, "US Surgeon General to Get Smallpox Shot," *Washington Post*, March 11, 2003, A21.
71. Ceci Connolly, "Smallpox Vaccination Campaign Bolstered," *Washington Post*, March 7, 2003, A31.
72. Several hundred federal health care workers at CDC and the Public Health Service Commissioned Corps, as well as rescue workers, would also be vaccinated.

Sheriff Fletcher, says County Director of Health Policy and Planning Norbin, "had done his own research on smallpox and smallpox vaccine... and was convinced that we needed to have a vaccinated first responder corps." The sheriff's department alone numbered 250 people. Even if only half of them qualified for the vaccine, that would be a large group to vaccinate. Norbin told the sheriff that MDH would let him know as soon as Phase 2 started, but he objected. "His response," recalls Norbin, "was 'Who do I have to call to get this going? I'm calling our state senators. I'll call the governor. This is unconscionable that public health would hold this up. They did themselves, and they won't do first responders?'"

When MDH heard about the Ramsey County request, not to mention Secretary Thompson's March 6 announcement, many reacted strongly against it. Deputy State Epidemiologist Danila was unambiguous about where he stood:

> Some of us are clearly drawing a line in the sand right now and we will not do that [Phase 2]. We certainly will not do that in the same way we've done Phase 1. We cannot maintain this pace that we've been on.

On March 10, Danila sent an e-mail to many of the state's top health officials, including Leitheiser, now back to being assistant commissioner for health protection. "Several of us," Danila began, "feel very strongly that we cannot continue at the current Phase 1 level of detail, quality of patient safety, and pace of operations beyond March 31."[73] Hospitals, too, he said, had told MDH they could not go beyond Phase 1. The pressing need now, he argued, was to evaluate: How many vaccinators have been vaccinated and where are they? How many disease investigators? How many patient care providers, at which hospitals? What Phase 1 gaps exist in Minnesota and how will they be addressed? Danila continued:

> We also feel strongly that we are becoming less prepared, not more prepared, for smallpox by focusing on vaccinating more persons rather than examining and exercising our post-smallpox event plans.

Hull agreed, noting that "promoting vaccination to create the illusion of preparedness doesn't take us any place." In addition, there were costs in terms of time and staffing requirements. "The attitude from Washington has been 'Well, we gave you $16 million, get on with it.' [But] that was for other purposes and it doesn't do anything to compensate the hospitals," says Hull.

At the same time, Assistant Commissioner Leitheiser was reporting via email to Susan Heegaard in the office of newly elected Republican Governor Tim Pawlenty. Pawlenty was close to the Bush Administration.[74] Heegaard was the governor's designated liaison

---

73. E-mail from Richard Danila to Aggie Leitheiser et al., March 10, 2003, 1:57 p.m., "Phase 2 Discussion."

74. Vice President Dick Cheney had asked Governor Pawlenty not to run for the US Senate in the fall 2002 elections so that Norm Coleman could run.

with the state departments of Health, Human Services, and Education. On Thursday, March 6, Leitheiser alerted Heegaard to the fact that the Ramsey County public health department was feeling pressure to vaccinate local law enforcement officials. She identified four problems with the request:

1. MDH had been approved by CDC to do public health/hospital teams, not general first responders.
2. There wasn't enough vaccine to do everyone.
3. The smallpox vaccination program had been expensive and staff intensive; there was neither the personnel nor money to do a wider program. The current need was for evaluation.
4. The federal government was working on a compensation package but nothing was in place yet.

MDH, Leitheiser reported, would be sending out a letter to all local public health departments asking that all smallpox vaccine be returned. That memo went out the next day, March 7.

By Monday, March 10, however, Heegaard was pushing back in support of the sheriff's request. The governor's chief of staff, Charlie Weaver—who as former public safety commissioner had close ties to law enforcement and fire officials—had said MDH should go ahead and vaccinate local law enforcement officials, starting with Minneapolis and St. Paul. According to Heegaard, the newly appointed commissioner of health, Dianne Mandernach, was in the room for the discussion. "Have you come up with a plan in light of the broad discretion given by the feds?" she asked, referring to Secretary Thompson's March 6 announcement that states could move to Phase 2 at will.

Leitheiser responded early on Thursday, March 13, trying once again to explain the MDH objections to moving to Phase 2 quickly. The department wanted, she said, to offer "Phase 2 in an organized way." She mentioned a number of outstanding issues: medical coverage, training and screening, whether MDH should provide bandages, review of the vaccine take. She reiterated that hospitals and local public health officials found the costs of expanding vaccinations to first responders "large and that the money isn't there." She reported that, nonetheless, each region had been asked to come up with a Phase 2 plan within a week. MDH would be meeting with local health planners shortly to coordinate activities.

But Leitheiser realized she could hold off for only a limited time. Later on Thursday, Leitheiser called a meeting that included Hull, Ehresmann, Einweck, Danila, and other MDH staff involved with the smallpox program. By the end of the meeting, she told them, they had to decide what to tell the Ramsey County public health department.

When Prevention Can Kill: Minnesota and the Smallpox Vaccination Program (Epilogue)

Kirsten Lundberg

A t the Minnesota Department of Health (MDH) meeting on March 13, 2003, the conversation was lively and wide-ranging. "If we say yes to Ramsey, then is every other county going to want to do this? You know, what are the implications?" then–MDH Immunization Section Chief Kristen Ehresmann recalls discussing. The group talked about staff burnout, the cost of taking on Phase 2, what kind of bandages to use, the deferral of other public health activities, and other topics. But the political reality, she adds, was clear to all of them:

> We had a new administration with whom we had not yet established a relationship, or our scientific credibility. We felt we had to consider the implications of refusing their first directive.

By the end of the meeting, the MDH staff had come to a consensus that balanced the political and scientific agendas. They agreed there was a need to evaluate Phase 1, but that it must be done quickly and while preparing for Phase 2. They decided to send each of the nine Minnesota regions an assessment form that would ask for an estimate of how many fire, police, and other emergency personnel might actually want to be vaccinated.

At the same time, MDH planners would schedule a conference for regional groups in the near future. The agenda would be to evaluate Phase 1, with an emphasis on ideas for

This epilogue was written by Kirsten Lundberg for Dr. Arnold M. Howitt, Director of the Executive Session on Domestic Preparedness and Executive Director, Taubman Center for State and Local Government, Kennedy School of Government. Funding was provided by the Volpe National Transportation Systems Center, US Department of Transportation, with additional assistance from the Robert Wood Johnson Foundation. (0803)

streamlining the time-consuming vaccination process. The conference would also try to specify just what preparedness should mean in the Minnesota public health context so that, next time around, it would be easier to know when success had been achieved. After the conference, MDH would draw up a plan that assessed whom to vaccinate in order to be prepared, how many numbers would be involved, and what gaps remained from Phase 1 that should be filled. The department would establish minimum standards for safety, draw up a vaccination plan, define first responders, and set a definite timeline for implementation.

But as for Ramsey County, the MDH officials at the meeting decided that the local public health department could go ahead and vaccinate public safety officials if it wanted to, on a timetable of its own choosing. So on March 26, a Ramsey County public health team vaccinated 11 people from the sheriff's office. On April 29, it vaccinated two firemen/medical technicians, and on May 11 one policeman. Response was low, as it developed, because public safety officials had a similar reaction to doctors and nurses when invited to volunteer for the vaccination.

Nationwide, by the end of May 2003, only 38,000 out of the anticipated 500,000 eligible health care workers had been vaccinated against smallpox.[1] Only a handful of public safety officials chose to take the vaccine. The Advisory Committee on Immunization Practices recommended in late May that only health care workers continue getting the shot after three vaccinees died from heart attacks in March. But Centers for Disease Control and Prevention Director Julie Gerberding responded that the continued threat of bioterrorism made the ongoing vaccinations necessary. Rather than limiting the program, states had started to screen out those at risk for heart disease.

---

1. David Wahlberg, "Smallpox Shots to Continue Despite Warnings," *Atlanta Journal and Constitution*, June 27, 2003, 5A.

IV. PUBLIC HEALTH SYSTEM ISSUES

The City of Chicago and the 1995 Heat Wave

Pamela Varley

EDITORS' INTRODUCTION

The heat wave that swept over Chicago for five days in July of 1995 was a severe public health crisis that, by the county Medical Examiner's tally, left 576 people dead in Cook County—mostly frail, elderly residents, many of them poor, living alone in non–air-conditioned apartments. But it was an emergency that caught city and county government substantially unaware until pressure on public agencies mounted to extraordinary levels, and the increasing number of bodies of the deceased literally compelled realization that something unprecedented was happening.

The two parts of this case study thus describe a clear example of an emergent crisis, one that began in ways that seemed routine but ultimately showed important elements of novelty that created critical challenges for those dealing with the crisis. As well, the second part of the case tells how Chicago reflected on the crisis at its conclusion and instituted changes in policy and practice intended to significantly improve the area's ability to handle future heat waves.

On Thursday, July 13, metropolitan area weather, already very hot, turned unusually brutal. By Friday, the strain on city and county agencies was becoming readily apparent. Ambulance services were nearly overwhelmed by calls for service that

This case was written by Pamela Varley, Kennedy School case writer, for Dr. Arnold Howitt, Director of the Kennedy School's Executive Session on Domestic Preparedness and Executive Director of the Taubman Center for State and Local Government. Funding was provided by the Office for State and Local Domestic Preparedness Support, US Department of Justice, and the Robert Wood Johnson Foundation. (0102)

spiked to 80% above normal. Fire trucks were pushed into improvised ambulance service. The capacities of hospital emergency departments, some also experiencing power outages, were strained near breaking; by Saturday, more than 25% were on bypass, meaning that they could no longer take additional patients arriving by ambulance. The police department was receiving more calls for handling the bodies of deceased individuals than it could readily process and transport to the morgue. For its part the county Medical Examiner's Office received 87 bodies on Saturday, surpassing its previous record of 35 and far exceeding the normal daily workload. Mutual aid from surrounding locales, usually helpful in handling surge demand for services, was insufficiently effective; as the heat consumed the region, all communities in the Chicago area were experiencing similar pressures and therefore couldn't provide much, if any, assistance to their neighbors.

Even as the pressure mounted, Chicago officials were slow to put together the separate pieces of the gathering crisis. The Public Health Department was not getting systematic data about the number of cases of heat-related illness and death; these were not reportable disease cases. The mayor's senior staff did not learn about the crisis conditions building up until late on Saturday, and the mayor himself did not know until Sunday morning. By the time the city declared a Heat Emergency on Sunday afternoon and mobilized for additional response, the heat wave was nearly tapering off.

Once the heat wave broke, a dispute broke out over the count of heat-related deaths, with the county medical examiner publicly declaring the heat wave impacts a disaster. In the aftermath of this public controversy and much criticism over the city's handling of the situation, the mayor appointed a commission to study what caused the heat wave, why so many people died, and how the city should prepare to cope with future bouts of extreme heat or cold. Among the reforms that the commission and separate work by various government agencies developed were an expansion of the conditions that health care providers would monitor and report to the Health Department, new procedures for getting surge capacity from private ambulance services during future crises to complement the Fire Department's ambulances, changes in the bypass protocols that allowed hospitals to temporarily shut down new ambulance deliveries of patients, and refinements in the methods that the city used to predict severe-heat weather.

Even more quickly, the city developed a Heat Emergency plan, which got an early test—but under less severe conditions—only a few weeks after the July heat wave. The city's preparations fit well with an ongoing project to create an Office of Emergency Communications that would include a command center in which top officials could assemble to manage any new crises. As the experience of the 1995 heat wave was assimilated, however, Chicago continued to look at additional ways to manage future crises.

DISCUSSION QUESTIONS

1. What factors made it difficult for city and county officials to grasp the full set of conditions that made the heat wave so deadly and challenged the government's ability to respond?
2. Why were responses to the developing crisis so fragmented?
3. Organization theorists would call the public health and health care systems of Chicago "loosely coupled" systems whose components operated with a great deal of independence. To what extent is this a disadvantage in times of crisis?
4. What methods of coordination should Chicago consider for more effectively managing future public health crises?

*   *   *

The heat wave that swept across the Great Plains and Midwest in mid-July 1995 was one of the deadliest in US history and one of the worst disasters ever to strike the City of Chicago, where it claimed 522 lives by one count and 733 by another; meanwhile, the death toll for all of Cook County, which included Chicago and several neighboring municipalities, was 576, according to the Cook County Medical Examiner. Yet, within Chicago, the 1995 heat wave was not recognized as a disaster, nor even as a serious event, until almost after the fact.

Those who lived through the five days of punishing heat knew at the time that the combination of high temperature, high humidity, and bright sun had created miserably uncomfortable conditions—far worse than the usual Chicago summer hot spells. But it was not until after the worst days of heat had passed that Chicago political leaders, journalists, and residents began to grasp the toll it had taken. In a macabre drama that drew national television coverage, residents of greater Chicago discovered that hundreds of their neighbors and relatives—mostly old, frail, and living in small, urban apartments—had died. Police wagons, carrying the deceased in body bags, lined up for several city blocks outside the Cook County[1] Medical Examiner's building, waiting to deliver the bodies into the custody of a small, overburdened staff of medical examiners. In the end, the Medical Examiner had to borrow ten refrigerated trucks to hold all the dead in the parking lot.

After the fact, it also came to light that hospital emergency departments (EDs) and Fire Department ambulances had been under severe strain during the heat wave, with resulting delays in medical treatment to residents suffering from the heat. The Illinois Department of Public Health later calculated that, of the 172 patients that had to wait at least 30 minutes for an ambulance, 12 were pronounced dead on arrival at the hospital. Whether they would have died anyway, no one ever knew for certain. By and large, the patients who called for emergency medical assistance did survive, though some

---

1. Cook County comprises all of Chicago and a number of adjacent municipalities.

suffered permanent adverse health affects. And the vast majority of the people who died of the heat never called for help at all. But, at the least, the delays in the delivery of ambulance and hospital services added to the distress of heat-sick patients and created grueling work conditions for emergency medical personnel. They also raised a flag about the way the emergency medical system was primed to recognize and respond to an unusual and unanticipated strain.

Once the heat had subsided and its toll on the city had grown clearer, the mayor and his administration were left with a number of sobering questions. Chicago prided itself on responding well to emergencies, yet this one had caught the city unaware. How had a crisis that had claimed the lives of hundreds of city residents gone unrecognized until almost after the fact? And what, if anything, could be done to prevent another unanticipated emergency from killing or injuring large numbers of people before the city recognized the crisis and mobilized its forces?

BRACING FOR A HOT SPELL

Chicago was not the only city to suffer from the 1995 heat wave, nor was the arrival of the heat, itself, unexpected. On July 5, and again on July 8, the National Weather Service (NWS) warned of a high-pressure system and suffocating air mass moving slowly eastward from the Great Plains, bringing temperatures above 100°F to the City of Chicago by Tuesday July 11 or Wednesday July 12. In fact, as they braced for the heat, Chicago's 2.7 million residents could observe its effect on the states just to the west of Illinois, where the heat wave had already hit. In Iowa, hundreds of livestock had died, and TV cameras showed bulldozers pushing the bodies into trucks for burning. In Nebraska, extreme heat caused a railway rail to buckle and that, in turn, caused a freight train to derail.

On paper, the City of Chicago did have a policy for dealing with extreme heat. The Chicago Forecast Office of the NWS issued a Heat Advisory whenever it forecasted at least two consecutive days with a peak heat index of 105°F or higher and a minimum heat index of 80°F or higher at night. (The heat index was the felt heat level when temperature and humidity were considered in combination.) The NWS issued a more urgent Heat Warning whenever the heat index reached 120°F. Whenever it issued either a Heat Advisory or a Heat Warning, the NWS notified the city's Weather Center, an office in the Department of Streets and Sanitation. In turn, the city's Department of Public Health could announce a formal citywide Heat Emergency. In fact, public health officials say the plan for responding to a Heat Emergency was sketchy—a page and a half in total length, with general instructions to open certain Department of Human Services buildings as "cooling centers" and to put out public advisories about coping with high heat—things the city did anyway during heat waves without a formal declaration of a Heat Emergency. Beyond these measures, "we didn't have a system set up to *do* anything if we declared it," says then–Public Health

Commissioner Sr. Sheila Lyne. In point of fact, she adds, the city had not declared a Heat Emergency in anyone's memory; few city officials knew the policy existed.

As City Hall prepared for the heat wave of 1995, therefore, the city did not declare a Heat Emergency, but city officials did take their usual hot weather precautions: The Department of Public Health put out flyers and public service announcements advising residents, for example, to drink plenty of water, stay inside during the heat of the day, and avoid strenuous activity.[2] The Department of Human Services announced that several emergency assistance buildings would be open as cooling centers for any residents who wanted to use them.

Chicago City Hall did have one overriding concern about the impending heat wave— and that was the problem of the city's 43,000 fire hydrants. In hot weather, residents in neighborhoods all across the city opened thousands of fire hydrants to create impromptu water sprays for children and teenagers. Under such conditions, the loss of water pressure could reach hazardous levels, leaving Chicago homes without running water just as they most needed it for drinking water and cooling showers. Even more worrisome was the possibility of inadequate water for Chicago hospitals and other medical facilities and, of course, inadequate water for firefighting. Anticipating that the coming five-day blast of heat would provoke a rash of hydrant-opening, the city mobilized large numbers of city Water Department employees to travel around the city closing the hydrants, in some cases, with a police escort, as neighborhood residents were sometimes hostile to hydrant closings.

A SPORTING ATTITUDE

Between Tuesday, July 11, and Wednesday, July 12, Chicago's high temperature rose from 89°F to 97°F, and the heat index hit 101°F. On Thursday, July 13, Chicago's official temperature was 104°F at O'Hare Airport, though in southwest Chicago, at Midway Airport,

---

2. The human body is designed to keep a steady temperature of about 98.6°F. Confronted by severe heat, the body of a healthy individual cools itself either by shedding heat to cooler air surrounding it via radiation or by sweat and evaporation. When air temperature is hotter than body temperature, radiative cooling no longer works. When humidity is high, evaporative cooling is much less effective. Thus, public health experts recommend that under conditions of high temperature *and* high humidity, people should try to go to a cooler environment in order to lower their core body temperature—ideally, spending at least two hours in an air-conditioned location or, at the least, taking a cooling bath. Furthermore, as the body ages, the mechanisms that maintain the body's internal temperature balance begin to break down. The body does not register temperature as well. Blood vessels are supposed to expand to cool down the body, but this requires the heart to pump the blood with more force—a stress that a compromised heart may not be able to withstand. The body has fewer sweat glands that work less efficiently. The hypothalamus does not respond as quickly to dehydration. And, if the patient is unable to care for himself or herself, has a history of alcoholism, uses tranquilizers, or uses any number of other medications, the risks may be far greater. (For example, if a patient is prescribed diuretics for a heart condition, this will exacerbate dehydration. If a patient is taking antipsychotic drugs, these can interfere with the body's physiological response to extreme temperatures.) If the body temperature rises to 105°F, the person is said to suffer from heat stroke, and the consequence is usually organ damage followed relatively quickly by death. Heat stroke can develop quickly. According to one CDC study, two-thirds of people to suffer heat stroke were reported to have been ill less than one day before hospitalization or death.

the mercury hit 106°F. What's more, the humidity was stultifying: the heat index for Thursday was 123°F. According to the NWS, July 13 was the hottest day in Chicago's recorded history.

Chicago was known for its weather extremes, however, and some city residents took a perverse pride in the excessive nature of this scorcher. *Chicago Sun-Times* columnist Richard Roeper and some friends decided, "as a lark," to spend time outside—in Roeper's case, in order to write "the definitive fun column on 'surviving' the hottest hour in our city's recorded history."

> We were almost giddy out there on the deck. It was the July equivalent of plunging into Lake Michigan on New Year's Day; we were all quite proud of ourselves for being right there in the middle of the white-hottest Chicago sun experience any of us had ever known.[3]

Thursday night brought little relief from the heat, with temperatures remaining in the 80s, and on Friday, the heat was still intense; the official high temperature was 100°F, and the heat index, 115°F. Mayor Richard Daley held a press conference about the heat wave but urged the media not to exaggerate the situation: "It's hot. It's very hot. We all have our little problems, but let's not blow it out of proportion. It's like getting real cold weather. Yes, we go to extremes in Chicago, and that's why people *like* Chicago…. Let's just all work together and calm down."[4]

HARBINGERS OF TROUBLE ON FRIDAY NIGHT

After the fact, the Department of Emergency Medicine at Cook County Hospital would estimate that on Thursday, 575 people went to Chicago-area hospital EDs complaining of some form of heat sickness, such as hyperthermia, heat stroke, heat exhaustion, heat cramps, or heat edema. On Friday, another 875 heat-sick patients went to hospital EDs, and 725 more arrived on Saturday.[5] At the time, however, no one in city or state government realized that, by the hundreds, people were falling ill and rushing to the hospital. The emergency medical personnel in individual hospital EDs knew they were under strain, but emergency patient load was, by nature, erratic. And it was no secret that the city was in the grip of a severe heat wave. Emergency workers therefore hunkered down and did their best to cope.

---

3. *Chicago Sun-Times*, July 17, 1995.
4. *Chicago Sun-Times*, July 18, 1995.
5. Robert J. Rydman, Associate Professor and Research Codirector, Department of Emergency Medicine, Cook County Hospital/Rush Medical College, School of Public Health, University of Illinois, Chicago, IL, "1995 Heat Crisis in Chicago: An Area Morbidity Study of Hospital Emergency Department Treated Prevalence," May 1998. With Dino Rumoro, Julio Silva, and Tess Hogan, Department of Emergency Medicine, Resurrection Medical Center, Chicago, IL.

One of those emergency workers was, in fact, the chief of Emergency Medical Services (EMS) for the Illinois Department of Public Health, Leslee Stein-Spencer. Stein-Spencer made it a practice to keep one foot in the trenches by moonlighting as an ED nurse. At 7 p.m. Friday night, she arrived at the ED of the Michael Reese Hospital near Chicago's South Side and was immediately struck by the crowded waiting room and long lines of patients awaiting treatment. "Our emergency department had an average waiting time just to be seen by an MD of 12 hours, and, amazing enough, people were waiting," she later wrote in a memo about the heat wave to the director of the Illinois Department of Public Health. Paramedics on Fire Department ambulances were becoming visibly exhausted, she noted. What's more, 11 of the city's 67 hospital EDs had announced a bypass, which meant that the EDs had judged themselves overwhelmed by patient demand and were temporarily closing their doors to new ambulance patients (though they still accepted walk-in patients, as required by law).

It was not rare for a Chicago hospital to call for a bypass. Years of cost cutting, coupled with the nationwide nursing shortage, meant that many hospitals lacked the medical equipment and staff resources to cope with unusually high numbers of emergency patients. For 11 hospitals to be on bypass at once did put an added burden on the other hospitals and on city ambulances, which had to travel farther to deliver their patients. Even so, "at that point, I didn't see it as a big issue," Stein-Spencer recalls.

Friday Night for the Cook County Medical Examiner

Emergency medical workers were not the only people in Chicago to see, first hand, the toll of the heat Friday night. In the office of the Cook County Medical Examiner, Friday was a slightly busier-than-average day. The job of the Medical Examiner was to determine the cause of death of any Cook County resident who had died violently, in a manner sudden or unexpected, or without medical attendants. On average, the county office examined 17 bodies a day, but on Friday, the Office of the Medical Examiner had received 23—including the sad case of two three-year-old boys who had died of the heat inside a closed sport utility vehicle. At home with his family at 9 p.m. Friday, Edmund Donoghue, chief medical examiner for Cook County, received a call from one of his medical examiners. "He said, 'Dr. Donoghue, we thought we should call you because we have 40 cases scheduled for tomorrow,'" Donoghue recalls. This stopped the doctor in his tracks. "Never in the history of the Medical Examiner's Office have we had more than 35 cases.[6] I said, 'What's happening?' He said, 'They're dying of the heat.'"

---

6. That is, the Medical Examiner's Office had never had more than 35 cases in a single day unless the city was in the throes of an obvious disaster, such as a train wreck or plane crash.

Friday Night for the Chicago Police

Whenever a dead body was discovered in Chicago, the first officials called to the scene were officers of the Chicago Police Department. After an initial investigation, the police dispatched a squad roll—a police wagon specially equipped with stretchers, body bags, and contamination gear—to the scene and transported the body of the deceased to the Cook County Medical Examiner. Like the Cook County Medical Examiner, therefore, the Chicago Police were seeing a marked increase in dead bodies Friday night. Frank Radke, deputy chief of patrol for the Chicago Police's Northwest Area, recalls that he was driving back from his son's freshman orientation at Michigan State University when, at 7 p.m., he got a call from a commanding officer in his area. His police officers, he learned, were responding to an unusually high number of calls reporting the discovery of dead bodies. In addition, responding to a number of requests for a well-being check on someone elderly or in poor health, police officers were finding the person dead on arrival (DOA). This spike in DOA calls had presented an unusual logistical problem: the police were running out of squad rolls. Across the city, there were about 25 squad rolls in active service; each of the city's 25 police districts was assigned one, which did double duty, transporting prisoners to and from jail or transporting dead bodies to the Medical Examiner.[7] Now, all were being used to transport bodies to the Medical Examiner's Office—and still, there were not enough.

A WILD WEEKEND

Chicago got little relief from the heat Friday night, with nighttime low temperatures in the 80s, and Saturday dawned hot and muggy. The NWS was reporting, however, that the worst was over. The heat index would hit 115°F on Saturday, but the high temperature would only reach 98°F. By Sunday, the heat index would fall to 107°F, and the temperature would drop to 93°F. On Monday, temperature and heat index were both forecasted in the livable mid-80s range. But for many emergency medical and public safety workers, the worst effects of the heat wave were yet to come.

---

7. The arrangement in Chicago—to have police responsible for transporting the bodies to the Medical Examiner—was unusual. In many communities, the Medical Examiner's Office, itself, provided this transportation. In fact, the City of Chicago had long wished that Cook County would take over the body transport job in Chicago as well. The county had steadfastly resisted this idea, however, and Donoghue argues that in the case of the 1995 heat wave, the involvement of the Chicago Police was crucial. "If we [in Cook County] had to take over body transport, we'd lucky if they gave us six vehicles to cover the whole city," Donoghue says. "The county will only budget you for what you routinely need—they don't budget for emergencies. The fact that these [police squad roll] vehicles have mixed use really protects the City of Chicago, because it allows you to have a lot more vehicles out there. If the police had not been involved in the transport [during the 1995 heat wave], this would have been a *disaster*."

HOSPITAL EMERGENCY DEPARTMENTS IN TROUBLE

By Saturday, hospital EDs—facing their third straight day of high patient loads—were severely overloaded, especially those that were suffering the power shortages affecting many parts of the city. Trinity Hospital, on Chicago's far South Side, for example, had already declared a bypass at 8:50 a.m. due to shortages of equipment and beds. Compounding this overload, the ED lost power at 11:30 a.m. and had to function without air conditioning, computers, elevators, dumbwaiters, or x-ray equipment. "Within 45 minutes, temperatures in the ED rose from 72 to 90," says Julie Novak, Trinity's EMS coordinator.[8]

> With our dumbwaiters out of service, blood and urine samples had to be rushed to the lab by staff members who hand carried the samples up and down five flights of stairs. Without the elevators, patients could not be transferred to their rooms. We were forced to place them in halls and waiting areas. Without computers, the staff had to hand-write all the information in the patients' charts.

Walk-in patients "continued to stream in," Novak continues. Despite spending 11 hours and 20 minutes on bypass, the Trinity Hospital ED treated 117 patients on Saturday, 54% more than its usual patient load. Novak says:

> The emergency department was forced to function as a MASH unit, with the staff focusing their energy on their patients and ignoring the conditions in which they were working. There was no time for the hospital staff to eat or take a break. Personnel were fighting off dehydration and heat exhaustion themselves.

Meanwhile, 63 blocks north at Reese Hospital, Stein-Spencer, again moonlighting as an ED nurse, arrived at 11 p.m. Saturday night to find the ED busier than the night before. To her dismay, she soon discovered that there were 18 Chicago-area hospital EDs on bypass simultaneously—about 25% of the EDs in the metro area. Virtually all the EDs on Chicago's South Side—a large, densely populated, low-income area of town—were on bypass. This meant patients and ambulances had to travel long distances to get to the nearest open ED. "Reese had just received a patient from 130th and Halsted [a distance about 100 blocks south of the hospital and 30 blocks west], as we were the closest available emergency department open," Stein-Spencer wrote in her summary of the event. Right away, "I knew I had a major issue." She swiftly shifted from her role as ED nurse to that of Illinois's chief of EMS.

To have 18 hospital ED on bypass was to plunge the city into dangerous territory. The more EDs on bypass, the more patient load shifted to the remaining EDs, increasing the likelihood that they, too, would collapse under the strain and have to declare a bypass.

---

8. Drawn from Julie Novak's testimony at a hearing of the Illinois Senate Public Health and Welfare Committee on July 26, 1995.

In addition to the domino effect on other hospitals, the bypass situation was by now putting enormous pressure on the city's ambulance crews, which were receiving far more calls than usual and having to spend far more than the usual amount of time on each hospital run. Stein-Spencer quickly called Chicago's deputy fire commissioner in charge of EMS, Cortez Trotter, to let him know about the bypass situation. Trotter was predictably horrified, she recalls in her report. "He told me to do something—that his ambulances could not be going all over the city." Stein-Spencer assured Trotter that she was going to get the hospital EDs back in operation as soon as possible. To do so, however, was to move into uncharted waters.

EMERGENCY DEPARTMENT BYPASS POLICY

Chicago-area hospitals had been granted the legal right to declare an ED bypass, or temporary resource limitation, under a policy adopted by the EMS Commission of Metropolitan Chicago in 1981. Before this policy change, hospital EDs had been required to accept and treat every patient who arrived by ambulance, by police transport, or by his or her own means. Overloaded hospitals had been permitted—after the initial emergency treatment—to transfer a patient to another, less burdened hospital, but this process was bureaucratically involved and often time-consuming. In adopting the 1981 policy, the commission had been persuaded that patient care would benefit if overwhelmed hospital EDs were allowed to call for a bypass, which rerouted ambulance patients to the next nearest, and presumably less burdened, hospital. The commission policy made it clear that hospitals were not to decide lightly to call for a bypass; but at the same time, the policy left the criteria for doing so "somewhat vague and open-ended," according to Stein-Spencer.

Over time, Chicago's hospital EDs developed personalities when it came to invoking a bypass. Some prided themselves on never doing so unless the facility was in extremis. For example, the ED might reluctantly call for a bypass if an adjacent section of the hospital was on fire but otherwise would stay open by any means necessary—pulling in staff, moving patients into other areas of the hospital, discharging patients early, turning the cafeteria into a waiting room, and lining up gurneys in the hall. Other hospitals, however, were far quicker to announce an ED bypass. Some called for a bypass if they were short of staff; nursing shortages in Chicago, as across the nation, had made it difficult to find replacements when staff members called in sick. Some called for a bypass because they had no more beds and nowhere to put additional patients. Some called for a bypass when ED patients had to wait several hours to see a doctor. It was always considered legitimate to call for a bypass when the ED had no access to cardiac-monitored beds, but there were gray areas. For instance, was it legitimate to call for a bypass if the ED had run out of monitored beds even though there were open monitored beds elsewhere in the hospital? That was unclear. What's more, some hospitals fudged on the monitored bed standard. "They'll say, 'All our monitored beds are full' but they've put a [patient with a] broken arm in a monitored bed, so it's really not a monitored *patient*," says Stein-Spencer. "Or they go on bypass because they want to hold [some monitored] beds for [the patients of] their private attending [physicians]." EDs that were thought to abuse the bypass policy were subject to grumbling from paramedics and other personnel in Chicago's emergency medical system. Some joked about EDs that would go on bypass "for the Christmas party."

Such debate and comment were almost entirely confined to the world of EMS workers, however. The bypass policy had provoked no public controversy except in 1992, when a hospital ED on bypass refused the urgent appeal of a nearby ambulance crew attending a three-month-old baby who was unconscious, near death, and in need of immediate care. The baby subsequently died. Whether swifter medical attention might have saved her life was never clear, but the case caused a public outcry. The state Department of Public Health's EMS division was called in to investigate the case and concluded that in the particular circumstances the hospital had been wrong to refuse the baby. After this case, the state legislature had given the Department of Public Health's division of EMS the authority to assess a hospital's decision to go on bypass, to revoke the bypass, and to levy fines up to $5,000 against hospitals that inappropriately called for a bypass (or up to $10,000 if the bypass could have caused imminent harm or death).

In reality, the Department of Public Health's EMS division used this authority on rare occasions to investigate a questionable bypass decision after the fact. Day to day, the EMS division had a minimal role in overseeing hospital bypass decisions. That responsibility fell to the three EMS Resource Hospitals—Illinois Masonic, Northwestern Memorial, and University of Chicago—which oversaw ambulance traffic from the scene of illness or injury to the 67 Chicago hospitals. Each hospital reported to one of these three Resource Hospitals, and each Resource Hospital governed a specific geographic region of the city. In a routine case, an ambulance was sent to the scene of illness or injury by an EMS 9-1-1 dispatcher. If the patient required hospital attention, the paramedics called the appropriate Resource Hospital to confer with a physician about the patient's condition and immediate care and to decide which hospital ED the ambulance should head for—usually, the nearest. A Resource Hospital telemetry operator then notified the ED to expect the patient. When a hospital declared its ED on bypass, it notified the appropriate Resource Hospital,[9] which kept an updated list of all the hospitals presently on bypass in the city. That way, if the paramedics were preparing to take a patient to a hospital that had just declared a bypass, the telemetry operators would divert them to the next nearest option.

---

9. The hospital on bypass also notified the EMS dispatchers for the Chicago Fire Department, so that paramedics, generally, knew all the hospitals on bypass in their territory. Because police officers sometimes brought patients to the ED as well, the hospital on bypass also notified the dispatchers for the Chicago Police Department.

Stein-Spencer believed the EMS medical directors, who were in charge of the EMS division of each Resource Hospital, should play a greater watchdog role, making sure that no more than one or two hospitals in any one region went on bypass at the same time. As a rule, however, the EMS medical directors were uncertain of their legal authority in this regard and reluctant to refuse to honor another hospital's bypass decision. Across town, over the telephone, it was hard to judge the situation on the ground in another hospital. To second-guess a fellow ED coordinator was seen as disrespectful and, perhaps, irresponsible.

In fact, the issue had never come to a head. Neither an EMS medical director nor the chief of the state's EMS division had ever forced a hospital to end a bypass. If push came to shove, no one was certain how hospitals would react to such an order. Thus, Stein-Spencer says, as she contemplated the need to reopen hospital EDs Saturday night, she tried to be "proactive… but political at the same time."

MANAGING BYPASS DURING THE HEAT WAVE

Stein-Spencer's biggest priority was to reopen EDs on Chicago's South Side, and she wanted to enlist the help of the South Side Resource Hospital—the University of Chicago Hospital—to do this. The hospital itself was on bypass, however, so Stein-Spencer's first move was to persuade it to reopen its own EDs and set an example for others. She decided, as a rule of thumb, to give hospitals two hours to reopen their EDs. "I didn't want to call them up and say, 'You have to go off bypass immediately,'" she says. "I wanted to give them time." The hospital reopened its ED at 2 a.m., and shortly thereafter, its attending physician agreed to help Stein-Spencer call the list of hospitals to find the reason for the bypass decision and tell them the state was requiring them to reopen.

While the ED directors did not flatly refuse to reopen, some did argue. In many cases, "The question came up, 'What are we supposed to do?'" Stein-Spencer says. The answer she gave them was, "Implement your internal disaster plan." Every hospital was required by law to have such a plan. That meant calling in extra staff, moving patients from one area of the hospital to another, discharging patients early to open up beds, halting elective surgery procedures, maybe even renting additional equipment—doing, in other words, whatever they judged necessary to make their ED fully operational.

Stein-Spencer did make certain allowances as a matter of judgment. For example, one hospital was suffering a power outage, and she allowed this ED to remain on bypass. Also, in some sections of town, only one hospital was on bypass. That did not cause hardship to the overall EMS system, so Stein-Spencer did not ask such hospitals to reopen to ambulance traffic.

By 7:30 a.m. Sunday, the list of hospitals on bypass was down to eight, with another two due to reopen by 10 a.m. After an exhausting night, Stein-Spencer reflected, the situation appeared to be under better control. But as the day wore on, she found that some hospitals were reinstating their bypass status, and some were going on and off bypass almost by the hour, which led to confusion, especially for ambulance crews. The Fire Department EMS division was pushing for a solution, and Stein-Spencer concluded that she needed to institute a new policy to get through the remainder of the heat wave. In consultation with the director of the Illinois Department of Public Health, she "made up a new policy on the fly." Under this stop-gap arrangement, hospitals could declare a bypass as they judged necessary, but—bypass or no—had to be prepared to accept ambulance patients in two circumstances: whenever a patient was critically ill and needed care urgently and whenever a Chicago Fire Department ambulance estimated that to honor the bypass and take a patient to the nearest open ED would take longer than 15 minutes. "I also said I wanted to be paged any time multiple hospitals were on bypass," Stein-Spencer says.

In deciding to circumscribe the bypass option of city hospitals, Stein-Spencer was aided by Patrick Finnegan, the director of Clinical, Administrative, Professional and Emergency Services for the Metropolitan Chicago Healthcare Council (MCHC), an advocacy organization for local hospitals. Though sympathetic to the pressures on the hospitals and adamant that bypass be respected for any hospital suffering a power failure, Finnegan also understood that in a citywide emergency, the state had to be able to limit the number of hospital EDs on bypass. Under the auspices of MCHC, he sent out a broadcast fax to all MCHC hospitals to signal, "The policy's been changed. Leslee's in charge." Although on the books Stein-Spencer had the authority to revoke any hospital bypass, "some hospitals believed it, others didn't," Finnegan adds. "Now it was clear-cut: She's got it. She's doing it. She's got final word."

The implementation of the new policy was not entirely trouble-free. As Stein-Spencer later wrote, "Someone from the Fire Department started calling around the Resource Hospitals, misrepresenting state policy, saying that the state had said there could be no more than five hospitals on bypass citywide, and if that occurred, the Chicago Fire Department didn't have to honor [anyone's] bypass. That got people upset." But, by and large, both hospitals and ambulances cooperated with Stein-Spencer's compromise policy. And, by the end of the day Sunday, the heat wave was lifting anyway. A study would later estimate that the number of patients arriving in city EDs with heat sickness dropped from about 725 on Saturday to 250 Sunday and was down to 150 by Monday.[10]

FIRE DEPARTMENT AMBULANCES: AN INCREASING STRAIN

For years, the Chicago Fire Department's EMS ambulance crews had complained that the city's fleet of 59 ambulances was insufficient to serve the steadily growing number of emergency medical calls in Chicago. During times of high call volume, the paramedics

---

10. Rydman, "1995 Heat Crisis in Chicago."

felt the pressure keenly. On Thursday, July 13, the Fire Department received 952 emergency medical calls—45% above the usual call volume. On Friday, July 14, there were 1238 calls—89% more than usual. On Saturday, July 15, there were 1196 calls—82% more than usual. The increasing number of Chicago hospital EDs on simultaneous bypass—5 on Thursday, 11 on Friday, and 18 on Saturday—compounded the problem, as it dramatically increased the time necessary to transport a patient to the hospital. Especially time-consuming were ambulance runs from Chicago's vast and sprawling South Side, where virtually no EDs were open, which meant ambulances sometimes had to travel several miles to the nearest hospital and then sometimes had to wait at the hospital until they could hand off the case to the ED staff.

As both call volumes and time spent per call increased, so too did ambulance response times. The state EMS Act defined a range of response times that any emergency ambulance provider was expected to meet: 4 to 6 minutes in primary coverage areas, 10 to 15 minutes in secondary coverage areas, and 15 to 20 minutes in outlying coverage areas. During the heat wave, however, a significant number of calls fell outside these parameters. In fact, the number of calls that did not receive an ambulance response for longer than 30 minutes increased from 18 on Thursday to 97 on Friday, then back down to 56 on Saturday and 3 on Sunday. The medical consequences of these delays were never certain, but statistics showed that of the 172 EMS patients that received an ambulance after a delay of 30 minutes between Thursday and Sunday, 12 were pronounced DOA when they reached the hospital and eight were diagnosed with cardiac arrest, a condition in which speed of response can be crucial.

The more ambulances were tied up and unavailable, the more the EMS dispatchers sent out fire trucks as a first response with ambulances to follow as soon as possible, as provided under the department's ambulance assistance program. On Thursday, 57% of EMS calls received a fire truck first. On Friday, the number had increased to 72%, and on Saturday, 94%. However, unlike the first responding program in place in some cities, the Chicago fire trucks were equipped only with first aid equipment, and the firefighters were trained only in first aid and cardiopulmonary resuscitation (CPR). Thus, many firefighters had neither the training nor the equipment necessary to stabilize the patients. According to testimony later presented at a state Senate subcommittee hearing, there was at least one case in which firefighters were in the position of performing CPR for longer than 40 minutes before ambulance backup arrived. Over the radios, the exchanges between the firefighters on the scene and the dispatchers grew testy at times, recalls Jeffrey Rodrigues, deputy director for fire operations of the Office of Emergency Communications. "[The firefighters would say,] 'We need an ambulance.' [The dispatchers would say,] 'We'll get you one when we can.' [The firefighters would persist,] 'What number ambulance are you going to send?' [The dispatcher would say,] 'We'll let you know.'" The frustration, he says, was evident.

One thing the Fire Department could have tried to do—but did not—was to call in additional ambulance help from the Chicago suburbs, under the area's mutual aid program, or from private ambulance companies in Chicago. Trotter, the Fire Department's top EMS official, has consistently maintained that the city did not call extra ambulances because it did not need extra ambulances. The EMS crews were able to handle the extra load, he says. Response times were sometimes long because of the number of hospital EDs on bypass. The answer to the problem was to get the EDs off bypass, he says—not to bring in more ambulances.

However, the fire commissioner at the time, Raymond Orozco, later indicated that EMS field supervisors were not alerting the Fire Department command staff to the problems in the field and intimated that the department might well have decided to bring in additional ambulance help if they had fully understood the situation. He would later tell a Senate panel: "My command staff was not aware that there were 18 hospitals on bypass.... Nobody indicated that we needed more personnel or supplies.... Our field supervisors told us, 'We're holding our own.'... We needed something to trigger the mechanism. Nobody pulled the trigger."[11]

Other observers in the Chicago EMS business, however, have suggested there were a number of reasons—philosophical, logistical, and political—that militated against the Fire Department bringing in extra ambulance help. One was that the Chicago Fire Department had more resources, sophistication, and experience than smaller suburban departments or private companies, and would not have thought to call on their smaller counterparts for help. "It's just not done," says Stein-Spencer. If anything, it was the smaller suburban companies that turned to Chicago when extra help was needed.

What's more, the mutual aid system among public fire departments had been created in anticipation of a specific emergency—for instance, an explosion—that caused mass casualties. The heat wave was not that kind of event. The entire metropolitan area was suffering through the heat wave, and EMS ambulances in the suburbs were under strain too.

Finally, although there was a general understanding among public sector fire departments that they could call on one another for emergency backup help, there was no system in place to make this an easy thing to do, says Rodrigues. If, for example, Chicago had decided it needed 30 extra ambulances, the Fire Department's EMS division would have had to "free wheel and try to come up with 30 departments in the [mutual aid network]. They would have had to call around and see who could go," he says. That was a cumbersome proposition. In addition, once they arrived, suburban ambulances would be unfamiliar with the city and would require extra guidance to navigate.

There was a different set of impediments to calling in the private companies. Private ambulance companies had developed a market niche providing nonemergency transport for patients—for example, moving them from one hospital to another or transporting them to a facility for medical tests. The Metropolitan Ambulance Association represented, together, some 300 basic and advanced life support ambulances in Chicago.

---

11. *Chicago Tribune*, July 28, 1995.

The private sector paramedics were not accustomed to emergency work, but they had received the same training as the Chicago Fire Department paramedics; their advanced life support ambulances were similarly outfitted and they were familiar with the city streets. Thus, they could reasonably be expected to provide backup emergency service if necessary. But the private companies operated by different rules and financial arrangements than did the public EMS. Both charged fees to patients for the service, but the Chicago Fire Department did not demand up-front payment and ultimately absorbed a high rate of nonpayment. By contrast, the private firms often did demand payment up front. They also charged patients according to different formulas. "The privates might charge by the mile, charge for each [piece of equipment] they use—it's a whole different ball game," says Stein-Spencer. Thus, if the Chicago Fire Department had asked private ambulances to help out during the heat wave, it was unclear what rules and protocols would apply.

Finally, the Fire Department's EMS crew had long felt like an embattled minority among firefighters who believed the Fire Department should not be in the EMS business to begin with. "We've been the bastard stepchildren of this department for 20 years," a paramedic had told a *Chicago Sun-Times* reporter in May 1994.[12] The EMS division had long insisted that it was understaffed and underequipped. The division also waged continuing battles against proposals to privatize EMS service altogether. In this context, the EMS division did not relish the idea of turning to nonunionized private companies for assistance. "There's always a certain amount of friction between the privates and the municipalities," says one well-placed observer in the EMS system. "It stems from a view that the privates are going to take over their jobs."

OVERLOAD AT THE MEDICAL EXAMINER'S OFFICE

When Cook County's chief medical examiner Edmund Donoghue had gotten the call Friday night, alerting him to the surprise arrival of 40 bodies, he decided he would work Saturday, although it was his day off. He also called in two other doctors and all the office's autopsy technicians. But when he arrived at the office Saturday morning, there were no longer 40 bodies awaiting him, there were 87. On Saturday, police would bring in another 110 bodies, and on Sunday, 100 more. This unprecedented situation—the sudden discovery of hundreds of dead bodies all across the City of Chicago[13]—created logistical problems for both the medical examiner and the Chicago Police. For Donoghue,

---

12. *Chicago Sun-Times*, May 27, 1994.
13. Under normal circumstances, the Cook County Medical Examiner examined about 25% of the bodies of those who died in Chicago; private physicians determined the cause of death in the great majority of cases. But the medical examiner examined the bodies of all those who died suddenly or without medical care, as had the vast majority of the heat wave victims.

the most pressing problem Saturday morning was the fact that he was fast running out of refrigerator space.

When a body arrived at the Medical Examiner's Office, it first went to a reception area, where the body was identified and the personal effects of the deceased were inventoried. The body was then stored in the Medical Examiner's refrigerator until the doctors performed the medical examination and determined the cause of death—a procedure that generally took about 30 minutes. Afterward, the body was wrapped and refrigerated until it was either claimed by family members or buried by the county. The refrigerator at the Medical Examiner's Office had a capacity of about 200 bodies, "but it had a tendency to run kind of full," Donoghue explains, as the bodies were kept for some time in hopes that someone would step forward to claim them. Unless Donoghue could find a way to expand his refrigerator capacity quickly, his operations would grind to a halt.

Donoghue knew from experience that a standard refrigerated truck would hold about 38 bodies. If he could borrow several of these trucks and park them in the office parking lot, he reasoned, the office could transfer bodies from its own refrigerator into the trucks and open up more space for incoming bodies. "So," he recalls, "we were making phone calls attempting to find refrigerated trucks on one of the hottest days in the history of Chicago." Donoghue's staff managed to find two trucks on its own but was eventually rescued by Chicago's Commissioner of Streets and Sanitation, Eileen Carey, who had rented refrigerator trucks for city festivals in the past. Donoghue asked her for two more trucks. She sent six. "She probably knew from [past] disasters that you don't know what's going on, you can always use more, and you can always send them back," says Donoghue. "That was a godsend. Eventually we ended up using 10 refrigerated trucks."

The next challenge was to bring in additional manpower. The Cook County Medical Examiner's office was a relatively small operation with a total staff of 120 and Donoghue did not want to work his autopsy staff round the clock, especially as he did not know how long the crisis would last. He did bring in all 15 doctors to work, without days off, until the emergency was over. The biggest need, however, was for simple manpower to wrap the bodies and move them from one place to another. To that end, he brought in volunteers from a local school of mortuary science over the weekend and volunteers from the county sheriff's community service program on Monday. In addition, to keep up with the paperwork on all the bodies, Donoghue asked some private sector funeral home directors to help, and he also asked for help from a group of dentists who had volunteered to be on-call for dental identification work during mass casualties. ("Dentists are real good on details," Donoghue notes.) As the crisis wore on and the visibly overwhelmed Cook County Medical Examiner's Office became a featured part of local and national television news reports, some private citizens walked in off the street to volunteer their help, Donoghue says, and the Salvation Army set up a canteen to support the Medical Examiner staff and volunteers. "The impact of that was the psychological boost," says Donoghue. "The food was okay. But the Salvation Army only goes out when important things are happening. You have to reassure your people that what they're doing is appreciated. There was also a camaraderie there. And fantastic press coverage—we were the center of attention—and that helps too."

THE BURDEN ON THE POLICE

For the Chicago Police, the challenges were parallel in nature. The first task for Deputy Chief Radke and his counterparts in other areas of town was to increase the number of squad rolls available for body transport. To this end, they pulled all the spare wagons they could from the Police Department's emergency pool, which effectively doubled the number of squad rolls in service. Even so, the number of bodies soon overmatched the transport capacity. In part, this was because a bottleneck had developed in the Medical Examiner's reception area. While Donoghue could bring in extra doctors to conduct the examinations and extra technicians and volunteers to prepare and move the bodies from one place to another, "there's not much capacity to expand reception," he says. "You can only take in bodies so fast. Their personal effects have to be inventoried, they have to be identified. If you have a mix-up on a body, people can be upset."

Soon there was a column of police wagons outside the Medical Examiner's Office, each waiting its turn to transfer custody of another body to the county. "We had our transport vehicles lined up for blocks. With decomposing bodies. With no air conditioning," recalls Radke.

This bottleneck had other ramifications for the police, as well. For one, the officers waiting in line were not available for other police duties. In addition, the squad rolls themselves were tied up in line. As the police continued to get new DOA calls, it took an increasingly long time for each squad roll to unload the last body and come for the next one. Officers initially dispatched to the scene were required by law to stay with the body until the squad roll arrived, which sidelined still more officers.

The spate of DOA calls, combined with the bottleneck at the Medical Examiner's Office and the limited number of squad rolls, created a significant manpower shortage for the police. In response, the police did several things, Radke says. If a two-person vehicle was assigned to a death investigation, they divided the team up, so that one officer stayed with the body and drove the squad roll while the other continued routine policing duties in the cruiser. As the weekend progressed, top police commanders took several other steps to increase police manpower. First, they extended the tour of duty for many officers from 8 to 12 hours. When that eventually proved insufficient, they cancelled days off and pulled in extra officers.

THE CHICAGO DEPARTMENT OF PUBLIC HEALTH

One of the responsibilities of the Chicago Department of Public Health was to be aware of any unusual outbreak of illness in the city, so as to minimize its spread and advise victims of the best course of medical care. On Thursday and Friday, an estimated 1,450 people had turned up in the EDs of area hospitals complaining of some form of heat sickness, and between 5 p.m. Friday night and 9 a.m. Saturday morning, 87 dead bodies, mostly heat victims, had been discovered across the city and delivered to the Cook County Medical Examiner. But none of this news had reached the Chicago Department of Public Health. On Saturday morning, John Wilhelm, the city's deputy health commissioner, was relaxing at home when he received a surprise mid-morning call from his department's public information director. One of the TV channels had called and wanted to send a reporter over to do an interview with Wilhelm about the heat wave. This request was perplexing to both Wilhelm and the public information director. All week, Wilhelm had been interviewed by reporters about the heat and had delivered the usual litany of advice—to stay hydrated, to limit exercise, to remain indoors during the heat of the day. It was not clear why, with the weather forecast showing a cooling trend, the heat wave was still a story. "But I was home, and they were coming to me, so it was no problem for me to go outside and talk," Wilhelm recalls.

> On camera, I went through hydration, and look-after-the-elderly, and then [the reporter] said, "Dr. Wilhelm, I've just come from the Medical Examiner's office, and there's 70 police wagons there with bodies." I never saw the interview, so I don't know what I looked like; but my eyes must have gotten very large. And what was racing through my head was, "Is there a gas leak in some neighborhood? Where did these bodies come from? Was it one city block? Was there an explosion?"

At the time, there was little Wilhelm could say, except, "I haven't talked to the Medical Examiner, so I really can't comment." But as soon as the interview was over, Wilhelm recalls, "I ran upstairs and called Ed Donoghue and said, 'What's going on?'"

Information Systems at the Chicago Department of Public Health

Since 1990, the Chicago Department of Public Health—previously devoted primarily to the delivery of clinical care—had shifted its focus to research, prevention work, and the dissemination of public information. As part of this shift, the department had made a point of improving its ability to detect an outbreak of either communicable disease or food-borne illness in Chicago at the earliest possible moment. To that end, the department's Communicable Disease division had forged relationships with the infection control divisions of local hospitals, and the hospitals were now "quite diligent" in fulfilling a state mandate to report any incidence of 54 specified diseases to the department, Wilhelm says. In addition, the Department's Food and Dairy section had developed relationships with Chicago's 14,000 restaurants. The department actively encouraged restaurants or citizens to call the department if someone became ill as a result of eating in a restaurant. If either the Communicable Disease division or the Food and Dairy division of the Public Health Department learned of an unusually high incidence of any illness in Chicago, they were instructed to inform the commissioner immediately.

Heat sickness, however, was neither a communicable disease nor a food-borne malady; it was simply a recognizable cluster of symptoms. Thus, although more than a thousand patients had turned up at hospital EDs all across Chicago with symptoms of heat sickness, Wilhelm says, "It wasn't a reportable condition—so it didn't get reported" through the department's established reporting mechanism. Nor had Wilhelm heard about the discovery of hundreds of dead bodies across the city from the mayor's staff in City Hall, because the mayor's staff did not learn about the dead bodies until late Saturday morning either.

THE OFFICE OF THE MAYOR

With the weather forecast indicating a lingering heat through the weekend but the worst of the heat wave over, Mayor Richard Daley had headed north to a lakeside vacation spot for the weekend of July 15 and 16. On Saturday, at about midday, the mayor's first deputy, Sarah Pang, who served as the mayor's liaison to the police, received a page from the first deputy for the police: "He said, 'We are getting a large number of dead bodies in apartments—senior citizens—we believe they are heat related,'" Pang recalls. "I said, 'What is a large number?' He said, 'A hundred. Climbing quickly.'"

Pang immediately paged the mayor's newly appointed chief of staff, Roger Kiley, who had been on the job only a few days when the heat wave hit. "He said, 'What is typical on a Saturday?'" Pang recalls. "I said, 'Well, nothing like this.' It was unbelievable." In addition, she could tell ambulance runs were up. "You could just hear sirens running in the street nonstop." Kiley and Pang quickly called in the mayor's staff, along with Police and Fire Department officials and tried to get a better purchase on what was happening. What was the pattern? Where were the deaths centered? Who was sick? Who was dying? City staffers were also preoccupied with complaints of power outages across the city. Commonwealth Edison, the local power company, experienced a substation fire and several equipment failures during the heat wave that left thousands of Chicago residents without power at one time or another—sometimes for less than an hour, sometimes for as many as 20 hours. The hardest hit were 41,000 North Side residents who lost electricity Friday night due to the substation fire. An estimated

8,500 did not have power restored until late in the day on Saturday. Power failures, too, had ancillary effects. For instance, if grocery stores lost power in their refrigeration units, food might spoil. The city needed to inspect food stores to be sure they were not trying to sell any potentially spoiled food.

Into the night Saturday and into Sunday, as well, the mayor's staff gathered information and responded to emergencies on an ad hoc basis. The role of Mayor Daley himself during this period was never made publicly clear. According to John Kass, City Hall reporter for the *Chicago Tribune*, the mayor did not learn of the scope of the crisis until Sunday morning.[14] In any event, the mayor did return to the city on Sunday and did call an emergency meeting of his cabinet on Sunday afternoon at 3 p.m. After that meeting, the mayor declared an official Heat Emergency and the city mobilized new resources. The commissioner of human services rounded up eight vans and 60 staff workers to respond, on an ad hoc basis, to citizens who called City Hall asking for help. Staff from the Department on Aging began combing through lists of residents who participated in its programs and calling as many as they could to see if they needed assistance. The Chicago Department of Public Health sent out inspectors to check on temperature conditions in the two Chicago nursing homes without air conditioning and the 12 with only limited air conditioning. The "senior citizen" officers for the Chicago Police—officers in each of the city's 25 districts with particular responsibility for elderly residents—began checking on the medically vulnerable residents on their own lists. In addition, the mayor held a press conference in which he made an impassioned plea to residents to check on relatives, neighbors, and friends who might be vulnerable. The city would do what it could, but the city could not do it all, he said.

Although the city set these responses in motion on Sunday afternoon, Pang notes that by this time, "It was cooling off. It was over from the point that you needed to respond to it. So it was unlike anything we had ever experienced before. It was as if nobody had ever heard of a tornado, and it came through and wiped out a thousand people, and then you thought, 'What the heck was that?'"

On Monday, July 17, Mayor Daley appointed an 18-member Commission on Extreme Weather Conditions, chaired by Wilhelm. The mayor gave the new commission several responsibilities: to determine the factors involved in making the 1995 heat wave so severe in Chicago; to develop an understanding of why so many people died, especially elderly people; and to develop a new plan for coping with extreme heat or extreme cold weather in the future.

---

14. John Kass, "In the Heat, Government Shouldn't Take Beating," *Chicago Tribune*, July 23, 1995.

The City of Chicago and the 1995 Heat Wave: The Aftermath of a Crisis

Pamela Varley

Mayor Richard Daley and his staff spent the week of July 17 regaining their moorings in the aftermath of Chicago's devastating heat wave. "It was obvious that none of us really knew what had happened," says Sarah Pang, the mayor's first deputy. "What were the conditions that led to this? Who were the people who died from it? Who were the people most at risk? How do we communicate with them next time we experience extreme heat?" It was not even clear at first what the scope of the tragedy had been. In the days immediately following the heat wave, the mayor and Cook County Medical Examiner Edmund Donoghue squared off in a heated public wrangle over the magnitude of the death toll.

DEATH TOLL AND DISBELIEF

Observers report that the dispute between Daley and Donoghue was born of a combination of factors: the mayor's genuine disbelief that the heat could have killed so many, City Hall's effort at political damage control, and confusion about the proper definition of a "heat-related death." Beginning Saturday, July 15, when the press— both national and local—began to report on the fatalities, the beleaguered office of

This case was written by Pamela Varley, Kennedy School case writer, for Dr. Arnold Howitt, Director of the Kennedy School's Executive Session on Domestic Preparedness and Executive Director of the Taubman Center for State and Local Government. Funding was provided by the Office of Justice Programs, US Department of Justice, and the Robert Wood Johnson Foundation. (0102)

the Cook County Medical Examiner had suddenly taken center stage. Donoghue had become Man of the Hour, giving reporters periodic updates about the number of bodies that had been discovered and the number of deaths his office had officially deemed heat-related.

Though Donoghue had kept a low profile in his two previous years as chief medical examiner, he pulled no punches in declaring the 1995 heat wave a "disaster." As he told a reporter for the *Chicago Tribune*, "This was a disaster in Chicago akin to the earthquake in Los Angeles, the floods in Mississippi, and Hurricane Hugo in Miami. We'd been struck with overwhelming forces of nature that we were not equipped to handle." Donoghue believed he had an obligation to speak plainly in order to alert the public to the potential deadliness of the heat and the fact that heat deaths were almost entirely preventable, if medically vulnerable people could find their way to an air-conditioned environment. Based on Donoghue's assessments and statistics, reporters all across the country were declaring the heat wave one of the deadliest in recorded history and were expressing bewildered amazement at the death toll in Cook County, which eventually climbed to 576,[1] far higher than anywhere else in the country.

Donoghue's figures were politically awkward for Mayor Daley, who had declared a Heat Emergency only on Sunday, four days after temperatures surged above 100°F. The mayor and his staff expressed incredulity—and frank skepticism—about Donoghue's figures and methodology. Surely the medical examiner was exaggerating the case? After all, the fact that people were dying on a hot day did not necessarily mean they were dying of the heat. "Every day people die of natural causes," Daley told the media. According to Daley, not every death could be attributed to the heat.[2] Chicago journalists, too, began to wonder out loud, "[W]as the Chicago disaster a freak of nature or a twist of statistics?" as one *Chicago Tribune* article put it.[3]

The debate was fed by the fact that there was disagreement among medical examiners nationwide over the proper definition of a "heat-related death"—a debate that unfolded in somewhat confused fashion in the Chicago press. If a healthy three-year-old child died after being enclosed in a car in 100°F heat, it was not difficult to identify the cause of death as the heat. But most of the Chicago residents who died during the heat wave were elderly, and many had medical problems to begin with. Thus, if someone with a history of heart failure was sitting in an apartment in stifling heat and died of a heart attack, what was the cause of death? Or if someone was found dead on Sunday morning with a very high blood-alcohol level and a very high core body temperature, what did he die of?

---

1. Cook County comprised all of Chicago and a number of adjacent municipalities. For Chicago, alone, the city Department of Public Health later calculated the death toll at 522.
2. The University of Chicago Press, "Dying Alone: An Interview With Eric Klinenberg," 2002, http://www.press.uchicago.edu/Misc/Chicago/443213in.html.
3. Cindy Schreuder and Peter Gorne, "Coroners Don't Always Agree on When Heat Kills," *Chicago Tribune*, July 18, 1995.

Or, as blunt-spoken Chicago columnist Mike Royko put the matter, "[O]ld people died. That's because old people inevitably die of one thing or another."[4]

To Donoghue, the question was whether any given individual would have died in mid-July of other causes regardless of the heat, or whether the heat had, in fact, played a crucial role in the death. Since 1978, the Cook County Medical Examiner had listed heat as either the primary or secondary cause of a death in three circumstances:

- If a body were examined soon enough after death to measure the core body temperature, heat was considered a factor if the core body temperature was 105°F or higher.
- If the body were found too long after death to measure core body temperature, heat was considered a factor if the body had been found in an environment with a temperature of 100°F or higher.
- In the case of a decomposed body, found substantially after the fact, heat was considered a factor if the individual had last been seen alive during the heat wave.

Over the duration of the 1995 heat wave, Donoghue listed heat as the primary cause of death in 68 cases. In 482 cases, he listed heat as a "contributing factor." In 276 cases, he concluded that heat had not been a factor at all. Using the same criteria, Donoghue had determined that in all of 1994, heat had been a primary or secondary cause of death in only eight cases; in 1993, three cases; in 1992, one case; in 1991, four cases; and in 1990, six cases.

Many medical examiners across the country, however, listed heat as the primary or secondary cause of death only when the core body temperature could be determined. Thus, Mayor Daley and other political leaders argued that Donoghue's figures were inflated, that his figures made the Chicago heat death toll look wildly out of line vis-à-vis other communities.

In epidemiological circles, however, the most up-to-date thinking ratified Donoghue's methods and definitions and regarded heat-related deaths, in general, as woefully underreported. According to one researcher, F. P. Ellis, who wrote on the topic in 1972, the number of actual deaths from heat was, in general, about 10 times greater than the number recorded.[5] Because of the variation of standards from one medical examiner to another, a growing number of epidemiologists favored another approach to figuring out the death toll from a heat wave: comparing the number of deaths during the heat wave with the number of deaths during a comparable number of "normal" days at the same time of year and in the same location. Such an approach nearly always indicated that

4. While it was true that 73% of the heat wave deaths were people aged 65 and older, 63% of deaths from all causes were aged 65 and older.
5. Stanley A. Changnon, Kenneth E. Kunkel, and Beth C. Reinke, "Impacts and Responses to the 1995 Heat Wave: A Call to Action," *Bulletin of the American Meteorological Society* 77 (1996).

there were far more excess deaths during a heat wave than doctors or medical examiners had attributed to the heat.

Given the controversy over Donoghue's figures in 1995, the Chicago Department of Public Health calculated excess deaths in Chicago during July 1995 and concluded that there had been 733—well beyond the final tally Donoghue had given. For practical purposes, this study served to vindicate Donoghue's work, and Mayor Daley, for his part, later told a reporter that his comments at the time had been misunderstood:

> What happened last summer was unbelievable to all of us. I simply questioned whether some of the deaths attributed to the heat might have been connected to other causes and, sadly, might have been inevitable because of the victims' existing medical conditions. I was in no way criticizing Dr. Donoghue or attacking his credibility. And I certainly was not minimizing the seriousness of a very real Chicago tragedy.[6]

REFORMS TO THE SYSTEM

At the same time that the debate over Chicago's heat death toll was taking its course, Mayor Daley created an 18-member Commission on Extreme Weather Conditions, chaired by John Wilhelm, deputy commissioner of the Chicago Department of Public Health. The Commission's task was to determine the meteorological factors that had made the 1995 heat wave so severe in Chicago; to develop an understanding of why so many people died, especially elderly people; and to recommend a new blueprint for coping with extreme heat or extreme cold weather in the future.

The Commission's research work, in tandem with a more general evolution of thinking that took place in Chicago after the 1995 shock, culminated in the development of the city's Extreme Weather Emergency Operations Plan in November 1995. In addition, fallout from the 1995 crisis reverberated for years and eventually contributed to several policy changes in the public health and emergency medical service (EMS) areas:

- The city Department of Public Health made changes to its disease monitoring system.
- The Fire Department developed protocols that made it easier to call in extra ambulance assistance in an emergency.
- The state Department of Public Health established a permanent policy that circumscribed the ability of a hospital emergency department (ED) to call a bypass—the process by which an ED judged itself overwhelmed and temporarily closed its doors to incoming ambulance patients.

---

6. Joel Kaplan, "Dead Right: How Medical Examiner Edmund Donoghue, Jr., Stood Up to Mayor Daley During Last Summer's Tragic Heat Wave," *Chicago*, May 1996.

Revisiting Disease Monitoring Protocols at the Chicago Department of Public Health

By the end of the second day of the infamous mid-July 1995 heat wave in Chicago, an estimated 1,450 patients had gone to Chicago-area hospitals with heat-related complaints and 87 dead bodies had been discovered across the city; yet not until the middle of the third day of the heat wave did the city's top public health officials learn of the heat-related sickness and deaths, and when they did learn of them, it was not from their own disease-monitoring system but from a television news reporter.

For the city Department of Public Health, that had been a shocking moment, and also an embarrassing one. After the heat wave, the department began to think about how it might alter its monitoring system to pick up more nebulous medical complaints—the kind that might arise not only from the heat but also from the accidental release of toxins in the environment or from a bioterrorist attack. In such situations, "you're going to see clusters of people coming in with some vague symptoms, and there are going to be clusters in many hospitals," says Wilhelm.

> We used the heat wave as an example of how something which was noncommunicable—it wasn't meningitis, it wasn't measles—was showing up. People were coming in with heat exhaustion. But no one put together that it wasn't just my emergency room—it was your emergency room—it was every emergency room in the city.... Somebody has to recognize that there's something going on here. And that's what *wasn't* happening in the summer of '95.

By state law, hospitals were required to inform the city only about the appearance of the 54 reportable diseases, but the Communicable Disease staff at the Department of Public Health began to work with the infection control staff at the hospitals in an effort to expand the universe of conditions they would voluntarily monitor and report to the city. Says Wilhelm:

> We're working with the infection control people and the emergency room people to say, "We're drawing up some syndrome complexes. If you see clusters of people coming in with these symptoms—even if it doesn't fit into a pigeon hole of a communicable disease—you need to call us [and say,] 'There's something odd going on.'"

If the Department of Public Health's Communicable Disease division were to hear of an unusual syndrome in the city's EDs, the staff members were instructed to let the commissioner know "immediately," Wilhelm says. "I would let the Mayor's office know," and the city would likely activate its emergency response system by calling together top-level city officials to a special Command Center to coordinate a response, he adds.

In addition, Wilhelm was "working out a relationship with the 9-1-1 center" in Chicago so that the Department of Public Health would receive logs of the 9-1-1 emergency and

3-1-1 nonemergency calls in the city.[7] That way, over time, the Department of Public Health could develop baseline data about the number of medical complaints that came in during a given season of the year, and would be in a position to notice any spikes— for instance, a sudden increase in respiratory complaints or skin rashes in a certain area of the city.

Arranging for Ambulance Assistance

Neither the mayor nor his Commission ever voiced public criticism of the Chicago Fire Department for choosing not to call in extra ambulance help during the mid-July 1995 heat wave, but the Commission plan did, quietly but specifically, call upon the Fire Department to monitor its call volume during any future Heat Warning and to call in extra ambulances if needed.

The Fire Department did, in fact, move quickly to develop a standing contract with private ambulance companies for use in emergencies. Although, in theory, the Chicago Fire Department had always been able to call in private ambulances in an emergency, private ambulance companies operated by a different set of rules and patient-billing arrangements than did the city. The new contract made it easier for the department to call in private ambulance help by clarifying, up front, the terms under which private ambulances would agree to assist the city's fleet in an emergency. When Chicago was hit with another, lesser heat wave two weeks after the deadly event of mid-July 1995, the Fire Department called in eight private ambulances.

In 2001, the Chicago-area Mutual Aid Box Alarm System (MABAS), the system by which public-sector fire departments in Chicago and the surrounding cities called on one another for help in an emergency, also revised its mutual aid protocols in order to make the system easier to use. Experts had long complained that the old system was logistically awkward; essentially, it required a fire department in need of assistance to call around to see which nearby fire companies or ambulances were available. Under the new system, any time a fire department needed help, it had only to decide how many extra fire trucks or ambulances it needed, and its MABAS disaster card listed, in order, 10 groups of 10 public ambulances from surrounding cities, geographically dispersed, that could be called into service. If one was unavailable, dispatchers would automatically move to the next. "We can get [up to] 100 ambulances in here at the drop of a hat—just by making a radio call," says Jeffrey Rodrigues, deputy director of Fire Operations at the Office of Emergency Communications. Once the MABAS system had been improved, it became the Chicago Fire Department's first recourse if it

---

7. The City of Chicago had created a central 3-1-1 hotline for residents to use either to report nonemergency concerns or to seek help and information from any city department.

needed to call in outside ambulance help, with private ambulance assistance a secondary option.

The question of bringing in outside assistance was a tense one in Chicago, as the EMS Division of the Chicago Fire Department had long insisted, with little success, that it needed more ambulances and paramedics to adequately serve the city. Over the next five years, however, the city did increase the EMS fleet from 59 Advanced Life Support ambulances to 86 Advanced Life Support ambulances and 12 Basic Life Support ambulances. In addition, the Fire Department began cross-training its firefighters to be paramedics and vice versa. Also, the Fire Department added the chief piece of equipment used to stabilize patients suffering from cardiac arrest—automatic external defibrillators—to 25 fire trucks so that they could more ably serve as first responders to emergency medical calls.

Amending Bypass Policy

In the course of the 1995 heat wave, which had strained hospitals all across the city as thousands of residents sought ED care for heat-related sickness, some 18 hospital EDs in the Chicago metropolitan area had at one point simultaneously declared an ambulance bypass. For so many hospitals to declare a bypass at once put great strain on the remaining hospitals and on Chicago Fire Department ambulances, which had to travel farther to deliver their patients. In combination with a limited supply of ambulances, this had led to a slowdown in ambulance response times.

In the wake of this crisis, the state legislature voted in 1995 and 1996 to strengthen the authority of the state EMS Division to regulate and, when necessary, curtail hospital bypass. During the formal comment period, hospitals fought the new bypass rules, arguing that each hospital needed to be able to make its own final judgment call about declaring a bypass. They lost the battle and decided to accept, rather than fight, the new policy. In part, says Leslee Stein-Spencer, chief of EMS for the Illinois Department of Public Health, the acquiescence came out of concern that the legislature might vote to forbid bypass altogether.

Under the new policy, hospitals had to report to the state EMS Division within 24 hours whenever they declared a bypass and to explain why. In addition, hospitals could only declare a bypass in two situations: when they had no available beds with cardiac monitors—not just in the ED but in the whole hospital—or when they faced an internal disaster, such as flood, fire, or power outage. Over time, these criteria were liberalized somewhat. "What we've allowed recently as an 'internal disaster' is if they've tried—and can verify to us that they've tried—to get additional nursing staff, and they can't get anyone in because there just is no one there," says Stein-Spencer. (The nationwide nursing shortage made it extremely difficult, and sometimes impossible, to find replacement staff in emergencies.)

At the same time, however, the state EMS Division was encouraging hospitals to proactively develop "a 'peak census' policy," Stein-Spencer says. Thus, if a hospital was down to just two or three available monitored beds or if 95% of inpatient beds were full, it would begin to take steps to reduce its census. That meant discharging patients early, transferring patients to other facilities, and canceling elective surgeries and elective admissions. According to Stein-Spencer, this policy was developed in response to comments from some ED physicians that hospital administrators tended to see the ED and the rest of the hospital as separate entities, rather than parts of a unified whole. In reality, it was impossible for a hospital both to operate at peak capacity and still be adequately available for emergencies, Stein-Spencer adds.

In addition to imposing stricter criteria on hospitals for calling an emergency bypass, the state EMS Division had the explicit authority to cancel a hospital's bypass if three or more hospitals in a single geographic area had declared a bypass. In addition, the state could waive an ED's bypass on a case-by-case basis if an ambulance's transport time to the next nearest hospital would be greater than 15 minutes or if the life of a particular patient might be endangered by the delay of traveling to another hospital.

For some hospitals, the new policy was, admittedly, a hardship. "They're afraid a patient will die in the ER," explains Stein-Spencer. "They say they're trying every means to get off [bypass] but they just can't. But I've told them, 'We don't have a choice.' The ambulances have to go somewhere with the patient—they can't be driving around the streets. There's really no answer. You're between a rock and a hard place."

As in the past, the state relied on the EMS medical directors in charge of emergency operations in Chicago's three Resource Hospitals to monitor and regulate hospital use of bypass day to day. And, as in the past, the EMS medical directors were reluctant to challenge a fellow-hospital's decision to call a bypass, according to Stein-Spencer. Increasingly, however, paramedics and some ED staff (usually from hospitals that were *not* on bypass and were under added pressure because other EDs were on bypass) did call the state EMS Division directly when they believed a particular ED was creating a strain on the overall EMS system, she added.

THE WORK OF THE MAYOR'S COMMISSION

The mayor created his Commission on Extreme Weather Conditions on July 17, and the group quickly decided to undertake two pieces of research work. The first piece, undertaken in cooperation with the National Weather Service (NWS), was to identify the particular combination of meteorological factors that had made the July 1995 heat wave so deadly. The second one, in concert with the Centers for Disease Control and Prevention (CDC), was to analyze the population that had died of heat-related causes in order to understand what risk factors had made them particularly susceptible to the heat.

These research projects were likely to take weeks or even months, however, and there were still many more weeks left in the summer of 1995; Chicago might be hit with another deadly heat wave before the Commission's work was complete. As its first task, therefore, the Commission created an interim plan. The interim plan laid out a three-tiered government response to the heat that depended on the forecasted heat index, the apparent temperature when air temperature and humidity levels were considered together.

An Early Test

The Commission presented its interim plan to the city on July 20, and the plan received a test run 10 days later, when the city was hit with another hot weather spike. By comparison to the mid-July heat wave, the late July event was both briefer—lasting only July 30 to July 31—and less severe. Official temperatures peaked at 95°F on July 30 with a heat index of 103°F—substantially lower than the mid-July temperature peak of 104°F and heat index of 123°F. Humidity levels were reportedly 25% lower than they had been in mid-July.

The city nonetheless rolled out its full Heat Emergency plan. According to a report in the *Chicago Sun-Times*, the city identified 150 public buildings as cooling centers during the two-day heat emergency, which were visited by 1,900 people. In addition, 753 elderly residents visited the Department on Aging Senior Centers. The Chicago Fire Department called into service its five reserve ambulances and another eight ambulances from private companies. Outreach workers with the Department on Aging visited 2,500 people in their homes. About 4,000 people called the Mayor's Office of Inquiry and Information with heat-related questions or problems. The shock and dismay that attended the mid-July heat wave mobilized private citizens as well. "City workers were calling [the elderly] and their children were answering, saying, 'Not to worry: I'm here with my mother. We're here to take her to our place in the suburbs,'" says Wilhelm.

For a combination of reasons—including the relative mildness of the heat wave itself—the July 30–31 heat emergency resulted in little heat-related sickness or death. Hospitals across the city reported that only 16 people were admitted for heat-related conditions, and another 22 were treated and released. Cook County Medical Examiner Edmund Donoghue reported that two people died of heat-related causes during the two-day heat emergency.[8]

A week later, on August 8, a day with a high temperature of 85°F, a 13-story elderly housing development with 240 tenants lost power and, consequently, air-conditioning, for several hours. Although the city did not declare a Heat Emergency, it did dispatch an impressive show of force to the scene of the power outage. Some 60 firefighters and police officers were sent to the high-rise, prepared to carry people out of the building and offer emergency medical assistance. During the course of the day, officials from the Department

---

8. *Chicago Sun-Times*, August 1, 1995.

of Human Services arrived at the building, along with Fire Commissioner Raymond Orozco. "Several dozen city workers stood nearly elbow to elbow in the complex's crowded lobby as others distributed water and periodically checked on the residents," the *Chicago Tribune* reported. The tenants, however, were apparently unperturbed by the outage. Almost all opted to remain in the building and only two requested medical assistance.

Four days later, on August 12, the city Department of Public Health again called a Heat Emergency, when temperatures reached 98°F, with a heat index of 114°F.

Overkill?

By early August, these frequent emergency responses were drawing a reaction of dismay from officials of the NWS, who were concerned that the city had set its threshold too low, and would be in the position of "triggering this thing every other day or every third or fourth day."[9] After the traumatic events of mid-July, the city was predisposed to err on the side of caution, but the NWS saw in the city's approach a new set of potential dangers: City staff and private citizens, alike, would become desensitized to the warnings. City staff would grow angry at repeated intrusions on personal time and repeated calls to work nights and weekends. Elderly and disabled residents might even grow peevish at repeated phone calls and visits from city workers asking how they were feeling. On August 14, the city's efforts also received a slap on the nose from the *Chicago Tribune*. "No question the city was caught napping last month," the paper editorialized. "But costly, over frequent heat alerts are no way to stay awake for the next real emergency."

The mayor told critics that the city's Extreme Weather Plan was still a "work-in-progress" and said that he planned to defer to the judgment of meteorological and public health experts in making final decisions about the criteria for declaring a Heat Emergency. The Mayor's Commission on Extreme Weather Conditions, meanwhile, redoubled its efforts to identify the particular heat wave conditions that most often led to illness and death.

THE METEOROLOGICAL STUDY

Before the mid-July heat wave, the policy of the Chicago Forecast Office of the NWS was to issue a Heat Advisory when, for two days in a row, the peak heat index was forecasted for 105°F or higher, and the minimum heat index was expected to fall no lower than 80°F

---

9. Paul Dailey, area manager for the NWS, as quoted in: John Kass, "City Warned of Risks in Heat Alerts," *Chicago Tribune*, August 8, 1995.

at night. The NWS issued a more urgent Heat Warning when the heat index reached 120°F or higher. These trigger points, however, had not been established on the basis of rigorous study comparing particular hot weather patterns with patterns of heat-related sickness and death. Thus, the Committee on Weather Conditions and Forecasting for the Mayor's Commission worked with NWS meteorologists and other experts to correlate 16 years of meteorological and epidemiological data.

Importantly, they found that not all heat waves were created equal. Even beyond the familiar variables of peak temperature levels and humidity, some heat waves were significantly more severe than others. Several factors had combined to make the mid-July heat wave especially severe in Chicago. One crucial factor was the impact of limited nighttime cooling—nights where the temperature never dipped below 80°F. The phenomenon of limited nighttime cooling was a particular liability of urban areas—a function of the so-called heat island effect. Roads, brick buildings, black tar, and asphalt on roads and roofs all soaked up the heat and radiated it back. In general, Chicago's heat island yielded temperatures about 5°F higher than in outlying areas.[10] Another important factor was the duration of the heat—the number of consecutive days with unbroken high temperatures. In the case of the mid-July heat wave in Chicago, the heat index was 100°F or higher for five consecutive days and was 115°F or higher two days in a row. While the heat peaked early in the heat wave—on July 13—the death rate peaked two days later; 346 people died on July 15, indicating that it was the duration as well as the harshness of the heat that proved fatal. A third factor was the intensity of the sun, measured as the percentage of sunshine. During the 1995 heat wave, sun intensity had approached 100 percent, according to Wilhelm.

To forecast the constellation of factors likely to produce a dangerous heat wave, therefore, meant capturing these other variables in addition to the stalwarts of air temperature and humidity. Eventually, the NWS hoped to refine the heat index measure so that it would reflect a broader range of variables; but in the meantime, the NWS developed four scenarios that it believed constituted heat conditions dangerous to human health, yet also rare enough to forestall an over-frequent emergency response from city government:

- One day with a heat index of 110°F or higher.
- Two consecutive days with a heat index between 105°F and 110°F.
- Three consecutive days with a heat index between 100°F and 105°F and sun intensity of at least 85% on at least two of the three days.
- Three consecutive days with a heat index between 100°F and 105°F and a minimum heat index of at least 75°F on each of the three days.

If any of these four sets of conditions were obtained, the NWS would declare a Heat Warning. When such conditions were forecasted more than two days in advance, the NWS would declare an Excessive Heat Outlook, and when they were forecasted

---

10. The eastern edge of Chicago that borders Lake Michigan was often spared the heat island effect, owing to lakefront cooling.

less than two days in advance, a Heat Watch. The Mayor's Commission recommended that the city align its own heat emergency plan with the new NWS terms and definitions. During an NWS Heat Watch, the city should "mobilize for an emergency response" and monitor assorted indicators of extreme heat, including ED visits, hospital admissions, 9-1-1 calls, and illegally opened fire hydrants and electrical power outages. During an NWS Heat Warning, the city should implement its emergency operations plan, which the Commission sketched and the city later fleshed out in greater detail.

IDENTIFYING WHO'S AT RISK

Anecdotal evidence and back-of-the-envelope calculations had shown, even in the midst of the mid-July heat crisis, that the majority of heat-related fatalities in the city were elderly residents. But the Mayor's Commission wanted a more detailed portrait of those who had died in order to tailor the city's response. The centerpiece of this research was a study done by CDC, which confirmed what everyone sensed—73% of the heat wave victims had been 65 or older. What's more, within this population, the risk increased with age. Thus, of people aged 65 to 74, 75 per 100,000 had died of heat-related causes in mid-July 1995. Of people aged 85 and older, 300 per 100,000 had died.

Poverty

The Chicago Department of Public Health also conducted a study of the deaths by neighborhood and discovered that the death rate varied greatly from one to another. In the city's 77 neighborhoods, the number of deaths ranged widely—from 0 to 90 per 100,000 residents. The highest risk neighborhoods were those with proportionately more elderly residents living alone, a higher homicide rate, lower income levels, lower education levels, and larger overall population. Citywide, 16% of Chicago residents 65 and older lived in poverty.

Race and Ethnicity

Very few Hispanic and Asian residents died in the 1995 heat wave—perhaps because very few elderly Hispanics and Asians lived alone. The heat-related deaths had been overwhelmingly non-Hispanic whites and non-Hispanic African Americans and were evenly divided between the two: 252 white and 253 black. The death rate among African Americans, however, was nearly double the death rate among whites.

Other Risk Factors

Overall, CDC found that the residents at greatest risk were elderly people who were both living alone and, more generally, socially isolated. They were less likely than other elderly residents to have friends, pets, or to participate in group activities. They tended to live on the upper floors of flat-roofed, unshaded apartment buildings, without air-conditioning. They tended to have no access to transportation. They tended not to take special precautions about the heat, such as drinking more liquids, taking cool baths, or deliberately spending time in air-conditioned buildings. Those who were bedridden, suffered heart or kidney conditions, or had mental health problems or alcoholism were at especially high risk. All things held equal, the greatest protective factor, according to CDC, was the presence of a working air conditioner in the home. "We estimate that more than 50 percent of the deaths related to the heat wave could have been prevented if each home had a working air conditioner," the CDC study concluded.

Other Issues

But even this detailed profile did not capture all of the particular vulnerabilities of the people who had died. For instance, some of the people who died of the heat actually did have working air conditioners in the home but did not turn them on because their thermoregulatory systems were impaired and they did not realize how hot they were, because they feared the utility bills, or because air-conditioning aggravated their other medical conditions—for example, arthritis or respiratory problems. Anecdotally, friends and relatives reported that many of the victims had been so fearful of crime that they adamantly refused even to open their windows or leave their apartments. In bygone days, Chicago's poor had sat outside in the evening to escape the heat or slept in parks or on lakefront beaches; few who were not already homeless would have dreamed of such a thing in 1995. And some of those who had been offered help by family members or social service workers had refused it. For some, that was a matter of misunderstanding their own precarious state, for others a matter of distrust or disinclination. Still others were bent on hiding from outside view their declining health or fading mental acuity. "They don't want to be detected and pushed into a nursing home," Bruce Rybarczyk, a clinical psychologist who specialized in treating the elderly, told a *Chicago Tribune* reporter. "They just hold on as if in a bunker."[11]

---

11. Barbara Brotman, "Elderly Guard Jealously Their Right to Be Wrong," *Chicago Tribune*, August 13, 1995.

THE COMMAND CENTER

The efforts of the Mayor's Commission to recommend the features of a new Extreme Weather Emergency Plan also took place in the context of another city project well underway and nearing completion: the creation of a new Office of Emergency Communications in Chicago. The new facility, due to begin operations in September 1995, had originally been conceived in 1989 to replace a 9-1-1 system built in the 1960s that resembled "a set out of *Adam 12*,"[12] according to one *Chicago Tribune* reporter.[13] By the mid-1990s, the 9-1-1 system was antiquated, divided among several locations, and teetering dangerously on the brink of collapse, according to city communications experts. The Office of Emergency Communications was an ambitiously conceived facility that would house an all-new, consolidated 9-1-1 system, connected to thousands of miles of telecommunications cables and an independent, fully redundant,[14] 176-mile network of fiber-optic cables running to 215 city buildings, including all Fire and Police Stations.

Of special relevance to the creators of the Extreme Weather Emergency Plan, however, was the fact that the elegant, tornado-proof Office of Emergency Communications would also house a Command Center. In times of real or potential emergency,[15] the city Fire Commissioner, in consultation with the mayor and the police chief, would call the top officials from relevant city departments to the Command Center. Under the direction of the Fire Commissioner, the agency heads and/or their deputies would remain at the center for the duration of the crisis. The center was outfitted with cots and a kitchen to sustain hundreds of people, if necessary. Within the center, top officials would monitor the emergency, exchange information, coordinate response activities with other city agencies, and mobilize the resources of their own agencies in response to sudden developments or changing conditions.

This setup, says Greg Bishop, executive director of the Office of Emergency Communications, promised to mark an important advance over the city's existing emergency response arrangements. Under the existing system, the mayor activated the city's disaster plan by summoning his top cabinet officials to a meeting at City Hall. The department heads shared information at this meeting, agreed upon a plan of action, and then each returned to his or her own agency to preside over the department's role in bringing the crisis under control. When agencies had to call on one another for

---

12. "Adam 12" was an NBC crime drama that aired from 1968 to 1975.
13. Andrew Martin, "911 Answers Some With Deadly Quiet: New System's Quirks Thwart Some Callers," *Chicago Tribune*, November 10, 1995.
14. A telecommunications network was "fully redundant" if network traffic had at least two ways of getting from any one point to another; thus, it was considered the state-of-the art way to deliver uninterrupted service.
15. The city would activate the Command Center during the 1996 Democratic Convention, for instance, in case of trouble.

assistance, which was commonplace, communication and coordination were often difficult. "Every agency had its own 'command center,'" says Jeffrey Rodrigues, deputy director of the Office of Emergency Communications for Fire Operations. "If I need Streets and San' [the Department of Streets and Sanitation] to do something, I pick up the phone and call Streets and San's command officer. It was center to center, agency to agency, at the communication center level. And they often didn't have the authority to right away order something—they had to go up their chain of command." In addition, each agency, focused on its particular purview, had a different view of any given emergency—"different people describing an elephant by touching what they could," says Rodrigues. "You had your own department and you knew from your own people what was going on—but that's *your* view of it." That partial view sometimes made it hard to understand the urgency of another agency's request, and difficult to prioritize the use of agency resources.

At the Command Center, only top agency personnel, authorized to make snap decisions, would be present. With instant access to the Police and Fire Department's computer-aided dispatch system, they would be able to see at a glance hot spots all across the city. They would be able to see the volume of 9-1-1 calls. They would have immediate access to the information of their colleagues around the table, all of whom would be receiving constant dispatches from their own agencies. Armed with this big picture, they would quickly grasp why they were receiving a request from another agency. Furthermore, the mayor's demonstrated personal commitment to the Command Center would send a clear signal that all agencies were expected to be responsive, delivering their agency resources immediately when needed. Says Rodrigues:

> If you're all in the same room, you're all getting reports in and you're all in touch—you have a better feel for what the other guy is asking you for, and you're able to respond right away. [In the old days,] you may have [had] the resources, you may have [had] the talent, but when you have the *mood* correct for what's going on, the spirit of cooperation is generally better.

COMPONENTS OF THE NEW PLAN

The fact that the city had already developed a prototype emergency response gave the Mayor's Commission a considerable leg up in developing its recommendations for the city's Extreme Weather Emergency Operations Plan. Once a Heat Warning had been declared, the city's need for central coordination and information exchange among agencies could be handled by activating the Command Center, in accordance with the city's more general emergency protocols. The challenge facing the Mayor's Commission, therefore, was to decide the exact procedures for calling a Heat Watch or Heat Warning into effect,[16] to decide what additional services the city should provide during each, and to assign specific responsibilities to the various city departments.

Invoking a Heat Watch or Heat Warning

The Chicago Forecast Office of the NWS in Romeoville, Illinois, issued two- and five-day forecasts for the Chicago area four times a day based on meteorological data collected at three Chicago airports—O'Hare, Midway, and Lakefront. Whenever conditions led the NWS to call a Heat Watch or Heat Warning, the Chicago Forecast Office used a direct telephone line to reach the city's Weather Center, which was situated in the Department of Streets and Sanitation. The Commissioner of Streets and Sanitation would then inform the fire commissioner, the mayor's chief of staff, and the director of the Mayor's Office of Inquiry and Information.[17] The fire commissioner would coordinate both Heat Watch and Heat Warning operations. The public information officer of the Mayor's Office of Inquiry and Information would then notify the other city departments.

As in the interim plan developed by the Mayor's Commission, the primary activities of the city during a Heat Watch were backstage moves to prepare city departments for emergency duty in the event of a Heat Warning, distribution of heat information and cooling tips through all city departments, and increased monitoring of hospital EDs for heat sickness and bypass status.

Heat Warning

When the Fire Commissioner announced a Heat Warning and activated the city's emergency response, he summoned the top officials from eight other city departments to join him at the Command Center: the Mayor's Office of Inquiry and Information, the Department of Public Health, the Department of Human Services, the Department of Streets and Sanitation, the Chicago Housing Authority, the Department on Aging, the Police Department, and the Water Department. (Other departments might be called as well, at the discretion of the fire commissioner. Although the nine designated city departments were most involved in responding to a Heat Warning, 28 city departments played

---

16. The Commission developed a parallel set of procedures for declaring a Wind Chill Advisory—also invoked on the basis of NWS criteria—and a parallel set of city services to cope with it. As this case study is concerned particularly with the city's changing response to extreme heat, these cold weather procedures and protocols have not been included here.

17. Later, as part of a City Hall reorganization, many of the duties of this office were replaced by the city's newly created 3-1-1 office—a nonemergency hotline and counterpart to the 9-1-1 system, through which city residents could ask questions or voice concerns.

a role of some kind under the city's emergency plan.) Over time, the fire commissioner began routinely requesting a representative of the local power company, Commonwealth Edison, to join the Command Center group, as power outages during Chicago heat waves were common and potentially dangerous but could be mitigated with up-to-the-minute information about where and when outages were expected to occur.

In recommending what particular services the city should provide, once its forces were mobilized, the Commission considered a number of options. For example, the Commission did briefly consider an initiative attempted in the City of St. Louis in the 1980s after a severe heat wave: giving air conditioners away to residents who met certain eligibility requirements. The Commission members soon became persuaded that the expense, logistical complexity, and potential for mishap in such a plan were too great, however. "In a city like Chicago, it would be incredible," says Commission Chair Wilhelm.

The Commission ultimately decided that the city's responsibility resided in several basic activities:

- Providing both broad and well-targeted public information about heat dangers, cooling tips, and city services.
- Providing places people could go to cool down.
- Checking on as many at-risk people as possible.
- Managing power outages.

Based on the Commission's report and recommendations, the city developed an Extreme Weather Operations Plan, which was completed in November 1995 and updated each spring, with minor changes that reflected, for the most part, minor reorganizations of responsibility within City Hall.

In the five years that followed the July 1995 heat wave, Chicago invoked its Heat Warning procedures at least once during most summers and sometimes two or three times. The most severe heat wave to strike Chicago in this period occurred at the tail end of July 1999. Afterward, the Chicago Department of Public Health asked CDC to evaluate the effectiveness of the city's heat wave response. Although CDC had a number of suggestions for future improvement, the organization gave the City of Chicago high praise for an "exemplary" effort and praised the plan itself as "sound" and an "excellent guide for other cities that develop heat wave response plans."

In the end, says Wilhelm, "To me, the lesson that was learned [from the 1995 heat wave and its aftermath] was a social lesson. That in a city the size of Chicago and probably other large metropolitan areas, people are isolated, especially seniors, living alone, who are medically fragile, who are in neighborhoods that have changed. It's layer upon layer—economic, social, medical isolation." In 1995, no one in the city had been prepared for the ramifications of this evolving social reality, when taken in combination with a weather system that put this same population of elderly people at particular risk, he adds.

In addition, Donoghue says, in 1995 the city was prepared to handle any number of disasters from explosions and riots to plane crashes and train wrecks. "The problem was, this [heat wave] wasn't an identifiable disaster." The illness and death that attended the heat wave were geographically diffuse and occurred over time—and no one figured out what was happening until it was nearly over. For workers out in the trenches, "nobody had been trained to recognize the rising water," he adds.

"Everyone was working hard, but nobody connected the dots," agrees Wilhelm. "But that will never happen again."

Keeping an Open Mind in an Emergency: CDC Experiments With Team B

Pamela Varley

EDITORS' INTRODUCTION

A defining characteristic of a crisis is that it contains a significant amount of novelty—whether in terms of its scale, its newness (unfamiliarity) for those experiencing it, or a combination of elements not seen before by the responders. Sometimes, this novelty is strikingly and immediately clear as in the case of the 2004 Indian Ocean Tsunami, with its massive size and extensive geographic reach. But people and organizations often have considerable difficulty in sensing, identifying, and responding to novelty (as seen in the account of the Chicago heat wave in Case 14). This is due in large part to cognitive and organizational biases that prompt us to think and behave in familiar ways, based on past experiences and amplified through established ways of operating. As useful as these biases may ordinarily be, they can also cause us to miss and misinterpret signs and data in the face of novel circumstances and, consequently, fail to perceive a developing crisis.

Organizations—especially those that play critical roles in emergency response and find themselves navigating crises more frequently than others—thus stand to benefit from developing systems and tools for identifying novelty and overcoming cognitive and organizational biases. There have been several notable examples of such an

This case was written by Pamela Varley, a senior case writer at Harvard Kennedy School of Government. It was sponsored by the two faculty co-directors of the Kennedy School's Program on Crisis Leadership: Prof. Herman B. "Dutch" Leonard, George F. Baker, Jr. Professor of Public Management at the Kennedy School, and Dr. Arnold M. Howitt, Executive Director of HKS's Taubman Center for State and Local Government. It was funded by Harvard's National Preparedness Leadership Initiative, a project sponsored by the US Centers for Disease Control and Prevention. The Kennedy School takes sole responsibility for the content of this case. (1108)

approach, including a series of efforts by the Centers for Disease Control and Prevention (CDC), which typically serves as the lead federal agency for public health emergencies.

As described in this case study, CDC began to make a concerted effort to address novelty in the early 2000s. By then, it found itself confronting a host of new public health threats, ranging from emergent infectious disease to bioterrorism. After struggling to respond to the 2001 anthrax attacks, CDC proceeded to experiment over the next several years with a method for better detecting and responding to threats that presented themselves in new and unanticipated ways. In particular, the agency formed what it referred to as "Team B." The first formal iteration of Team B was in support of CDC's response to a 2002 outbreak of West Nile virus. Consisting of a small group of subject matter experts, the team discussed issues relevant to the outbreak investigation and provided response leaders with summaries of its discussions but—importantly—did not intervene in the actual investigation.

CDC reconstituted Team B in different forms and with different leaders and members over the next several years, seeking to bring additional voices to the table and to apply outside-the-box thinking as it organized responses to a series of difficult events, including the 2003 severe acute respiratory syndrome (SARS) outbreak and the 2003–2004 flu season. Despite the advantages CDC leadership saw in having additional insight from Team B, however, many at the agency remained confused about the group's role and responsibilities, which seemed to evolve from one event to the next. Was it intended to play an advisory role and ultimately answer to the officials charged with leading the response? Or was it supposed to function as an independent body that would provide alternative courses of action to the CDC director and other senior leadership? And, if the latter, how would response leaders react should their own recommendations be superseded by Team B's?

These core questions had not been resolved when in 2004—after existing until then on an ad hoc basis—Team B was made a permanent entity and positioned within the director's office. Yet even with its elevated positioning, Team B continued to struggle to find its place and influence responses.

DISCUSSION QUESTIONS

1. What are the main obstacles CDC officials encountered in trying to organize and operate their various iterations of Team B?
2. If you were a senior official at CDC, what recommendations would you make to improve Team B's effectiveness?
3. CDC is involved in responses to a range of public health emergencies, including but not limited to infectious disease and bioterrorism. Should mechanisms like Team B be configured and organized in different ways for different types of

events and threats? If so, how? And what challenges do you foresee in creating and maintaining such an adaptive entity?

4. Is the Team B approach broadly applicable to different types of organizations, professional domains, and sectors, or do you think it more effective for some— such as in the military and intelligence communities—and less so for others?

* * *

By the early 2000s, the Centers for Disease Control and Prevention (CDC) had to face a disturbing new reality. One of the agency's most important public protection roles, to investigate and contain disease outbreaks, was becoming progressively more difficult— and, almost certainly, the worst was yet to come.

As recently as the 1970s, public health experts had believed that deadly infectious diseases were very nearly a thing of the past, successfully vanquished by a combination of vaccines, antibiotics, and modern sanitation techniques. But new, resurgent, and drug-resistant pathogens emerged as a serious health threat in the 1980s and 1990s.[1] Global trade and travel allowed for their rapid spread. The September 11, 2001, terror attacks revealed the determination of the United States' terrorist enemies, and the subsequent anthrax attacks demonstrated that, if they chose to do so, terrorists could wreak havoc with the deliberate release of deadly or weaponized pathogens.

In the midst of CDC's anthrax investigation, and in its immediate aftermath, it became painfully apparent to CDC leadership that the agency's traditional approach to managing an emergency response, which had served CDC well for years, was not always well suited for the new class of public health emergencies—those that involved novel pathogens, that were instigated by terrorists, or that were widespread and protracted. But CDC leaders were divided about how radical a change was needed and about how to design a new model that preserved CDC's strengths while increasing its capacity and flexibility.

CDC's chief response in a public health emergency was to undertake a high-speed scientific investigation—combining epidemiological, clinical, and laboratory data—in order to come up with strategies to prevent, contain, and cure the ailment in question. In the perilous new landscape, CDC was faced with intense pressure to reach conclusions quickly without succumbing to the kind of tunnel vision that could lead investigators to miss something unfamiliar in an outbreak—a deliberately altered pathogen, for instance; a simultaneous disease outbreak in animals; or a pathogen that was geographically out of place. Traditionally, "we would look at the event and say, 'okay, how does this fit into *what we know*?'" explains one CDC official. But how to make room for the possibility of something new or unforeseen?

---

1. Disease outbreaks in this period included AIDS, Lyme disease, Legionnaire's disease, Ebola, hantavirus, West Nile virus, tuberculosis, and variant Creutzfeldt-Jakob disease (colloquially known as "mad cow disease").

Some CDC strategists began to discuss adding a new feature, called "Team B," to emergency investigations, at least in the case of large or unusual incidents. Team B would be made up of people inside CDC and outside, with expertise in the topic at hand, but without significant responsibilities in the investigation itself. This group would convene regularly over the course of the emergency investigation to review the latest developments in the outbreak and—essentially—to brainstorm about them. In particular, the members of Team B would ask themselves whether there were alternative interpretations of the data, or concurrent developments, that the principal investigating team had missed.

The first Team B was one created midway through the 2002 West Nile outbreak. It was followed, a few months later, by a more elaborate Team B created at the start of the 2003 severe acute respiratory syndrome (SARS) investigation. In the succeeding 18 months, CDC would convene a Team B in each of two smaller-scale emergencies as well. But its role and its reception within the agency would vary considerably from one incident to the next. The CDC executive team would ultimately have to decide whether Team B was an idea worth refining or whether another approach would serve the agency better.[2]

NO NEW THING UNDER THE SUN?

The idea of calling in outside experts during a public health emergency was not, per se, new at CDC; lead scientists had often done so. For example, Jim Hughes, director of CDC's National Center for Infectious Diseases (NCID) from 1992 to 2005, had led CDC's 1993 investigation into a mysterious respiratory disease first spotted on a Navajo reservation in New Mexico. In that case, CDC laboratory scientists made a surprising finding: the disease appeared to be a previously unrecognized hantavirus. This was unsettling, as there was no evidence that a hantavirus had ever before caused acute disease anywhere in the western hemisphere. Hughes therefore arranged for a 90-minute teleconference with "five or six" internationally recognized hantavirus experts and virologists and presented them with CDC's data. They listened and agreed with CDC's conclusions; however unlikely on its face, the cause of this new outbreak did, in fact, show all signs of being a new hantavirus. "It was extremely useful in raising our level of confidence," Hughes recalls.

Deciding when, how, and on what scale to call in outside experts, however, had traditionally been left to the discretion of individual research scientists and response leaders. In retrospect, CDC insiders questioned whether disinterested outside input might

---

2. One source of confusion within CDC was the fact that the term "Team B" was, at different times, used by various agency leaders to refer to different things. "Team B in the CDC is a shape-shifting creature," says Joe Henderson, director of CDC's Office of Terrorism Preparedness and Response from August 2002 to August 2004. In 2002, for example, Henderson himself used the term "Team B" to refer to the creation, at the start of an emergency response, of a special, short-term group to help the agency make the shift from business-as-usual operations to its emergency management model. This case confines itself to describing CDC's experiences with Team B when the term referred, as described here, to a group tasked with maintaining a big picture view of an emergency while others in the agency were absorbed with the demands of running the emergency investigation.

have saved responders from making mistakes in certain investigations—for example, West Nile or anthrax.

West Nile

Before its appearance in New York in 1999, the West Nile virus had never been reported in the western hemisphere. Based on certain lab findings, CDC scientists initially believed the New York outbreak to be St. Louis encephalitis (SLE). Though SLE had never before appeared in the northeast, it had appeared in other parts of the country. As the investigators set to work to verify this hypothesis, however, they skated past reasons, apparent in retrospect, to doubt the SLE theory. In addition, the CDC investigators initially paid little attention to a concurrent veterinary investigation into an avian disease outbreak in the same geographic area. Had they been persuaded to pay more attention, some observers believe they would have discovered the true, albeit surprising, virus behind both human and avian outbreaks more quickly.[3]

Anthrax

CDC made a different kind of misjudgment during the 2001 anthrax attacks—this one more consequential and politically costly for the agency.[4] On October 15, when an anthrax-laced letter arrived in the office of Senate Majority Leader Tom Daschle, there were immediate concerns about the safety of Senate staff, followed closely by concerns about whether postal workers along the letter's route from Trenton, New Jersey, to Washington, DC, might have been exposed. CDC quickly issued an assurance that postal workers were in no danger. Within a few days, however, four postal workers had been diagnosed with inhalation anthrax linked to the letter, and two had died. Another two postal workers were diagnosed with the less serious cutaneous (skin) anthrax.[5]

CDC's initial judgment had been made without an opportunity to analyze the anthrax sample in the Daschle letter (which was in military custody) and had been based on the prevailing wisdom about anthrax:

- Traces of anthrax were not thought to be a health risk.
- Anthrax spores were thought to be too heavy and sticky to escape through the pores of an envelope.
- Heavy taping on the envelope's seams was thought to have kept any of the spores from leaking out around the edges.

---

3. See Case 4.
4. See Case 11.
5. The other two inhalation anthrax victims in this event, and the two skin anthrax victims, recovered.

"There was a lot of dogma about anthrax—what it was, what its characteristics were, and what they weren't—some of which proved to be wrong," says one CDC veteran, in retrospect. Jurisdictional issues certainly complicated the case, but could a group of outside experts, sifting through the data, have spared CDC this mistake? A thoughtful group might have urged caution, he suggests—might have said, "Wait a minute. How do you know? Here's what we think we know—are we sure?"

CDC would create its first Team B during the 2002 West Nile outbreak, but two precursors in the anthrax investigation helped to set the stage.

PRECURSORS TO TEAM B: THE 2001 ANTHRAX INVESTIGATION

The Meta-Epi Group

One evening, several weeks into the anthrax emergency, after a long day in the trenches, about a half dozen team leaders in the CDC's investigation gathered together to review what they each had learned over the preceding day or two. Julie Gerberding, then acting deputy director of CDC's NCID, led the discussion. "As I recall, Dr. Gerberding even went to a board, or a flip chart, and got some things down on paper," says Jay Butler, coleader of the State Team in the anthrax response.[6] "We all came away saying, 'That was helpful,' because each of us knew something that the others didn't know, and it gave us a bigger understanding of the situation." All agreed to meet periodically for this purpose throughout the remainder of the investigation.

The "Meta-Epi Group," as some called it, did meet several more times, Butler adds, but the meetings were "frequently disrupted because everybody was doing other things. Cell phones were always going off. Julie Gerberding led the meetings, but frequently had to come late and then got called out." In the end, the general consensus of the group was that the exercise was useful, but that, realistically, the leadership team for the investigation was unable to sustain the function. In Butler's words, "You can't be on the ground and up on the observation deck at the same time."

The Clinical Training Group

One of the problems that arose during the anthrax attacks was the fact that most practicing physicians did not know how to test patients for anthrax exposure and the associated illnesses. CDC therefore decided to create a special task group of CDC staff, academics,

---

6. The job of the State Team was to field inquiries from state and local health authorities and dispatch research teams to investigate reports of suspected anthrax samples.

and physicians to focus on the creation of Web-based instruction to clinicians. In a deliberate move to shelter the task group from the pressures of the larger investigation, the members held their meetings not on the CDC campus but at nearby Emory University.

After the anthrax emergency was over, when the CDC reviewed what had gone well and badly in the anthrax response, this task group stood out as a particular success, according to Joe Henderson, then assistant director of the Division of Bioterrorism Preparedness and Response in CDC's NCID.

TEAM B: WEST NILE, SUMMER OF 2002

A few months later, in the spring of 2002, the West Nile virus began an ominous spread. Between 1999 and 2001, there had been 149 reported cases of West Nile in the United States altogether, resulting in 18 deaths. In 2002, there would be 4,155 cases, resulting in 284 deaths. The upsurge was apparent in the spring, with cases reported in new locations—Louisiana and Georgia—as well as in the northeast. CDC set up an emergency response.

By this point, CDC was already in the midst of an uncertain transition in the way it organized itself during an emergency. In the past, CDC's emergency investigations had been managed by whichever center held the appropriate scientific expertise. For disease outbreaks, that usually meant NCID or one of its divisions. The CDC director was always free to weigh in. Other personnel in other parts of the agency might be recruited to the effort. But as a practical matter, NCID was in charge. This system had the advantage of allowing personnel who knew each other well and were expert in a particular field to work together, efficiently and with common assumptions, in familiar environs, with familiar equipment. But for large, protracted, or complex emergencies, the resources of a single center were insufficient, critics argued; day-to-day work in the center invariably ground to a halt; the system depended too heavily on particular individuals; and it failed to take advantage of significant resources and complementary kinds of expertise elsewhere in the agency. Thus, there was a move afoot to move CDC toward an agency-wide Incident Management model,[7] in hopes that this approach would do better at tapping the resources of the whole agency.

In the 2002 West Nile outbreak—and for many years to come—CDC's emergency response was an amalgam of the old system and the new. In the case of West Nile, that meant that, in the main, the investigation was managed the "old" way, by NCID's Division

---

7. The Incident Management System featured a preestablished organizational template that had the advantage of being simple, consistent, and flexible. A basic structure was prescribed, but the pieces of the structure could be expanded, contracted, or eliminated to adapt to emergencies of varying sizes and types. The Incident Management System was originally created to eliminate chaotic management of large fires that crossed jurisdictional lines. Whether the template was appropriate for public health emergencies had been a longstanding topic of debate.

of Vector-Borne Infectious Diseases.[8] But a wider cast of characters did participate in the daily emergency operations briefings, including the CDC director and representatives of other complementary research areas within CDC. New participants, with their different backgrounds and perspectives, had new suggestions. The investigating teams took these "under consideration," but, for the most part, lacked the time, resources, and/or inclination actually to pursue them.

In the summer of 2002, newly appointed CDC Director Julie Gerberding asked Rima Khabbaz, NCID's associate director of epidemiological science, to play a bigger role in the West Nile investigation. Until this point, Khabbaz had played a peripheral, supporting role in the response, but she had attended enough of the emergency response meetings to be well informed about the issues in the investigation. Gerberding asked her to create something she called a Team B.[9] "I said, 'Wonderful,'" Khabbaz recalls. "What is a 'Team B'?"

Gerberding's idea—building on the experiences of the anthrax response—was to pull together a group of people, inside CDC and outside the agency, with expertise relevant to the West Nile outbreak, to get their thoughts about the outbreak, the investigation, and the new ideas that had come up in CDC's emergency briefings. It was quite open-ended, Khabbaz recalls, and the director of the 2002 West Nile investigation was initially skeptical, asking, "Is this group going to second-guess us? Who are you going to bring into it?" Khabbaz understood the concern and tried to reassure him: "I said, 'Look, my understanding is the idea is to try to help you.'" It might be a way to get a quick outside reading on questions that the investigators had run across but did not have time to explore, she suggested. She also asked his advice about whom to include in the group.

Khabbaz assembled a group of four to five people with expertise in vector-borne illness, virology, and entomology and held weekly teleconferences. At these, she updated the group on the investigation and posed questions raised either in the investigating teams or the emergency operations briefings. "We'd just have a very fluid discussion, and people would give opinions."

It was relatively easy to assemble the group, Khabbaz says, and she believes the team enjoyed the discussions. "I don't think there's any problem getting people to be on Team B":

> They're interested. They're not out there having to [manage the investigation] and put in the long hours, and yet they're kept involved. I sent them little summaries of what was happening week to week—the numbers, the questions, the issues. And they had some good discussions. It was fun.

---

8. A vector-borne disease is one transmitted by blood-feeding arthropods, such as mosquitoes, ticks, and fleas. West Nile is spread by mosquitoes.

9. The origins of the name are a little uncertain. According to one report, a former high-level CDC administrator had advocated that CDC follow the example of the Central Intelligence Agency's Team B, employed selectively to provide agency executives with a second opinion of staff assessments. Most people who worked on CDC's Team B, however, were reportedly unaware of the CIA's Team B. Some believed the "B" stood for "brainstorming." Others assumed the "B" was meant simply to distinguish the team from the "A" teams that were actually running the response.

Khabbaz was less sanguine about Team B's impact, however. "It left me thinking [that] it was an interesting exercise, [but] in terms of making a difference in the response—I'm not sure it made a huge difference," she says. After each Team B discussion, Khabbaz wrote up a brief summary, which she gave to the leadership team for the investigation; to Hughes, as infectious disease director; and to Gerberding. "There were a few nice ideas here and there, but I don't think there were any earth-shattering things that people [running the investigation] had overlooked," Khabbaz adds.

A few months later, Team B would get its first full-scale outing.

TEAM B: SARS, MARCH–MAY 2003

The severe and often deadly respiratory disease that would soon be named SARS became visible in China's Guangdong Province, Hong Kong, and Hanoi, Viet Nam, in late February and early March 2003. On March 12, the World Health Organization issued a global alert about the new disease and two days later, Canadian authorities announced an apparent SARS cluster in Toronto.[10] The disease was suddenly close to home, and CDC jumped into the investigation at full throttle. NCID Director Hughes led the investigation himself. As he assembled his investigative teams, he also called upon two of his nine division directors—Butler, director of the Arctic Investigations Program, and Jon Kaplan, director of the Division of STD, HIV, and TB Laboratory Research—to create and manage a Team B for the SARS investigation.

What, exactly, was Hughes looking for? He remembers it this way:

> The way I think of Team B is—people with expertise relevant to a particular problem, who are not actively involved in the investigation, so they have the ability to reflect upon the evolving investigation and think about the evidence that's accumulating. And equally important—think about what other things might be going on here that aren't appreciated by people that are caught up in the middle of the investigation. Is there anything that we're missing, or we're not thinking of, that we should be? To me, that's the value of Team B.

Like Khabbaz, Butler and Kaplan found it relatively easy to recruit members to Team B. Within CDC, they asked infectious disease experts without major responsibility for the investigation to participate. In addition, team leaders in the response were welcome to participate whenever they could. From outside the agency, they chose people they knew and respected who were working in academia or in public health systems at the state level. All were well known in the infectious disease world, and all had associations of long standing with CDC. As scientific investigators across the world learned more about the nature of SARS, the Team B coleaders added new scientific and technical

---

10. See Case 5.

experts, some as permanent members of the team and some as guest speakers for a session or two. For example, once SARS was identified as a coronavirus—more common as a cause of disease in cats and birds than in people—the Team B coleaders pulled in some veterinary virologists. These scientists contributed interesting pieces of information—for example, different patterns of illness depending whether the virus entered an animal's body via airways or the digestive track. This was provocative, as there were anomalies in the pattern of symptoms reported in the human version of the disease that scientists were still trying to explain.

On average, about a dozen people joined in the Team B discussions. Those invited were generally more than willing to participate, the coleaders report. SARS was a compelling medical mystery—a race between a deadly spreading virus and the virologists on its trail. In this high-stakes context, they were eager to help if they could. Also, to serve on Team B was to be "in the loop," where they would hear the latest reports from the front lines.

Early on, Butler was concerned about how to keep Team B well enough informed about the fast-moving investigation to be of help—and about how to convey the thoughts and perspectives of Team B members back to the CDC investigative teams in a useful form. Within the first few meetings, Butler, Kaplan, Hughes, and Mitch Cohen, director of the NCID's Division of Bacterial and Mycotic Diseases, who became an active Team B member,[11] settled on a modus operandi similar to Khabbaz's approach during West Nile: one of the Team B coleaders would attend the daily—and often twice-daily—emergency operations briefings. In this way, the coleaders would keep abreast of the latest issues, in order to report them to Team B. In turn, they would report any relevant contributions from Team B at the emergency operations briefings.[12] The emergency leaders would have the chance to ask follow-up questions or to ask the team to consider other issues as they arose. The team was also free to decide, on its own, where to focus its attention. One of the things Team B was specifically told *not* to do, however, was to make more work for the investigating teams by proposing new tasks or chores. Team B was to operate at a higher level—analyzing the outbreak and the thinking behind the response.

As in the West Nile experience, the members of Team B were dispersed across the country, so Butler and Kaplan arranged meetings via teleconference three times a week (twice a week in the final month of the investigation). All members of the team were busy professionals and some were highly placed state officials. Out of respect for their time, the Team B coleaders agreed to keep the meetings to one hour—which meant the discussions

---

11. A few weeks into the SARS investigation, Kaplan withdrew from Team B to resume his responsibilities as division director and Cohen took his place for the remainder of the investigation.

12. Notes from each Team B teleconference were also condensed to a concise, one-page summary, using bullet points to telegraph the key ideas quickly. These summaries were distributed at the briefings and posted to a secure area of CDC's computer network, along with other information about the investigation.

had to be focused and disciplined. In addition, they decided not to ask the team members to do any outside reading or preparation—though some did so anyway on their own.

Each teleconference began with a briefing or an update of about five minutes, followed by a discussion focused on one or two predetermined questions. One of the coleaders' responsibilities, Cohen notes, was to set the right atmosphere. The forums were a place to get new ideas out on the table—not a place to subject them to withering scrutiny. For one thing, there was not enough time to pull each idea apart but, in addition, the coleaders wanted to create an atmosphere of safety, a brainstorming session in which anyone could throw out an idea without risk to his or her credibility. "Scientists are really sensitive about expressing their lack of knowledge about something," Cohen notes.

The planning and coordination work involved in arranging such teleconferences did take more time than anyone had imagined, Butler says. He estimates that he and the other coleaders ended up spending "80 to 90 percent" of their time on Team B, while the SARS investigation was underway.

Assessing Success or Failure

Participants both in SARS Team B and in the SARS investigation came away with a positive view of the experiment. For one thing, many of the 28 teleconferences were stimulating conversations that fully engaged the participants. One of the most exciting, Butler recalls, was a session that featured a CDC investigator in Hong Kong looking into a confusing development—the rapid spread of SARS, by uncertain means, through the residents of an apartment building called Amoy Gardens. The prevailing hypothesis at the time held that SARS was spread by droplets—relatively good news, if true, as it meant close physical contact was necessary to spread the disease. But the droplet theory did not seem to explain the pattern of transmission at Amoy Gardens. By including an investigator on the ground in Hong Kong, the Team B coordinators were able to create "an opportunity for someone who was very knowledgeable about the situation, and was going to be involved in trying to interpret it and make policy recommendations, to tap into some other opinions and perspectives," Butler says. Some 27 people participated in that session.

Did this or any other Team B conversation provide the investigation with critical insights? Certainly, the team did not come up with any idea so new and radical that it altered the course of the investigation, but was that the appropriate measure of success? "You're not going to hit a home run every time you're at bat," Butler says. Perhaps the importance of Team B was in providing the "at-bat opportunity," he adds. "To me, [the Amoy Gardens discussions, in particular] fit well with what I thought Team B had the potential to do."

Team B was one of many sources of input for investigators, notes Khabbaz, who also participated in the SARS Team B; it was probably difficult—maybe impossible—for the investigators to know, after the fact, how much they were influenced by one source or another, especially if all were pointing in more or less the same direction. For his part, Hughes says that he regarded SARS Team B as a useful addition. Hughes left the CDC in 2005, but says that if he were to lead another SARS-type investigation, he would not hesitate to create another Team B.

A Harbinger of Future Trouble?

There was a nagging concern about one aspect of Team B's job in the SARS outbreak—an issue that had also arisen in the West Nile response and that would come into greater focus when Team B was created again in subsequent emergency response investigations. Was the team to be fundamentally advisory, answering to the scientific director of the investigation—in this case, Hughes—in the manner of a consultant? Or was the team expected to be more independent than that? Was the team, in fact, being asked to sec-ond-guess Hughes—to challenge him—if the members thought he was off track? Put another way, was Team B intended to provide Hughes and his team with thoughts and perspectives that they, in turn, were free either to consider or ignore? Or was Team B intended to provide the CDC director with a second opinion that could potentially lead her to overrule the director of the investigation and order a different approach? This distinction was particularly freighted in the context of CDC's shift from a center-centric to an agency-wide emergency response system.

In the SARS investigation, Team B leaned toward the former. Hughes had requested the creation of Team B, had assigned trusted colleagues to assemble the group and over-see it. The CDC director was privy to the Team B reports, by virtue of attending the emergency operations briefings. In that sense, Butler says, SARS Team B ended up play-ing both roles. But the potential conflict between these two roles never materialized during the SARS investigation—perhaps because, in general, CDC's conduct of the investigation was not controversial. By all reports, the Team B members, while eager to help in the investigation, were not inclined to take issue with it; their deliberations were characterized by a spirit of collegial good will.

TEAM B: THE FLU, DECEMBER 2003–JANUARY 2004

About six months after the SARS Team B was disbanded, in December 2003, CDC began to receive alarming reports about the seasonal flu. For one, it appeared to be getting an early start. For another, anecdotal reports indicated a high number of pediatric deaths.

Further complicating the picture, by early indications, the flu vaccine was not well matched to the year's prevailing flu strain.[13] Finally, there was an anticipated shortage of inactivated flu vaccine (the flu shot). It might be possible to make up for the shortage with live attenuated influenza vaccines (the nasal spray flu vaccine), but these were more expensive and, in some recipients, set off symptoms (albeit mild) of the flu itself. CDC considered them a fine option for healthy, not-pregnant people between the ages of 5 and 49. But for high-risk groups—the same groups for whom flu vaccination was considered most important[14]—CDC recommended the inactivated flu shot. What should the agency recommend this year, however, if the flu proved more virulent than usual, especially for children; if the vaccine proved less effective than usual; and if the safest version of the vaccine proved less available than usual?

CDC launched an investigation to get a better handle on the issues. Cohen suggested to Hughes that he convene another Team B to assist in the effort and enlisted Butler's help in running it. The pair re-engaged many of the same outside experts who had participated in the SARS investigation. The cast of characters within CDC was different, however, featuring staff with specific expertise in influenza and influenza vaccines.

In retrospect, Butler and Cohen give this Flu Team B a mixed review. On the one hand, as in the SARS investigation, the team rolled up its sleeves and engaged the issues with energy and dedication, even participating in a teleconference on Christmas Eve. But Butler and Cohen agree that Flu Team B ended up being significantly more disputatious than SARS Team B. Butler notes that there were some basic differences between the two investigations. In the case of SARS, no one knew much about the disease—an inherently humbling state of affairs that perhaps led to more open exchanges. Flu, though, was a different matter. Flu was not mysterious. What's more, in the flu world, there was a set of well-worn and recurring disputes about the illness and the flu vaccine. For instance, should the public be encouraged to get a flu vaccine if it was poorly matched to the flu strains in circulation? Some said yes, because even a poorly matched vaccine would offer some measure of protection that might save lives, especially of people in the high-risk groups. Some said no, because if people got the vaccine and then came down with the flu anyway, they might lose faith in flu vaccines, generally.

Neither Butler nor Cohen recall the specific points of difference that arose in the Flu Team B discussions, but they do recall that there was a sharp difference of views between

---

13. Each year, flu experts chose one flu strain in each of three broader categories to include in the vaccine. The vaccine for 2003–2004 protected against A/Panama flu but not against A/Fujian flu, which was emerging as the most prevalent strain in circulation. (A/Fujian was similar enough to A/Panama that experts hoped the vaccine would provide partial protection. In addition, it was possible that, in the course of the year's flu season, A/Fujian would fade and another strain would become more prominent.)

14. The groups at highest risk for complications from influenza, and therefore most strongly advised to get a yearly flu shot, were children between the ages of six months and five years; adults older than 49; pregnant women; people of any age with certain chronic medical conditions; and people who resided in long-term care facilities or nursing homes.

the CDC participants, on one side, and one of the outside participants, on the other, over a particular matter of CDC policy. Were the CDC participants overly defensive? One observer notes, "People think [Team B] is an intriguing concept until the first time it tells them something they don't want to hear." On the other hand, was the critical member of Team B out of line? What were the extent and limits of Team B's purview? Butler recalls telling the Team B members, "You know, we haven't been asked to completely *change* [the CDC] approach—we've been asked to *critique* this approach," but he also respected the perspective of the Team B critic. "His answer was, 'Well, it's the *wrong approach!*'" Butler says. The day after this meeting, an article appeared in the *New York Times* reporting the results of an unpublished study (itself controversial) that drew into question the effectiveness of the 2003–2004 flu vaccine.[15] Team B had been privy to the study, and some believed the Team B critic had leaked the story to the press. Tensions escalated—within Team B and between Team B and the CDC team in charge of the flu response—but fate intervened to ease the strain. By mid-January, it was clear that the 2003–2004 flu season was lifting early; effectively, the concerns over the flu vaccine were moot.

That same month, a few human cases of a particularly worrisome strain of avian flu, H5N1, were diagnosed in Asia. Virologists were concerned that, at some point, this virulent and lethal virus would mutate to a form that could be transmitted from person to person, perhaps leading to the world's next flu pandemic. Butler and Cohen proposed that Team B shift its attention to H5N1. Somewhat to their surprise, however, the team showed little appetite for taking up the question. Perhaps, they later surmised, the combination of people on Team B was not especially well matched to the issue. Perhaps, in the absence of person-to-person transmission, the threat was too hypothetical. Perhaps the group had grown weary and disaffected by the flu vaccine discussions. In any event, Butler and Cohen disbanded Flu Team B at the end of January, disappointed that it had not gone better, yet uncertain what lessons to draw from the experience.

CREATING A PERMANENT TEAM B

Although the Team B model was more formal and structured than past CDC efforts to consult with outside experts during an emergency response, Team B had been, to this point, assembled and disassembled on an ad hoc basis. In any given emergency investigation, large or small, the director of the scientific investigation, the director of one of the CDC centers at the heart of the investigation, or the CDC director herself could set up a Team B if it seemed useful.

In the spring of 2004, however, CDC began to implement a sweeping agency reorganization, known as the Future's Initiative. In addition, Gerberding continued to move

---

15. Lawrence K. Altman, "Vaccine Is Said to Fail to Protect Against Flu Strain," *New York Times*, January 15, 2004.

CDC's emergency response model away from the center-centric approach of old and toward the agency-wide Incident Management System.

As a part of the larger organizational overhaul, Gerberding created a new position: a permanent Team B director. This position was situated within her own executive office of Strategy and Innovation. The idea was that, during an emergency response, the Team B coordinator would assemble and manage a Team B along the lines of those set up during West Nile, SARS, and the 2003–2004 flu. Like the previous Teams B, the new Teams B would walk the delicate line between serving and second-guessing the research teams involved in the investigation and response. Ultimately, though, they would answer to the director's office rather than to the scientific director of the investigation.

Under Gerberding's plan, Team B would also play a role in the agency between major emergencies. At her direction, the Team B coordinator would set up a Team B to offer a second look at significant, nonemergency agency projects. If the agency were to retool its approach to obesity, for example, a Team B might be established to assist, advise, or challenge the CDC public health staff who were working on the issue. If the CDC were to rethink how to handle growing public concern over vaccine safety—a hot political issue for the agency—a Team B might be formed to offer an outside view.

In September 2004, Gerberding appointed Suzanne Smith as the first permanent Team B coordinator. Most recently, Smith had served as acting director of the Public Health and Practice Program Office (PHPPO). PHPPO—CDC's point of contact for state and local health departments, professional organizations, and academic institutions—had been divided up and redeployed under the reorganization. Before that, Smith had worked in several roles, over a 20-year period, spending the greatest time in the areas of injuries and chronic diseases. Smith had not sought the Team B position; like most people in the agency, she had never heard of Team B. She recalls that Gerberding explained the position as "the person who challenges the conventional wisdom." Though uncertain what that would mean day to day, Smith was ready to roll up her sleeves and figure it out.

As a starting point, Gerberding suggested that she talk to Butler, Cohen, and others in the Infectious Disease area who had worked on the SARS Team B. Smith listened with interest to their description. She came away with a mixed impression. It seemed clear that those involved had found the SARS Team B to be positive and helpful. The participants already knew and trusted one another. Smith imagined that the sessions—though conducted via teleconference—had the flavor of a relaxed brainstorming session over a beer with friends. That had some real advantages, she says: "It was a model that was acceptable to the internal scientists and comfortable culturally and there wasn't a lot of dispute." But it did not strike her as a disinterested second look at the outbreak or at CDC's investigation. "Did you get a wide variety of input? Did you have any reactors from the outside, testing or validating what you were saying? Well ... no."

Smith did some further research and learned that the Central Intelligence Agency (CIA) had created its own version of a "Team B" several decades earlier. Under the CIA approach, the agency's senior leaders had periodically assembled a group of experts outside the agency to provide a second opinion about the CIA's own in-house assessment of a selected security threat. The most famous CIA Team B, constituted during the Cold War, asserted that the Soviet arsenal was a far greater threat than the CIA's own analysts believed. Though influential at the time, this appraisal was, in retrospect, seen by many as suspect, inspired more by anti-Soviet ideology than by a rigorous review of the data. Concerned about this politically loaded association, Smith tried to persuade the CDC executive team to rename Team B but was unsuccessful. She also looked into a strategy developed in the US Navy to create in-house "red teams," which participated in selected Navy operations and reported observations to high-level officers—essentially, providing a "second opinion" to the reports that came up through the traditional chain of command.

TEAM B: THE VACCINE SHORTAGE, OCTOBER 2004

In September 2004, while Smith was researching the CIA's Team B and the Navy's red teams, a new vaccine problem was brewing. Authorities in Great Britain announced that, owing to safety concerns, the British pharmaceutical company Chiron, responsible for producing half of the annual US supply of flu vaccine, would be shut down for several months. This meant Chiron would not be able to deliver its flu vaccines to the United States for the 2004–2005 flu season. Other manufacturers might be able to boost their production a little bit, to compensate, but it was too late to avert a dramatic shortfall. In early October, when Smith had been in her new job just nine days, CDC launched an emergency response to the vaccine shortage. This response effort involved the newly created Coordinating Center for Infectious Diseases and the National Immunization Program. Gerberding assigned Mitch Cohen, director of the Coordinating Center for Infectious Diseases, to take charge of the response. The goal was to try to make sure the existing vaccines were dispensed to people across the country at the highest risk for hospitalization and death due to the complications of flu. This was easier said than done, because CDC directly controlled only about 10% of the vaccine supply. The rest was bought and sold on the private market—and about a third of the vaccine had already been distributed when Chiron's shutdown was announced.

Cohen invited Smith to sit in on his staff meetings for the response, and Gerberding included Smith in the daily emergency response briefings to provide a Team B perspective. At the first emergency response briefing Smith attended, she received Team B's task list, which took her by surprise, as it was focused not on the day-to-day response effort, per se, but on contingency planning. What if, on top of the vaccine shortage, there was an outbreak of avian flu, for example? Or, in event of an exceptionally bad 2004–2005 flu season, how should CDC think about whether to close schools and businesses? And—though it was too late to affect the present situation—could Team B think about how CDC should, in the future, respond to a manufacturing shortfall? The broad nature of these questions worried Smith. She knew, for instance, that there was already a major effort afoot in CDC's parent agency, the Department of Health and Human Services, to plan for an avian flu outbreak. Was Team B really supposed to take up this question, starting from scratch?

Smith asked Cohen his thoughts. He suggested that she talk to CDC staff in the National Immunization Program (NIP) to see what kind of assistance they thought would be most useful from Team B. The NIP group was most concerned about the distribution of the existing vaccine, Smith says: "The vaccine was sitting in certain pockets and localities. It was particularly rich in places that had had the good fortune not to buy Chiron vaccine—and CDC had no way of knowing where that was," especially with respect to private health care providers. Might Team B work with the National Association of County and City Health Officials to see if they could help, the NIP staff wondered? This question was far more specific than the contingency planning questions and, to Smith, more manageable.

Smith's first order of business, though, was to create a Team B. In this respect, she was aware of starting at a disadvantage compared to her predecessors in the 2003 SARS and 2003–2004 flu responses. By virtue of their background and professional contacts, Butler, Kaplan, and Cohen—division directors in the Center for Infectious Diseases—had known, reflexively, whom to recruit for the SARS and Flu Teams B. They were known personally in the infectious disease world. They were also acting at the direct behest of Hughes, who was a prominent and powerful figure in that field. These facts quickly telegraphed to ranking public health officials that Team B was a distinguished advisory group, worthy of their time.

Smith was supposed to assemble a team—presumably that meant a team of flu and vaccine experts—but she had never worked in these areas at CDC and was not an insider in these professional circles. While she did work for Gerberding, she did not report directly to Gerberding and was not part of the CDC executive leadership team. What's more, there were growing tensions between the Coordinating Center for Infectious Diseases, NIP, and Gerberding's office over the reorganization and the shift to an agency-wide Incident Management model. Smith found that she was not able to persuade CDC staff already busy with the response to participate reliably on the team. "They didn't know me," she says. "I had no currency."

Nor did she know on her own which outside experts to recruit for Team B. The people in the best position to advise her were involved in the response, she says, and too busy to help. She therefore sought advice from Butler and others in the infectious disease area, who gave her a list of suggestions. That was a help, but "I had to persuade these people that this was a legitimate effort," she recalls. "Some of them knew me, but they knew

I didn't work in this area." Smith did succeed in pulling together a group of about six or eight people for a few sessions, and she did report back on their comments at the emergency response briefings. Her reports, however, met silence at the briefings. Meantime, the Team B participants themselves grew dubious about the effort, she says: "These are smart people. I think they sorted out quickly that I wasn't really being listened to—that I didn't have a seat at the Big Table." Smith recalls vividly the moment when one prominent member of the group said, "Suzanne, I'm just going to call Julie myself."

> People wanted to talk to Jim Hughes, or Mitch Cohen, or Julie Gerberding. These are the people they're used to dealing with. They knew that if those three people were serious about their input, they would call and talk to them themselves—that this must be of far less importance or urgency.

After a few sessions, Smith says, "I chucked that approach as futile." But by this time, she had developed some independent thoughts about the nature of the response and about what sort of Team B would be useful. She had come to agree with the perspective of NIP staff that the key issues were about the location and distribution of the vaccine, rather than the vaccine itself. Unlike the SARS outbreak, which had enlisted infectious disease experts worldwide to identify and characterize a mysterious and threatening new disease, the vaccine shortage was, at base, a health systems problem: "It was a health services delivery issue. It was a distribution issue. It was a communications issue," Smith says.

> I'm going to call in my own group of people that I know will actually stay on the calls. I'm not going to pretend to get people who are big players in the infectious disease world. But I will get people who I think can give the response teams a lot of wrap-around experience that, frankly, I think they're missing the boat on, and that [in this situation] is more valuable than the technical information about flu or the vaccine.

Smith's Team B, which held its first teleconference October 21, included about a dozen state health officers, service providers, consultants, and business people. This group talked, via teleconference, twice a week for about four to six weeks, she estimates, and discussed a range of topics that had arisen in the emergency response briefings. For instance, Team B members weighed in with some suggestions about how CDC might piece together information about where the vaccine had already been distributed. The team also raised issues that were not being discussed at CDC, Smith says. A pet peeve from the field, for example, had to do with CDC's communications about the vaccine shortage to the public, which always included the suggestion that citizens take their further questions to their local health department. To small health departments, this was an entirely unmanageable burden. "They were livid," she says, "They would say, 'Don't tell them to call us! Tell them to call the CDC!'"

Smith also learned that in late October, another division of CDC was sponsoring a meeting in Washington, DC, for business and labor organizations about how to cultivate a healthier workforce. She was able to piggyback on this event to hold a town hall–style conversation about the vaccine shortage, about how a severe flu season would affect businesses, and about how CDC might work more effectively with businesses with respect to a serious flu outbreak.

Smith reported on this meeting and on the Team B sessions at the daily emergency operations briefings and entered her notes in the secure part of the computer network devoted to the vaccine shortage response. But she recalls that these reports were consistently met with silence and she was not aware that the CDC response teams acted on any of the suggestions.

Cohen, the director of the response, says he does not any longer remember the Team B reports clearly. Though a partisan of the Team B idea, then and later, he does not recall that it was particularly useful in this situation. In retrospect, he thinks a different approach might have been more helpful. For example, once CDC had identified health care providers with a relative vaccine oversupply, the agency wanted to redistribute it to those who had no vaccine. Many providers were willing to do so in theory but, as Cohen discovered partway into the response, were barred from doing so by the US Food and Drug Administration (FDA) regulations.[16] It would have been helpful, Cohen reflects, if, early on, the Team B coordinator had gathered together a group of knowledgeable regulators to discuss the various hurdles to vaccine redistribution. At the time, however, no one thought of using Team B in this way.

By December, "it hadn't developed into a bad flu year," Smith says. At that point, the vaccine shortage became a less worrisome issue, and "I got to the point where I felt I couldn't any longer use up the time of those on the outside who were participating in these conference calls," she says. "I recognized, after weeks of this, that no one was even reading the reports." Thus, she quietly disbanded the team. In January 2006, however, she did help to set up two different planning groups—one with school officials and one with business officials—to exchange perspectives with CDC officials about the pros, cons, and ramifications of shutting down schools or businesses in the event of a serious influenza outbreak.

---

16. The FDA did later suspend some of its regulations to permit some vaccine redistribution.

Keeping an Open Mind in an Emergency: CDC Experiments With Team B (Sequel)

Pamela Varley

The Centers for Disease Control and Prevention (CDC) continued to experiment with the Team B idea after the 2004 vaccine shortage but, by January 2007, its star had fallen. During those years, CDC tried out variations on the Team B concept to provide outside perspectives on important nonemergency issues facing CDC. In some instances, the CDC staff reportedly viewed Team B as a useful resource. In others, however, they reportedly viewed it as a vote of no confidence in their own work.

CDC also created a Team B to assist in its emergency response to Hurricane Katrina, which made landfall in southeast Louisiana at the tail end of August 2005. By that point, CDC Team B Director Suzanne Smith had retired. CDC Director Julie Gerberding asked the CDC Office of Strategy and Innovation (OSI) to create a Team B for the Katrina response. OSI Director Lonnie King asked David Bell, a senior CDC medical officer on special assignment to OSI, to head up the effort. According to Bell, the team—which included no experts from outside the agency but did include public health experts from about eight CDC departments—focused less on advising the response teams about the Katrina response, per se, and more on big picture questions. For example, the team identified public health problems that arose when a major city became nonfunctional and provided ideas about how CDC might consider preparing itself to deal with such dilemmas in the future. In particular, Team B considered the question of whether it was a good idea to

This case was written by Pamela Varley, a senior case writer at Harvard Kennedy School of Government. It was sponsored by the two faculty co-directors of the Kennedy School's Program on Crisis Leadership: Prof. Herman B. "Dutch" Leonard, George F. Baker, Jr. Professor of Public Management at the Kennedy School, and Dr. Arnold M. Howitt, Executive Director of HKS's Taubman Center for State and Local Government. It was funded by Harvard's National Preparedness Leadership Initiative, a project sponsored by the US Centers for Disease Control and Prevention. The Kennedy School takes sole responsibility for the content of this case. (1108)

set up temporary laboratory facilities near the areas of hurricane damage. Bell and his team researched the issue, conducted some interviews outside the agency, and provided a brief written analysis about the pros and cons of deploying laboratories versus airlifting medical specimens out of the area and transporting them to existing laboratories.

After the Katrina response, Bell and Team B assisted an outside consultant in preparing an after-action report about CDC's Katrina response. Bell also wrote up a proposal for creating an expanded Team B—called a Learning, Analysis and Perspective Team (LAPT)—with a director and three to five other permanent, full-time staff members. Under the proposal, the LAPT would "inform CDC response operations, and other operations as requested by the CDC Director, by conducting during- and after-action assessments involving people with diverse expertise who are not directly implementing the response" in order to ensure "continuous improvement of CDC response processes, procedures, and structural alignments." This proposal was never funded, however.

Bell's assignment to OSI ended in February 2006. After his departure, the position of Team B director was never refilled. Some of the functions that had previously been assigned to Team B were incorporated into CDC's Incident Management model, however. For example, the model included the option of creating a group to consider future planning as part of the response effort, and another group to consider ethical concerns.

According to Brad Perkins, CDC's chief strategy and innovations officer, the thinking in CDC's executive office evolved in this period. The agency's leadership remained committed to the initial goals of Team B—to provide a big-picture perspective, with a lot of outside information, from a variety of sources, usefully synthesized—but was inclined to meet them in new ways. For one thing, he says, CDC had been working to incorporate "greater outreach to the public and partners as part of our daily business."

In addition, as of January 2007, CDC's executive staff was moving forward with a proposal—under consideration for some time—to create a centralized CDC health threat assessment unit. Perkins cautioned that the design of the unit was a work in progress, but, as conceived, it would be a resource for the CDC director that would, at all times, collect and synthesize intelligence data, biosurveillance data (emergency room visits across the country, the purchase of over-the-counter pharmaceuticals, etc.), and more traditional sources of public health information. "In an emergency, they'd be doing the same thing with the volume turned up and more directed," Perkins says. The unit would not only inform CDC's own emergency responses but also would allow the CDC director to provide information quickly to the top decision makers in the federal government. Unclassified information would also flow, back and forth, from the health threat assessment unit to the various CDC programs.

"The central recognition here, I think, is that we need to get professional about our intelligence gathering and our intelligence interpretation," says Perkins. The agency's scientific program knowledge would continue to be an important part of the whole, "but it can't possibly be fully informed by all the possible streams of intelligence that we have, and that we anticipate creating."

Moving People Out of Danger: Special Needs Evacuations From Gulf Coast Hurricanes

David W. Giles

EDITORS' INTRODUCTION

The US Gulf Coast regularly experiences hurricanes and tropical storms, the worst of which cause extensive damage and inflict terrible suffering on the local population. In an effort to protect area residents, states and localities in the region have, on occasion, organized mass evacuations of millions of individuals prior to a storm's landfall. But evacuating, sheltering, and caring for large numbers of people is a complex and costly undertaking, especially when it involves special needs individuals— that is, people requiring various forms of assistance to relocate, such as hospital patients, nursing home residents, the homebound, and the carless. Because moving these individuals can result in significant upheaval and undermine their well-being, some institutions charged with their care have embraced alternative strategies, such as "sheltering in place." Yet this approach has its own dangers, exposing those who have stayed behind to the potentially deadly consequences of a storm.

This case study describes the evolution of special needs evacuation procedures in two Gulf Coast states—Texas and Louisiana—detailing how health, social services,

This case was written by David W. Giles, Assistant Director, Program on Crisis Leadership, for Dr. Arnold M. Howitt, Executive Director of the Ash Center for Democratic Governance and Innovation at the Harvard University John F. Kennedy School of Government. Funds for case development were provided by the Robert Wood Johnson Foundation as part of its State Health Leadership Initiative. Additional funding was provided by the US Department of Transportation through the New England University Transportation Center. HKS cases are developed solely as the basis for class discussion. Cases are not intended to serve as endorsements, sources of primary data, or illustrations of effective or ineffective management.

and public safety officials struggled to protect the most vulnerable citizens from a series of storms over a four-year period, from Hurricanes Katrina and Rita in 2005 to Gustav and Ike in 2008. Opening with an overview of New Orleans's experience with Katrina, the case first focuses on the fate of the many special needs residents who were unable to evacuate in advance of the storm. It recounts how, as floodwaters overtook much of New Orleans, thousands of residents were forced to flee to locations ill-equipped to provide shelter, while hospital patients suffered deplorable conditions in facilities that had lost power and, consequently, the ability to care for them.

Eventually, those stranded in New Orleans were airlifted and bussed to shelters in a number of host states. Although they finally made their way out of the disaster zone, relocating across state lines brought its own challenges. For instance, traveling with little to no documentation, some evacuees went missing for several weeks as their loved ones struggled to determine their whereabouts. Further complicating matters, just a few weeks after Katrina, Hurricane Rita bore down on the Houston–Galveston area, where a number of evacuees from Louisiana had taken refuge. Although Texas officials managed a relatively orderly airlift of hospital patients to interior parts of the state, the evacuation of the general population quickly devolved into a crisis in its own right. With the horrors of Katrina fresh in their minds, millions of area residents flocked to the roads, desperate to escape the looming storm. They soon found themselves mired in gridlock, however, and dozens of people, including nursing home residents and medical patients, died while stuck in the traffic.

In Katrina and Rita's wake, officials at all levels of government revamped plans for moving and sheltering special needs populations. The second half of this case study describes many of the ensuing reforms, including the creation of various tracking systems that Louisiana, Texas, and federal authorities developed to keep tabs on the location of evacuees. The remainder of the case explores how these plans performed once put to the test in 2008 when Hurricane Gustav threatened New Orleans and Hurricane Ike bore down on the Houston–Galveston region. It illustrates several significant improvements since 2005, including how, in advance of Gustav, tens of thousands of New Orleanians requiring transportation assistance benefited from a massive government-led prestorm evacuation effort. And in Texas, post-Rita reforms helped the region avoid gridlock during the general evacuation.

All the same, the region continued to experience problems with large-scale evacuations. In New Orleans, the surge of people taking part in the operation overwhelmed efforts to register and track them. Even more disturbingly, an initial shortage of appropriately equipped airplanes caused delays in evacuating hospital patients out of Gustav's path, leading to the deaths of several patients waiting to depart. In Texas, because thousands of Galveston residents had decided not to evacuate in advance of Ike, officials had to organize a major search-and-rescue effort amidst highly dangerous conditions.

As this case study illustrates, important progress was made between 2005 and 2008, but the Gustav and Ike experiences reveal that moving large numbers of people, especially those requiring assistance and specialized care, is a complex challenge with serious consequences for those in the danger zone. In the face of considerable uncertainty, public officials must determine the level of risk each approaching storm poses and then the costs and benefits of having the most vulnerable stay in place or relocate.

DISCUSSION QUESTIONS

1. The evacuations profiled in this case involve many different localities, multiple states, and various federal agencies. What are some of the challenges of moving people, especially those with special needs, when so many jurisdictions and organizations are involved?
2. Based on your understanding of how the 2008 evacuations played out, do you think that the reforms implemented following Katrina and Rita were sufficient, taking into account perceived and actual risk, along with financial constraints and other considerations?
3. What is the appropriate role of the federal government in mass evacuations and related activities (sheltering, medical support, etc.)?
4. Different parts of the country experience different types of natural disasters. Do the challenges encountered by the Gulf states when moving, sheltering, and tracking special needs individuals apply to other parts of the country and to different disaster scenarios?

* * *

Toward the end of the 2005 hurricane season, Hurricanes Katrina and Rita delivered a one-two punch to the United States' Gulf Coast, causing unprecedented destruction and taking the lives of more than 1,000 people. Both storms also triggered large-scale evacuations of major metropolitan areas: New Orleans in the case of Katrina and the Houston–Galveston region in advance of Rita. Involving the relocation of millions of people, the evacuations proved extremely challenging, and jurisdictions throughout Louisiana and Texas encountered enormous difficulties in moving so many people out of harm's way—particularly those with medical and other special needs.[1] This was especially the case in New Orleans, where tens of thousands of individuals who had not

---

1. "Special needs" is a broad term, but in the context of evacuation planning essentially refers to any individual or group that requires assistance to relocate away from danger. This includes people with disabilities and medical conditions, the elderly, the institutionalized, the homebound, and people without access to cars or other means of transportation.

evacuated in advance of Katrina found themselves stranded in their homes, in hospitals and long-term care facilities, and in "shelters of last resort" as water from nearby Lake Pontchartrain rushed through breached levees and into the city. Hundreds of New Orleanians died as a result of the flooding. Those who were eventually rescued, including many with preexisting medical conditions, endured a chaotic post-storm evacuation that often entailed exhausting journeys of several days through multiple states and via varying means of transportation.

Public safety authorities and elected officials at all levels of government implemented a series of ad hoc measures in an attempt to move, shelter, and care for individuals affected by the post-Katrina flooding, as well as those subsequently threatened by Rita. But resources were repeatedly overwhelmed and plans upended. And because there was little capacity at the time for keeping track of evacuees, host states frequently had little idea of who was arriving at their shelters and hospitals and what types of special needs they might have. Moreover, many individuals became separated from their families, friends, and neighbors, a particularly troubling predicament for those with serious health problems, who relied on others for care and for assistance in advocating their needs. While the damages caused by the storms were consequential (and in the case of Katrina, absolutely devastating), the failure to make adequate arrangements for relocating the regions' most vulnerable residents, including those with serious medical needs, proved to be one of the most significant shortcomings of the emergency responses to Hurricanes Katrina and Rita.

For a chronology of events and a cast of characters, see Exhibits 16A-1 and 16A-2.

EVACUATING NEW ORLEANS

Hurricane Katrina moved across the Gulf of Mexico during the final days of August 2005, gathering strength as it headed ever closer to the United States' Central Gulf Coast.[2] As the storm continued to grow in power and size, fears quickly escalated that it could very well devastate large swaths of the coastline, including the historic city of New Orleans, home to approximately 455,000 people.[3] Forecasters predicted that Katrina would make landfall late Sunday, August 28, or early Monday, August 29; and as the hurricane approached, officials in Louisiana and in neighboring coastal states

---

2. For a detailed account of New Orleans's experience with Hurricane Katrina, see: Esther Scott, *Hurricane Katrina (B): Responding to an 'Ultra-Catastrophe' in New Orleans,* Kennedy School of Government Case Program, 1844.0, 2006. See also: US Senate, Committee on Homeland Security and Governmental Affairs, *Hurricane Katrina: A Nation Still Unprepared* (Washington, DC: GPO, 2006; hereafter, Senate Report); and US House of Representatives, Select Bipartisan Committee to Investigate the Preparation for and Response to Hurricane Katrina, *A Failure of Initiative* (Washington, DC: GPO, 2006; hereafter, House Report).
3. US Census Bureau, *Annual Estimates of the Resident Population for Counties of Louisiana: April 1, 2000 to July 1, 2008* (CO-EST2008-01-22), March 19, 2009.

hastened to implement a series of measures that they had designed to safeguard residents from the storm's wrath, including plans for evacuating hundreds of thousands of area inhabitants.

On Saturday, August 27, Louisiana Governor Kathleen Babineaux Blanco and New Orleans Mayor Ray Nagin held a midday news conference at which they warned the public about the seriousness of the threat posed by Katrina. "This is not a test. This is the real deal. Things could change, but as of right now, New Orleans is definitely the target for this hurricane," Nagin declared.[4] All the same, the mayor did not call for a mandatory evacuation of the city. Instead, he announced a voluntary evacuation, effective for the remainder of the day and Sunday.

For its part, the state had taken steps earlier in the day to begin implementing the Southeast Louisiana Emergency Evacuation Plan (LEEP).[5] Finalized just a few months earlier, the plan was an attempt to overcome the failures experienced during the Hurricane Ivan evacuation a year before, when multiple jurisdictions had evacuated at the same time, bringing contraflow traffic to a standstill.[6] Consequently, LEEP laid out a phased evacuation process in which lower-lying parishes (primarily those farthest to the south) would begin evacuating first, followed by the metropolitan New Orleans area. Contraflow would only go into effect once Orleans and Jefferson parishes were set to evacuate.[7]

In the lead up to Katrina, it appeared that the state's plan was working. Low-lying parishes (such as Plaquemines, St. Bernard, and St. Charles) initiated mandatory evacuations throughout Saturday, well in advance of New Orleans and its suburbs.[8] Although some of the approximately one million people who took to the roads experienced traffic delays lasting up to several hours, the evacuation was, in the words of one post-event assessment, "a great improvement over the Hurricane Ivan evacuation," when travel times had lasted up to 15 hours.[9]

Still, the prestorm evacuation of southern Louisiana encountered some serious difficulties. No doubt deciding whether and when to issue and implement an evacuation order, and determining its scope, can be a challenging process for public authorities in any jurisdiction. And as Dr. Rosanne Prats, Director of Emergency Preparedness for the Louisiana Department of Health and Hospitals (DHH), pointed out, making this decision in the face of a hurricane threat can be particularly difficult, given the high degree of uncertainty involved. (For instance, a forecasted storm's intensity can increase or decrease at any moment and its projected trajectory can easily shift course.) While calling for an evacuation might end up saving countless lives, it could just as well

---

4. Senate Report, 247.
5. Ibid., 67–68.
6. Contraflow is the practice of redirecting traffic along multiple lanes of roadway for travel in a single direction, rather than the normal bidirectional traffic flow.
7. Senate Report, 243–245.
8. House Report, 107; Scott, *Hurricane Katrina;* Senate Report, 245–247.
9. Senate Report, 243–244.

unnecessarily uproot thousands, if not millions, of people, disrupt commerce and other essential activities, and entail the costly allocation of resources.[10]

As Katrina approached, New Orleans officials delayed making a decision about whether to call for a full-scale evacuation until the very last minute, even as forecasters continued to warn of the storm's potentially devastating impact. The city had never before issued a mandatory evacuation order, and Nagin's administration struggled to resolve a series of outstanding legal issues, such as who could be included under such a decree.[11] Only on Sunday morning, with the storm's landfall less than a day away, did Nagin put the mandatory evacuation order into effect. In doing so, he told residents remaining in the city, "We are facing a storm that most of us have feared. I do not want to create panic. But I do want citizens to understand that this is very serious, and it's of the highest nature."[12]

Although the vast majority of New Orleanians ultimately heeded Nagin's advice and evacuated by the end of the day Sunday, tens of thousands remained behind. Those that stayed did so for a variety of reasons: some were simply unwilling to leave their homes; others lacked access to vehicles (more than a quarter of New Orleans residents did not own a car[13]) or had disabilities or medical conditions that made it impossible to drive; others yet had been receiving treatment in hospitals or were otherwise institutionalized. Unfortunately, the government provided little evacuation assistance to those who may have wanted to leave but couldn't. Even though officials in New Orleans had explored options for utilizing buses and Amtrak trains to move special needs individuals to shelters elsewhere in Louisiana, plans remained incomplete in the lead up to the 2005 hurricane season.[14] And despite increasing concern regarding Katrina's potential effect on the New Orleans area, state and federal officials made no effort in the weekend preceding landfall to obtain additional transportation assets in support of a last-minute evacuation of the city.[15]

As a result, those who remained in New Orleans on Sunday had just two options: shelter in their residences or host institutions, with the hope that they could survive on their own, or get to the Louisiana Superdome, a sports complex in downtown New Orleans that the city had designated as a "refuge of last resort."[16] And so, throughout Sunday, with Katrina nearing Louisiana's coastline, buses crossed the city, gathering and carrying thousands of elderly, ill, home-bound, and transportation-disadvantaged residents to the facility.[17]

10. Telephone interviews with Dr. Rosanne Prats, May and September 2009. Unless noted, all subsequent quotations from and attributions to Prats are from these interviews.

11. Senate Report, 248.

12. House Report, 109–110.

13. John L. Renne, Thomas W. Sanchez, and Todd Litman, *National Study on Carless and Special Needs Evacuation Planning: A Literature Review*, 2008, http://planning.uno.edu/docs/CarlessEvacuationPlanning.pdf.

14. Senate Report, 248–249.

15. Ibid., 254, 257–259.

16. Ibid., 243.

17. House Report, 113.

Although authorities failed to organize a large-scale, prestorm evacuation of medical special needs and transportation-disadvantaged individuals, they did make some arrangements for sheltering residents at the Superdome. The Federal Emergency Management Agency (FEMA) and the Louisiana National Guard, for instance, brought in food and water supplies,[18] while state and city health and social service workers established a section to support individuals with medical special needs. But, according to one state employee on scene that weekend, they were ill-prepared to adequately process the hundreds of nursing home residents, chronically ill, and disabled who arrived by the hour. Among other things, they soon ran out of intake forms, which severely limited their ability to quickly identify shelterees and keep track of their medical needs. As a result, those staffing the special needs section were often hard-pressed to connect patients with family members or friends who arrived looking for them. "What does the person look like?" workers asked, in a desperate and often futile attempt to help reunite loved ones. Perhaps they were still at the Superdome or perhaps they had been moved on to a hospital or some other shelter. Perhaps they had never arrived in the first place.[19]

The Rescue

Following Hurricane Katrina's landfall at around 6 a.m. Monday, August 29, it at first appeared that New Orleans had escaped the horrific devastation many had feared in advance of the storm. Katrina's surge had decimated smaller cities elsewhere along the coast, but New Orleans and its residents had emerged relatively unscathed. Just hours later, however, an all-out crisis engulfed the city. With multiple breaches in the area's levee system, floodwaters from neighboring Lake Pontchartrain were pouring through New Orleans's streets.[20]

Had the levees held, life would likely have returned to normal fairly quickly, and the actions taken to safeguard the city and its remaining residents would have presumably proven adequate. Instead, those remaining behind faced a horrific nightmare. Stranded in the midst of a disaster zone, they fought desperately to reach safe shelter. In the process, many sustained injuries, developed illnesses, or endured rapidly worsening health conditions. Hundreds died in the process.[21] Most would survive, but their journeys out of New Orleans would leave them exhausted and disoriented. Moreover, thousands would

18. Ibid., 117.
19. Jed Horne, *Breach of Faith: Hurricane Katrina and the Near Death of a Great American City* (New York: Random House, 2006), 50–53.
20. Scott, *Hurricane Katrina.*
21. A conservative estimate of Katrina-related deaths in Louisiana put the number at just under 1,000. See: Joan Brunkard, Gonza Namulanda, and Raoult Ratard, "Hurricane Katrina Deaths, Louisiana, 2005," *Disaster Medicine and Public Health Preparedness* 2 (2008): 215–223.

become separated from family and companions, lost for days, even weeks, in the chaos of the mass exodus.

With the floodwaters continuing to rise, residents who had ridden out the storm at home were forced to escape onto their rooftops. Some waited for help to arrive; others took to the flooded streets, navigating past debris in search of higher ground. Meanwhile, a slew of government agencies—including the Louisiana Department of Wildlife and Fisheries, local police forces, the Louisiana National Guard, the US Coast Guard, and FEMA Urban Search and Rescue teams—began deploying boats, helicopters, trucks, and ambulances in an effort to bring stranded residents to safety.[22] Over the next several days many New Orleanians gathered at "lily pads," or highway overpasses the city had predesignated as collection points; thousands more made their way to the Superdome and, eventually, to the city's Ernest N. Morial Convention Center.[23]

The Superdome, however, was already straining to accommodate the 10,000 to 15,000 people who had taken shelter in advance of Katrina.[24] When the storm had passed over New Orleans Monday morning, its strong winds had badly battered the facility. Jed Horne, metro editor of the *New Orleans Times-Picayune*, vividly recounted the scene there:

> The wind that had contented itself with shredding the flags and chevrons circling the Dome's exterior terraces tore loose two air vents and then began to peel away long sheets of the rubberized weather-proofing from the convex twelve-acre rooftop that gave the Dome its name. Rain had begun to fall through the disintegrating roof and onto the floor of the stadium, when suddenly the lights went out, to screams and groans from the thousands of people encamped on the gridiron or sprawling in the tiered seats; the air-conditioning died, and it was as if the giant spacecraft that was the Louisiana Superdome had settled onto the dark side of a planet too near the sun.[25]

Yet despite their discomfort and growing anxiousness, those sheltering at the Superdome still had enough food and water to meet their needs.[26] And with conditions elsewhere in flooded New Orleans far worse, throughout Monday and Tuesday, more and more residents arrived at the now damaged "shelter of last resort." By mid-week, as many as 30,000 people had gathered at the Superdome—double the complex's population sheltered before the storm.[27]

Meanwhile, as early as Monday night, stranded residents had also begun appearing at the Convention Center. Up to 19,000 people eventually sheltered there, but the scene

---

22. House Report, 104, 116.
23. Ibid., 117; Senate Report, 363.
24. Senate Report, 359.
25. Horne, *Breach of Faith*, 55–56.
26. House Report, 117.
27. Senate Report, 364.

soon became even more unbearable and dangerous than that at the Superdome. As was the case at facilities throughout the city, there was no electricity, air conditioning, or lighting. Moreover, because the city had never planned on using the Convention Center as a shelter, it had made no arrangements to provide even the most basic necessities such as food, water, and medical supplies—much less a system for triaging and registering individuals.[28]

As tens of thousands continued to languish at the Superdome, Convention Center, and elsewhere across the city, widespread confusion and extensive miscommunication among public authorities seriously hampered efforts to finalize and implement an evacuation strategy.[29] Only on Wednesday, August 31, did plans for relocating those stranded within the city really begin to move forward, with Governor Blanco putting responsibility for managing the evacuation into the hands of the newly formed Joint Task Force Katrina. On Thursday, the Task Force, which was coordinating relief efforts of active duty federal troops, arranged for the evacuation of the Superdome and some lily pads. The Convention Center was secured Friday and evacuated a day later.[30]

In an attempt to bring some order to what promised to be a tumultuous journey, health care workers scrambled to generate paper medical records for the special needs evacuees leaving the Superdome. But this last ditch effort was largely for naught, as many of the documents soon disappeared amidst the chaos of the ensuing evacuation.[31] Confusion would reign over the next several days and weeks, as evacuees ended up at shelters and hospitals far removed from New Orleans. Who was who, and what were their medical needs?

Hospitals and Nursing Homes

Nightmare scenarios played out at hospitals and nursing homes as well. With hospital personnel and patients exempted from the city's mandatory evacuation order,[32] many medical facilities had opted to shelter in place, believing that an evacuation would be too taxing for their most fragile patients. Moreover, adds Rosanne Prats of the state's DHH, many New Orleans hospitals were centuries old and, unlike medical facilities in the more storm-vulnerable parishes farther to the south, had never before evacuated due to a storm. Given this history, they were reluctant to believe, even amidst alarming forecasts, that the risk posed by Katrina necessitated the advance relocation of patients—an

---

28. Ibid.; House Report, 118, 280–281.
29. House Report, 121; Senate Report, 362–363.
30. Senate Report, 364–365; Brigadier General Mark Graham, "Testimony to the Senate Committee on Homeland Security and Governmental Affairs Committee," February 1, 2006.
31. House Report, 280.
32. Senate Report, 248.

expensive and potentially life-threatening endeavor. As a result, there were still about 2,500 patients in New Orleans on Sunday night as the hurricane bore down on the city.[33]

Among the facilities still housing patients was Charity Hospital, one of just two major trauma centers in the entire state.[34] Four hundred fifty patients, 46 in critical condition, remained at the downtown facility, as did hundreds of staff members and relatives.[35] At around 8 a.m. Monday, Charity lost power.[36] Jed Horne captures the challenges medical staff suddenly faced:

> Elevators froze in place, air-conditioning died along with the refrigerators critical to the maintenance of medicines, plasma, food, and the corpses in the hospital morgue.... Power packs in the portable blood-sugar monitors couldn't be recharged. Blood pressure cuffs were electronic, not to mention the dialysis machines. Even the pill dispensers were electronic, though they could be busted open with a screwdriver.[37]

A similar scene played out at medical facilities across the city, including University Hospital, which also lost power Monday morning.[38] Despite the urgency of the situation, however, patients would have to wait days for relief. By Tuesday, Charity and University, along with much of the rest of New Orleans, were stranded in a sea of floodwater, and the hospitals' staffs struggled to provide care to their critically ill patients. But it was a nearly impossible task in the absence of electricity and running water,[39] and dozens of hospital patients perished before help finally arrived.[40]

Desperate to evacuate, the hospitals asked DHH for assistance in tracking down transportation assets. But state health officials soon discovered that search-and-rescue teams had become completely consumed by the massive rescue operations taking place across the city. Dr. Jimmy Guidry, DHH's Medical Director, detailed the frustration he experienced in trying to link the hospitals to search and rescue:

> The calls started coming saying ... "We got to get them out of here. We got to get them out of here. We got to get them out of here." And I was asking for the resources to move them. Search and rescue [was] going to have to move them.... So the Hospital Association is coming to me in tears, the folks there are in tears trying to help their folks and I'm beating my head to try to get the help. And you've got the search and rescue that's trying to get people out of water and rooftops and out of hospitals. And that's all the competing needs for the limited assets.[41]

---

33. Although nursing homes were not exempt from Nagin's evacuation order, many also decided to shelter in place. See: Senate Report, 248, 399.
34. Senate Report, 399.
35. Horne, *Breach of Faith*, 133–139.
36. House Report, 285.
37. Horne, *Breach of Faith*, 137.
38. House Report, 285.
39. Horne, *Breach of Faith*, 132–133, 137–139.
40. Brunkard et al., "Hurricane Katrina Deaths, Louisiana, 2005." In total, close to 150 bodies were recovered from New Orleans hospitals in the aftermath of Katrina. Another 70 or more individuals died in nursing homes in Orleans, St. Bernard, and Jefferson Parishes.
41. Senate Report, 402.

After several abortive attempts, the US Coast Guard, along with the Louisiana Department of Wildlife and Fisheries and city and state police, finally began evacuating both Charity and University on Friday, September 2.[42] Moving patients was no easy task, however, as many, in the words of one account, "required continuous, individual medical care."[43] As at the Superdome, hospital staff attempted to provide departing patients with identifying documentation and medical records, pinning the forms to their clothing.[44] But this was hardly an organized process, nor would much of the paperwork survive the arduous journey lying ahead.

The Scene at Louis Armstrong Airport

By the time help arrived at Charity and University, the federal government had already activated its National Disaster Medical System (NDMS) to transport rescued hospital patients out of New Orleans and on to medical facilities located outside the disaster zone.[45] In the early morning of Wednesday, August 31, three NDMS Disaster Medical Assistance Teams (DMATs)[46] had arrived at Louis Armstrong New Orleans International Airport to triage and provide medical assistance to arriving patients who were eventually airlifted out of the city on planes belonging to the US Air Force, the National Guard, and private carriers. Initially under the impression that they would be working with about 2,500 patients, DMAT members quickly learned that this estimate was considerably off the mark.[47] The surge in arriving evacuees was rapid and extreme, according to Hemant Vankawala, one of the first DMAT physicians on scene. Within the first 15 hours, he said, "We watched our population grow from 30 DMAT personnel taking care of six patients and two security guards [to] around 10,000 people."[48]

Helicopters arriving as often as every 15 seconds delivered thousands of hospital patients and nursing home residents, as well as people rescued from rooftops, overpasses, and other ad hoc gathering places. As Vankawala put it, "It was a non-stop, never-ending, 24-hour-a-day operation."[49] Those in need of medical attention were triaged and grouped

42. Ibid.; House Report, 285–286.

43. Senate Report, 403.

44. Horne, *Breach of Faith,* 143–144.

45. Senate Report, 414.

46. DMATs are groups of regionally based volunteer medical professionals that, as part of the National Disaster Medical System, can be called up by the federal government and deployed in the event of an emergency. See: Senate Report, 411; US House of Representatives Committee on Government Reform Minority Staff, "The Decline of the National Disaster Medical System," December 2005.

47. Christopher Sanford, et al., "Medical Treatment at Louis Armstrong New Orleans International Airport after Hurricane Katrina: The Experience of Disaster Medical Assistance Teams WA-1 and OR-2," *Travel Medicine and Infectious Disease* 5 (2007): 230–235; Senate Report, 414.

48. Hemant Vankawala, "A Doctor's Message From Katrina's Front Lines," *National Public Radio,* September 7, 2005, http://www.npr.org/templates/story/story.php?storyId=4836926.

49. Ibid.

according to the severity of their condition. Although some of the evacuees cared for at the airport had been injured during the storm, most were suffering acutely from disruptions to treatments for chronic illnesses. Diabetics had gone for days without insulin, while patients suffering from renal failure had been unable to access dialysis services. Evacuees with hypertension had suffered strokes and heart attacks after losing or running out of their medications.[50] With the number of people requiring assistance so dramatically outnumbering DMAT personnel, the physicians and nurses at Louis Armstrong strained to provide even basic medical care. As for the most serious cases, Vankawala said, "We watched many, many people die. We practiced medical triage at its most basic—'black-tagging' the sickest people and culling them from the masses so that they could die in a separate area."[51] In total, 26 patients died at Louis Armstrong.[52]

Conditions within the airport bordered on the unbearable. Never intended to serve as a medical staging facility or care center, the complex lacked basic necessities such as blankets, potable running water, and sufficient supplies and facilities for accommodating sanitary needs.[53] Vankawala reported, "We were so short on wheelchairs and litters we had to stack patients in airport chairs and lay them on the floor. They remained there for hours, too tired to be frightened, too weak to care about their urine- and stool-soaked clothing, too desperate to even ask what was going to happen next."[54] Flies swarmed around trash cans and piles of litter.[55] And with the air-conditioning down, the indoor air temperature soared to 100 degrees.[56] One horrified DMAT member observed, "Evacuees were being taken from a very dehumanizing experience [and] placed into an equally dehumanizing environment at the airport.... The situation was very similar to those found in the Third World."[57]

Amidst the chaos of receiving, processing, and treating the thousands of individuals passing through Louis Armstrong, record keeping was, in the words of DMAT personnel "at best intermittent."[58] A DMAT after action report deemed the documentation of medical care and needs "dismal,"[59] and there was no comprehensive system in place for tracking

---

50. Sanford et al., "Medical Treatment at Louis Armstrong."
51. Vankawala, "A Doctor's Message."
52. Senate Report, 412. But although he admitted that conditions were deplorable, Captain Art French, one of the NDMS doctors on scene, believed that these patients would have likely died in almost any well-functioning hospital.
53. Sanford et al., "Medical Treatment at Louis Armstrong"; Anne Hull, "At an Airport Turned Field Hospital, Urgent Arrivals," *Washington Post*, September 4, 2005, A25.
54. Vankawala, "A Doctor's Message."
55. Hull, "At an Airport Turned Field Hospital."
56. Sanford et al., "Medical Treatment at Louis Armstrong."
57. Helen Miller, Joel McNamara, and Jon Jui, *Hurricane Katrina—After Action Report, OR-2 DMAT*, September 25, 2005, https://www.hsdl.org/?view&did=766144.
58. Sanford et al., "Medical Treatment at Louis Armstrong."
59. Miller et al., *Hurricane Katrina—After Action Report*.

individuals as they moved through Louis Armstrong and to points beyond.[60] NDMS physician Captain Art French described the rudimentary tracking process: "We wrote down their names, where they were going, and with whom on a piece of paper. Those pieces of paper I hope are still there."[61]

Moreover, family members who had managed to stick together throughout the horrors of the flooding in the city below were suddenly separated from one another at the airport, triaged into separate groups, and, in many cases, sent on to different states for shelter and care. Anne Hull, a *Washington Post* reporter, observed one such heartbreaking scene: Shirley Kenner had patiently sat waiting for medics to finish treating her husband Joseph—to whom she had been married for 50 years—only to be informed that he had already been airlifted to a hospital in Lafayette without her. Although Shirley was eventually flown to Lafayette, thousands of others were not so lucky.[62]

A Word About the National Disaster Medical System

In the end, more than 3,000 patients were airlifted from Louis Armstrong Airport to receiving hospitals via the NDMS patient evacuation process.[63] A federally coordinated program involving the US Departments of Health and Human Services (HHS), Defense, Veterans Affairs, and Homeland Security (DHS), NDMS was founded in 1984 to help support the evacuation of US nationals injured or otherwise affected in overseas conflicts. The program's mission was subsequently expanded to include medical support in the event of a natural disaster or act of terrorism within the United States. Originally administered by HHS, it was, following the passage of the Homeland Security Act of 2002, moved to DHS.[64]

Designed to "temporarily supplement" federal, tribal, state, and local public health and medical capabilities, the program performed three main functions: (1) to

---

60. Only a small number of evacuees moving through Louis Armstrong were entered into any type of robust tracking system—data on the approximately 1,800 patients that were transported by US military aircraft (other patients were flown out by National Guard or on private planes) were logged into the NDMS's patient tracking program. See: Senate Report, 414.

61. Senate Report, 412.

62. Hull, "At an Airport Turned Field Hospital."

63. Sanford et al., "Medical Treatment at Louis Armstrong." Other estimates are even higher (see for example: Senate Report, 414), and thousands more individuals not requiring hospitalization were also evacuated from Louis Armstrong (House Report, 287–288).

64. Dan Niederman, "The National Disaster Medical System, Can It Respond to a Major Southern California Earthquake?" November 11, 2008, http://ezinearticles.com/?The-National-Disaster-Medical-System,-Can-it-Respond-to-a-Major-Southern-California-Earthquake?&id=1677932; Senate Report, 410–411; US House of Representatives Committee, *The Decline of the National Disaster Medical System*. In January 2007, following post-Katrina reforms to the organization of the federal emergency management apparatus, NDMS was returned to HHS, where it was placed under the Assistant Secretary for Preparedness and Response.

provide medical response assistance in the event of a disaster, (2) to move patients from disaster areas, and (3) to provide "definitive medical care" through NDMS-affiliated hospitals.[65] DMATs, such as those that reported to Louis Armstrong Airport, formed the core of NDMS. Organized at the regional level, DMATs consisted of volunteer doctors, nurses, and other medical care professionals and support personnel, who conducted triage and emergency medical care services when deployed to the scene of a disaster.[66]

According to Dr. Guidry and Dr. Prats of Louisiana's DHH, it was only in the year leading up to Katrina that utilizing NDMS to evacuate hospital patients in the event of a major disaster was first discussed seriously within the state.[67] In early summer 2004, local, state, and federal officials had participated in a five-day exercise, dubbed Hurricane Pam, which simulated a catastrophic hurricane pummeling the greater New Orleans region. Conceived as a slow-moving Category 3 hurricane, Pam featured high winds, heavy precipitation, and a large storm surge. The scenario envisioned the overtopping of levees, widespread structural damage, and the almost complete collapse of transportation and communication networks. Local response capacity would be overwhelmed.[68] Among other things, the Pam exercise led to the development of the Temporary Medical Operations and Staging Areas (TMOSA) plan, which laid out how Louisiana and its federal partners, including NDMS, were to rescue and evacuate residents and medical patients stranded by a storm of a similar scale. According to the plan, search and rescue would first round up and deliver people requiring medical attention to base-of-operation sites. From there, a mix of volunteer, state, and federal assets would bring victims to TMOSAs, where they would be registered and assessed. Evacuees would then be transported by the state or the federal NDMS system to areas outside the disaster zone.

When NDMS was activated for the post-storm evacuation of New Orleans, it played a critical role in getting thousands of hospital patients out of the flooded city and on to secure facilities elsewhere in the country. In fact, NDMS evacuation operations at Louis Armstrong and elsewhere represented the largest air evacuation in US history.[69] Still, Rosanne Prats noted that even with the Pam exercise and the formation of the TMOSA plan, the state had been given little more than "an introductory discussion" on how it could utilize NDMS. Nor had Pam prompted an extended discussion regarding how the

65. US Department of Health and Human Services, "National Disaster Medical System," http://www.phe.gov/Preparedness/responders/ndms/Pages/default.aspx.

66. Niederman, "The National Disaster Medical System"; Senate Report, 411; US House of Representatives Committee, *The Decline of the National Disaster Medical System*.

67. Telephone interview with Drs. Jimmy Guidry and Rosanne Prats, May 2009. Unless noted, all subsequent quotations from and attributions to Guidry and Prats are from this interview and a follow-up interview in September 2009.

68. FEMA, "Hurricane Pam Exercise Concludes," July 23, 2004, https://www.fema.gov/news-release/2004/07/23/hurricane-pam-exercise-concludes; Rosanne Prats, personal communication, September 9, 2009.

69. Sanford et al., "Medical Treatment at Louis Armstrong."

state could use NDMS to facilitate a hospital evacuation *in advance* of a storm. Because it was the first time the system had been utilized in such a manner, Louisiana public health officials said they faced a steep learning curve in understanding how it operated. As Coletta Barrett, Vice President of Resource Development and Member Services for the Louisiana Hospital Association observed, "A lesson learned was that we really do need to have a better understanding of how the federal system works." According to Barrett, Louisiana health officials were particularly frustrated by their inability to monitor the whereabouts of the thousands of people evacuated via NDMS. "When patients were taken into the NDMS system and flown out of our state, we had no idea where they went," she said.[70]

ON TO THE HOST STATES

With tens of thousands of rescued New Orleanians requiring shelter in the immediate aftermath of Katrina, public officials were forced to look beyond Louisiana's borders. As General Russel Honoré, the commander of Joint Task Force Katrina, declared, "Baton Rouge is full. Shreveport is full. Jackson, Mississippi, is full. There's no more capacity in the state."[71] Although Katrina evacuees eventually ended up in communities throughout the United States, large numbers found themselves in neighboring Arkansas and Texas. Evacuating to both states made sense for several reasons. For one thing, their geographic proximity to Louisiana meant that an evacuation to either state would take less time than to almost anywhere else in the country. Additionally, because Arkansas was completely landlocked and Texas had a large interior, they could shelter evacuees safely away from the most extreme effects of a storm. Dr. William Mason, head of emergency preparedness and response for the Arkansas Department of Health, described his state's sheltering role bluntly: "Basically, Arkansas is like an empty ward in a hospital.... We're kind of the surge state for Louisiana and the rest."[72]

The first wave of evacuees to arrive in both Arkansas and Texas consisted of those who had the ability and means to leave Louisiana in the days leading up to Katrina. Some of these prestorm evacuees had relatives with whom they could stay, while others were willing to pay to stay in hotels and motels. The second wave was an altogether different matter. These were the people who evacuated post-storm. First rescued from their homes, the city's streets, hospitals, and nursing homes, they were then dropped off at lily pads, the Superdome, and the Convention Center. Some were also diverted to

---

70. Public Health Grand Rounds, "Learning From Katrina: Tough Lessons in Preparedness and Emergency Response," March 31, 2006.
71. Senate Report, 366.
72. Telephone interview with Dr. William Mason, April 2009. Unless noted, all subsequent quotations from and attributions to Mason are from this interview.

triage points such as the one set up at Louis Armstrong. Ahead of them lay yet more travel, as they boarded buses and planes for transport to safe shelter in host states like Arkansas and Texas. Mason commented on their exhausting and oftentimes disorienting odysseys:

> The people were traveling a long time.... When they got off the bus, sometimes it would be in the middle of the night. And they would come out from New Orleans or wherever they were evacuating [from], and then they would wake up or get out in the morning in the middle of the Ozarks. No idea where they were. Some thought they were in Arizona. They did not know where they were.

For their part, authorities in the host states usually knew next to nothing about the evacuees showing up at their doorstep. The chaos in New Orleans had led to the breakdown of registration systems, and the ad hoc efforts to provide special needs individuals and hospital patients with identification and medical records proved insufficient. Nor did the host states receive much information from public officials in Louisiana or the federal government regarding the evacuees' identities or their medical histories. "We had no idea [about] the medical condition of those people that were coming in," Dr. Paul Halverson, Director of the Arkansas Department of Health, said. "They might have been in a hospital, they might have been in a nursing home.... We just didn't know where they were coming from or what their condition was.... It was a real hodge-podge."[73]

Dr. David Lakey, subsequently Commissioner of the Texas Department of State Health Services, faced a similar experience while working with shelters in and around Tyler, a city of just under 90,000 in east Texas. Echoing Halverson, he said:

> We had no idea what was going to arrive on those buses.... You'd have folks that would step off the bus and were in obvious distress and had to get immediate attention. And then you had a lot of people that had some injuries that we could handle there in the shelters, but we didn't know what was coming on those buses.[74]

Communication from Louisiana was sporadic at best, according to Halverson and Mason; authorities there were simply too overwhelmed dealing with the crisis immediately at hand to be of much help in addressing the initial confusion in the host states.

In an effort to bring some order to the daunting task of receiving the thousands of evacuees pouring into Arkansas (in total, the state processed more than 30,000 individuals),[75] authorities there set up a massive reception and sheltering operation at Fort Chaffee, a former US military base and now a training facility for the Arkansas National

---

73. Telephone interview with Dr. Paul Halverson, April 2009. Unless noted, all subsequent quotations from and attributions to Halverson are from this interview.
74. Telephone interview with Dr. David Lakey, April 2009. Unless noted, all subsequent quotations from and attributions to Lakey are from this interview.
75. Association of State and Territorial Health Officials, *Arkansas' Response to the Hurricanes of 2005.*

Guard in the western part of the state.[76] Health officials and volunteers, led by Dr. Bryan Clardy of the just-formed Western Arkansas River Valley Medical Reserve Corps, triaged and treated incoming evacuees. [77] Those with serious medical conditions were sent on to area hospitals, while healthier individuals were either sheltered on-site or transferred to dozens of church camps throughout the state.[78] When all was said and done, approximately 12,000 people passed through Chaffee, roughly three times as many evacuees as Arkansas had been prepared to handle at the base.[79] Clardy summed up the scale of the operation at Chaffee, saying simply, "Katrina happened, and we kind of had to speed it up.... It was a big, huge effort."[80]

The number of people taking shelter in Texas, however, dwarfed that in Arkansas, with approximately 137,000 evacuees from New Orleans alone ending up in the state.[81] Although Texas had no central processing site like Arkansas's Fort Chaffee, cities such as Houston and Austin served as major hubs; a number of smaller communities also took in evacuees.[82] The pace of arrivals was intense across the board. According to one account, so many evacuees were arriving in Houston, that by the evening of Thursday, September 1, buses were "wrapped around Reliance Center [sic] ... scores of buses, forty or fifty at a time."[83] Soon, the complex, which includes the Astrodome, was home to some 27,000 evacuees—enough people to warrant it having its very own zip code.[84] As evacuees continued to show up, authorities there were eventually forced to turn additional buses away.[85] Many of these buses, said Halverson and Mason, ended up driving on into Arkansas—very much to the state's surprise.

For the evacuees staying on in Houston, the accommodations were a dramatic improvement over what they had left behind. As one evacuee, a pregnant mother who had waded through the flooded streets of New Orleans and then stayed for four days at the Superdome, said of the Reliant Center, "It was good. Air—fresh, clean air—food,

---

76. Chaffee had sheltered large groups of displaced persons several times in the past, including Vietnamese and Cuban refugees. See: Steven Strode, Bryan Clardy, and Aubrey Hough, "AHECs, Medical Reserve Corps, and Coping With Disasters: AHEC Fort Smith Response to Hurricanes Katrina and Rita," *The National AHEC Bulletin* 22 (2006): 36–38.
77. The Medical Reserve Corps, founded in the aftermath of 9/11, is sponsored by the US Office of the Surgeon General. Corps members include volunteer physicians and nurses, as well veterinarians and other medical and public health professionals. The Arkansas Medical Reserve Corps was formed less than a month prior to Katrina making landfall. See: Carolyne Park, "Reservists Critical to Medical Network," *Arkansas Democrat-Gazette*, January 28, 2008; Strode et al., "AHECs, Medical Reserve Crops, and Coping With Disasters."
78. Strode et al., "AHECs, Medical Reserve Corps, and Coping With Disasters."
79. AmyJo Brown, "Lessons of Katrina a Help With Gustav; State Plans for Evacuees Seen as Success," *Arkansas Democrat-Gazette*, September 7, 2008; Park, "Reservists Critical to Medical Network."
80. Park, "Reservists Critical to Medical Network."
81. Horne, *Breach of Faith*, 183.
82. Ibid., 190–191.
83. Ibid., 187.
84. Thomas Gavagan et al., "Hurricane Katrina: Medical Response at the Houston Astrodome/Reliant Center Complex," *Southern Medical Journal* 99 (2006): 933–939; US Department of Transportation, *Catastrophic Hurricane Evacuation Plan Evaluation: A Report to Congress*, 2006, http://www.fhwa.dot.gov/reports/hurricanevacuation/rtc_chep_eval.pdf.
85. Horne, *Breach of Faith*, 188.

water."[86] Such basic amenities made a world of difference for thousands like her. Many had arrived badly dehydrated, delirious, and physically and mentally distressed, and for the first time since Katrina, they were also able to access a medical clinic, which local public health authorities had established at the center. More than 11,000 patients were treated at Reliant's "Katrina Clinic" in the two weeks immediately following Katrina.[87]

For its part, Austin took in an additional 4,000 Katrina evacuees, most arriving by air from New Orleans's Louis Armstrong Airport.[88] Dr. Adolfo Valadez, subsequently Assistant Commissioner for Prevention and Preparedness Services at the Texas Department of State Health Services, was medical director for the Austin/Travis County Health and Human Services Department at the time. Like Houston, he said, the city experienced an intense surge of evacuee arrivals. "[They] were just airlifted out at the last minute," he observed, "and it was kind of like a plane was landing at our airport every 15 minutes for 36 hours."[89] From the airport, evacuees were brought to a central shelter established by the city and the American Red Cross at the Austin Convention Center. There, as in Houston, a medical clinic provided essential care to the evacuees, nearly half of whom arrived showing signs of acute illnesses.[90]

Incomplete Records, Desperate Searches

Frustrated by the lack of information they had initially received about arriving Katrina evacuees, authorities in Arkansas and Texas did their best to keep tabs on the individuals they hosted and the medical care provided to them. In Arkansas, said Halverson and Mason, charts and lists were maintained by the staff and volunteers at Chaffee, the hospitals, and the church camps sheltering evacuees, but the state did not collect and integrate that information into a comprehensive tracking system. A similar scenario played out in Texas, where shelters also attempted to keep lists of the evacuees they took in. But the practice was not uniform. For instance, while authorities at the Reliant Center registered individuals receiving medical care at the Katrina Clinic, there was no system in place for the shelter at large. The absence of such a system had significant consequences, with one review concluding that it "caused difficulties in measuring the population and its demographics and ensuring that patients received the services they required."

---

86. Michael Perry et al., *Voices of the Storm: Health Experiences of Low-Income Katrina Survivors* (Menlo Park, CA: Henry J. Kaiser Family Foundation, 2006), 32.

87. Gavagan et al., "Hurricane Katrina: Medical Response at the Houston Astrodome."

88. Joshua Vest and Adolfo Valadez, "Health Conditions and Risk Factors of Sheltered Persons Displaced by Hurricane Katrina," *Prehospital and Disaster Medicine* 21 (2006): 55–58.

89. Telephone interview with Dr. Adolfo Valadez, May 2009. Unless noted, all subsequent quotations from and attributions to Valadez are from this interview.

90. Vest and Valadez, "Health Conditions and Risk Factors."

Moreover, the review continued, "the lack of identification also made it difficult to reunite families with relatives."[91] As in Arkansas, Texas had no state-wide system in place to aggregate data collected at individual shelters.[92]

Despite the best efforts of some shelters in Arkansas and Texas—as well as of the workers in places like Charity and University Hospitals and at the Superdome—thousands of evacuees, many with serious medical conditions, went missing during the massive upheaval following Katrina. Where tracking systems did exist, they were primarily paper-based and proved largely inadequate for keeping tabs on the rapidly swelling diaspora of Katrina evacuees.[93] And even as the public's attention slowly moved on from the disaster, some families continued to grapple with the most personal and trying of challenges for weeks on end, calling multiple state and federal agencies and nonprofit organizations in an increasingly frustrating search for lost relatives and loved ones. [94]

THEN CAME RITA

And still, yet another mass relocation of residents along the Gulf Coast was to take place just a few weeks later, further complicating efforts to shelter, care for, and locate those displaced by Katrina. By mid-September, Hurricane Rita, a powerful storm churning across the Gulf, was on target to make a direct landfall on the Houston–Galveston region. Although Texas had taken the task of sheltering Katrina evacuees in stride, it was now suddenly desperate to move them, along with millions of its own residents.[95]

Throughout the week of September 18, political leaders and public safety officials encouraged residents across eastern Texas to evacuate the region. With the trauma of Katrina fresh in their minds, they were determined to get as many citizens out of the storm's path as possible. Speaking in the starkest terms, Governor Rick Perry declared to the public at large, "Homes can be rebuilt, lives cannot. If you're on the coast between Beaumont and Corpus Christi, now's the time to leave."[96] And as he issued evacuation

---

91. Gavagan et al., "Hurricane Katrina: Medical Response at the Houston Astrodome."

92. Lakey, personal communication, April 22, 2009.

93. Barbara Pate, "Identifying and Tracking Disaster Victims," *Family and Community Health* 31 (2008): 23–34.

94. The US Senate found that more than 13,500 adults were reported missing to the National Center for Missing Adults following Katrina; another 5,000-plus children were reported missing to the National Center for Missing and Exploited Children (Senate Report, 366). According to congressional testimony, state and federal governments were inundated with calls from people searching for these missing individuals. The state of Mississippi alone handled more than 10,000 such calls (US Department of Transportation, *Catastrophic Hurricane Evacuation Plan Evaluation.*).

95. For a more extensive discussion of the Hurricane Rita evacuation in Texas, see: David W. Giles, *Gridlock in Texas (A): Evacuating the Houston Galveston Region in Advance of Hurricane Rita,* Program on Crisis Leadership, Harvard Kennedy School (2017).

96. Ceci Connolly and Sylvia Moreno, "Texas Coast Braces for Rita; 1.1 Million Ordered to Evacuate Homes," *Washington Post,* September 22, 2005, A1.

orders for low-lying parts of his city on Wednesday, September 21, Houston Mayor Bill White warned ominously, "Don't follow the example of New Orleans."[97] At the same time, the state engineered a massive airlift of special needs individuals out of coastal areas, moving some 9,000 people from the cities of Houston and Beaumont on Thursday, September 22, alone. State Emergency Management Coordinator Jack Colley emphasized the importance of getting these residents, in particular, to safety. "Whatever we have to do, do not turn anyone back," he instructed state workers.[98]

But the evacuation quickly spiraled out of control. Instead of the 1.25 million people authorities had expected to take to the roads, at least double that number fled, including many individuals who lived well beyond the danger zone.[99] As a result, traffic stalled along evacuation routes, causing massive and prolonged gridlock. Unable to endure the oppressive heat, dozens of people died along the way, including fragile nursing home residents and medical patients. Frustrated by the traffic jams, a large number of evacuees chose to turn around and take their chances waiting out the storm in their homes. Those who continued the journey arrived at shelters already filled to capacity.[100]

Processing and Sheltering Special Needs Evacuees

In Tyler, Texas, Dr. David Lakey and his colleagues shifted gears, as the state designated a community gymnasium as a medical special needs shelter in support of the Rita evacuation.[101] Most of those who arrived came from East Texas nursing homes where evacuation plans had failed.[102] (When Rita did eventually make landfall near Sabine Pass, Texas,

---

97. Ralph Blumenthal and David Barstow, "'Katrina Effect' Pushed Texans Into Gridlock," *New York Times*, September 24, 2005, A1.

98. Chuck Lindell and Tony Plohetski, "Forecast: Disaster; Road Weary; Thousands Hurry Up and Wait in Flight From Coast; Widespread Devastation; Storm Won't Spare Inland Areas, Forecasters Say; No Way Out?; Some Still Stuck in Houston With Few Options," *Austin American-Statesman*, September 23, 2005, A1.

99. Blumenthal and Barstow, "'Katrina Effect' Pushed Texans Into Gridlock."

100. Patrick Driscoll, "The Good, the Bad and the Ugly of Rita," *San Antonio Express-News*, October 4, 2005, A1; Mike Ward, "Gustav Could Give Texas' New Evacuation Plan First Real Test," *Austin American-Statesman*, August 30, 2008, A17.

101. In Texas, medical special needs shelters are intended to accommodate "persons who need assistance with medical care administration," including those who require monitoring by a nurse or assistance with medications, who are dependent on equipment, or who have mental health disorders. See: City of Austin, Travis County, and Williamson County Offices of Emergency Management, *Capital Area Shelter Hub Plan*, 2006.

102. A review by the *Houston Chronicle* revealed that there had been extraordinarily lax oversight of nursing home disaster planning in advance of Rita throughout the state of Texas. This was largely due to the fact that the Texas Department of Aging and Disability Services, which regulates nursing homes across the state, lacked the authority to adequately enforce compliance with emergency planning procedures. Consequently, dozens of nursing homes in the greater Houston area and elsewhere were ill-prepared to facilitate the evacuation of residents in the lead up to Rita, and many elderly residents were simply absorbed into the excruciatingly slow general evacuation that slogged along through the brutally hot and humid conditions See: Roma Khanna, "Nursing Home Evacuation Plans Largely Unimproved; Despite Rita's Chaos, Dozens of Facilities Are Still Relying on Flimsy Arrangements," *Houston Chronicle*, September 17, 2006, A1.

on Saturday, September 24, its impact was primarily limited to this corner of Texas and western Louisiana; the Houston–Galveston region was largely spared.) According to Lakey, many of the 300 individuals who sheltered in Tyler's gymnasium were seriously ill, suffering from, among other things, heart conditions, lung disease, and cancer. Lakey observed, "We were able to get through it and care for those individuals. [But] a lot of times it wasn't pretty." He added, "A lot of times we didn't have the staffing that we needed." Lakey explained that authorities relied on volunteers to staff the shelter and provide medical care, and that many had day jobs to perform as well. A good number had also just participated in the exhausting process of sheltering and caring for Katrina evacuees.

With Rita coming so rapidly on the heels of Katrina, there was little change in how evacuees and their medical needs and care were tracked and recorded, and procedures continued to vary from one shelter to the next. In Austin, authorities managed to put in place an evacuee registration system, while health workers collected information regarding medical needs and conditions.[103] As for Tyler, said Lakey, "We did try to create, on-the-fly, some health records for the folks to send back with them. But, it really wasn't that organized.... [It] was more a record for the patients while they were in the shelter versus a permanent medical record that would be able to go with them in the future." Despite efforts by individual shelters like those in Tyler and Austin, there had simply been no time since Katrina to implement a more comprehensive tracking system.

Once again, thousands more families found themselves separated, and locating evacuated individuals remained a serious challenge.[104] In one extreme instance, more than 1,000 nursing home patients were temporarily lost by authorities when they were airlifted out of Beaumont and Houston in advance of Rita. One of these evacuees, Ouida Richardson, went missing for several days, until her daughter located her in a nursing home in Oklahoma City. Richardson, a 92-year-old Alzheimer's patient, had been unable to provide those evacuating her with her name or any information regarding her caregivers, family, or medical history.[105]

In the ensuing months, authorities in Louisiana and Texas continued to respond to a slew of ongoing issues related to Katrina and Rita. But at the same time, they—along with their partners in neighboring states and in the federal government—also had to begin thinking ahead about how they could improve preparedness in advance of the next hurricane season. The storms of 2005 had served as a tragic reminder that major metropolitan regions along the United States' Gulf Coast were very much vulnerable to

103. Jessie Patton-Levine, Joshua Vest, and Adolfo Valadez, "Caregivers and Families in Medical Special Needs Shelters: An Experience During Hurricane Rita," *American Journal of Disaster Medicine* 2 (2007): 81–86.
104. Lakey, personal communication, April 22, 2009; Motorola, *State of Texas Deploys Special Needs Evacuation Tracking System*, 2007, http://media.govtech.net/Digital_Communities/Motorola/SNETS_RC-99-2161.pdf; Lise Olsen and Roma Khanna, "Hurricane Aftermath: Fleeing the Storms Was Just the Start of Troubles for the Elderly, as Many Are Isolated From Their Families and Have No Home Left," *Houston Chronicle*, November 28, 2005, A1.
105. Lise Olsen and Roma Khanna, "Hurricane Aftermath."

large-scale and potentially catastrophic hurricanes, and it was now abundantly clear that the plans put in place prior to 2005 were woefully inadequate.

Developing measures to effectively relocate individuals with special needs was a particularly high priority, given the glaring inability of government at all levels to safeguard this population during both Katrina and Rita. To this end, authorities had their work cut out for them. Among other things, appropriate and secure shelters would have to be established and maintained; transportation assets would have to be identified in advance; coordination and communication among all partners in the evacuation process would have to be drastically improved; and systems would have to be designed to easily identify, keep track of, and locate the thousands of people moving with government assistance across multiple jurisdictions. Nobody knew if another Katrina or Rita would strike again anytime soon. But it was clear to everyone that public authorities could—and certainly needed to—do better.

Exhibit 16A-1. Chronology of Events: Hurricane Katrina and Rita Evacuations, August–September 2005

Saturday, August 27

- With Hurricane Katrina approaching, Louisiana Governor Kathleen Babineaux Blanco and New Orleans Mayor Ray Nagin held a midday news conference. Mayor Nagin issued a voluntary evacuation order for New Orleans.
- Louisiana's southern low-lying parishes began evacuating, followed by those in the greater New Orleans area. Evacuation traffic flowed relatively smoothly.

Sunday, August 28

- Mayor Nagin issued a mandatory evacuation order, less than a day before Katrina was projected to make landfall.
- Special needs individuals and others remaining in New Orleans began arriving at the Louisiana Superdome, the city's "shelter of last resort."
- New Orleans hospitals and many nursing homes prepared to shelter in place instead of evacuating their patients and residents in advance of the storm.

Monday, August 29

- Katrina made landfall at around 6 a.m., initially sparing the city the very worst, but still battering the Superdome and causing damage to hospitals and nursing homes housing patients and residents.
- Breaches appeared in levees protecting New Orleans, unleashing floodwaters into the city.
- Stranded residents scrambled to rooftops to escape the rising floodwaters. Others began making their way to the Superdome, the city's Ernest N. Morial Convention Center, and highway overpasses.

Tuesday, August 30

- Residents continued to arrive at the Superdome, Convention Center, and overpasses.
- Surrounded by floodwaters, Charity and University hospitals struggled to provide care to their patients. Despite requesting evacuation assistance, they remained almost completely isolated for several days.

Wednesday, August 31

- Early Wednesday morning, after the federal government activated its National Disaster Medical System (NDMS), Disaster Medical Assistance Teams (DMATs) arrived at the Louis Armstrong New Orleans International Airport to triage, provide medical care, and help evacuate residents rescued from New Orleans.
- Later in the day, Governor Blanco requested that the Department of Defense's Joint Katrina Task Force take control over efforts to evacuate the city.

Thursday, September 1

- The Joint Task Force arranged for the evacuation of the Superdome and highway overpasses. Evacuees began arriving in the Houston area and other host sites outside Louisiana.

Friday, September 2

- The Convention Center was secured.
- Charity and University hospitals were evacuated.

Saturday, September 3

- The Convention Center was evacuated.

Early–mid September

- Shelters across the country took in and cared for Katrina evacuees.
- Families of thousands of Katrina evacuees struggled to locate their loved ones.

Wednesday, September 21

- With Hurricane Rita tracking toward the Houston–Galveston region, Houston Mayor Bill White issued evacuation orders for parts of his city. Millions took to the roadways throughout southeastern Texas, triggering massive gridlock.

Saturday, September 24

- Hurricane Rita made landfall near Sabine Pass, Texas, causing significant damage but sparing the Houston–Galveston area.

Exhibit 16A-2. Cast of Characters: Hurricane Katrina and Rita Evacuations, August–September 2005

State of Arkansas
- Dr. Paul Halverson, Director, Arkansas Department of Health
- Dr. William Mason, Director, Preparedness and Emergency Response, Arkansas Department of Health

State of Louisiana
- Kathleen Babineaux Blanco, Governor
- Dr. Jimmy Guidry, Medical Director, Louisiana Department of Health and Hospitals
- Dr. Rosanne Prats, Director of Emergency Preparedness, Louisiana Department of Health and Hospitals

State of Texas
- Jack Colley, State Emergency Management Coordinator
- Rick Perry, Governor

City of New Orleans, LA
- Ray Nagin, Mayor

City of Austin, TX
- Dr. Adolfo Valadez, Medical Director, Austin/Travis County Health and Human Services Department (and subsequently Assistant Commissioner, Prevention and Preparedness Services, Texas Department of State Health Services)

City of Houston, TX
- Bill White, Mayor

City of Tyler, TX
- Dr. David Lakey, Associate Professor of Medicine, University of Texas Health Center, Tyler, and a lead physician for the Tyler area's medical response to Katrina and Rita (and subsequently, Commissioner, Texas Department of State Health Services)

Western Arkansas River Valley Medical Reserve Corps
- Dr. Bryan Clardy, Unit Commander

Moving People Out of Danger: Special Needs Evacuations From Gulf Coast Hurricanes

David W. Giles

In the aftermath of Hurricanes Katrina and Rita, which wreaked havoc along the United States' Gulf Coast in 2005, review after review condemned the emergency responses to the two storms, including the mismanagement of the evacuation of two of the region's largest metropolitan areas: New Orleans and Houston.[1] In particular, the reviews heavily criticized the woefully inadequate safeguarding of individuals with medical and other special needs, who generally require extra attention throughout the evacuation and sheltering process.[2] Consequently, over the next several years, localities and states along the coast spent considerable time and effort overhauling their response plans and building systems that, they hoped, would allow them to more effectively carry out future mass evacuations and ensure the safe movement of their most vulnerable residents.

This case was written by David W. Giles, Assistant Director, Program on Crisis Leadership, for Dr. Arnold M. Howitt, Executive Director of the Ash Center for Democratic Governance and Innovation at the Harvard University John F. Kennedy School of Government. Funds for case development were provided by the Robert Wood Johnson Foundation as part of its State Health Leadership Initiative. Additional funding was provided by the US Department of Transportation through the New England University Transportation Center. HKS cases are developed solely as the basis for class discussion. Cases are not intended to serve as endorsements, sources of primary data, or illustrations of effective or ineffective management.

1. See, for example, reports by the US House of Representatives (*A Failure of Initiative*) and the US Senate (*Hurricane Katrina: A Nation Still Unprepared*), which catalogue a litany of shortcomings and failures at all levels of government.
2. "Special needs" is a broad term, but in the context of evacuation planning, it essentially refers to any individual or group that requires assistance to relocate out of harm's way. This includes, among others, people with disabilities and medical conditions, the elderly, the institutionalized, the homebound, and people without access to cars or other means of transportation. For a detailed exploration of the challenges of evacuating special needs individuals during Katrina and Rita, see Case 16A.

This included identifying ways to keep track of and locate special needs evacuees, so that unlike in 2005, they would not become "lost" to their loved ones and primary caregivers for weeks on end; acquiring sufficient and appropriate transportation assets for carrying these residents out of the danger zone in a timely manner; and ensuring effective communication with partners at all levels of government and in the private sector.

The opportunity to demonstrate that the region's evacuation preparedness had indeed improved came during a particularly intense 2008 hurricane season that saw 16 named storms, including five hurricanes of Category 3 strength or greater.[3] In an eerie echo of 2005, two of these storms, Hurricanes Gustav and Ike, threatened to make direct hits on New Orleans and the Houston–Galveston area, respectively. Once again, millions of individuals would have to relocate, including tens of thousands of medical and special needs individuals who required varying forms of government assistance to do so. But this time around, there were significant differences in how the evacuations were carried out, as states and localities put their new plans into action.

For a chronology of events and a cast of characters, see Exhibits 16B-1 and 16B-2.

EVACUATION PLANS REVISITED

Determined to avoid their ultimate nightmare—a repeat of the 2005 evacuations—authorities in Louisiana and Texas responded quickly to the impending threats posed by Gustav and Ike. In the days leading up to the storms' expected landfalls, they raced to implement their revamped evacuation plans, predeploying resources, relocating special needs populations to inland shelters and hospitals, and launching systems they had spent the past three years designing to keep track of evacuees' whereabouts. But as the hurricanes edged ever closer to land, a central question remained: Had Louisiana and Texas done enough in the intervening years? Or were these states doomed, yet again, to endure the chaos, confusion, and suffering that had so memorably characterized the last go-around?

Louisiana Seeks to Avoid Another Katrina

In designing its post-Katrina evacuation plans, Louisiana placed particular emphasis on utilizing public transportation assets to move special needs populations, including individuals lacking access to cars, as well as those with medical conditions requiring specialized evacuation and sheltering assistance.[4] New Orleans's City Assisted Evacuation Plan, for instance, called for residents who could not evacuate via their own means to gather at

---

3. Michael Kunzelman, "Storm Planners Reflect on Busy Hurricane Season," *Associated Press,* November 29, 2008.
4. Cain Burdeau, "La. Grapples With Fresh Pot of Hurricane Logistics," *Associated Press State & Local Wire,* November 24, 2008; US Department of Transportation, *Catastrophic Hurricane Evacuation Plan Evaluation: Report to Congress,* 2006, http://www.fhwa.dot.gov/reports/hurricanevacuation/rtc_chep_eval.pdf.

17 pick-up sites, where Regional Transit Authority buses would collect and then deliver them to the city's main train station, Union Passenger Terminal. There, they would be processed for evacuation out of the city by bus or Amtrak train. Residents who were unable to get themselves to collection points were encouraged to contact a 3-1-1 call center to register for pick-up at home.[5] New Orleans's new plan also eliminated "shelters of last resort"—that is, places people remaining in the city could report to at the last minute. Neither the Superdome nor the Convention Center, both of which had been the scene of so much chaos and despair during Katrina, would be open to shelter residents in the event of another major storm.[6]

Meanwhile, determined to overcome the state's frustrating inability to track and locate evacuees during Katrina, the Louisiana Department of Social Services (DSS) procured the software for [EWA]Phoenix crisis management tools—a Web-based system that would allow DSS and its partners to electronically register and monitor the location of Louisiana residents evacuating with state assistance.[7] Operating Phoenix seemed straightforward. State and parish workers would register individuals as they arrived at collection points, entering into an electronic database the name of and contact information for each evacuee. During registration, evacuees would receive barcode wristbands, which would allow the state to track evacuees individually over the course of their journey. (Accompanying pets would be tagged and tracked through Phoenix as well.) Manifests would be generated for each vehicle transporting evacuees, and the evacuees' arrival at in-state shelters would also be recorded. Finally, when it came time to transport evacuees back to their homes, officials could electronically sort shelter lists and swiftly group returning evacuees by zip code.[8]

Louisiana's Department of Health and Hospitals (DHH) also worked hard in the aftermath of Katrina to improve evacuation processes for individuals with special needs, focusing largely on critical care hospital patients. In 2005, when multiple levees breached in the aftermath of Katrina, hundreds of individuals had been stranded in hospitals besieged by floodwaters and operating without electricity. Because it was impossible to provide basic medical care in these conditions, the patients had to be evacuated post-storm through the disaster zone. The process took days to organize and proved enormously difficult to implement—not to mention extremely taxing for the patients themselves. In an effort to avoid a similar scenario in the future, DHH developed its Medical Institution Evacuation Plan to coordinate logistics and the flow of information among parties likely to be involved in future pre-event medical evacuations,

5. Mark Schleifstein and Michelle Krupa, "Gustav Has State on Alert; Evacuations Could Start Early as Friday," *Times-Picayune,* August 27, 2008, 1; The US Conference of Mayors, "New Orleans Mayor Nagin Develops Pioneering Evacuation Plan," *U.S. Mayor Newspaper,* September 15, 2008.
6. Rick Jervis and Donna Leinwand, "New Orleans on Top of Gustav to Avoid 2005 Repeat; Hurricane Plans Were Set in Motion Earlier in Week to Ensure Response," *USA Today,* August 29, 2008, 5A.
7. State of Louisiana Department of Social Services, "DSS Offers First Look at Hurricane Evacuee-Tracking System," May 30, 2008.
8. Ibid.; State of Louisiana Governor's Office of Homeland Security and Emergency Preparedness, *After-Action Report and Improvement Plan: Hurricanes Gustav and Ike,* 2009.

including the state, evacuating hospitals, and the federal National Disaster Medical System (NDMS), which would airlift patients to affiliated hospitals outside the threatened area.[9] The plan also established timeframes for emptying the hospitals.[10]

Putting together a workable plan was by no means easy. At Congress's behest, DHH originally attempted to work out a system for evacuating all of Louisiana's hospitals in advance of an incoming storm, a hugely expensive and time-consuming process, according to DHH's Director of Emergency Preparedness, Dr. Rosanne Prats, who spearheaded the planning effort:

> You would need 10 days to evacuate everybody in all these institutions. Well you might as well, you know, evacuate them now ... I mean we're trying to put this plan in place for a *"maybe"*...[11]

Prats elaborated, explaining that almost the entire US Gulf Coast could be included in the "cone of error" (the area at potential risk) 10 days out from a storm's projected landfall. At that point, she noted, the potential scenarios are still numerous, with a high degree of uncertainty as to exactly when, where, and at what intensity the storm will hit. She continued:

> So it's taken a lot, a lot, of meetings with NDMS partners to get that plan fine-tuned.... You're looking at 48 to 50 hours to get all those planes there, get all the personnel to operate those planes, the backup hospitals to receive those patients, and airports.

According to Prats, the state continued to develop a post-event evacuation plan as well. But because there were so many unknowns as to exactly what would be affected and to what degree, a good part of an after-the-fact evacuation would still have to rely on significant improvisation and on-the-ground reconnaissance work. Extensive flooding could certainly necessitate a full-blown evacuation like that following Katrina, but given how straining evacuations could be for patients and other victims, the delivery of generators and basic supplies could be just as appropriate, depending on the severity of conditions.

Texas Moves Forward From Rita

Meanwhile, in Texas, authorities worked to improve their ability both to receive evacuees from neighboring states and to manage their own internal evacuations. On one hand, Texas's experience during the 2005 hurricane season had highlighted the challenges it

---

9. Based out of the US Department of Health and Human Services, NDMS is a federally coordinated program that provides assistance to states during emergencies. Among other things, it can help states evacuate hospital patients out of a disaster zone. See Case 16A for a more detailed description of NDMS.

10. For more on the Medical Institution Evacuation Plan, see: Louisiana Hospital Association, *Hurricane Information for Hospitals.*

11. Telephone interviews with Dr. Rosanne Prats, May and September 2009. Unless noted, all subsequent quotations from and attributions to Prats are from these interviews.

faced as a host state. (For instance, in the immediate aftermath of Katrina, when it took in hundreds of thousands of individuals from Louisiana, Texas had struggled to identify and keep track of evacuees, while also caring for their needs.) Yet, on the other hand, Hurricane Rita, which followed Katrina by just a few weeks, forced the state to grapple with managing a large-scale evacuation within its own borders. Although Rita had not resulted in an all-out catastrophe on the scale of Katrina, the prestorm evacuation it triggered had been disastrous in itself. In a desperate attempt to flee the storm, more than 2.5 million residents of the Houston–Galveston region had taken to the roads. Fortunately, Rita eventually changed course, making landfall along the more rural Texas–Louisiana border, but not before evacuees endured massive traffic jams in extreme heat and humidity. In the end, more Texans died as a result of the evacuation than from hurricane-related injuries.[12]

Among the many changes implemented by Texas in the intervening years were the creation of a system for ensuring that fuel would be available to evacuating drivers; the establishment of roadway comfort stations that would provide evacuees with food, water, and medical assistance; and the implementation of a staggered evacuation process, which, officials hoped, would bring more order and clarity to who should evacuate when. The state also refined plans for evacuating residents with medical and other special needs, establishing special needs registries and identifying in advance fleets of buses, ambulances, and planes for transporting these individuals from coastal cities to predetermined host communities—or so-called Sister Cities—further inland. (Under this program, evacuees from Galveston, for example, would be sheltered in Austin.)[13]

As in Louisiana, Texas also went to work on establishing an electronic evacuee tracking system in an effort to drastically cut down on the number of special needs individuals who were "lost" to their families and loved ones as they moved out of their communities and reported to shelters across the state.[14] To this end, Texas contracted with AT&T to design the state's Special Needs Evacuation Tracking System (or SNETS, for short).

SNETS was designed to operate in a similar fashion to Louisiana's Phoenix system. As individuals seeking state transportation assistance arrived at local evacuation centers (collection points) throughout coastal Texas, they would be given wristbands equipped with barcodes and Radio Frequency Identification (RFID) technology. Texas National Guardsmen would then scan each wristband and enter information about the evacuee

---

12. Anthony Zachria and Bela Patel, "Deaths Related to Hurricane Rita and Mass Evacuation," *CHEST* 130 (2006): 124S.

13. Mike Ward, "Gustav Could Give Texas' New Evacuation Plan First Real Test," *Austin American-Statesman*, August 30, 2008, A17; Mike Ward, "In Early Assessment, State Earns Praise for Its Hurricane Planning," *Austin American-Statesman*, September 21, 2008, A1; Texas House of Representatives, *Hurricane Ike Devastation, Interim Report*, 2009, http://www.house.state.tx.us/_media/pdf/committees/reports/80interim/Hurricane-Ike-Devestation-to-the-Texas-Gulf-Coast.pdf.

14. Dr. David Lakey, personal communication, April 22, 2009; Motorola, *State of Texas Deploys Special Needs Evacuation Tracking System*, 2007, http://media.govtech.net/Digital_Communities/Motorola/SNETS_RC-99-2161.pdf.

into a corresponding electronic database, including what medical equipment, pets, and relatives accompanied each person. Upon arrival at reception centers (or shelters), evacuees would be rescanned (or would walk collectively through RFID portals) and the central database updated wirelessly. Family members could access their relative's location remotely by contacting the state's 2-1-1 information service hotline.[15]

Texas also put in place several measures to cut back on confusion during transit. Before departing the evacuation centers, bus drivers would be provided with manifests generated from the electronic registration process. Additionally, the state outfitted buses with Global Positioning System (GPS) devices, so that the state emergency operations center could pinpoint their location and redirect them if necessary. According to Dr. David Lakey, Commissioner of the Texas Department of State Health Services (DSHS), this action was taken as part of an effort to reduce the uncertainty surrounding the whereabouts of the many phantom buses that had reportedly traveled across eastern Texas, in desperate search of shelter, in 2005.[16]

The Feds Get Involved

A number of changes were made at the federal level as well. In reaction to the failures and confusion that marred the responses to the 2005 storms, Congress passed the Post-Katrina Emergency Management Reform Act (PKEMRA) of 2006.[17] PKEMRA brought significant organizational changes to the federal emergency management apparatus, particularly to the Federal Emergency Management Agency (FEMA) and its parent organization, the US Department of Homeland Security. It also better clarified the federal government's role in regard to mass evacuations. Although some have argued that the Stafford Act and the Homeland Security Act of 2002 had provided for a federal role in carrying out evacuations at the time of Katrina and Rita, federal officials had generally deferred to local and state authorities when it came to managing evacuations.[18] PKEMRA, along with the issuance of the National Response Framework in early 2008, significantly expanded the federal government's role in evacuation planning and implementation,

15. John Burnell, "Texas Turns to RFID for Emergency Evacuation System," *RFID Update,* January 3, 2008; Motorola, *State of Texas Deploys Special Needs Evacuation Tracking System.*

16. Telephone interview with Dr. David Lakey, April 2009. Unless noted, all subsequent quotations from and attributions to Lakey are from this interview.

17. For more on PKEMRA, see: US Government Accountability Office (GAO), *Actions Taken to Implement the Post-Katrina Emergency Management Reform Act of 2006,* GAO-09-59R (Washington, DC: GAO, 2008), http://www.gao.gov/new.items/d0959r.pdf; Title VI of the Department of Homeland Security Appropriations Act, Public Law 109-295, 120 Stat. 1355 (2006), http://www.gpo.gov/fdsys/pkg/PLAW-109publ295/pdf/PLAW-109publ295.pdf.

18. US Senate, Committee on Homeland Security and Governmental Affairs, *Hurricane Katrina: A Nation Still Unprepared* (Washington, DC: GPO, 2006), 258–260.

especially in regards to catastrophic events (such as Katrina), when local and state governments would likely be overwhelmed.[19]

Following the passage of PKEMRA, FEMA also began exploring ways to improve evacuee tracking and locating capabilities. But unlike Louisiana and Texas's self-contained efforts, the agency sought to design a system that could be used more broadly on the national level, recognizing that during Katrina, evacuees had traveled through multiple states multiple times before reaching long-term shelter. (According to one analysis, families displaced by Katrina moved an average of 3.5 times—some as many as nine times across state lines.)[20] As it explored its options, FEMA decided to create a set of three tracking systems, known collectively as the National Mass Evacuation Tracking Systems (NMETS). Although each version was to collect the same basic identifying information and to link evacuees to other family members, their pets, luggage, and medical equipment, they varied dramatically in terms of their technological complexity.

Using RFID technology similar to that used in the Texas system, FEMA's advanced evacuation support tool was designed to capture the most data the most quickly. Operators would be able to collect evacuee information in the field via hand-held scanners, which would then wirelessly transmit data back to a central processing site. Participating states could then access the collected information via an electronic database. Designed as an open-source system, the software could also be adapted to meet the specific needs of individual states. For example, although the system was not configured to collect data on medical care provided to evacuees, a state could add additional fields to collect that information as needed.

John Bischoff, of FEMA's Mass Care Unit, noted, however, that because fully automated tracking systems require hand-held scanners and other peripheral equipment, they could be too costly for some states, especially for those with an infrequent need for mass evacuations.[21] With this cost issue in mind, FEMA created two other versions of NMETS. Featuring Microsoft Access software, the low-tech evacuation support tool would allow states to capture information electronically without having to invest large sums of money in equipment. States would still be able to share information with one another, albeit in a more cumbersome manner, by uploading, encrypting, and e-mailing their databases to one another. FEMA also designed a paper-based system, which, according to Bischoff, made sense for several reasons. "Electronic systems may fail due to power outages, connectivity problems, or equipment or staff shortages," he explained. "If a system goes down, it's crucial to have a fallback solution."

---

19. Unlike its predecessor, the National Response Plan, the Framework featured an annex specific to mass evacuations (http://www.fema.gov/pdf/emergency/nrf/nrf_massevacuationincidentannex.pdf).

20. Barbara L. Pate, "Identifying and Tracking Disaster Victims," *Family and Community Health* 31 (2008): 23–34.

21. Telephone interview with John Bischoff, May 2009. Unless noted, all subsequent quotations from and attributions to Bischoff are from this interview.

EVACUATING FROM GUSTAV: KATRINA REDUX?

As it turned out, FEMA would not be ready to deploy NMETS during the 2008 hurricane season. But when Hurricane Gustav and then Hurricane Ike threatened two of the Gulf Coast's largest metropolitan areas in late summer that year, the ability to move special needs populations effectively and track and locate their whereabouts became paramount. Consequently, as Gustav moved ever closer to New Orleans and Ike to the Houston–Galveston region a few weeks later, all eyes turned to Louisiana and Texas in the hopes that their revamped evacuation plans and newly designed tracking systems would prove effective. (See Exhibits 16B-3 and 16B-4 for maps depicting the tracks of Hurricanes Gustav and Ike.)

The Gustav Evacuation Ramps Up

When Hurricane Gustav made landfall the morning of Monday, September 1, as a Category 2 storm in Cocodrie, Terrebonne Parish, Louisiana—about 90 miles southwest of New Orleans—its 110 mph winds, along with torrential rain and flooding, caused extensive damage throughout the state.[22] But even with Gustav resulting in 48 deaths and about $2 billion in insured losses in Louisiana, the storm's toll paled in comparison with that of Hurricane Katrina, which took the lives of approximately 1,000 Louisiana residents and resulted in tens of billions of dollars worth of property damage.[23] Moreover, this time around, New Orleans emerged largely unscathed, escaping the massive flooding that overtook the city in 2005. All the same, in the lead up to the storm's arrival, forecasters, the media, and public leaders warned of an altogether different scenario.

As Gustav moved across the Gulf the week of August 24, meteorologists predicted that it could very well reach Category 5 strength and decimate coastal Louisiana with storm surges of up to 20 feet.[24] Moreover, they cautioned, ever-vulnerable New Orleans lay within the storm's "cone of error," meaning that there was a chance that Gustav could make a direct hit on the city.[25] With warnings about Gustav intensifying throughout the week, Louisiana Governor Bobby Jindal issued a statewide Declaration of Emergency on Wednesday, August 27, telling residents, "Be ready ... this is a serious storm."[26] Three days

---

22. State of Louisiana Governor's Office of Homeland Security and Emergency Preparedness, *After-Action Report*.

23. John Beven and Todd Kimberlain, *Tropical Cyclone Report: Hurricane Gustav,* January 22, 2009, http://www.nhc.noaa.gov/data/tcr/AL072008_Gustav.pdf; Richard D. Knabb, Jamie R. Rhome, and Daniel P. Brown, *Tropical Cyclone Report: Hurricane Katrina,* December 20, 2005, http://www.nhc.noaa.gov/data/tcr/AL122005_Katrina.pdf.

24. Adam Nossiter and Shaila Dewan, "Mayor Orders the Evacuation of New Orleans," *New York Times,* August 31, 2008, A1; State of Louisiana Governor's Office of Homeland Security and Emergency Preparedness, *After-Action Report*.

25. Schleifstein and Krupa, "Gustav Has State on Alert."

26. Ibid.

later, when announcing a mandatory evacuation order for New Orleans, Mayor Ray Nagin used far more dramatic language. "Ladies and gentlemen, I must tell you—this is the mother of all storms," he said. "This could be the most horrific thing that happened in this country," the mayor continued, dubbing Gustav the "storm of the century."[27] Making clear that those who stayed behind did so at their own peril, Nagin also noted that they would have no access to emergency services in the immediate aftermath of the storm.[28] Jindal's and Nagin's warnings proved more than effective. Taking part in the most extensive evacuation in Louisiana history, almost 2 million people moved away from the state's coastline in advance of Gustav—far more than the number that had taken to the roads prior to Katrina three years earlier.[29]

By the time Nagin's order went into effect at 8 a.m., Sunday, August 31, the evacuation of New Orleans was actually well under way. Hundreds of thousands of New Orleans-area residents had left the city via their own means. And by Saturday, individuals requiring transportation assistance had begun showing up at Union Passenger Terminal. From there, some 30,000 people were placed on Amtrak trains bound for Memphis, Tennessee, and on buses and planes that then transported them to shelters in northern Louisiana and beyond.[30] In contrast to 2005, when approximately 25,000 people waited out Katrina in the Superdome and thousands more struggled against the floodwaters in their homes or in hospitals and nursing homes, just 10,000 people—or about 3% of the city's population—remained in the city when Gustav made landfall.[31] As Brad Harris, FEMA's Deputy Federal Coordinating Officer for Louisiana during Gustav, observed, "New Orleans was pretty much a ghost town by the time the storm hit." Harris gave much of the credit to Nagin's forceful words, saying, "Despite what everybody might think [Nagin] did a tremendous job in helping that city evacuate; he scared those people to death, is basically what he did, and that really helped to get people out of there."[32]

The plans for evacuating transportation-disadvantaged residents were almost derailed, however, when Landstar System, a transportation logistics company that had contracted with the state to provide 700 buses, failed to deliver more than half of the pledged vehicles.[33] "We had to scramble," Mark Cooper, Director of the Governor's Office of Homeland Security and Emergency Preparedness admitted afterward.[34] With Gustav edging ever

27. Allen M. Johnson, "Nagin Orders Mandatory Evacuations," *The Advocate,* August 31, 2008, A4.

28. Kunzelman, "Storm Planners Reflect."

29. Rick Jervis, Marisol Bello, and Andrea Stone, "New Storm, New Lessons; Fear of Another Katrina Heightened Sense of Urgency," *USA Today,* September 2, 2008, 1A; State of Louisiana Governor's Office of Homeland Security and Emergency Preparedness, *After-Action Report.*

30. Johnson, "Nagin Orders Mandatory Evacuations;" Nossiter and Dewan, "Mayor Orders the Evacuation of New Orleans;" Burdeau, "La. Grapples With Fresh Pot of Hurricane Logistics."

31. Jervis et al., "New Storm, New Lessons"; Helen Kennedy, "We're Ready for You, Gustav," *Daily News,* September 1, 2008, 3.

32. Telephone interview with Brad Harris, May 2009. Unless noted, all subsequent quotations from and attributions to Harris are from this interview.

33. Burdeau, "La. Grapples With Fresh Pot of Hurricane Logistics."

34. Jervis et al., "New Storm, New Lessons."

closer, the state successfully improvised, filling the gap by procuring school buses and assigning National Guardsmen to drive them.[35]

(Re)turning to the National Disaster Medical System

Gustav represented the first opportunity to see whether the DHH's newly drafted Medical Institution Evacuation Plan would lead to improvements in the prestorm relocation of hospital patients. In terms of the number of individuals evacuated, the operation was certainly impressive. Beginning Saturday, August 30, ambulances carried all types of patients—from the critically ill to newborn babies—to airports in southern Louisiana, where they were then put on military planes and sent on to NDMS-partner hospitals outside the danger zone.[36] As Governor Jindal proudly noted in Gustav's aftermath, "The evacuation of patients that took place even before the storm made landfall was the largest medical evacuation in our nation's history."[37] In total, roughly 1,000 medical patients were evacuated out of Louisiana hospitals, hundreds of whom were airlifted across state borders.[38]

The operation was not without serious complications, however. Alarmingly, as ambulances poured into New Orleans's Lakefront Airport and other departure points Saturday, they encountered a serious shortage of planes.[39] Dr. Jimmy Guidry, DHH's Medical Director, detailed the frustrating scene at the airport:

> We worked real hard in the past few years to come up with a plan on how to open up an airport to move patients of hospitals by the NDMS system. [But] as we got the patients lined up … and got the patients out to the tarmac ready to get on the plane, the planes weren't showing up. The Department of Defense for some reason hadn't had the communication, didn't get the planes that were necessary. [And] planes started showing up that didn't have the medical equipment to care for these very sick patients, or the critical care team.[40]

---

35. Ibid.; Robert Travis Scott, "Jindal Takes Full Command in Crisis; Governor Pushes Bureaucracy Aside," *Times-Picayune*, September 7, 2008, 1.

36. CNN, "Governor Bobby Jindal Holds Press Conference," *CNN Newsroom*, September 2, 2008, http://transcripts.cnn.com/TRANSCRIPTS/0809/02/cnr.02.html; William L. Mason, "The Incomplete Circle of the National Disaster Medical System: What Arkansas Hospitals Learned From Hurricane Gustav," *Biosecurity and Bioterrorism* 8 (2010): 183–191; David Montgomery and Philip Rucker, "Hospitals Evacuating High-Risk Patients," *Washington Post*, September 1, 2008, A8; Scott, "Jindal Takes Full Command in Crisis."

37. CNN, "Governor Bobby Jindal Holds Press Conference."

38. Ibid.; Laura Maggi, "B.R. Hospital to Send Patients to N.O.; Five Facilities on Back-up Power," *Times-Picayune*, September 3, 2008, 4; Mason, "The Incomplete Circle"; Montgomery and Rucker, "Hospitals Evacuating High-Risk Patients." Another 8,000 or more nursing home residents were successfully moved in the lead up to Gustav throughout southern Louisiana as well. See: Jervis et al., "New Storm, New Lessons"; Marsha Shuler, "Plans Urged for Hospital, Nursing Home Evacuations," *The Advocate*, September 30, 2008, A1.

39. Scott, "Jindal Takes Full Command in Crisis."

40. Office of the Assistant Secretary for Preparedness and Response (ASPR), US Department of Health and Human Services, *Public Health Emergencies: When Nature Rages*, November 18, 2008, http://videocast.nih.gov/Summary.asp?File=14777.

Knowing that flights would likely be grounded within the next 24 hours, Governor Jindal convened a meeting of his emergency command group at 2 a.m. Sunday morning to address the problem. "You could see it in his eye[s]," said Alan Levine, Secretary of DHH. "He didn't want any bureaucracy to get in the way."[41] Jindal tasked Levine with the job of obtaining additional aircraft, and following a flurry of early morning calls, Levine's team eventually managed to acquire enough planes—mainly C-130s from federal partners, other states, and Canada—to relieve the bottleneck at Lakefront. When the governor reviewed the airlift in person later on Sunday, he observed a vastly improved operation. Planes continuously loaded patients (350 people in total) and took off roughly every 30 minutes until 8:30 p.m., when the arrival of tropical storm–force winds grounded flights.[42]

Still, Guidry said, with the evacuation of these critically ill patients having come dangerously close to collapsing, health authorities had faced a particularly challenging quandary: should patients stay at the airport, awaiting airlifts for hours on end; should they be flown out on ill-equipped planes; or should they be sent back to hospitals that could very well experience a direct hit by a major hurricane?[43] None of these options was optimal, and the state was fortunate that the additional air assets finally arrived, bringing the crisis to an end. All the same, several patients died waiting on the tarmac and en route to receiving hospitals. Clearly, communication among NDMS partners still needed considerable work, despite the many hours local, state, and federal authorities had spent hammering out the Medical Institution Evacuation Plan.[44]

In the lead up to Gustav, Louisiana hospitals also continued to grapple with what to do with patients not evacuating through NDMS. Seeking to empty out as many beds as possible, a number of facilities discharged non–critical care patients, many of whom were left to their own devices for finding evacuation assistance.[45] But even with the memory of what institutions like Charity and University hospitals had endured during Katrina still fresh, a good number of hospitals did not evacuate completely. At Tulane Medical Center, for instance, around 500 patients and staff remained as Gustav bore down on the city. Reflecting on the complex challenge of moving hospitalized individuals, with their varying degrees of mobility and oftentimes extensive medical needs, Robert Lynch, the hospital's chief executive, told the *Washington Post*, "It'd be nice to get to zero, but I don't think we will."[46] At least those staying behind were better protected against the storm's potential effects than patients had been in 2005. To avoid the power failures that plagued

41. Scott, "Jindal Takes Full Command in Crisis."
42. Ibid.
43. ASPR, *Public Health Emergencies.*
44. Following Gustav, Rosanne Prats noted that DHH had begun reviewing why so many more airlifted patients died than those evacuating via ground transport and how, in the future, authorities could better determine which patients could endure the stress and complications of an air evacuation.
45. Montgomery and Rucker, "Hospitals Evacuating High-Risk Patients."
46. Ibid.

hospitals in the aftermath of Katrina, generators had been moved to higher ground and were now protected from floodwaters by newly installed submarine doors.

Tracking Evacuees: A Work in Progress

Although the state had tested its newly designed tracking system in several exercises, it was not until Gustav that it was able to deploy Phoenix on a mass scale. But the state quickly learned that implementing the system was not an easy process. As Dr. Rosanne Prats of DHH said, "You would think it would be such a simple system to put in place, but it becomes very complicated." FEMA's Brad Harris elaborated, "It's not something that is just intuitive, it does require some knowledge, it requires that laptops be ready to go, and it requires some familiarity with the equipment, how to use it."

Phoenix's shortcomings proved to be extensive, and as a result, the state once again encountered problems keeping track of some of its evacuating residents, although nowhere near the levels of 2005.[47] Problems included the lack of backup modes of registration, connectivity issues—especially among wireless systems (hardwire connections proved more durable)—and little redundancy in communications systems. Although these problems flared up in multiple parishes throughout the state, the system's failure was perhaps most vividly illustrated at the Union Passenger Terminal collection point in New Orleans. There, things initially appeared to be proceeding smoothly: evacuees were registered, and manifests for trains, buses, and planes were being generated. But with Gustav swirling ever closer and more and more people congregating at the station, the registration process collapsed. This was due in large part, state officials said, to an inability to handle surge. DHH's Dr. Jimmy Guidry explained, "When there are large volumes of people, like there was, and we didn't have enough registration tables, it became unmanageable, because it couldn't be done quickly enough."[48] Consequently, when city officials saw the backed-up lines, said Brad Harris of FEMA, they panicked and demanded that Phoenix be abandoned in order to expedite the evacuation.

Rosanne Prats articulated the dilemma that confronted officials. Registering evacuees on the front-end—at collection points—she said, "helps you provide answers on the back-end later, as to how many people are on [a bus or train or plane] and [who] the individuals are.... But the time it takes to register individuals can be up to 2 minutes.... So on the front-end, it could take a lot of time but [it helps to] answer questions on the back-end." The drawback, she continued, is that it could take "so much time to collect all that needed information on the front-end, [that] you have a huge stall in trying to get people out quickly." All the same, Brad Harris believed that officials in New Orleans

---

47. State of Louisiana Governor's Office of Homeland Security and Emergency Preparedness, *After-Action Report.*
48. Telephone interview with Dr. Jimmy Guidry, May 2009. Unless noted, all subsequent quotations from and attributions to Guidry are from this interview.

shouldn't have had to shut Phoenix down, asserting that the real problem was that Louisiana's DSS, which managed the system, had simply not prepared sufficiently for game day. "If there had been training and a commitment to the system, it would have worked," he asserted.

Another limitation to Phoenix was that although shelters in states hosting evacuees could now obtain manifests as planes, trains, and buses arrived at their doors, officials in these states, such as Arkansas and Texas, could not directly access the system. That meant that they could not fully monitor evacuee movement, nor could they input data into the database if the status of an evacuee changed. And even within Louisiana itself, Phoenix was not used at all shelters. Dr. Prats observed that the system was far more robust at state-operated facilities than at those run by parishes, many of which, she said, continued to do simple headcounts of evacuees. Dr. Guidry put it even more bluntly, saying, "Tracking for those other shelters at the local level still needs a lot of work."

Tracking Medical Special Needs Evacuees: Multiple Systems

A final complicating factor for effectively tracking evacuees during Gustav was that Louisiana continued to employ different systems for monitoring different populations and for collecting different types of data. DSS used (or, better put, tried to use) Phoenix for registering and tracking evacuees transported to state-run critical transportation needs shelters and medical special needs shelters.[49] But because the system was designed to collect a limited amount of data—the basics for generating manifests, registering evacuees at shelters, and facilitating repatriation—the recording and tracking of medical information was left largely to the state's DHH, according to Dr. Guidry and Dr. Prats. Thus, in a process altogether separate from Phoenix, DHH collected only the data it considered necessary for effectively running a medical special needs shelter: for instance, whether an evacuee required medical equipment, like oxygen tanks or dialysis machines, or had certain mental health conditions. DHH's method for collecting this information, however, was based on a fairly rudimentary paper-based system, as opposed to the electronic program that federal Disaster Medical Assistance Teams were using to good effect in the same shelters.[50]

---

49. Shelters run by the State of Louisiana included critical transportation needs shelters, which accommodated citizens unable to evacuate by their own means of transportation, and medical special needs shelters, which shelter individuals requiring special medical attention and are operated jointly by DSS and Louisiana's DHH. General population shelters, meanwhile, were largely operated at the local level, often in conjunction with the American Red Cross. See: Kristy H. Nichols, "Assessment of Louisiana's Disaster Sheltering Plan and Operations Post Hurricanes Gustav and Ike," Louisiana Department of Social Services, September 22, 2008.

50. According to Dr. Guidry, DHH subsequently began exploring whether to adopt an electronic system such as that used by the federal Disaster Medical Assistance Teams.

Hospital patients, meanwhile, were handled by yet another set of systems. DHH worked with medical facilities throughout southern Louisiana to maintain manifests of patients evacuating via NDMS, but once patients were loaded onto military aircraft, an NDMS-specific tracking system coordinated by the US Department of Veterans Affairs took over. On top of this, the Louisiana Hospital Association launched its own online patient locator tool to help families more easily trace evacuated patients,[51] and FEMA offered still another Web-based program, the National Emergency Family Registry and Locator System (NEFRLS). Through NEFRLS, medical patients and others displaced during Gustav could voluntarily self-report their location and condition online or to a toll-free number.[52]

According to Waddy Gonzalez, Chief of FEMA's Mass Care Unit, there were several challenges in implementing NEFRLS during Gustav. "We certainly tried very hard to get [evacuating patients] to register in NEFRLS," he said, "[but] we had all kinds of issues because of the condition of the patients who were evacuated." He elaborated: "Critical patients are the ones who have to be moved during evacuations, and many of them are unable to communicate, making it difficult, if not impossible, to capture the information necessary to inform their families of their location."[53] Although patient advocates were sometimes able to access patient files and reach family members, FEMA was not included in the process. This left the agency unaware of the reunification needs of evacuated patients, a critical issue, as some of the evacuated patients were released into host communities without support from family members.

Rosanne Prats said that Louisiana officials have looked at ways to integrate some of the different systems, but she added that having multiple methods of registering, tracking, and locating different evacuees is not necessarily a bad thing as long as the information stored by each system is easily accessible. She explained,

> I'm not sure if hospitals will want to know everything that's in a shelter [or] a shelter will want to know everything that's in a hospital. So there are certain systems that are fairly closed, but one has got to be able to at least know that the other one exists, or be able to, if they need to find somebody, know where to go to get that information. Because then you're just looking at a lot of data overload. It just makes the response effort more distracting when you've got too much data coming at you.

And certainly during Gustav, the multiple systems largely proved to be more of an advantage than a disadvantage, given the significant problems that arose with registering and tracking individuals through the Phoenix system. In fact, while DHH's efforts to monitor the whereabouts of evacuated medical patients ran relatively smoothly,

---

51. Montgomery and Rucker, "Hospitals Evacuating High-Risk Patients."
52. FEMA, "Disaster Assistance Directorate Fact Sheet," 2009.
53. Telephone interview with Waddy Gonzalez, May 2009. Unless noted, all subsequent quotations from and attributions to Gonzalez are from this interview.

DSS received extensive criticism in the weeks following the storm for the collapse of the Phoenix registration process (as well as for shortcomings related to a range of other evacuation and sheltering functions).[54] In response, Governor Jindal removed much of the department's top leadership—including its secretary, Ann Williamson—declaring that it had "fundamentally failed" to meet its obligations.[55] Williamson's successor, Kristy Nichols, acknowledged the department's mistakes and announced that for the remaining few weeks of the 2008 hurricane season, Orleans and Jefferson parishes would put Phoenix aside and revert back to a manual registration process. Nichols assured residents, however, that DSS was dedicated to making sure "people have a way of finding their loved ones."[56]

BACK TO ARKANSAS

As Louisiana grappled with its revamped evacuation plans, Arkansas once again found itself in a familiar role, playing host to thousands of evacuees. A little more than 2,300 ended up in Fort Chaffee's barracks, the home for so many Arkansas-based Katrina evacuees three years earlier. But this time around, according to David Maxwell, Arkansas's Director of Emergency Management, "it was a much more controlled evacuation," due in large measure to Arkansas and Louisiana having agreed in advance to limit the number of evacuees Arkansas would host.[57]

Even though evacuation and sheltering processes had been significantly improved, Arkansas authorities still encountered problems, many of which they were able to overcome with relative ease. For instance, the state had not planned for Chaffee to host evacuees with medical special needs in 2008, but a number of people staying at the base ultimately required medical attention. As in 2005, Dr. Bryan Clardy and the Western Arkansas River Valley Medical Reserve Corps responded by organizing a triage operation at the complex, sending the most critically ill evacuees on to nearby hospitals, and setting up a clinic to treat the rest on site.[58]

---

54. Burdeau, "La. Grapples with Fresh Pot of Hurricane Logistics"; Michelle Millhollon, "Gustav-Related E-mails Reveal Disorganization," *The Advocate*, November 9, 2008, A1.

55. Burdeau, "La. Grapples with Fresh Pot of Hurricane Logistics."

56. Bill Barrow, "Evacuation Shelter Plans Upgraded; Gustav Lessons Used to Add Confidence," *Times-Picayune*, October 10, 2008, 2.

57. AmyJo Brown, "Lessons of Katrina a Help with Gustav; State Plans for Evacuees Seen as Success," *Arkansas Democrat-Gazette*, September 7, 2008. In total, Chaffee provided shelter to around 2,300 state-assisted evacuees, while another 3,000 or so self-evacuees stayed at additional state and county shelters. Thousands more found private accommodations. See: Association of State and Territorial Health Officials (ASTHO), *State Public Health Agencies Respond–Hurricane Gustav* (Arlington, VA: ASTHO, 2009).

58. Arkansas Department of Health, *The Public Health Response to Hurricanes Gustav and Ike,* September 19, 2008; Adam Wallworth, "Planes Due to Fly Evacuees Home from Fort Smith," *Arkansas Democrat-Gazette*, September 7, 2008.

More difficult was Arkansas's experience with hosting 225 hospital patients evacuated by NDMS from southern Louisiana.[59] Problems arose from the very start. As planes began to deliver medical evacuees to Little Rock late in the evening of Saturday, August 30, the state health department was ready to coordinate the matching of patients with NDMS-affiliated hospitals in the area.[60] But, said Dr. Paul Halverson, Director of the Arkansas Department of Health, "We had to really work hard with the NDMS folks to get a coordination clarification because they essentially wanted to move patients in here— but without any real coordination by the state health department." He emphasized, "You can't just come in and take over a major portion of bed capacity without coordination."[61]

While state and federal officials soon resolved that issue, keeping tabs on medical evacuees remained problematic. Despite the systems put in place by Louisiana and the federal government, Arkansas hospitals reported receiving confusing and misleading information about arriving patients. Moreover, the problem of keeping families connected to evacuated patients persisted. Staff at host hospitals said they were "inundated" by people calling in, desperately seeking relatives who had been evacuated out of Louisiana.[62] And Laurie Driver, a spokesperson for the Central Arkansas Veterans Healthcare System, which helped coordinate the transportation of the patients, acknowledged, "Communications back to the family is one of the issues we're trying hard to improve."[63] Noting that "there are always going to be a few glitches here and there," she said that NDMS had not received accurate manifests for patients evacuating out of Louisiana hospitals.

Of perhaps greatest frustration to health officials and hospital administrators in Arkansas, however, were two interrelated issues: (1) the lack of any system for moving patients back to Louisiana and (2) the length of time evacuated patients ended up staying in-state. For instance, days after Gustav had swept through the region, St. Vincent Infirmary Medical Center in Little Rock, which had accepted 63 Gustav evacuees, was still struggling to arrange transportation for some of the patients it had discharged. The president and CEO of St. Vincent, Peter Banko, complained, "I don't think the federal folks thought about how to get people home."[64] Paul Halverson elaborated,

> There was a lot of thought in regard to getting patients out of harm's way, but no real plan for getting them back home. And no payment mechanism had been worked out. So essentially what we have are hospitals that really went out of their way to take care of these patients, and

---

59. Mason, "The Incomplete Circle." As a largely rural state, Louisiana has little hospital capacity outside of greater New Orleans. Thus, Rosanne Prats explained, when a large swath of the state is evacuated, as was the case during both Katrina and Gustav, Louisiana must turn to its neighbors for assistance in caring for displaced medical patients.

60. Arkansas Department of Health, *The Public Health Response to Hurricanes Gustav and Ike*.

61. Telephone interview with Dr. Paul Halverson, April 2009. Unless noted, all subsequent quotations from and attributions to Halverson are from this interview.

62. Brown, "Lessons of Katrina."

63. Ibid.

64. Ibid.

now all of a sudden they're left holding the bag. There's millions of dollars that are left outstanding in terms of the costs of care and a lot of people wanting to make it right but it's just not happening.

With hospitals eager to resume their routine services, they turned to the state for help in finding a way to get the patients back to Louisiana, or at least off of their hands. As a result, said Dr. William Mason, head of preparedness and emergency response at the Arkansas Department of Health, state health officials basically had to step in and facilitate the repatriation of these medical evacuees. Mason said, "So we became the tracking system for the patients, everything you can think of, trying to get these patients out of the hospitals."[65]

From Louisiana's perspective, however, repatriating evacuees—especially those with serious medical conditions—was simply not possible in the days immediately following Gustav, as tens of thousands of households remained without power and debris blocked major roadways. In fact, New Orleans Mayor Ray Nagin originally announced that residents would not be allowed to return until Thursday, September 4, a full three days after Gustav's landfall. (But, with thousands of anxious residents gathering along the city's edge, he eventually moved reentry up by a day.)[66] Perhaps most concerning of all, another storm—Hurricane Ike—had appeared on the horizon, again threatening Louisiana's coast. Dr. Jimmy Guidry of Louisiana's DHH said, "Let's be clear. We had another storm out there.... The patients we moved out, we couldn't readily take them back because we had another storm coming a week behind, coming right down our neck—so we could not tell them that it was safe to come back."

But other issues contributed to the delay in repatriating hospital patients back to Louisiana as well. Drs. Guidry and Prats noted that after Katrina there had been plenty of time to move patients back into New Orleans and other affected areas, given that for months, few facilities were capable of receiving them. They said that because the private contractor hired to return patients in 2008 based its repatriation plans on the Katrina experience, it was unprepared to swiftly transport the hundreds of patients waiting to return to Louisiana in the immediate aftermath of Gustav, which had affected hospitals to a far lesser degree than had Katrina.

Guidry feared that another round of delayed repatriation could have a serious effect on the willingness of host states and hospitals to welcome Louisiana's evacuee surge. He said, "So literally that extended visit, getting that paid for ... my worry is that [after] all that help we received, are they going to be there the next time after this experience?"[67]

---

65. Telephone interview with Dr. William Mason, April 2009. Unless noted, all subsequent quotations from and attributions to Mason are from this interview.
66. Adam Nossiter and Anahad O'Connor, "New Orleans Residents Can Return, Mayor Says," *New York Times,* September 4, 2008; Robert Tanner and Vicki Smith, "Gustav Only Sideswipes New Orleans," *Pittsburgh Tribune Review,* September 2, 2008.
67. ASPR, *Public Health Emergencies.*

IKE HITS TEXAS

Louisiana officials' decision to delay repatriation proved sound, as Ike indeed triggered widespread power outages and significant flooding throughout coastal parts of the state.[68] But the storm's real impact was felt in neighboring Texas, where it made landfall over Galveston Island at 2:10 a.m. on Saturday, September 13, at Category 2 strength. Slow-moving and massive in size—at its largest, Ike measured more than 500 miles across—the hurricane severely affected much of the state's coastline.[69] It flooded Galveston City, destroyed towns like Gilchrist and Bridge City, and pummeled the greater Houston area, shattering skyscraper windows and disrupting transportation and utility systems. Around two million Texans lost power, and some residents of the Houston area remained without electricity for weeks.[70] With total damages at an estimated $30 billion (and a death toll of more than 70), Ike ranked as the third most destructive hurricane in US history at the time.[71]

From the outset, authorities in Texas faced considerable challenges in implementing the plans they had spent so much time fine-tuning in the aftermath of Rita. With forecasters predicting that the enormous storm could make landfall anywhere between Corpus Christi to the south and Galveston to the north,[72] public officials had no choice but to start moving people out of harm's way well in advance of Ike's projected arrival. Governor Rick Perry declared a state of emergency on Monday, September 8, and throughout the remainder of the week, the state marshaled and deployed more than 1,000 buses, along with ambulances, planes, and paramedic vehicles, in support of medical and other special needs evacuations taking place in localities up and down the coast.[73]

Although most special needs individuals were eventually delivered to predesignated shelters on buses, those with critical medical conditions required a higher level of care throughout the evacuation process. And so, on Wednesday, September 10, Texas turned to its federal NDMS partners to help airlift approximately 200 hospital patients out of

68. State of Louisiana Governor's Office of Homeland Security and Emergency Preparedness, *After-Action Report*.

69. Vanessa Chris and Pat Moore, *A Real Test: What Did We Learn?*, February 2009, http://www.disaster-resource.com/articles/08r&r_p06.shtml.

70. Ibid.; FEMA, *Hurricane Ike Impact Report*, 2008, http://www.fema.gov/pdf/hazard/hurricane/2008/ike/impact_report.pdf; James C. McKinley, "Amid Rubble of Storm, Rescue Teams Scour Ravaged Texas Coastline," *New York Times*, September 15, 2008, A21.

71. Bobbie Berg, *Tropical Cyclone Report Hurricane Ike*, 2009, http://www.nhc.noaa.gov/data/tcr/AL092008_Ike.pdf; Houston–Galveston Area Council Transportation Department (HGAC), "Ike Strikes Houston-Galveston Region," *The Vision*, October 2008.

72. Anahad O'Connor, "Thousands Flee as Hurricane Churns Toward Texas," *New York Times*, September 11, 2008, A21.

73. Chris and Moore, *A Real Test*; FEMA, *Hurricane Ike: From Disaster to Recovery*; "Update on Texas Preparations for Hurricane Ike Sept. 10, 2008," *State News Service*, September 10, 2008.

coastal cities to hospitals further inland.[74] But unlike in Louisiana, where hospital capacity was far less extensive, the state aimed, in the words of Dr. Adolfo Valadez, Assistant Commissioner for Prevention and Preparedness Services at DSHS, to keep all "Texans in Texas" throughout the entire evacuation and sheltering process.[75] For the most part, the state managed to do just that, although Dr. David Lakey, Texas Health Commissioner, noted that repatriation of medical patients still remained an enormously complicated process.[76]

Also on Wednesday, the City of Galveston issued a mandatory evacuation order for residents of its West End neighborhood, as it had become clear by midweek that landfall would happen somewhere in the Houston–Galveston area. Houston and Harris County followed a day later, but orders there were limited to select zip codes, as per the evacuation plans designed in the aftermath of Rita. Desperate to avoid the gridlock caused by that storm, city and county officials urged millions living outside of vulnerable neighborhoods to stay put.[77] In the end, many residents did as advised, resulting in far less gridlock and dramatically reduced travel times.[78] Although 1.9 million Texans evacuated in advance of Ike, the number fell well short of the close to 3 million people who took to the roadways during Rita.[79]

All the same, the significant decrease in the number of Texans evacuating was not entirely good news. It also meant that upwards of 100,000 people living in coastal communities had ignored evacuation orders, electing to wait out the storm in their homes. As a result, many found themselves struggling to survive in Ike's immediate aftermath in conditions reminiscent of New Orleans in 2005. Speaking of the task that now confronted the state, Andrew Barlow, a spokesman for Governor Perry, observed, "The unfortunate truth is we're going to have to go in and put our people in the tough situation to save people who did not choose wisely.... We'll probably do the largest search and rescue operation that's ever been conducted in the state of Texas."[80] Indeed, public safety officials went to extensive lengths in the days following Ike to save those stranded in flooded areas, including the 20,000 or more residents of Galveston City who had remained behind.[81] Thousands of Texas National Guardsmen, along with the US Coast Guard and

74. "HHS Provides State Assistance in Preparing for Hurricane Ike, Recovering from Hurricane Gustav," *Business Wire*, September 11, 2008.

75. Telephone interview with Dr. Adolfo Valadez, May 2009. Unless noted, all subsequent quotations from and attributions to Valadez are from this interview.

76. ASPR, *Public Health Emergencies*.

77. Chris and Moore, *A Real Test*; HGAC, "Ike Strikes Houston-Galveston Region"; Juan Lozano and Chris Duncan, "Devastating Hurricane Ike Swamps Texas, Louisiana," *Associated Press*, September 13, 2008.

78. Eric Berger, "Hurricane Ike, the Aftermath; Compared to Rita, Ike Evacuation Called Breeze," *Houston Chronicle*, October 2, 2008, B2.

79. FEMA, *Hurricane Ike: From Disaster to Recovery*; HGAC, "Ike Strikes Houston-Galveston Region."

80. Eva-Marie Ayala, Aman Batheja, and Evan S. Benn, "Texas Mounts Massive Search for Those Who Defied 'Ike' Warning," *McClatchy-Tribune News Service*, September 13, 2008.

81. Chris and Moore, *A Real Test*.

other first responders, poured into the affected area, conducting door-to-door searches and bringing thousands of survivors to safety.[82] Moreover, once rescue operations came to an end, many affected areas remained closed off for weeks as public authorities struggled to remove debris and bring utilities back online. It was not until Wednesday September 24, for instance, that Galveston residents were allowed home.[83]

Tracking Special Needs Evacuees

With at least 12,500 special needs individuals evacuating with state assistance,[84] Ike provided the state with its first opportunity to implement its electronic special needs evacuee tracking system, SNETS, on a large-scale. (Although Texas had prepared to deploy SNETS during Hurricane Dean in 2007, plans were called off when it became clear that the storm was not going to seriously affect the state.)[85] In some ways, say officials, SNETS led to improvements in keeping track of evacuees traveling and sheltering with state assistance. In particular, noted Dr. David Lakey, Texas's health commissioner, the state was able to eliminate the problem of lost buses by placing GPS units on all vehicles transporting evacuees. "We were able to see when a bus made the wrong turn or if they were going the wrong way. We knew exactly who that bus driver was and we were able to contact them and get them pulled back into play," he explained.

But Texas authorities also admitted that they continued to encounter difficulties with tracking evacuees. In fact, many of the problems were strikingly similar to those experienced in Louisiana during Hurricane Gustav. As with the Phoenix system, SNETS was not always able to keep up with the pace of people reporting to evacuation centers. Adolfo Valadez of DSHS acknowledged, "We think it could have worked a lot better. Some of these storms moved too quickly and as we registered evacuees, it just wasn't a very effective system." According to Valadez, a significant reason for registration delays was that some receiving jurisdictions often lacked the proper equipment for scanning evacuee wristbands and for inputting data into the electronic database. SNETS experienced other complications as well, such as when some evacuees removed their wristbands due to discomfort or when others left state shelters for hospitals, hotels, and other facilities that were not integrated into the system.[86] As Valadez put it, "On paper and in theory, it seems like it could work. But as I always reiterate, people are not packages, and so it's a little harder to track sometimes."

---

82. Ayala, Batheja, and Benn, "Texas Mounts Massive Search."
83. HGAC, "Ike Strikes Houston-Galveston Region."
84. Keith Richburg and Joel Achenbach, "Texans Take Shelter, Feel First Effects of Ike," *Washington Post,* September 13, 2008, A6.
85. John Burnell, *"Texas Turns to RFID."*
86. David Lakey, personal communication, April 22, 2009.

The tracking process was also complicated by the fact that as in Louisiana, Texas used several different systems for registering and locating evacuees. For example, although SNETS performed the main registration and data-collection functions, the state turned to an altogether different program, WebEOC, to report evacuees' whereabouts. Moreover, Valadez pointed out, some localities and counties used entirely different systems (such as EMTrack) that could not share data with SNETS, WebEOC, or with one another. Texas also experienced compatibility issues with the NDMS tracking processes, as had Louisiana and Arkansas during Gustav. Although the state offered its staff to help hospitals navigate NDMS's electronic patient tracking program, that tool was not integrated with Texas's own systems.

Following Ike, the state moved to overcome some of these challenges, allocating funds to support the integration of its various tracking systems. It also investigated ways to coordinate more closely with NDMS so, in the words of Valadez, patient tracking could be "a little more seamless." Moreover, having recognized that other states may need access to its systems and databases in the event of another large-scale disaster and evacuation, Texas began exploring how it could make evacuee data available to partners outside of Texas. Despite their "Texans in Texas" policy, state officials acknowledged that a uniform tracking system needed to be a national priority, given that mass evacuations often cross state lines. Even if Ike did not scatter people across the country as did Katrina, they recognized that another catastrophic hurricane anywhere along the Gulf Coast could require the mass movement of individuals to places far beyond their home states.

A NATIONAL TRACKING SYSTEM ON THE HORIZON?

In fact, FEMA's efforts to develop a multistate tracking system continued to move along throughout the 2008 hurricane season. As they refined their NMETS, FEMA officials paid close attention to how Phoenix and SNETS functioned during the Gustav and Ike evacuations. Particularly concerned by Phoenix's collapse in New Orleans, they became further committed to developing systems with varying levels of technological complexity, including an entirely paper-based tool. As Waddy Gonzalez, head of FEMA's Mass Care Unit, emphasized, "One of the critical things required is a printed manifest for all flights and trains that the Federal government provides."

Also based on experiences during Gustav, FEMA offered to make NMETS available to the US Department of Health and Human Services (HHS), which coordinated the NDMS evacuation process. Although NDMS maintained its own tracking system, Gonzalez asserted that greater integration of the different tools in use and in development is critical.[87] "Our experience in Gustav was that patients do not always remain patients throughout an evacuation," he explained. "If they are released by a 'host' hospital before they are transported back by air ambulances, they become the responsibility of FEMA. HHS is not responsible [anymore] because they're no longer patients." But, according to Gonzalez, HHS and FEMA encountered multiple obstacles in exchanging patient data due to the Privacy Act and the Health Insurance Portability and Accountability Act (HIPAA). "So," he continued, "at this point, we're working with them as we continue developing a completely automated tracking system, and we hope that HHS will adopt our system when it is ready for use."

FEMA officials were quick to point out that they were not looking to impose their systems on other agencies or on individual states. With the legal authorities for managing evacuations and the related sheltering and care services distributed across multiple jurisdictions and public bodies, any approach would have to be collaborative in nature. As Gonzalez emphasized, "We just want to have a common process with systems that can communicate with one another. At the end of the day, it is imperative that the same information is captured and can be shared across state lines, no matter what system is used."

Despite their independent efforts, authorities in Louisiana, Texas, and at the federal level all shared the same aim as the 2009 hurricane season moved into high gear: to have in place working systems for managing the mass relocation of people, so that they would never again have to experience the chaos and confusion of the Katrina and Rita evacuations. 2008 had been a step in the right direction, but public officials at all levels of government realized that they still had a long way to go. Speaking to Louisiana legislators in the aftermath of Gustav, Jerry Sneed, New Orleans's director of emergency preparedness, made clear the need for continued improvement. "Gustav was not a Katrina," Sneed said. "If we keep patting ourselves on the back, I think we're missing the point, because when a worse storm comes, we might not fare so well."[88]

---

87. A September 2008 report assessing the effectiveness of NDMS determined that there was a "critical need to integrate" patient tracking systems, concluding that "an integrated patient tracking system would assist in connecting and reuniting individual patients and families who are separated due to disasters." See: Disaster Medicine Working Group, *Strategic Improvements to the National Disaster Medical System,* September 2008.
88. Bill Barrow, "Hurricane Evacuation Strategies Assessed; Legislators Hear from Local Officials," *Times-Picayune,* February 19, 2009, 2.

Exhibit 16B-1. Chronology of Events for the Hurricane Gustav and Ike Evacuations: August–October 2008

Wednesday, August 27
- Louisiana Governor Bobby Jindal issued a state-wide emergency declaration as Hurricane Gustav moved closer to the Louisiana coast.

Saturday, August 30
- New Orleans Mayor Ray Nagin announced a mandatory evacuation of the city, which went into effect the following day.
- Individuals requiring evacuation assistance arrived at collection points throughout Louisiana. They were registered into the state's electronic Phoenix tracking system, triaged, and assigned to various means of transportation.
- At New Orleans's Union Passenger Terminal collection point, the registration process was soon overwhelmed. City leaders in New Orleans ordered that Phoenix be abandoned.
- The state rushed to acquire buses to help evacuate residents when the company it had contracted with failed to deliver half the vehicles it had promised to supply.
- Ambulances began delivering hospital patients to airports in southern Louisiana for evacuation via the National Disaster Medical System (NDMS). At New Orleans's Lakeview Airport, state officials were surprised to learn that their federal partners had failed to arrange for enough planes.
- NDMS evacuees began arriving in Arkansas and other host states.

Sunday, August 31
- 2 a.m. Governor Jindal convened a meeting to address the plane shortage at Lakeview.
- Throughout the early morning, a team led by Louisiana's Secretary of Health and Hospitals, Alan Levine, scrambled to obtain additional aircraft.
- 8 a.m. The mandatory evacuation order for New Orleans went into effect.
- Beginning mid-morning, substitute aircraft arrived at Lakeview, and patients were evacuated throughout the remainder of the day.
- 8:30 p.m. The last medical airlift took off from Lakeview.

Monday, September 1
- 10 a.m. Hurricane Gustav made landfall in Louisiana as a Category 2 storm.

Tuesday, September 2
- New Orleans and Louisiana officials struggled to restore utilities and clean up debris in Gustav's wake. They were reluctant to immediately repatriate evacuees.

Wednesday, September 3
- New Orleans residents were allowed to return to their homes, but some patients who were evacuated out of state via NDMS remained in host hospitals for many more days.

Monday, September 8
- Texas Governor Rick Perry declared a state of emergency in advance of Hurricane Ike, freeing state assets to assist localities requiring assistance with evacuations.

Wednesday, September 10
- Texas began coordinating with federal NDMS partners to evacuate hospital patients away from the coast.
- The City of Galveston issued a mandatory evacuation order for its West End neighborhood.
- Special needs individuals reported to evacuation centers along the coast, registering with the state's Special Needs Evacuation Tracking System and boarding buses for transportation to inland shelters.

Thursday, September 11
- Evacuation orders were issued for targeted zip codes in Houston and Harris County.

(Continued)

Exhibit 16B-1. (Continued)

Saturday, September 13

- 2:10 a.m. Hurricane Ike made landfall on Galveston Island, Texas, as a Category 2 storm, causing tremendous damage there and in other parts of northeast Texas. Significant damage was also experienced throughout the Houston area.
- The Texas National Guard, the US Coast Guard, and other first responders began search-and-rescue operations in coastal areas throughout Texas, including Galveston City, where approximately 20,000 remained behind.

Wednesday, September 24

- Galveston City residents were allowed to return home.

October 2008

- Louisiana's Acting Secretary of Social Services, Kristy Nichols, announced that the Phoenix system would not be used for the remainder of the 2008 hurricane season.

Exhibit 16B-2. Cast of Characters: Hurricane Gustav and Ike Evacuations, August–October 2008

State of Arkansas
- Dr. Paul Halverson, Director, Arkansas Department of Health
- Dr. William Mason, Chief, Preparedness and Emergency Response, Arkansas Department of Health

State of Louisiana
- Mark Cooper, Director, Governor's Office of Homeland Security and Emergency Preparedness
- Dr. Jimmy Guidry, Medical Director, Department of Health and Hospitals
- Bobby Jindal, Governor
- Alan Levine, Secretary, Department of Health and Hospitals
- Dr. Rosanne Prats, Director of Emergency Preparedness, Department of Health and Hospitals

State of Texas
- Dr. David Lakey, Commissioner, Department of State Health Services
- Rick Perry, Governor
- Dr. Adolfo Valadez, Assistant Commissioner, Prevention and Preparedness Services, Department of State Health Services

City of New Orleans
- Ray Nagin, Mayor
- Jerry Sneed, Emergency Preparedness Director

Federal Emergency Management Agency
- John Bischoff, Mass Care Unit
- Waddy Gonzalez, Chief, Mass Care Unit
- Brad Harris, Deputy Federal Coordinating Officer for Louisiana during Gustav

Exhibit 16B-3. Map Indicating Track of Hurricane Gustav: August 25–September 4, 2008

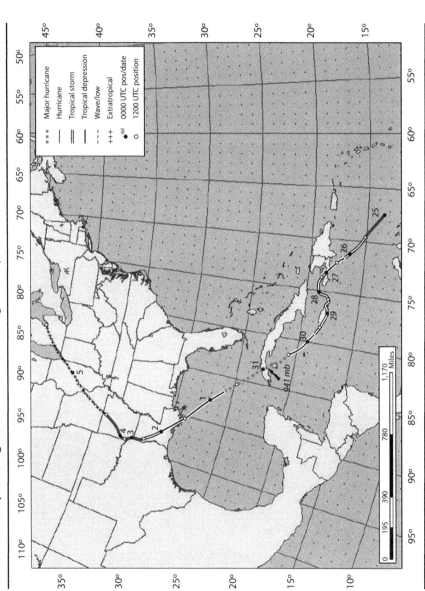

Source: Adapted from John L. Beven and Todd B. Kimberlain, *Tropical Cyclone Report: Hurricane Gustav*, January 22, 2009, http://www.nhc.noaa.gov/data/tcr/AL072008_Gustav.pdf.

Exhibit 16B-4. Map Indicating Track of Hurricane Ike: September 1-14, 2008

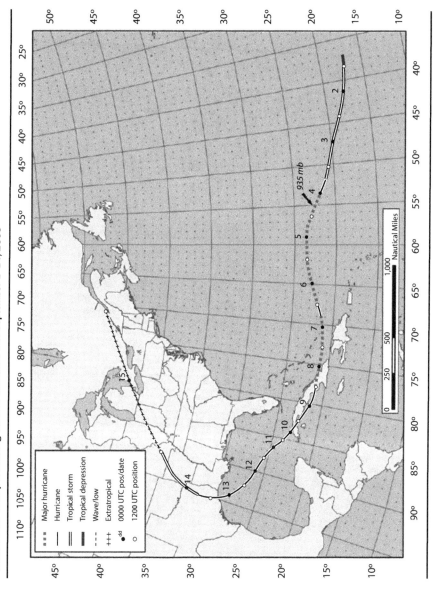

Source: Adapted from Robbie Berg, *Tropical Cyclone Report: Hurricane Ike,* January 23, 2009, http://www.nhc.noaa.gov/data/tcr/AL092008_Ike.pdf.

Contributors

John Buntin is a staff correspondent at *Governing Magazine*. A graduate of Princeton University's Woodrow Wilson School of Public and International Affairs, he first began writing about public safety as a case writer at Harvard's Kennedy School of Government. Buntin has written for *Slate*, the *New York Times Magazine*, the *Washington Post*, the *Wall Street Journal*, *City Journal*, and the *Crime Report*. He is also the author of the book *LA Noir: The Struggle for the Soul of America's Most Seductive City*, which was recognized by the *Los Angeles Times* as one of the year's outstanding books. He lives in Nashville, Tennessee.

Daniel J. Collings was formerly a case writer for Harvard Kennedy School.

David W. Giles is Associate Director and Senior Research Associate, Program on Crisis Leadership, at the John F. Kennedy School of Government, Harvard University. He co-edited *Natural Disaster Management in the Asia-Pacific: Policy and Governance* (2015) and *Managing Crises: Responses to Large-Scale Emergencies* (2009) and has authored a number of Harvard Kennedy School case studies. Previously, he worked as a staff researcher at the Institute of Medicine and served for two years as a Peace Corps volunteer in Romania. He received his BA from Vassar College and his MA from the Elliott School of International Affairs at The George Washington University.

Arnold M. Howitt is Senior Adviser of the Ash Center for Democratic Governance and Innovation and Faculty Co-Director of the Program on Crisis Leadership at the John F. Kennedy School of Government, Harvard University. Previously, he served for many years as Executive Director of the Taubman Center for State and Local Government and then of the Ash Center. Among other writing, Dr. Howitt is co-author and editor of *Natural Disaster Management in the Asia-Pacific: Policy and Governance* (2015), *Managing Crises: Responses to Large-Scale Emergencies* (2009), and *Countering Terrorism: Dimensions of Preparedness* (2003). He received his BA degree from Columbia University and his MA and PhD degrees in political science from Harvard University.

Herman B. "Dutch" Leonard is George F. Baker, Jr. Professor of Public Management at Harvard Kennedy School and Eliot I. Snider and Family Professor of Business Administration at Harvard Business School. At Harvard Kennedy School, he is Faculty

Co-Director of the Program on Crisis Leadership, and at Harvard Business School, Co-Chair of the Social Enterprise Initiative. He teaches leadership, organizational strategy, crisis management, and financial management. His current research concentrates on crisis management, corporate social responsibility, and performance management. Among other writing, he is co-author and editor of *Managing Crises: Responses to Large-Scale Emergencies* (2009). He received his PhD in economics from Harvard University.

Kirsten Lundberg owns the Boston-based Lundberg Case Consortium, which produces case-based curriculum for professional education. She formerly created and directed the Case Consortium @ Columbia (University) and the Knight Case Studies Initiative. She was a senior writer for many years and acting director of the Case Program at Harvard Kennedy School. Before that, she worked for United Press International as a correspondent in Brussels, London, Stockholm, and Moscow.

Esther Scott was a senior case writer at Harvard Kennedy School for many years. She grew up in Cambridge, Massachusetts, and is a graduate of Harvard College.

Wendy Robison has a background in education, international development, and technology. She focuses on adult learning, leadership development, and organizational learning in the workplace. Her work includes strategic planning, program design, curriculum development, and using data to create, refine, and scale learning initiatives across for- and non-profit organizations. She has a bachelor's degree from the University of Virginia and master's and doctoral degrees from Harvard University.

Pamela Varley is an award-winning senior case writer and case writing consultant at Harvard Kennedy School. She has written a broad array of teaching materials in the course of her 25 years at Harvard Kennedy School and consults with faculty and freelance writers about the case writing process. She began her career in journalism and continues to write and edit on a freelance basis, including editing a book on international labor standards, *The Sweatshop Quandary: Corporate Responsibility on the Global Frontier.*

Index